Adult and Family
Nurse Practitioner

Certification Review Book

Comprehensive Outline and Study Guide

Amelie Hollier, MSN, APRN, BC, FNP

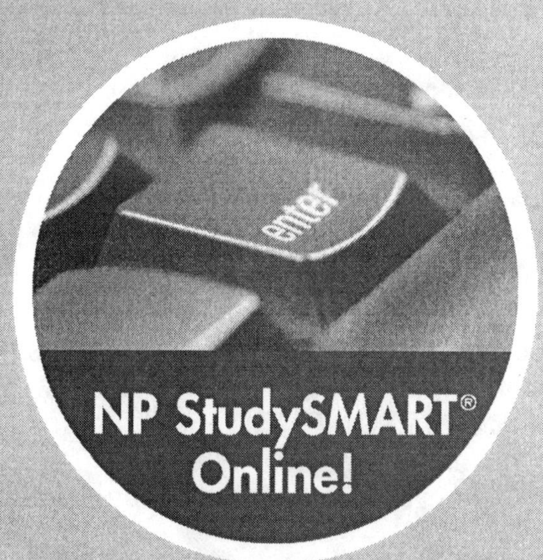

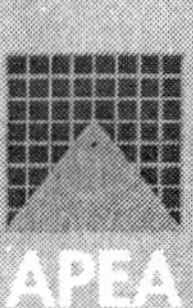

Advanced
Practice
Education
Associates

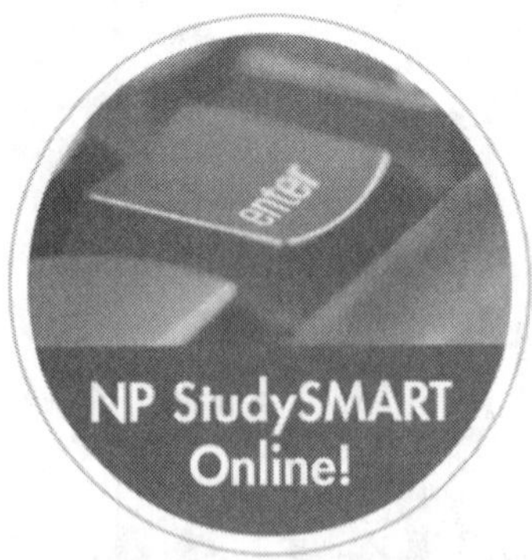

NP StudySMART® Online:

Test your readiness for your nurse practitioner certification exam with your exclusive access to practice questions!

Thank you for purchasing APEA's *Adult and Family Nurse Practitioner Review Book: Comprehensive Outline and Study Guide*!

Your purchase entitles you to an online practice test. The test consists of 60 multiple choice questions, comparable to those on the AANP and ANCC certification exam. After you answer each question, you'll receive immediate feedback. You may take the test at any time after you register this copy of the book.

Access to the online practice questions will terminate with the next edition of this book.

HOW TO REGISTER

1. Log on to www.apea.com
2. Click on NP StudySMART®
3. Register your username and password
4. Follow instructions on screen
5. Contact us for any questions at info@apea.com

Your user name: ***npstudysmart*** (case sensitive)
Your password: ***acethetest*** (case sensitive)

Access to online tests is strictly for the *original* individual purchaser and is not to be shared, sold, or otherwise circulated. **SHARING OF PASSWORDS IS STRICTLY PROHIBITED** and failure to comply with this may restrict the purchaser's use of the online tests. This book cannot be returned once the online practice questions have been accessed.

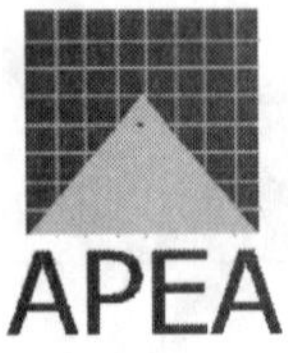

APEA

Advanced Practice Education Associates
103 Darwin Circle
Lafayette, LA 70508
800-899-4502
www.apea.com

Adult and Family

Nurse Practitioner Certification Review Book

Comprehensive Outline and Study Guide

Amelie Hollier, MSN, APRN, BC, FNP

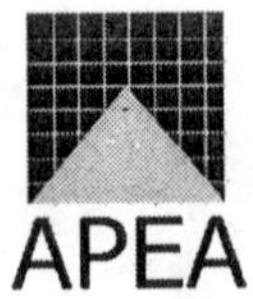

Advanced
Practice
Education
Associates

Adult and Family Nurse Practitioner Certification Review Book

Amelie Hollier, MSN, APRN, BC, FNP

Published by: Advanced Practice Education Associates, Inc.
103 Darwin Circle
Lafayette, LA 70508 U.S.A.

ISBN 1-892418-13-4

Printed in the United States of America.

Contents

FOREWORD

Methods of certification review for nurse practitioners were a planned project in the mind of the author during her student practitioner days and have grown to a comprehensive, concise, scholarly source of essentials in her review books. The Adult and Family Nurse Practitioner Certification Review Book is now in its 4th edition, written again for the student and the novice, and with currency, additions and improvements. This intellectual manuscript assists the student in bridging the gap from student to certified practitioner and then to progress forward to the role of expert. Learning and building knowledge are lifetime activities and this review book serves as a base for these treasured behaviors. The information provided will have a major impact on the learner and on the role played in advanced practice nursing. The content will be used for review prior to writing certification examinations and as the novice practitioner begins patient assessments and interventions. Review books are often just review books, however, Adult and Family Review is an immeasurable guide to success as it includes strategies on the use of evidence-based information, critical thinking and decision making skills. The concisely written materials allow independent study and pursuit of knowledge. The book includes the body systems and chapters on health promotion for adults and children, lactation, pregnancy, men's and women's health, sexually transmitted diseases and professional issues for advanced practice nursing. Each chapter is organized to highlight the critical problems related to the disease entities. In exploring the cardiovascular disorders valuable subject matter is easily identified. Each topic is completely discussed in relation to a definition, etiology, risk factors, assessment factors, diagnostic studies, prevention, pharmacological and non-pharmacological management, criteria for consultation and referral, and considerations during pregnancy. Well organized tables with significant data are used frequently throughout the chapter. The pharmacology tables list the name and action of the agent and in the comments column tips regarding dosage, when to avoid, diagnostic tests to order, and other prescribing red flags are found. The pharmacology tables are, in reality, a tool, which can be used for prescribing medications.

Plato said: "You know that the beginning is the most important part of any work especially in the case of a young and tender thing for that is the time at which the character is being formed and desired impressions

are more readily taken" (Bennett 1996). The present is a splendid and exhilarating time for advanced practice nurses, nursing and the profession. The 21st Century offers many opportunities for practice, advancement, impact on health care delivery, legislation, and for individual practitioners in their own practice. Advanced practice nurses are in prime positions for research, teaching, identifying evidenced-based practice, writing, and publishing. The author of Adult and Family Review practices Plato's wise statement and provides mentoring through her writings and review books which provide an outstanding base; create an environment of learning, and emphasize the rapid changes in health care, medications, and treatments necessitating the need for currency of information. The author stresses the need to always question and accentuates the need for quality practice and patient management.

Certification for nurse practitioners is required, but it also provides credibility to them and to their practice. Assisting nurse practitioners to earn certification is essential but that is only one of the purposes of this comprehensive, scholarly resource. The second purpose is to provide an accurate guide for practice for the novice and again the goal is accomplished. Nurse practitioner students who utilize this book to enter their profession and practice will find fear and apprehension rapidly disappearing and instead will find an understandable and helpful guide to practice.

The Adult and Family Nurse Practitioner Certification Review Book-4th edition is outstanding and will assist in certification and informing nurse practitioners about quality, comprehensive management of health-related problems for clients of all ages.

Mary B. Neiheisel, BSN, MSN, EdD, CNS, APRN-FNP-C, GNP
Professor of Nursing
U. L. Foundation Distinguished Professor
Pfizer/Ardoin Endowed Professorship

Reference

Bennett, W. J. (1996). *The book of virtues*. New York: Simon and Schuster.

Acknowledgments

This book would have been impossible without the never-ending patience, encouragement, and confidence of my family. I am especially grateful to Jeanie Doucet for her support, encouragement, and everything else she did to help get this book in print.

A special thank you to Julie A. Siracusa for sharing her artistic gift in the design of the cover of this book.

This book is dedicated to my family, both young and old.

Amelie Hollier

Disclaimer

NOTICE:

The author, reviewers, and publisher of this book have taken extreme care to insure that the information contained within this book is correct and compatible with standards of care generally accepted at the time of publication. Sources were used which were believed to be complete and accurate. If by human error or changes in standards of care, the information contained herein is not complete or is not accurate, the authors, reviewers, publisher, or any other party associated with this publication cannot accept responsibility or consequences from application of the material contained within. Readers and users of this publication are encouraged to check the information with other sources. **If you are unwilling to be bound by the above, please contact the publisher.**

1

CARDIOVASCULAR DISORDERS

Cardiovascular Disorders

**Denotes pediatric diagnosis*

HYPERTENSION
(High Blood Pressure, Pregnancy-Induced Hypertension)

DESCRIPTION

Systolic and/or diastolic blood pressure which is higher than expected for age or pregnancy status. A presumptive diagnosis can be made if the average of 3 measurements exceeds 140 mm Hg systolic or 90 mm Hg diastolic. Hypertension is classified as either primary (essential) or secondary.

Target BP:
General population: <140/90 mm Hg
Diabetics: <130/80 mm Hg
Renal disease/proteinuria: 125/75 mm Hg

ETIOLOGY: ADULT

Causes of Primary Hypertension
No known cause in 90% of cases

Causes of Secondary Hypertension	
Renal	Acute glomerular nephritis Chronic renal failure Polycystic kidney disease Pyelonephritis
Vascular	Coarctation of the aorta Renal artery stenosis
Endocrine	Pheochromocytoma Cushing's syndrome Neuroblastoma Hyperthyroidism
Neurological	Increased intracranial pressure
Pharmacological	Oral contraceptives Corticosteroids Cocaine NSAIDs Decongestants Sympathomimetics
Stress	"White coat hypertension" Alcohol abuse

ETIOLOGY: PEDIATRIC

Causes of Primary Hypertension
In children > 10 years, usually is primary, but secondary causes must be ruled out

Causes of Secondary Hypertension	
Renal	80% due to this
Vascular	Coarctation of the aorta (5-10% due to this)
Endocrine	Adrenal dysfunction Hyperaldosteronism Hyperthyroidism
Neurologic	Increased intracranial pressure Sleep apnea
Pharmacological	Oral contraceptives Corticosteroids Cocaine NSAIDs Decongestants Sympathomimetics

INCIDENCE

- Nearly 25% of U.S. population is hypertensive
- Reported rates of hypertensive children vary from 2-13% (highest in African- and Asian- American children)
- African-American adults have higher incidence than general population
- Males > Females
- Typically appears between 30-55 years
- Increased prevalence in the elderly
- 5-10% of all pregnancies

RISK FACTORS

- Family history
- Excessive alcohol intake
- Cigarette smoking
- Physical inactivity
- Dyslipidemia
- Microalbuminuria

- Age (>55 yrs. males; > 65 yrs. females)
- Obesity is single most important factor in children; important in adults as well
- Stress
- Excessive dietary intake of sodium
- Pregnancy

ASSESSMENT FINDINGS

- Asymptomatic
- Occipital headaches
- Headache on awakening
- Blurry vision
- Exam of optic fundi (may see AV nicking)
- Left ventricular hypertrophy (after long standing hypertension)
- Pregnancy with hypertension and proteinuria, edema, and excessive weight gain

ADULT CLASSIFICATION OF HYPERTENSION

Normal	SBP <120 mm Hg AND DBP < 80 mm Hg
Pre-hypertension	120-139 mm Hg SBP OR 80-89 mm Hg DBP
Stage 1	SBP 140-159 mm Hg OR DBP 90-99 mm Hg
Stage 2	SBP ≥160 mm Hg OR DBP ≥100 mm Hg

Note. From "JNC VII" National Institutes of Health, 2003.

PEDIATRIC CLASSIFICATION OF HYPERTENSION

High Normal	90th – 94th percentile for age
Significant	95th – 99th percentile for age
Severe	>99th percentile for age

Classified according to age and height

DIFFERENTIAL DIAGNOSIS

- Secondary hypertension
- Hypertension worsened by pregnancy
- Pregnancy-induced hypertension (PIH)

DIAGNOSTIC STUDIES

- Hematocrit
- Urinalysis: may reveal proteinuria
- Electrolytes, creatinine, calcium
- Fasting lipid profile
- Fasting blood glucose
- Electrocardiogram (ECG)
- Other studies depending on history and physical exam
- Measure BP twice; 5 minutes apart; patient should be seated with proper cuff size and application (always assess contralateral arm to confirm elevated reading)

Goal of diagnostic studies is to identify target organ damage, an underlying cause, and/or additional risk factors.

PREVENTION

- Maintenance of healthy weight and BMI
- Smoking cessation
- Regular aerobic exercise
- Alcohol in moderation (2 drinks per day for males; one drink per day for females)
- Stress management
- Compliance with medication regimen

NONPHARMACOLOGIC MANAGEMENT

- Initiate lifestyle modifications (see below) with abnormal BP readings
- DASH (Dietary Approaches to Stopping Hypertension) eating plan
- Compliance with medication regimen, diet, reduction or abstinence from alcohol intake, exercise, weight loss, and sodium restriction
- Identification and management of stressors
- Counseling about elimination of other cardiovascular risks (e.g., smoking cessation)
- Treatment of underlying disease, if applicable
- Twice weekly blood pressure checks during pregnancy if elevated
- Do not restrict salt intake during pregnancy
- Patient education regarding disease, treatment, prevention of complications, long term implications, diet changes, and lifestyle modifications

PHARMACOLOGIC MANAGEMENT

- A variety of agents may be used in adult, pediatric, and nonpregnant patients:
  - ◊ Diuretics
  - ◊ Angiotensin-converting enzyme inhibitors (ACE inhibitors)
  - ◊ Angiotensin II receptor blockers (ARB)
  - ◊ Beta blockers
  - ◊ Calcium channel blockers
  - ◊ Vasodilators
  - ◊ Combination of the above
- In pregnant patients:
  - ◊ Beta blockers
  - ◊ Methyldopa (Aldomet®)
  - ◊ Vasodilators
  - ◊ Avoid ARB and ACE inhibitors

AGENT	ACTION	COMMENTS
Diuretics ***Thiazide diuretics*** *Examples:* HydroDIURIL® hydrochlorothiazide chlorthalidone (Hygroton®)	Increase excretion of sodium and chloride and thus water; Decreases circulating plasma volume	Monitor for hypokalemia, (check potassium level about 2 weeks after initiation & with increase in dose). Maintain potassium 4 mm/L. Considered first line for most patients. May worsen gout and elevate blood glucose and lipid levels.
Loop diuretics *Examples:* furosemide (Lasix®) bumetanide (Bumex®) torsemide (Demadex®)	Inhibit absorption of sodium, chloride in proximal/distal tubules, and loop of Henle	More potent diuretic action than thiazides. Monitor for dehydration, electrolyte imbalances, and hypotension. May be used for patients who develop fluid overload.
Potassium-Sparing diuretics *Examples:* spironolactone (Aldactone®) triamterene (Dyrenium®)	Enhance the action of thiazide & loop diuretics and counteract potassium loss by these agents	Monitor for hyperkalemia and hypotension. May be used in patients who develop hypokalemia.
Angiotensin Converting Enzyme Inhibitors (ACEI) *Examples:* benazepril (Lotensin®) captopril (Capoten®) enalapril (Vasotec®) lisinopril (Prinivil®) ramipril (Altace®)	Inhibit the action of angiotensin converting enzyme (ACE) which is responsible for conversion of angiotensin I to angiotensin II; Angiotensin II causes vasoconstriction & sodium retention. Prevents breakdown of bradykinin.	End in "pril". Dry cough is common side effect; monitor for first dose hypotension, hyperkalemia, acute renal failure. Angioedema is rare but more common in African-Americans. Monitor for renal failure and worsening chronic heart failure. Preferred in patients with diabetes and CHF. Avoid use in patients with bilateral renal artery stenosis. Do not use in sexually active females.
Angiotensin II Receptor Blockers (ARB) *Examples:* candesartan (Atacand®) losartan (Cozaar®) eprosartan (Teveten®) olmesartan (Benicar®) valsartan (Diovan®)	Block vasoconstriction and sodium retention affects of AT II (angiotensin II) found in many tissues.	End in "sartan". Does not effect bradykinin; therefore no cough as seen in ACE inhibitors. Good venoprotective action; therefore good alternative in diabetics who cannot tolerate ACE inhibitors. Monitor for hypotension and possible renal failure. Do not use ARB in sexually active females.

AGENT	ACTION	COMMENTS
Beta Blockers		*Consider post-MI, in CHF, ischemic heart disease.* *Should be avoided (or used cautiously) in patients with airway disease, heart block.* *Should be used with caution in diabetics (may mask the symptoms of hypoglycemia) and in those with peripheral vascular disease.* *May cause exercise intolerance.*
Cardioselective beta blockers *Examples:* acebutolol (Sectral®) atenolol (Tenormin®) bisoprolol (Zebeta®) metoprolol (Lopressor®, Toprol®)	Block stimulation of the $beta_1$ receptors in the heart causing decreased heart rate, decreased blood pressure, and cardiac output	End in "lol". Low doses of these agents are cardiac selective but in moderate to high doses, may block stimulation of $beta_2$ receptors in the lungs. Common side effect is bradycardia, exercise intolerance, and fatigue. May mask signs/symptoms of hypoglycemia. Monitor for reflex tachycardia if discontinued too quickly.
Non-cardioselective beta blockers *Examples:* nadolol (Corgard®) penbutolol (Levatol®) pindolol (Visken®) propanolol (Inderal®)	Block stimulation of both $beta_1$ (heart) and $beta_2$ (lungs) receptors causing decreased heart rate, blood pressure, and cardiac output ($beta_1$) as well as decreased central motor activity, inhibition of renin release from the kidneys, reduction of norepinephrine from neurons, and mild bronchoconstriction ($beta_2$)	End in "lol". Contraindicated in patients with broncho constrictive disease (i.e. asthma, COPD, etc.) Cautious use in diabetics because of masking signs and symptoms of hypoglycemia (tachycardia, blood pressure changes). Nonspecific beta blockade helpful in patients with tremors, anxiety, and migraine headaches.
Calcium Channel Blockers ***Dihydropyridine (DHP)*** *Examples:* amlodipine (Norvasc®) felodipine (Plendil®) nicardipine (Cardene®) nifedipine (Procardia®) nisoldipine (Sular®)	Inhibit movement of calcium ions across the cell membrane and vascular smooth muscle which depresses myocardial contractility and increases cardiac blood flow	End in suffix "pine". Does not cause bradycardia. Monitor for hypotension and worsening of CHF, ankle edema. Good choice in diabetics with proteinuria, patients with ISH (isolated systolic hypertension), for migraine prophylaxis, and in patients with stable angina. Serious drug interactions with grapefruit juice. Long acting DHP calcium channel blockers preferred for isolated systolic hypertension.
Non-DHP *Examples:* diltiazem (Cardizem®, Dilacor®, Tiazac®) verapamil (Calan®, Covera® HS, Isoptin®, Verelan®)	Inhibit movement of calcium ions across the cell membrane which depresses myocardial contractility, impulse formation and conduction velocity	Watch for conduction defects. Decreases heart rate. Use cautiously or avoid with use of beta blockers. Monitor for worsening of CHF, hypotension, bradycardia, constipation. Consider in patients with atrial fibrillation with rapid ventricular response, in patients with angina, and in diabetics with proteinuria. Serious drug interactions with grapefruit juice.

SPECIAL PHARMACOLOGICAL CONSIDERATIONS

- If patient has Stage 2 hypertension, consider initiating therapy with 2 drugs
- Selection of antihypertensives in children is similar to adults

CONSULTATION/REFERRAL

- Referral to cardiologist for children with significant or severe hypertension
- Refer as needed for secondary causes of hypertension

FOLLOW-UP

- Monthly, until patient reaches goal; then every 3-6 months as appropriate

EXPECTED COURSE

- Only 25% of patients who are treated for hypertension are actually at goal; expect complications if inadequately managed

POSSIBLE COMPLICATIONS

- Stroke
- Coronary artery disease
- Myocardial infarction
- Renal failure
- Chronic heart failure
- Eclampsia (seizures)
- Pulmonary edema
- Hypertensive crisis

CHRONIC HEART FAILURE
(CHF)

DESCRIPTION

The inability of the heart to pump blood to meet the metabolic needs of the tissues

ETIOLOGY

- Systolic and/or diastolic failure due to
  - ◊ Left ventricular dysfunction
  - ◊ Volume overload
  - ◊ Myocardial infarction
  - ◊ Cardiomyopathy
  - ◊ Coronary artery disease
  - ◊ Cardiac drugs
  - ◊ Arrhythmias (especially atrial fibrillation)
  - ◊ Valvular abnormalities
  - ◊ Hyperthyroidism/hypothyroidism

INCIDENCE

- Depends on etiology
- Males > Females until age 75 years, then Males = Females
- More common in the elderly
- Most frequent cause of cardiac hospitalization in the U.S.

RISK FACTORS

- Underlying heart disease
- Noncompliance with medication and/or dietary modifications
- Pregnancy or postpartum cardiomyopathy
- Fluid or sodium excess
- Hyperthyroidism
- Long-standing hypertension
- Use of negative inotropic medications

ASSESSMENT FINDINGS

Mild failure symptoms	Crackles in lung bases S_3 gallop Jugular vein distention Dyspnea on exertion Nocturia Tachycardia Diminished exercise capacity Fatigue and/or weakness Peripheral edema Weight gain
Moderate failure symptoms	Cough, especially nocturnal Crackles in bases Paroxysmal nocturnal dyspnea Tachypnea/shortness of breath (especially at rest) Tachycardia Hepatomegaly/ascites Edema (extremities, presacral, and scrotal)
Severe failure symptoms	Ascites Cyanosis Decreased level of consciousness Frothy sputum and/or pink sputum Hypotension

DIFFERENTIAL DIAGNOSIS

- Chronic obstructive pulmonary disease
- Asthma
- Cirrhosis
- Peripheral vascular disease with edema
- Dependent edema
- Pulmonary embolism

DIAGNOSTIC STUDIES

- BNP (B type natriuretic peptide): > 100 pg/ml
- Transthoracic echo and 2-D Doppler flow studies: mechanically evaluates heart and establishes ejection fraction; if < 35-40%, then CHF
- 12 lead EKG
- Chest x-ray: establishes heart size, presence of pulmonary edema, pulmonary disease
- CBC: assesses anemia, infection
- Electrolytes: potassium, calcium, sodium, magnesium
- BUN/Creatinine: elevated Cr indicates renal failure and volume overload
- Urinalysis: proteinuria (less than one gram)

New York Heart Association Functional Classification	
Functional Class I	physical activity does not cause limitations
Functional Class II	physical activity brings about "slight limitation" (fatigue, palpitations, dyspnea, anginal pain)
Functional Class III	physical activity brings about "marked limitations"; symptoms brought about by "less than ordinary activity"
Functional Class IV	unable to participate in any physical activity without discomfort; symptoms at rest

Note: From New York Heart Association Classification for CHF, by American Heart Association, 2003.

PREVENTION

- Appropriate management of underlying conditions which can lead to CHF

NONPHARMACOLOGIC MANAGEMENT

- Surgery for underlying valve problems or other correctable etiologies
- Avoid smoking, alcohol
- Sodium restriction
- Fluid restriction when appropriate
- Daily weights for early identification of fluid overload
- Patient education regarding self-care, medication, diet, exercise, disease process
- Encourage exercise except in severe disease

PHARMACOLOGIC MANAGEMENT

AGENT	ACTION	COMMENTS
ACEI *Examples:* captopril (Capoten®) enalapril (Vasotec®) fosinopril (Monopril®) lisinopril (Prinivil®) ramipril (Altace®)	Decrease pulmonary systemic vascular resistance, decrease preload and afterload, increase cardiac output and exercise tolerance Decrease morbidity and mortality of CHF	Commonly used post-MI for systolic dysfunction or in patients with clinical symptoms of CHF (SOB, fatigue, exercise intolerance). Monitor potassium levels: goal is 4-5 mmol/L. Assess renal function and serum potassium within 1-2 weeks of drug initiation and after each dose change. Start at low dose and titrate in 2-4 week increments. Improvement of clinical symptoms is desired effect. Preferred in patients with diabetes and CHF.
Loop Diuretics *Examples:* furosemide (Lasix®) bumetanide (Bumex®) torsemide (Demadex®) ethacrynic acid (Edecrin®)	Inhibit absorption of sodium and chloride in the loop of Henle & can produce profound diuresis	Use in patients with evidence of moderate to severe fluid retention. Produce rapid improvement in symptoms. Monitor for hyponatremia, hypokalemia, hypomagnesemia, dehydration & hypotension.
Beta Blockers *Examples:* metoprolol (Toprol XL®) carvedilol (Coreg®)	Decreases sympathetic stimulation by beta blockade in the heart	Do not prescribe in an unstable patient or in patients with fluid overload; cautious use or avoid use in respiratory patients. Used in conjunction with ACEI, diuretics with/without digoxin; titrate dose to improve clinical symptoms. Decreases morbidity and mortality associated with CHF.
Digoxin Digoxin (Lanoxin®)	Increases intracellular concentration of calcium which increases force of myocardial contraction; decreases activation of the sympathetic nervous system Improved quality of life but no decrease in mortality	Use in patients with CHF secondary to poor myocardial contractility. Correct hypokalemia before prescribing. Do not use with heart block. Cautious use with agent which decreases heart rate (beta blocker). Monitor for toxicity, anorexia, nausea, muscle weakness. Consider in patients with atrial fibrillation with rapid ventricular response. Use in conjunction with ACEI, diuretic, beta blocker.

SPECIAL PHARMACOLOGICAL CONSIDERATIONS

- Most patients are managed on a combo of 3-4 drugs
- Symptom relief may take several weeks once drug therapy begun
- Diuretics will provide quickest relief from CHF symptoms but should be used in combination with other drugs
- Monitor potassium levels on patients taking diuretics and ACE inhibitors
- Monitor renal function and potassium 1-2 weeks after initiating ACE inhibitor, after dose increases; then periodically
- Initiate beta blockers at very low doses in a stable patient without evidence of fluid overload

- Do not initiate beta blockers or ACE inhibitors if systolic BP < 80 mm Hg; consider referral

PREGNANCY/LACTATION CONSIDERATIONS

- Do not restrict sodium in diet
- Requires immediate referral

CONSULTATION/REFERRAL

- Consult according to severity and patient objectives

FOLLOW-UP

- Variable depending on patient circumstances, but, generally daily, until exacerbation resolves, then 1-2 weeks until patient is symptom free; then, every 3-6 months.

EXPECTED COURSE

- Chronic disease with frequent exacerbations
- Common diagnosis associated with frequent hospital admission
- 15% die within first year of diagnosis

HYPERLIPIDEMIA

DESCRIPTION

An elevated level of blood lipids: cholesterol, cholesterol esters, phospholipids, and/or triglycerides

ETIOLOGY

- Inherited disorder of lipid metabolism
- High intake of dietary lipids
- Obesity
- Inactivity
- Diabetes mellitus
- Hypothyroidism
- Steroid use
- Hepatic disorders: hepatitis, cirrhosis
- Renal disorders: uremia, nephrotic syndrome
- Stress
- Drug induced: thiazide diuretics, beta blockers
- Alcohol and caffeine
- Metabolic Syndrome: characterized by hypertension, glucose intolerance, obesity, dyslipidemia, and/or coagulation abnormalities

INCIDENCE

- Hypercholesterolemia >200 mg/dL
  120 million people in U.S.
- Hypercholesterolemia >240 mg/dL
  60 million people in U. S.
- Male > Females
- Incidence increases as age increases

RISK FACTORS

- Family history of CHD
- Physical inactivity
- Smoking
- Age: men >45 years, women >55 years or premature menopause without estrogen replacement
- Obesity
- Diet high in saturated fat
- HDL <40 mg/dL
- Diabetes

ASSESSMENT FINDINGS

- Xanthomata
- Xanthelasma
- Corneal arcus prior to age 50 years
- Bruits
- Angina pectoris
- Myocardial infarction
- Stroke

DIFFERENTIAL DIAGNOSIS

- Primary or secondary causes

DIAGNOSTIC STUDIES

- Fasting lipid profile (9-12 hours of fasting)

- Urinalysis (for detection of nephrotic syndrome)
- TSH (for detection of hypothyroidism which may cause hypercholesterolemia)

PREVENTION

- Adults and children > 2 years of age: reduce dietary intake of fats to < 30% of total calories; < 7% should be from saturated fat (estimated 10% reduction in LDL with this low fat diet)
- Total cholesterol intake < 200 mg/day
- Minimize use of trans fatty acids
- Increase intake of fiber, vegetables, fruits, and other whole grains
- Decreased intake of fat is *not* recommended for children < 2 years of age
- Identify and eliminate risk factors in children and adults
- Encourage an active lifestyle in children (decreases likelihood of obesity); adults should exercise at least 2.5 hours per week (sustained aerobic activity increases HDL, decreases total cholesterol)
- Weight control and avoidance of tobacco products
- Appropriate management of systemic diseases (e.g., diabetes mellitus, hypothyroidism, hypertension)

NONPHARMACOLOGIC MANAGEMENT

- Therapeutic lifestyle changes (TLC): Nutrition, weight reduction, increased physical activity (*See* Prevention)
- Patient education regarding risk factors, lifestyle modifications, diet, exercise, etc.

INDICATIONS FOR PHARMACOLOGICAL MANAGEMENT

- 3 risk categories delineate treatment options based on "CHD 10 year risk" calculation from Framingham *and* presence of major risk factors
- Primary lipid target is LDL

ATP III Classification of LDL, Total, and HDL Cholesterol (mg/dL)	
LDL Cholesterol	
< 100	*Optimal*
100-129	*Near or above optimal*
130-159	*Borderline high*
160-189	*High*
≥ 190	*Very high*
Total Cholesterol	
< 200	*Desirable*
200-239	*Borderline high*
≥ 240	*High*
HDL Cholesterol	
< 40	*Low*
≥ 60	*High (negative risk factor)*
Source: Adult Treatment Panel III, 2004	
Pediatric patients	
Total Cholesterol	
< 170 mg/dl	*Desirable*
LDL Cholesterol	
< 110 mg/dL	*Desirable*

Lipid Screening Recommendation
Screen every 5 years beginning at age 20 for those who smoke, have diabetes, or have a history of heart disease.
Screen every 5 years beginning at age 35 (men) and at age 45 (women).

Note: From U.S. Preventive Services Task Force Guide to clinical preventive services, 1996.

Major Risk Factors
Age (men ≥ 45 years or females ≥ 55 years
Family history of premature CHD (first degree relatives, CHD in males < 55 yrs or females < 65 years)
Cigarette smoking
Hypertension (BP ≥ 140/90 mm Hg or on antihypertensive therapy)
HDL < 40mg/dl, triglycerides > 200 mg/dl
Metabolic syndrome
Established CHD (history of MI, stable/unstable angina, previous CAD interventions
CHD risk equivalents (Peripheral artery disease, abdominal aortic aneurysm, carotid disease, diabetes)

Note: From Third Report of the Expert Panel on Detection, Evaluation, and Treatment of High Blood Cholesterol in Adults (Adult Treatment Panel III) by the National Cholesterol Education Program (NCEP), 2004.

Summary of 2004
ATP III Updated Guidelines

Risk	Demographics	Lipid Goals/Pharmacologic Intervention
Low	0-1 risk factors and 10 year risk of CHD < 10%	Goal LDL < 160 mg/dl: if > 160, then trial of TLC; if goal not reached after trial, consider medication
Moderate	2+ risk factors; and 10 year CHD risk 10-20% or 10 year CHD risk < 10%	Goal LDL < 130 mg/dl; if > 130, then trial of TLC, if unable to achieve, then medication
High	2+ risk factors and 10 year CHD risk > 20%, established CHD or CHD equivalents	Goal LDL < 100 mg/dl (optional goal 70 mg/dl); if not at goal, initiate TLC and medication

Note: From Third Report of the Expert Panel on Detection, Evaluation, and Treatment of High Blood Cholesterol in Adults (Adult Treatment Panel III) by the National Cholesterol Education Program (NCEP), 2004.

Framingham Scales

Age

Age (yr)	Male	Female
20-34	-9	-7
35-39	-4	-3
40-44	0	0
45-49	3	3
50-54	6	6
55-59	8	8
60-64	10	10
65-69	11	12
70-74	12	14
75-79	13	16

Total Cholesterol

TC (mg/dL)	Age 20-39 M	20-39 F	40-49 M	40-49 F	50-59 M	50-59 F	60-69 M	60-69 F	70-79 M	70-79 F
< 160	0	0	0	0	0	0	0	0	0	0
160-199	4	4	3	3	2	2	1	1	0	1
200-239	7	8	5	6	3	4	1	2	0	1
240-279	9	11	6	8	4	5	2	3	1	2
≥ 280	11	13	8	10	5	7	3	4	1	2

Systolic BP (mmHg)

Systolic BP mmHg	Male Treated	Male Untreated	Female Treated	Female Untreated
< 120	0	0	0	0
120-129	1	0	3	1
130-139	2	1	4	2
140-159	2	1	5	3
≥ 160	3	2	6	4

Smoking Status

Age	Non-smoker	Male Smoker	Female Smoker
20-39	0	8	9
40-49	0	5	7
50-59	0	3	4
60-69	0	1	2
70-79	0	1	1

HDL-Cholesterol

HDL mg/dL	Male	Female
≥ 60	0	-1
50-59	0	0
40-49	1	1
< 40	2	2

POINT TOTAL

10-Year CHD Risk Assessment

Male Point Total	Male 10-yr Risk %	Female Point Total	Female 10-yr Risk %
<0	< 1	< 9	< 1
0	1	9	1
1	1	10	1
2	1	11	1
3	1	12	1
4	1	13	2
5	2	14	2
6	2	15	3
7	3	16	4
8	4	17	5
9	5	18	6
10	6	19	8
11	8	20	11
12	10	21	14
13	12	22	17
14	16	23	22
15	20	24	27
16	25	≥ 25	≥ 30
≥ 17	≥ 30		

10-Year Risk ______ %　　　10-Year Risk ______ %

M = Male　　F = Female

Note: From Framingham Heart Study Risk Chart and Adult Treatment Panel III by National Heart, Lung, & Blood Institute.

PHARMACOLOGIC MANAGEMENT

SUMMARY OF LIPID LOWERING AGENTS			
AGENT	**↓ LDL**	**↑ HDL**	**↓ TRIGS**
Statins	19-54%	5-15%	7-30%
Bile Acid Sequestrants	15-30%	3-5%	Insignificant
Nicotinic acid	5-25%	15-35%	20-50%
Fibric acids	5-7%	10-20%	20-50%
Cholesterol absorption inhibitor	15-18%	3-3.5%	Insignificant

LIPID LOWERING AGENTS		
AGENT	**ACTION**	**COMMENTS**
HMG-CoA Reductase Inhibitors ("Statins") *Examples:* atorvastatin (Lipitor®) fluvastatin (Lescol®) lovastatin (Mevacor®, Altocor®) pravastatin (Pravachol®) simvastatin (Zocor®) rosuvastatin (Crestor®)	Inhibit HMG-CoA, the enzyme which is partly responsible for cholesterol synthesis	Perform liver function tests before initiating therapy, at 6 and 12 wks, and after each dose increase, then periodically. To be used in conjunction with diet, exercise, & weight reduction in overweight patients. Watch for myopathy, rhabdomyolysis. Watch for drug interactions, especially with grapefruit juice and lovastatin, simvastatin, and atorvastatin.
Bile acid sequestrants *Examples:* cholestyramine (Questran®) colesevelam (WelChol®) colestipol (Colestid®)	Bind bile acids in the intestine which prevents their absorption. These insoluble bile acid complexes are excreted in the feces	In conjunction with diet, are used to lower LDL. All are taken twice daily. May prevent absorption of fat soluble vitamins A, D, E & K. Watch for constipation, flatulence. May reduce absorption of many oral medications.
Fibric Acids *Examples:* gemfibrozil (Gemcor®) fenofibrate (TriCor®)	Increase lipolysis and elimination of triglyceride rich particles from plasma. This results in lowering of LDL	Gemfibrozil and statins concomitantly can produce rhabdomyolysis and acute renal failure. Increases risk of gallstone formation. Monitor liver function studies and glucose during therapy; both may be elevated.
Niacin *Examples:* Niacor®, Niaspan®	Not well understood but thought to decrease hepatic VLDL production. VLDL is converted to LDL. Also, may decrease lipoprotein production in the liver	Monitor liver function studies before initiation of treatment, at 6 & 12 weeks after treatment, with each dosage increase, and periodically. Poorly tolerated. Causes flushing & hypotension. Take at bedtime with an aspirin to improve tolerability. Monitor for myalgias & rhabdomyolysis.
Cholesterol Absorption Inhibitor *Example:* ezetimibe (Zetia®)	Inhibit absorption of cholesterol by the small intestine. Does not inhibit cholesterol synthesis (statins) or increase bile acid excretion	May be given as monotherapy or in conjunction with a statin. Not necessary to monitor liver function tests unless administered concurrently with another drug requiring LFT monitoring. No evidence of myopathy when used alone. GI complaints are most common.

PREGNANCY/LACTATION CONSIDERATIONS

- Cholesterol levels are usually elevated during pregnancy
- Treatment contraindicated

CONSIDERATIONS FOR SPECIAL POPULATIONS

- *Elderly:* Benefits seen with total cholesterol and LDL reduction
- Statins typically well tolerated by elderly
- *Diabetics:* Aggressive management of hyperlipidemia needed

CONSULTATION/REFERRAL

- Dietitian
- Refer to lipid specialist for children with hyperlipidemia not responsive to dietary and conservative measures

FOLLOW-UP

- Evaluate lipid values every 5 years starting at age 20 if normal values obtained

EXPECTED COURSE

- Depends on etiology and severity of disease
- 1% decrease in LDL value decreases CHD risk by 1%

POSSIBLE COMPLICATIONS

- Coronary artery disease
- Cerebrovascular disease
- Peripheral vascular disease

STABLE ANGINA

(Angina Pectoris)

DESCRIPTION

A symptom which results when myocardial oxygen demand is greater than myocardial oxygen supply. Some patients may not be symptomatic.

ETIOLOGY

- Coronary artery disease
- Coronary artery vasospasm
- Coronary thrombosis
- Aortic stenosis/insufficiency

INCIDENCE

- Males > premenopausal females
- Males = Females after menopause
- Most common in fifties, sixties, seventies

RISK FACTORS

- Family history of coronary artery disease
- Hypertension
- Hypercholesterolemia
- Diabetes mellitus
- Tobacco/cocaine use
- Obesity
- Advancing age

TYPES OF ANGINA

Classic angina	reproducible and predictable, no increase in frequency, severity, or duration
Prinzmetal's angina	results from coronary artery vasospasm; occurs in typical patterns
Unstable angina:	recent onset, or an increase in severity, frequency or duration from usual, symptoms at rest, or nocturnal symptoms

ASSESSMENT FINDINGS

- Change in symptoms warrants further investigation
- Heaviness, discomfort, pressure, pain, ache radiating to back, chest, arms, jaw, teeth
- May be precipitated by exercise, stress, cold temperature, ingestion of a heavy meal, smoking
- Pain/discomfort relieved after nitroglycerin administration
- Shortness of breath with or without activity
- Asymptomatic ("silent ischemia")
- Nausea
- Perspiration
- Palpitations

DIFFERENTIAL DIAGNOSIS

- Esophagitis/esophageal spasm
- Gastritis/peptic ulcer disease/GERD
- Pericarditis
- Pulmonary emboli
- Costochondritis
- Pneumothorax
- Chest wall syndrome
- Cholecystitis

DIAGNOSTIC STUDIES

- Electrocardiogram: may demonstrate ST segment changes
- Chest x-ray: new or worsening CHF
- Lipid level measurements: may demonstrate hyperlipidemia
- Echocardiogram if on medication affecting conduction, syncopal episode, dysrhythmia, new or worsening valvular disease
- Treadmill exercise test (if stable)
- Stress radionuclide imaging
- Coronary angiography

PREVENTION

- Modify coronary artery disease risk factors
- Adhere to antianginal medication schedule
- Consumption of low fat diet
- Monitoring and control of hypertension, hyperlipidemia, and diabetes mellitus
- Smoking cessation
- Regular, aerobic exercise

NONPHARMACOLOGIC MANAGEMENT

- Cardiac rehabilitation program if appropriate
- Modify coronary artery disease risk factors
- Adhere to antianginal medication schedule
- Stress management
- Consumption of low fat diet
- Smoking cessation
- Regular, aerobic exercise
- Attain/maintain ideal body weight
- Patient education regarding disease, treatment, lifestyle changes, reporting of change in symptoms, etc.

PHARMACOLOGIC MANAGEMENT

AGENT	ACTION	COMMENTS
Nitroglycerin *Examples:* sublingual (Nitrostat®), sustained release (Nitrong®), translingual spray (Nitrolingual®)	Produce arterial and venous dilation by relaxing vascular smooth muscle	Tolerance develops; therefore a daily nitrate free period should occur. May produce severe headache. Monitor for hypotension, palpitations. Sublingual spray for immediate relief of symptoms.
ACEI *Examples:* Captopril (Capoten®), lisinopril (Prinivil®), ramipril (Altace®)	Suppress renin-angiotensin aldosterone system; attenuate catecholamine release from adrenergic nerve endings	Recommended for secondary prevention of MI. Improves morbidity and mortality from MI.
Beta Blockers *Examples:* acebutolol (Sectral®), atenolol (Tenormin®), bisoprolol (Zebeta®), metoprolol (Toprol®), propanolol (Inderal®)	Block beta receptors in the heart which depresses myocardial contractility and decreases sympathetic stimulation	Monitor for hypotension, bradycardia, and CHF. Abrupt withdrawal can precipitate reflex tachycardia. Can worsen symptoms of peripheral artery disease by decreasing cardiac output.
Calcium channel blockers *Examples:* Amlodipine (Norvasc®), diltiazem (Cardizem®), nicardipine (Cardene®), verapamil (Calan®), nifedipine (Procardia®)	Depress myocardial contractility and increases cardiac blood flow	Monitor for arrhythmias, hypotension. Occasionally there is worsening of anginal symptoms. May cause ankle edema. Significant drug interaction can occur with grapefruit juice.
ASA	Prevent platelet aggregation and exert anti-inflammatory effect in vessels by inhibiting prostaglandin synthesis	Monitor for bleeding, tinnitus, GI irritation. Cautious use in asthmatics due to hypersensitivity reactions.
HMG-CoA Reductase Inhibitors ("Statins) *Examples:* atorvastatin (Lipitor®), fluvastatin (Lescol®), lovastatin (Mevacor®, Altocor®), pravastatin (Pravachol®), simvastatin (Zocor®), rosuvastatin (Crestor®)	Inhibit HMG-CoA, the enzyme which is partly responsible for cholesterol synthesis	Perform liver function tests before initiating therapy at 6 and 12 weeks, and after each dose increase, then periodically. To be used in conjunction with diet, exercise, and weight reduction in overweight patients. Watch for myopathy, rhabdomyolysis. Watch for drug interactions-especially with grapefruit juice and lovastatin, simvastatin, and atorvastatin.

Combinations of the above (ACE inhibitor, aspirin, beta blocker, and statin) have shown to reduce the incidence of MI and other adverse ischemic events in patients with previous MI.

CONSULTATION/REFERRAL

- Refer to cardiologist for initial symptoms or symptoms which increase in intensity, severity, duration
- For suspected myocardial infarction, give an aspirin and transfer to nearest emergency facility

FOLLOW-UP

- Depends on frequency and severity of symptoms
- Patients with stable angina should be clinically assessed every 4-6 months for the first year; then at least annually and for any change in symptoms

EXPECTED COURSE

- Depends on severity of disease, age, gender, and left ventricular function

POSSIBLE COMPLICATIONS

- Myocardial infarction
- Chronic heart failure
- Arrhythmias
- Cardiac arrest
- Death

ACUTE CORONARY SYNDROME (ACS)

DESCRIPTION

A set of closely related disorders resulting in atheromatous plaque disruption within the coronary arteries and subsequent intravascular clot formation. Myocardial ischemia results that is sufficient to cause damage to the cardiac musculature.

CLASSIFICATIONS OF ACS	
Unstable angina	UA
Non-ST segment MI	NSTEMI
ST segment MI	STEMI

ETIOLOGY

- Coronary thrombosis (plaque rupture)
- Coronary artery vasospasm

INCIDENCE

- 1.8 million hospital admissions annually
- Males > Females under age 70 years; then Males = Females

RISK FACTORS

- Family history of premature CAD (prior to age 60 years)
- Hyperlipidemia
- Age (men over 40 and post-menopausal women)
- Cigarette smoking
- Hypertension
- Sedentary lifestyle
- Diabetes mellitus
- Stressful lifestyle

ASSESSMENT FINDINGS

- Ache, pain, tightness, discomfort, or pressure in chest, arm(s), jaw, teeth, epigastrium or neck usually lasting longer than 20 minutes; often unrelieved by nitroglycerin
- Escalating severity of angina
- Nausea, vomiting, diaphoresis
- Weakness, syncope
- Feeling of impending doom
- Hypertension/hypotension
- Silent (occurs about 20% of the time often in diabetics, women, the elderly)

DIFFERENTIAL DIAGNOSIS

- Esophageal spasm
- Gastritis
- Pericarditis
- Costochondritis
- Pulmonary emboli
- Anxiety

DIAGNOSTIC STUDIES

- Troponin I: detectable 3-6 hrs after MI (if negative, consider repeating at 8-12 hours), peaks at 16 hrs, declining levels over 9-10 days (best marker of cardiac damage, more sensitive and specific than CK MB)

- Electrocardiogram: may show elevation/depression of ST segment; presence of Q waves
- CK-MB isoenzymes: presence in serum indicative of myocardial infarction
- Coagulation studies: PT & INR
- Chest x-ray: helps identify cardiomegaly, CHF, and pulmonary diseases which may mimic or exacerbate cardiac disease
- Angiography: demonstrates narrowed coronary artery by atherosclerotic lesion
- Echocardiogram: 2 D and M mode
- Others: CBC, glucose, metabolic and lipid panels, TSH, and as indicated by history

PREVENTION

- Modify coronary artery disease risk factors
- Consumption of low fat diet
- Smoking cessation
- Regular, aerobic exercise
- Stress reduction/management
- Aspirin daily

NONPHARMACOLOGIC MANAGEMENT

- Re-establish coronary perfusion via angiographic/surgical means ASAP
- Low sodium, low fat diet
- Patient education regarding disease, treatment, lifestyle changes, medications
    - ◊ Anticoagulants/antiplatelets: precautions for bleeding
    - ◊ "Cardiac cocktail" (ACEI, ASA, beta blocker, statin)
    - ◊ Blood pressure lowering
    - ◊ Lipid-lowering medications: GI side effects of nausea, vomiting, and diarrhea

PHARMACOLOGIC MANAGEMENT

- Acute phase
    - ◊ Intravenous thrombolytic drugs
    - ◊ Heparin, aspirin, other anticoagulants
    - ◊ Nitrates
    - ◊ Beta blockers
    - ◊ Antiarrhythmics
    - ◊ Oxygen
    - ◊ Analgesics
- Post-MI
    - ◊ β-blockers or calcium channel blockers
    - ◊ ACE inhibitors
    - ◊ "Statins" and/or fibrates or niacin for lipid abnormalities
    - ◊ Nitrates as needed
    - ◊ Anticoagulants/antiplatelets

AGENT	ACTION	COMMENTS
Nitroglycerin *Examples:* sublingual (Nitrostat®) sustained release (Nitrong®) translingual spray (Nitrolingual®)	Produce arterial and venous dilation by relaxing vascular smooth muscle	Tolerance develops; therefore, a daily nitrate free period should occur. May produce severe headache. Monitor for hypotension, palpitations.
ACEI *Examples:* captopril (Capoten®) lisinopril (Prinivil®) ramipril (Altace®)	Suppress renin-angiotensin aldosterone system; attenuate catecholamine release from adrenergic nerve endings	Recommended for secondary prevention of MI. Improves morbidity and mortality from MI.
Beta Blockers *Examples:* acebutolol (Sectral®) atenolol (Tenormin®) bisoprolol (Zebeta®) metoprolol (Toprol®) propanolol (Inderal®)	Block beta receptors in the heart which depress myocardial contractility and decreases sympathetic stimulation	Monitor for hypotension, bradycardia, and CHF. Abrupt withdrawal can precipitate reflex tachycardia. Can worsen symptoms of peripheral artery disease by decreasing cardiac output.
Calcium channel blockers *Examples:* Amlodipine (Norvasc®) diltiazem (Cardizem®) nicardipine (Cardene®) verapamil (Calan®) nifedipine (Procardia®)	Depress myocardial contractility and increases cardiac blood flow	Monitor for arrhythmias, hypotension. Occasionally there is worsening of anginal symptoms. May cause ankle edema. Significant drug interactions can occur with grapefruit juice.
ASA	Prevent platelet aggregation and exerts anti-inflammatory effect in vessels by inhibiting prostaglandin synthesis	Monitor for bleeding, tinnitus, GI irritation. Cautious use in asthmatics due to hypersensitivity reactions.
HMG-CoA Reductase Inhibitors ("Statins) *Examples:* atorvastatin (Lipitor®), fluvastatin (Lescol®), lovastatin (Mevacor®, Altocor®), pravastatin (Pravachol®), simvastatin (Zocor®), rosuvastatin (Crestor®)	Inhibit HMG-CoA, the enzyme which is partly responsible for cholesterol synthesis	Perform liver function tests before initiating therapy at 6 and 12 weeks, and after each dose increase, then periodically. To be used in conjunction with diet, exercise, and weight reduction in overweight patients. Watch for myopathy, rhabdomyolysis. Watch for drug interactions-especially with grapefruit juice and lovastatin, simvastatin, and atorvastatin.

CONSULTATION/REFERRAL

- Immediate referral to nearest emergency department (give aspirin, O_2, nitroglycerin, and transport)

FOLLOW-UP

- Per cardiologist
- Encourage participation in cardiac rehab program

EXPECTED COURSE

- Dependent on severity, underlying coronary artery disease, age, response time to emergency facility

POSSIBLE COMPLICATIONS

- Death
- Chronic heart failure
- Dysrhythmias
- Left ventricular aneurysm, thrombus
- DVT, pulmonary embolism
- Mitral regurgitation
- Ventricular rupture
- Acute mitral regurgitation

VARICOSE VEINS

DESCRIPTION

Veins in which valves become incompetent and allow blood flow in the reverse direction resulting in dilated, tortuous, elongated veins.

ETIOLOGY

- Faulty valves at the saphenofemoral junction
- Previous deep venous thrombophlebitis (DVT)
- Pregnancy
- Obesity
- Prolonged standing
- Ascites

INCIDENCE

- Females > Males (2:1)
- 20% of U.S. adults

RISK FACTORS

- Prolonged standing
- Pregnancy
- Family history
- Constrictive garments (e.g., girdles, knee-high stockings)

ASSESSMENT FINDINGS

- Leg aching/burning/cramping
- Fatigue
- Orthostatic edema
- Visibly dilated and tortuous veins in lower extremities
- Symptoms may be worse during menses

DIFFERENTIAL DIAGNOSIS

- Peripheral neuritis (diabetic or alcoholic neuropathy)
- Lumbar nerve root compression or irritation
- Deep vein thrombosis
- Osteoarthritis of the hip
- Arterial insufficiency

DIAGNOSTIC STUDIES

- Usually none except inspection
- Trendelenburg's test: demonstrates retrograde blood flow past incompetent saphenous valves (leg is lifted above level of heart to empty vein, then leg is quickly lowered to observe refilling; the more quickly the veins refill, the more likely severe disease)
- Venography to rule out DVT

PREVENTION

- Leg elevation when symptomatic
- Support hose
- Avoid restrictive clothing (e.g., knee-high stockings, girdles)

NONPHARMACOLOGIC MANAGEMENT

- Support hose (best if applied before getting out of bed)
- Avoid long periods of standing in one place
- Surgical ligation and stripping
- Endovenous saphenous vein obliteration (shorter recovery time than ligation and stripping)
- Weight loss if obese
- Patient education regarding standing, use of support hose, etc.

PHARMACOLOGIC MANAGEMENT

- Usually none unless sclerotherapy is used (sclerosant is injected into intracapillary region)

PREGNANCY/LACTATION CONSIDERATIONS

- Support hose recommended
- Nonpharmacologic management as described above

CONSULTATION/REFERRAL

- Usually none needed
- Surgeon for recurrent, painful varicosities

FOLLOW-UP

- Usually none needed except to reinforce patient education

EXPECTED COURSE

- Chronic problem

POSSIBLE COMPLICATIONS

- Edema
- Venous stasis ulcers
- Pigmentation
- Phlebitis

DEEP VEIN THROMBOSIS (DVT)

DESCRIPTION

The presence of a blood clot in the venous system of the extremities or the pelvis which may migrate to the lung

ETIOLOGY

Hypercoagulable states	Oral contraceptive use Blood dyscrasias Malignant tumors (particularly prostate cancer) Pregnancy
Stasis	Postoperative period Postpartum Pregnancy
Trauma	Injury to the epithelium of the vein Hypercoagulability Stasis
Septic states	Especially from the placement of an indwelling catheter in a vein

INCIDENCE

- Male > Female (1.2: 1)
- Mean age is 60 years
- Causes 50,000 deaths per year

RISK FACTORS

- Immobility
- Malignancy
- Trauma, especially crush injuries
- Obesity
- Pregnancy with hypertension, eclampsia
- Increasing age
- Oral contraceptive use
- Smoking
- Postoperative status
- Placement of an indwelling catheter

ASSESSMENT FINDINGS

- Asymptomatic; especially initially
- Pain, warmth, erythema, tenderness, swelling of effected extremity
- Swelling without tenderness of the extremity
- Palpable cord over the involved vein

- Positive Homan sign (calf pain with dorsiflexion of the foot); low sensitivity and specificity

DIFFERENTIAL DIAGNOSIS

- Cellulitis
- Trauma
- Superficial thrombophlebitis
- Muscle strain

DIAGNOSTIC STUDIES

- D-dimer: If negative, DVT, PE highly unlikely (most authorities do not follow up with US)
- Ultrasound: inability to compress affected venous segment is diagnostic of thrombus
- Contrast venography
- CBC: elevated white count in sepsis

PREVENTION

- Depends on etiology
- Minimize or eliminate risk factors as described above

NONPHARMACOLOGIC MANAGEMENT

- Hospitalization required for acute DVT for anticoagulation therapy (heparin or IV unfractionated heparin until patient is transitioned to Coumadin)
- Patient education regarding disease, treatment, etc.

PHARMACOLOGIC MANAGEMENT

- Heparin, unfractionated heparin, or low molecular weight heparin
- Antibiotics if sepsis is suspected

PREGNANCY/LACTATION CONSIDERATIONS

- Warfarin and NSAIDs are contraindicated
- Heparin is a large molecule and does not cross the placenta

CONSULTATION/REFERRAL

- Refer to specialist for DVT, septic thrombophlebitis, hypercoagulable states

FOLLOW-UP

- Patient usually on oral anticoagulation therapy for 3-12 months depending on etiology

EXPECTED COURSE

- Good prognosis for aseptic thrombophlebitis
- Superficial thrombophlebitis is generally not associated with DVT
- Pulmonary embolism more likely if thigh veins are involved; less likely if calf veins are involved

POSSIBLE COMPLICATIONS

- Pulmonary embolism from DVT
- Sepsis

PERIPHERAL ARTERIAL DISEASE (PAD)
(Arteriosclerosis obliterans)

DESCRIPTION

A systemic disease which leads to impedance of arterial blood flow to the lower extremities. The upper extremities can be involved, but this is not usual.

ETIOLOGY

- Arterial atheromatous plaques develop in vessels of the lower extremities secondary to systemic atherosclerosis

INCIDENCE

- 20% of patients older than 70 years have PAD, 5% of these patients are symptomatic
- Males > Females (2:1)

RISK FACTORS

- Advancing age
- Elevated serum lipids
- Hypertension
- Cigarette smoking (a major risk factor)
- Diabetes mellitus
- Obesity
- Family history

ASSESSMENT FINDINGS

- Intermittent claudication (earliest manifestation): pain in legs with exercise; relief with rest
- Pain, ache, cramp, or tired feeling in extremity, foot, hip, thigh, or buttocks with exercise/activity (narrowed lumen produces characteristic pain distal to site)
- Lack of hair growth on lower legs
- Thickened toenails
- Pain at rest (signifies severe disease)
- Diminished or absent pulse distal to the lesion
- Bruits in abdominal, femoral or popliteal areas
- Pale, cool extremities
- Shiny, hairless skin
- Dependent rubor (signifies severe disease)
- Prolonged capillary fill time

DIFFERENTIAL DIAGNOSIS

- Varicose veins
- Spinal stenosis
- Thromboangiitis obliterans (TAO): seen in young, male smokers
- Lumbar disk disease

DIAGNOSTIC STUDIES

- Doppler and 2D ultrasound
- Segmental blood pressure measurements: expect reduction in pressure
- Ankle-brachial index: $\leq$0.9 indicative of disease (measure brachial pressure with blood pressure cuff and compare to ankle pressure using blood pressure cuff and Doppler)
- Arteriography

PREVENTION

- Eliminate/minimize risk factors as described above

NONPHARMACOLOGIC MANAGEMENT

- Exercise, stop when it hurts, but start again when relieved (exercise training shown to be beneficial in symptom relief; regression of relief if exercise stopped)
- Prophylactic foot care
- Percutaneous transluminal angioplasty (PTA) with or without stent placement
- Bypass surgery
- Patient education regarding disease, treatment options, etc.

PHARMACOLOGIC MANAGEMENT

AGENT	ACTION	COMMENTS
Anti-platelet *Examples:* Cilostazol (Pletal®)	Inhibit platelet aggregation and produce mild vasodilation	Drug interactions with grapefruit juice. Monitor for hypotension, bleeding. Antiplatelet therapy used to prevent ischemic events
Blood viscosity reducer *Examples:* pentoxifylline (Trental®, Pentoxil®)	Mechanism is unclear but thought to reduce blood viscosity	Monitor for bleeding and hypotension.

To prevent claudication: pentoxifylline, cilostazol.
Avoid beta blockers: may worsen claudication.
Nitrates have not proven helpful.

CONSULTATION/REFERRAL

- Refer to vascular surgeon for persistent symptoms or moderate or severe ischemia
- Refer if exercise and meds have not helped after 3-6 months (75% of patients will improve on this regimen)
- Refer all nonhealing ulcers

FOLLOW-UP

- As dictated by patient condition

EXPECTED COURSE

- Mild disease may be managed conservatively
- PTA has 95% success rates in iliac vessels
- Lower rates in thigh and calf vessels
- Poor prognosis for diabetics and smokers
- High incidence of coronary disease, stroke, and CHF in patients with arteriosclerosis obliterans

POSSIBLE COMPLICATIONS

- Amputation
- Intractable pain
- Immobility
- Ischemia → necrosis → gangrene

CONGENITAL HEART DISEASE (CHD)

DESCRIPTION

Disease of the cardiovascular system that occurs prenatally and becomes evident at birth, infancy, or young adulthood. May be cyanotic or acyanotic disorders.

ETIOLOGY

- Multifactorial and too complex to identify a specific factor

INCIDENCE

- 8-10 per 1000 births
    - ◊ 33% have critical symptoms
    - ◊ 33% have symptoms in childhood
    - ◊ 33% have no symptoms
- 8-10% of CHD is due to or associated with chromosomal abnormalities
- Overall Males > Females
- Most common CHD is ventricular septal defect (30%)
- Patent ductus arteriosus (PDA) and atrial septal defect (ASD) more common in females
- Coarctation of the aorta, tetralogy of Fallot, and transposition of the great vessels are more common in males

RISK FACTORS

- Family history
- Premature birth

- Maternal exposure to alcohol, coxsackie B, cytomegalovirus, influenza, isotretinoin, lithium, mumps, rubella, thalidomide, x-ray exposure during pregnancy, or other substances
- Associated with some chromosomal abnormalities (trisomy 21, 13, 18)
- Maternal age over 40 years
- Prenatal or perinatal fetal distress
- CHD in other siblings

TYPES OF CONGENITAL HEART DISEASE

Acyanotic diseases	Atrial septal defect (ASD) Atrioventricular septal defect Ventricular septal defect (VSD) Patent ductus arteriosus (PDA)
Cyanotic diseases	Transposition of the great vessels (arteries) Tetralogy of Fallot Tricuspid atresia
Obstructive lesions	Aortic stenosis Pulmonic stenosis Coarctation of the aorta

ASSESSMENT FINDINGS

SUMMARY OF MURMURS

Murmur	Timing	Characteristics
Atrial septal defect (ASD)	Mid-systolic ejection	Asymptomatic early in life Accentuation of tricuspid valve closure Wide, fixed S2 Arterial pulses = bilaterally Grade I-III/VI harsh Easy fatigability Prone to respiratory infections May have delayed growth and development
Atrioventricular septal defect	Systolic and mid-diastolic	Frequent respiratory infections Delayed growth and development, poor weight gain Widely split S_2 Usually diagnosed in first year of life; often associated with trisomy 21
Ventricular septal defect (VSD)	Holosystolic	Frequent respiratory symptoms Easy fatigability Delayed growth and development; poor weight gain Chronic heart failure frequently present; S_3 audible Grade II-VI/VI murmur depending on severity Palpable left sternal border thrill

SUMMARY OF MURMURS		
Murmur	**Timing**	**Characteristics**
Patent ductus arteriosus (PDA)	Systolic and diastolic	Poor weight gain Diaphoretic during feedings May present as soft, localized at left clavicle Murmur progresses to harsh, continuous, rumbling murmur Bounding pulses
Transposition of the great arteries	Systolic and diastolic	Cyanosis Chronic heart failure (CHF) Large for gestational age, but delayed growth and development
Tetralogy of Fallot	Systolic ejection	Cyanosis CHF "Tet" spells: cyanotic episodes precipitated by crying, feeding, other activities Poor growth and development Squatting after exertion Easy fatigability Pale skin, poor turgor, clubbing Grade III-VI/VI harsh, murmur at 2nd ICS, left sternal border, with a thrill
Tricuspid atresia	Holosystolic	Cyanosis Tachycardia Grade III-VI/VI harsh, murmur at left sternal border Poor growth, development, poor feeding, easy fatigability
Aortic stenosis	Systolic ejection	Grade III or IV/VI harsh murmur at upper right sternal border, right neck, apex Weak peripheral pulses Easy fatigability CHF
Pulmonic stenosis	Mid to late systolic ejection	Cyanosis CHF Grade III-IV/VI harsh, murmur heard at the upper left sternal border, transmission into both lungs, left neck
Coarctation of the aorta	Systolic	Decreased blood pressure in lower extremities (upper extremity hypertension, lower extremity hypotension) Diminished pulses in lower extremities compared to upper extremities

DIFFERENTIAL DIAGNOSIS

- Innocent heart murmur
- Pulmonary disease
- Cyanotic vs. acyanotic disease
- Metabolic abnormalities
- Thyrotoxicosis
- Dysrhythmias

DIAGNOSTIC STUDIES

- Chest x-ray
- Electrocardiogram
- Echocardiogram
- Arterial blood gases
- Angiographic studies

PREVENTION

- Elimination of risk factors described above

NONPHARMACOLOGIC MANAGEMENT

- Depends on severity
- Activity restriction
- Surgical repair
- Patient/family education regarding disease, treatment, prognosis, etc.

PHARMACOLOGIC MANAGEMENT

- PDA: indomethacin (Indocin®) helps constrict and close PDA
- Transposition of the great arteries: prostaglandin E_1 to delay closure of the ductus until surgery

CONSULTATION/REFERRAL

- Innocent murmurs need no referral
- Refer to cardiologist all murmurs which are not innocent

FOLLOW-UP

- Depends on severity, age, and type of defect
- Careful attention to murmur at each visit; consider referral to pediatric cardiologist for changes in murmur

EXPECTED COURSE

- Many congenital heart defects are amenable to surgery
- Depending on severity, many may be medically managed
- Small VSD may close spontaneously during childhood

POSSIBLE COMPLICATIONS

- Cyanosis with hypoxemia
- Delayed growth and development
- Shortened lifespan
- Death

HEART MURMURS

DESCRIPTION

The sound detected when there is turbulent blood flow through the heart or the great vessels

ETIOLOGY

Organic	Due to cardiovascular disease
Functional	Disturbances produced within the cardiovascular system but which are due to other causes (e.g., anemia, thyrotoxicosis, pregnancy)
Innocent murmurs	Disturbances which may or may not be cardiac in origin, but no cardiac disease is recognized as the cause

INCIDENCE

- 30%-50% of children on random auscultation will have an innocent murmur
- True rates of congenital and acquired murmurs are unknown
- Systolic murmurs during the 3rd trimester of pregnancy are very common

RISK FACTORS

- Age (very common in children, elderly)
- Fever
- Anemia
- Pregnancy
- Thyrotoxicosis
- Hypertension
- Rigid carotid arteries
- Myocardial infarction
- Atrial tumor or thrombus (usually causes "tumor flop")
- Congenital heart disease
- Valvular disease

ASSESSMENT OF MURMURS

Timing	Systolic or diastolic, position in systole or diastole (early, mid, late, pan)
Site	Point of maximal intensity, point of propagation
Loudness	(*see* Grading of Murmurs)
Quality	Blowing, harsh, musical, soft
Shape	Decrescendo, crescendo, plateau, diamond

GRADING OF MURMURS

Grade 1	Barely audible with intense concentration
Grade 2	Faint, but audible immediately
Grade 3	Moderately loud, no thrill palpable
Grade 4	Loud with a palpable thrill
Grade 5	Very loud, audible with part of the stethoscope off the chest, thrill palpable
Grade 6	Audible without a stethoscope on the chest wall, thrill palpable

ASSESSMENT FINDINGS

SUMMARY OF INNOCENT MURMURS

Examples	Characteristics
Still's	Most frequently detected in children and adolescents
Venous hum	Soft, short, systolic, no other evidence of abnormality
Systolic ejection	May be musical or vibratory (e.g., Still's)
	Able to alter by maneuvers (e.g., standing, lying, deep respiration, posture change): diminishes when in supine position
	Varies in loudness from visit to visit
	Does not affect growth and development
	Left lower sternal border (LLSB) or pulmonic area are most common sites
	Normal S_1 and S_2, normal vital signs

SUMMARY OF SYSTOLIC MURMURS

Murmur	Timing	Characteristics
Aortic stenosis	Systolic ejection (mid systole)	Most frequently heard in elderly patients Heard best in 2nd intercostal space (ICS) to the right of the sternum Sound radiates to right clavicle and transmitted to both carotid arteries Systolic thrill may be present
Hypertrophic obstructive cardiomyopathy (HOCM)	Late systolic	Best heard at the lower left sternal border Increases with Valsalva maneuver, standing Crescendo/decrescendo murmur Usually does not radiate to neck, but biphasic carotid pulse
Pulmonic stenosis	Mid systolic	Heard best at 2nd ICS left sternal border Does not radiate like aortic murmur Variable click audible
Mitral valve insufficiency	Systolic	Mitral valve prolapse may not produce murmurs (mid to late systolic cycle) Mitral regurgitation is holosystolic. Best heard at apex of heart with patient in left lateral decubitus position Radiates toward left axilla Varies in intensity
Tricuspid regurgitation	Systolic	Best heard at left lower sternal border, over the xiphoid, sometimes over the liver Increases in intensity with inspiration Regurgitant "v" waves in the neck veins
Ventricular septal defect	Holosystolic	Holosystolic murmur Best heard at left sternal border, 4th ICS Often harsh The greater the gradient, the louder the murmur

SUMMARY OF DIASTOLIC* MURMURS

Murmur	Timing	Characteristics
Mitral stenosis	Mid-diastolic	Low-pitched apical murmur Best heard after mild exercise and patient in left lateral decubitus position May be isolated to the apex beat site Does not radiate
Tricuspid stenosis	Early diastolic	Best heard in the 4th or 5th ICS left of the sternum, xiphoid, or apex Increased in duration and intensity by exercise, inspiration, sitting forward Decrescendo murmur
Aortic regurgitation	Early diastolic	Blowing, high-pitched, decrescendo murmur Best heard at left sternal border and toward the apex
Pulmonic regurgitation	Diastolic	High-pitched decrescendo murmur Radiates to apex Heard loudest at 2nd ICS at sternal border

**Always considered abnormal.*
**Tend to be softer than systolic murmurs. Best heard with the bell of the stethoscope because low pitched.*

SUMMARY OF CONTINUOUS MURMURS

Examples	Characteristics
Patent ductus arteriosus (PDA)	Heard throughout systole and diastole Bounding pulses – PDA
Coarctation of the aorta	Weak femoral pulses – coarctation of the aorta

DIFFERENTIAL DIAGNOSIS

- Systolic vs. diastolic vs. continuous murmurs
- Pulmonary disease

DIAGNOSTIC STUDIES

- Electrocardiogram
- Chest x-ray
- Doppler echocardiography
- Angiography

PREVENTION

- Depends on etiology
- Avoidance/elimination of risk factors listed above

NONPHARMACOLOGIC MANAGEMENT

- Surgical repair (palliative)
- Patient and family education regarding disease, treatment options, etc.

PHARMACOLOGIC MANAGEMENT

- Dependent on etiology

PREGNANCY/LACTATION CONSIDERATIONS

- Murmurs due to high flow state of pregnancy usually require no intervention
- Pathological murmurs present prior to pregnancy should be managed by obstetrician/cardiologist

CONSULTATION/REFERRAL

- Refer all new, non-innocent murmurs to cardiologist

FOLLOW-UP

- Depends on severity and etiology

EXPECTED COURSE

- Murmurs associated with pregnancy disappear when pregnancy ends (2-6 weeks after delivery)
- Innocent murmurs of childhood disappear as child matures
- Other murmurs may be managed medically or surgically depending on severity
- Consider antibiotic prophylaxis prior to dental procedures or tooth cleaning for non-innocent murmurs (specific guidelines available online American Heart Association @ www.aha.org)

POSSIBLE COMPLICATIONS

- Exercise intolerance
- Chronic heart failure
- Thrombotic events
- Hypoxia

RHEUMATIC FEVER

DESCRIPTION

An immune response to Group A β-streptococcal infections involving the heart, joints, skin, and central nervous system

ETIOLOGY

- Untreated Group A β-streptococcal infections of the upper airways (e.g., pharyngitis, sinusitis)

- Rheumatic fever is not a sequela of streptococcal skin infections

INCIDENCE

- 0.1-0.3% of untreated streptococcus infections in U.S.
- Most frequently occurs in 5-15 year olds
- Recurrences are common
- Some familial component

RISK FACTORS

- Untreated/incompletely treated Group A β-streptococcal infections

ASSESSMENT FINDINGS

- Jones criteria used to diagnose patient: 2 major and 1 minor criteria must be present as well as evidence of recent streptococcal infection

Major Criteria

- Carditis: 65% have with murmurs
- Polyarthritis: 75%
- Chorea: 15%
- Erythema marginatum: 5% (macular rash with an erythematous border)
- Subcutaneous nodules: 5-10%

Minor Criteria

- Fever (101-104°F or 38.3-40.0°C)
- Arthralgias (cannot use if arthritis was a major criteria)
- Previous rheumatic fever
- Elevated ESR, C-reactive protein
- Prolonged PR interval demonstrated on electrocardiogram

DIFFERENTIAL DIAGNOSIS

- Juvenile rheumatoid arthritis
- Lyme disease
- Kawasaki syndrome
- Carditis
- Huntington's chorea
- Congenital heart defects/innocent murmurs
- Septic arthritis

DIAGNOSTIC STUDIES

- Throat culture
- ESR, C-reactive protein
- ASO titer
- Electrocardiogram
- Chest x-ray
- CBC with differential

PREVENTION

- Prompt treatment of Group A β-streptococcal pharyngitis
- Bacterial endocarditis prophylaxis for dental procedures

NONPHARMACOLOGIC MANAGEMENT

- Supportive therapy
- Bedrest during acute episode of carditis
- Limited physical activity in patients with carditis
- Patient education regarding disease, treatment, etc.

PHARMACOLOGIC MANAGEMENT

- Treat Strep infection: Penicillin (may use erythromycin or first-generation cephalosporin depending on severity of penicillin allergy)
- Treat inflammation: Aspirin/NSAIDs for joint pain
- Prednisone for severe carditis
- Prophylactic treatment with penicillin for patients with carditis until at least age 21 years, possibly for life
- Prophylactic treatment with penicillin for patients without carditis until age 21 years

CONSULTATION/REFERRAL

- Refer new cases to cardiologist as soon as suspected or diagnosed

FOLLOW-UP

- Cardiology follow-up for patients with carditis
- For patients without carditis, assess closely for first 2-3 weeks to assess for carditis

EXPECTED COURSE

- Depends on severity
- Acute phase lasts 2-6 weeks

- 90% of symptoms resolved by 12 weeks

POSSIBLE COMPLICATIONS

- Chronic heart failure
- Recurrent rheumatic fever
- Endocarditis
- Valvular or myocardial disease

KAWASAKI SYNDROME
(Mucocutaneous Lymph Node Syndrome)

DESCRIPTION

An acute, febrile, self limited disease of young children characterized by vasculitis and multisystem involvement

ETIOLOGY

- Unknown
- Association with recent use of carpet cleaning agents or exposure to new carpet is unsubstantiated

INCIDENCE

- Most children are <4 years old
- Average age of patients is 2.3 years
- More prevalent in Japan
- 10 cases/100,000 non-Asian children
- 44 cases/100,000 Asian children

RISK FACTORS

- Unknown because etiology is unknown

ASSESSMENT FINDINGS

Acute (1-2 weeks)
- High fever (103-105F) for at least 5 days, toxic appearing
- Oral mucosal lesions may last 1-2 weeks
- Perineal rash
- Non-tender cervical adenopathy (1.5 cm or > may be unilateral)
- Painful rash and edema of the feet
- Diagnosis requires fever for 5 days and 4 of these criteria:
  - ◊ Edema or erythema of the hands and feet
  - ◊ Conjunctival injection (bilateral)
  - ◊ Cervical adenopathy
  - ◊ Rash (non vesicular and polymorphous)
  - ◊ Exudative pharyngitis, diffuse oral erythema, strawberry tongue, crusting of lips and mouth

Subacute (2-8 weeks after onset)
- Without treatment: desquamation of palms, feet, periungual area, perineal area, coronary artery aneurysms, joint aches and pains
- Acute myocardial infarction may be seen
- Pancarditis
- Diarrhea, jaundice, hepatosplenomegaly
- Aseptic meningitis
- Sterile pyuria

DIFFERENTIAL DIAGNOSIS

- Infection with other Group A streptococcal organisms
- Measles
- Epstein-Barr virus, Adenovirus, roseola
- Toxic shock syndrome
- Rocky Mountain spotted fever
- Stevens-Johnson syndrome
- Juvenile rheumatoid arthritis

DIAGNOSTIC STUDIES

- WBC: shift to the left
- Elevated platelet count: 50% have greater than 450,000 mm^3
- Erythrocyte sedimentation rate (ESR): >100 mm/hour
- C-reactive protein: positive
- Electrocardiogram: prolonged PR intervals, decreased QRS voltage, flat T waves, ST changes
- Chest x-ray: dilated heart

- Echocardiogram: effusion, coronary aneurysms
- Pyuria/mild proteinuria

NONPHARMACOLOGIC MANAGEMENT

- Comfort measures
- Bedrest and limited physical activity
- Isolation of patients not necessary
- Patient education regarding disease, treatment, prognosis, etc.

PHARMACOLOGIC MANAGEMENT

- Intravenous immunoglobulins may shorten acute phase, but thought to decrease risk of coronary artery aneurysms
- Aspirin: high dose initially; decreased over the next 6-8 weeks
- If coronary aneurysms form: aspirin or other antiplatelet agents
- Corticosteroids are CONTRAINDICATED. They may increase rate of coronary aneurysm formation.

CONSULTATION/REFERRAL

- Consult pediatric cardiologist immediately for suspected cases

FOLLOW-UP

- Depends on severity
- Per cardiologist

EXPECTED COURSE

- Acute phase lasts 1-2 weeks from onset of symptoms
- Subacute phase lasts 2-8 weeks after onset (gradual improvement during this phase)
- Convalescent phase lasts months to years depending on severity

POSSIBLE COMPLICATIONS

- Myocardial infarction
- Development and rupture of coronary artery aneurysms
- Myocardial dysfunction
- Heart failure

References

ACC/AHA key data elements and definitions for measuring the clinical management and outcomes of patients with chronic heart failure (2005). *Journal of the American College of Cardiology, 46*. 1170-1207.

Barloon, T.J., Bergus, G.R., & Seabold, J.E. (1997). Diagnostic imaging of lower limb deep venous thrombosis. *American Family Physician, 56*, 791-801.

Bedinghaus, J., Leshan, L., and Diehr, S. (2001). Coronary artery disease prevention: What's different for women? *American Family Physician,* 63: 1393-400, 1405-6.

Bickley, L.S., & Szilagyi, P.G. (2003). *Bates' guide to physical examination and history taking* (8th ed.). Philadelphia: Lippincott Williams & Wilkins.

Branch, W.T. (2003). *Office practice of medicine* (4th ed.). Philadelphia: Saunders.

Braunwald, E., Zipes, D.P., & Libby, P. (Eds.). (2001). *Heart disease: A textbook of cardiovascular medicine* (4th ed.). Philadelphia: W.B. Saunders.

Burns, C.E., Brady, M.A., Blosser, C., Starr, N.B., & Dunn, A.M. (2004). *Pediatric primary care: A handbook for nurse practitioners* (3rd ed.). Philadelphia: W.B. Saunders.

Dambro, M.R. (2005). *Griffith's 5 minute clinical consult.* Philadelphia: Lippincott Williams & Wilkins.

Coy, V. (2005). Genetics of essential hypertension. *Journal of the American Academy of Nurse Practitioners, 16,* 219-224.

Crowther, M. McCourt, K. (2005). Venous thromboembolism: A guide to prevention and treatment. *The Nurse Practitioner, 30*(8), 26-43.

Executive Summary of the Third Report of the National Cholesterol Education Program (NCEP) Expert Panel on Detection, Evaluation, and Treatment of High Blood Cholesterol in Adults (Adult Treatment Panel III). (2004). *Journal of the American Medical Association, 285,* 2486-2497.

Fowles, R. E. (1995). Myocardial infarction in the 1990's. *Postgraduate Medicine, 97*(5), 135-146.

Graber, M.A., & Lanternier, M.L. (Eds.) (2001). *The family practice handbook.* (4th ed.). St. Louis: Mosby.

Gutgesell, H.P., Barst, R. J., Humes, R. A., Franklin, W.H., & Shaddy, R.E. (1997). Common cardiovascular problems in the young: Part I. Murmurs, chest pain, syncope, and irregular rhythms. *American Family Physician, 56*, 1825-1830.

Gutgesell, H.P, Atkins, D.L., & Day, R.W. (1997). Common cardiovascular problems in the young: Part II. Hypertension, hypercholesterolemia and preparticipation screening of athletes. *American Family Physician, 56*, 1993-1998.

Hahn, R.G., Knox, L.M., & Forman, T.A. (2005). Evaluation of poststreptococcal illness. *American Family Physician, 71,* 1949-1954.

Hanna, I.R., & Wenger, N.K. (2005). Secondary prevention of coronary heart disease in elderly patients. *American Academy of Family Physicians, 71,* 2289-2296.

He, J., & Whelton, P. K. (1997). Epidemiology and prevention of hypertension. *Medical Clinics of North America,* 81(5), 1077-1098.

Hunt, S.A., Baker, D.W., Chin, M.H., et al. (2001). ACC/AHA guidelines for the evaluation and management of chronic heart failure in the adult: executive summary: A report of the American College of Cardiology/American Heart Association task force on practice guidelines. *J Am Coll Cardiol*, 38:2101-13.

Kasper, D.L., Braunwald, E., Fauci, A.S., Hauser, S.L., Longo, D.L., Jameson, J.L., et al. (2004). *Harrison's principles of internal medicine* (16th ed.). New York: McGraw-Hill.

Kelechi, T.J., & Edlund, B. (2005). Chronic venous insufficiency. *Advance for Nurse Practitioners, 13*(7), 31-34.

Kliegman, R.M., Greenbaum, L.A., & Lye, P.S. (2004). *Practical strategies in pediatric diagnosis and therapy* (2nd ed.). Philadelphia: W.B. Saunders.

Lambing, A. (2005). Clearing the way: Treating venous thromboembolism and deep vein thrombosis. *Advance for Nurse Practitioners, 13*(6), 24-30.

Mangion, S. (2000). *Physical diagnosis secrets.* Philadelphia: Hanley and Belfus.

Marriott, H.J. (1993). *Bedside cardiac diagnosis.* Philadelphia: J.B. Lippincott.

Mason, C.M. (2005). The nurse practitioner's role in helping patients achieve lipid goals with statin therapy. *Journal of the American Academy of Nurse Practitioners, 17*, 256-262.

Mellion, M.B., Putukian, M., & Madden, C.C. (2002). *Sports medicine secrets.* (3rd Ed.). Philadelphia: Hanley and Belfus.

Mladenovic, J. (Ed.). (2003). *Primary care secrets.* (3rd Ed.). Philadelphia: Hanley and Belfus.

Moody, L.Y. (1997). Pediatric cardiovascular assessment and referral in the primary care setting. *The Nurse Practitioner, 22*(1), 120-134.

Moredich, C., Kark, D., & Keresztes, P. (2005). Implications of LDL subclass B in patients at cardiovascular risk. *The Nurse Practitioner, 30*(7), 16-29.

National Institutes of Health. (2003). *The seventh report of the joint national committee on prevention, detection, evaluation, and treatment of high blood pressure.* http://www.nhlbi.nih.gov/nhlbi/cardio/hbp/prof/jncintro.htm.

O'Brian, J.G., Chennubhotla, S.A., & Chennubhotla, R.V. (2005). Treatment of edema. *American Family Physician, 71,* 2111-2117.

Rakel, R.E. (Ed.). (1998). *Essentials of family practice.* (2nd ed.). Philadelphia: WB Saunders.

Reynolds, E., & Baron, R.B. (1996). Hypertension in women and the elderly. *Postgraduate medicine, 100*(4), 58-70.

Schwartz, M.W. (Ed.). (2002). *The 5 minute pediatric consult.* (2nd ed.) Philadelphia: Lippincott Williams & Wilkins.

Thomas-Kvidera, D. (2005). Heart failure from diastolic dysfunction related to hypertension: Guidelines for management. *Journal of the American Academy of Nurse Practitioners, 17*, 168-175.

Tobin, L.J. (1999). Evaluating mild to moderate hypertension. *The Nurse Practitioner*, 24(5): 22-41.

Uphold, C.R., & Graham, M.V. (2003). *Clinical guidelines in family practice.* (4th ed.). Gainesville, FL: Barmarrae Books.

U.S. Preventive Services Task Force. (1996). *Guide to clinical preventive services.* (2nd ed.) Washington, D.C.: Office of Disease Prevention and Health Promotion, U.S. Government Printing Office.

Wise, G.R., & Schultz, T.T. (1996). Hyperlipidemia. *Postgraduate Medicine, 100*(1), 138-149.

Zellner, C., & Sudhir, K. (1996). Lifestyle modifications for hypertension. *Postgraduate Medicine, 100*(4), 75-83.

Zollo, A.J., Jr (Ed.). (2004). *Medical Secrets.* (4th ed.), St. Louis, MO: Mosby-Year Book.

2

DERMATOLOGIC DISORDERS: ADULT

Dermatologic Disorders: Adult

SKIN CANCER

DESCRIPTION

Malignant tumors of the skin arising from various skin layers

ETIOLOGY

- Almost always due to overexposure of the skin to ultraviolet rays

INCIDENCE

- Squamous cell: 20% of all skin cancers
- Basal cell: 900,000 cases annually (most common skin cancer)
- Malignant melanoma: <5% of all skin cancers

RISK FACTORS

- Exposure to ultraviolet rays, thermal burns, or radiation
- Fair skin; blondes and redheads
- Light blue or green eye color
- Improper and infrequent use of sunscreen
- Blistering sunburn in adolescence
- Intense, episodic sun exposure
- Living in sunny climates

ASSESSMENT FINDINGS

- *Squamous cell carcinoma (SCC)*
  - ◊ Common on sun exposed areas of the skin
  - ◊ Lower lip is common location in smokers
  - ◊ Nodule has indistinct margins; surface is firm, scaly, irregular and may bleed easily
- *Basal cell carcinoma (BCC)*
  - ◊ Common in 40 to 60 year olds
  - ◊ Most common sites are head (tip of nose) and neck
  - ◊ Usual appearance is pearly domed nodule with overlying telangiectatic vessels; later, central ulceration and crusting
- *Malignant melanoma*
  - ◊ Usual age is early forties
  - ◊ *ABCDE* characteristics of any lesion

***A* = asymmetry**
***B* = border is irregular**
***C* = color variegation**
***D* = diameter >6 mm (size of pencil eraser)**
***E* = elevation above level of skin**

  - ◊ Hypo or hyperpigmentation, bleeding, scaling, texture, or size change of an existing mole or lesion
  - ◊ Common in Caucasians on back, lower leg
  - ◊ Common in African Americans on hands, feet, nails

DIFFERENTIAL DIAGNOSIS

- Molluscum contagiosum
- Actinic keratosis
- Seborrheic keratosis
- Dysplastic nevi
- Basal cell vs. squamous cell vs. malignant melanoma

DIAGNOSTIC STUDIES

- Removal of lesion
- Surgical biopsy

PREVENTION

- Actinic keratosis is a scaly patch of red or brown skin which often becomes SCC
- Avoidance of sun exposures
- Frequent total body skin examination every 3-6 months after diagnosis of melanoma
- Teach importance of avoidance of sunlight at peak hours, use of sunscreen to patients, especially adolescents
- Hats, long sleeve shirts while exposed to sunlight

NONPHARMACOLOGIC MANAGEMENT

- Surgical biopsy
- Surgical removal of lesion

- Lymph node excision in melanoma

PHARMACOLOGIC MANAGEMENT

- Chemotherapy/immunotherapy for melanoma

PREGNANCY/LACTATION CONSIDERATIONS

- Melanoma may be spread to the fetus via the placenta
- Melanoma patients are encouraged to wait two years after no evidence of malignancy before attempting pregnancy

CONSULTATION/REFERRAL

- Dermatologist
- Surgeon

FOLLOW-UP

- By dermatologist or surgeon

EXPECTED COURSE

- Squamous cell: may metastasize
- Basal cell: slow-growing, rarely metastasizes; often there is recurrence within 5 years at another site
- Malignant melanoma: accounts for over 60% of skin cancer deaths, metastasizes to any organ

POSSIBLE COMPLICATIONS

- Metastatic spread
- Local recurrence
- Disfigurement

ALLERGIC CONTACT DERMATITIS (ACD)

DESCRIPTION

Acute inflammation of the skin due to contact with an external substance or object

ETIOLOGY

- Chemical irritants: nickel, turpentine, soaps, detergents (usually produces immediate discomfort)
- Plants (rhus-urushiol): poison ivy or oak (delayed hypersensitivity reaction produces discomfort within 4-12 hours)

INCIDENCE

- Common

RISK FACTORS

- Family history
- Continued contact with an offending substance: plants, chemicals, soaps.

Fluid in blister NOT able to spread reaction.

- Topical drugs: neomycin, thimerosal, paraben
- Occupation: gloves

ASSESSMENT FINDINGS

- Redness, itching, bullae, and/or surrounding erythema
- Lines of demarcation with sharp borders
- Papules and/or vesicles
- Scaling, crusting, or oozing
- Initially, the dermatitis may be limited to the site of contact, but may later spread
- Palms and soles less likely to exhibit reaction
- Thin skin areas may be more sensitive (e.g., antecubital space, eyelids, genitalia)

DIFFERENTIAL DIAGNOSIS

- Seborrheic dermatitis
- Eczema
- Herpes simplex if appearance vesicular

DIAGNOSTIC STUDIES

- Usually none
- Patch test with offending substance

PREVENTION

- Avoid contact with offending substance
- Use protective items (e.g., gloves, long sleeves)

NONPHARMACOLOGIC MANAGEMENT

- Avoid contact with offending substance
- If contact with substance occurs, wash skin immediately (within 15 minutes) with soap and water and rinse liberally
- Soaks with cool water may help burning and/or irritation
- Tepid bath may help with pruritus
- Emollients to prevent drying if chronic inflammation
- Monitor for bacterial secondary infection

PHARMACOLOGIC MANAGEMENT

- Corticosteroids: topical, oral and/or injectable
- 3 factors affect potency of topical corticosteroids: steroid, concentration, and vehicle (vehicle = lotion, cream, etc.)
- Absorption increases based on the vehicle: lotion< cream< gel< ointment
- Calamine lotion for itching
- Moisture barrier: zinc oxide
- Antihistamine: topical and/or oral
- Topical or oral antibiotics if secondarily infected

AGENT	ACTION	COMMENTS
Topical Corticosteroids Low potency (various) Medium potency (various) High potency (various) Very high potency (various)	Exert anti-inflammatory effect nonspecifically thru mechanical, chemical and immunologic means	Use lowest potency steroid cream that produces desired effect. Skin atrophy is common with long-term steroid use. Areas most susceptible are the face, groin, and axillae. Topical steroids will worsen skin infections. Systemic absorption is usually minimal, but broken skin will absorb significantly more steroid.

PREGNANCY/LACTATION CONSIDERATIONS

- Prudent use of medications

CONSULTATION/REFERRAL

- Dermatologist for slow to respond lesions
- Allergist

FOLLOW-UP

- Depends on severity

EXPECTED COURSE

- Self-limited

POSSIBLE COMPLICATIONS

- Secondary bacterial infection
- More severe subsequent reactions

ATOPIC DERMATITIS
(ECZEMA)

DESCRIPTION

Chronic, pruritic skin eruption with acute exacerbations appearing in characteristic sites. Eczema is often used interchangeably with atopic dermatitis, but the word eczema describes acute symptoms associated with atopic dermatitis.

Commonly seen in patients with other atopic illnesses (e.g., asthma, allergic rhinitis).

ETIOLOGY

- Multifactorial: genetic, physiological, immunologic, and environmental factors

INCIDENCE

- Effects 5% of all children
- Begins after 2 months of age, resolves by 3 years (50% continue into adulthood)
- Males = Females

RISK FACTORS

- Family history of atopic diseases
- Skin infections
- Stress
- Temperature extremes
- Contact with irritating substances (wearing new clothing prior to washing)

ASSESSMENT FINDINGS

- General: pruritus, erythema, dry skin, facial erythema, infraorbital folds (Dennie Morgan folds)
- Infants
    - ◊ Lesions on extensor surfaces of arms and legs, cheeks
    - ◊ Lesions are erythematous and papular
    - ◊ Vesicles may ooze, form crusts
- Children
    - ◊ Lesions common in wrists, ankles, and flexural surfaces
    - ◊ Presence of scales and plaques; lichenification occurs from scratching
- Adults
    - ◊ Flexural surfaces are common sites, dorsa of the hands and feet
    - ◊ Often reappears in adulthood after absence since childhood
    - ◊ Lichenification and scaling are typical

DIFFERENTIAL DIAGNOSIS

- Contact dermatitis
- Seborrheic dermatitis
- Scabies
- Psoriasis

DIAGNOSTIC STUDIES

- Usually none needed
- Skin biopsy to rule out other skin disorders

PREVENTION

- Prevent dry skin (essential for good control)
- Avoid any known precipitating factors (stress, wool clothing, fragrance-free detergents, etc.)

NONPHARMACOLOGIC MANAGEMENT

- Limit bathing (do not use hot water) to avoid further drying of skin
- Prevent skin trauma (sunburns, etc.)
- Soak for 20 minutes in warm water before applying emollient (when possible)
- Wet compresses (Burrow's solution) if lesions are weeping or oozing
- Patient education regarding disease process, self-care, and precipitating factors

PHARMACOLOGIC MANAGEMENT

- Topical corticosteroids are the mainstay of therapy (use lowest potency which controls symptoms)
- Topical immune modulators: Elidel®, Protopic®
- Antihistamines (oral and topical) for itching
- Emollients 2-3 times per day or as needed to correct dry skin (Eucerin®, Lubriderm®, Cetaphil®)
- Oral corticosteroids may be used for severe cases. Due to the chronic nature of this disease, this should be reserved and only used in short bursts.
- Intralesional steroid injections

AGENT	ACTION	COMMENTS
Topical immune modulators *Examples:* tacrolimus (Protopic®) pimecrolimus (Elidel®)	Potent immune modulators which inhibit T-lymphocyte activation	Do not use on infected skin. Infection will significantly worsen eczema. Potential for systemic absorption may increase formation of tumors.

CONSULTATION/REFERRAL

- Dermatologist for severe cases or those not responding to treatment

FOLLOW-UP

- Individualize based on patient severity

EXPECTED COURSE

- Exacerbations and remissions expected

POSSIBLE COMPLICATIONS

- Bacterial secondary infections from topical steroid use and scratching
- Atrophy or striae if high potency medications are used on the face
- Lichenification

PSORIASIS

DESCRIPTION

A chronic, pruritic, inflammatory skin disorder characterized by rapid proliferation of epidermal cells. Have frequent remissions and exacerbations.

There are several variants, but the most common form occurs with plaque type lesions.

ETIOLOGY

- Unknown, but family history present in one-third of cases
- Following streptococcal infections in children (acute guttate psoriasis)

INCIDENCE

- 1/1000 persons in U.S.
- Males = Females
- Peak ages of onset: 16-22 years and 57-61 years

RISK FACTORS

- Streptococcal infection
- Family history
- Stress
- Local trauma or irritation

ASSESSMENT FINDINGS

- Silvery, white scales on erythematous base
- Pruritus
- Common distribution to elbows, knees, scalp
- May also appear on eyebrows, ears, trunk
- Nails may be pitted
- Positive Auspitz sign (pinpoint bleeding occurs when lesions are scraped)

DIFFERENTIAL DIAGNOSIS

- Seborrheic dermatitis
- Pityriasis rosea, tinea corporis (guttate psoriasis)
- Squamous cell carcinoma
- Candidal infections
- Contact dermatitis
- Eczema

DIAGNOSTIC STUDIES

- Usually none needed, but if uncertain, then biopsy

- May order streptococcal swab if guttate psoriasis is suspected
- KOH to rule out fungal infection
- ESR: often increased
- If joint involvement: rheumatoid factor

PREVENTION

- Avoid sunburn which may precipitate exacerbations
- Avoid known precipitants
- Avoid sudden withdrawal of steroids
- Avoid stimulating drugs: ACE inhibitors, beta-blockers, NSAIDs, penicillin, salicylates, sulfonamides, tetracycline

NONPHARMACOLOGIC MANAGEMENT

- Warm soaks to remove thickened plaques
- Solar radiation, ultraviolet radiation
- Oatmeal bath for itching
- Wet dressings (Burrow's solution) for itching

PHARMACOLOGIC MANAGEMENT

- Emollients (Eucerin®, Lubriderm®, Cetaphil®) to hydrate skin
- Topical steroids (*see topical corticosteroid table Allergic Contact Dermatitis*): consider plastic occlusion in adults and older children (with caution) to hasten resolution; increases skin penetration 10-fold
- Intralesional steroid injections
- Tar solutions alone or in combination with topical steroids
- Salicylic acid gel or ointment as a keratolytic agent
- Ultraviolet lamps and sunlight
- Methotrexate, Etanercept (Enbrel®): used for severe cases

PREGNANCY/LACTATION CONSIDERATIONS

- Ultraviolet radiation may be safest
- Avoid coal tar preparations, systemic and topical steroids

CONSULTATION/REFERRAL

- Dermatologist for severe cases and those that are slow to respond to treatment

FOLLOW-UP

- Individualize per patient

EXPECTED COURSE

- Remissions and exacerbations are expected
- May be refractory to treatment

POSSIBLE COMPLICATIONS

- Thinning of skin, striae due to topical steroids
- Rebound after steroids are withdrawn

SEBORRHEIC DERMATITIS
(Cradle Cap, Seborrhea)

DESCRIPTION

Chronic, superficial disorder affecting the hairy areas of the body where many sebaceous glands are present (e.g., scalp, eyebrows, face).

ETIOLOGY

- Multifactorial: genetics, environment
- *Pityrosporum ovale* thought to be a causative agent

INCIDENCE

- Common throughout lifespan
- Males > Females

RISK FACTORS

- Emotional stress
- Family history
- Parkinson disease

- HIV infection (early cutaneous manifestation)

ASSESSMENT FINDINGS

- Infants
  - ◊ Mild disease presents as fine, white or yellow greasy scale on an erythematous base (usually resolves by 1 year of age)
  - ◊ Severe disease presents as dull, red plaques with thick white or yellow scale on an erythematous base
  - ◊ "Cradle cap" when occurs on scalp
  - ◊ Diaper rash
  - ◊ Axillary rash
  - ◊ Mild erythema
- Adults
  - ◊ Greasy, scaling rash
  - ◊ Commonly found in scalp, eyebrows, nasolabial area, ear canals, upper back/anterior chest
  - ◊ Erythema
  - ◊ Rash is usually symmetrical and bilateral
  - ◊ No loss of hair

DIFFERENTIAL DIAGNOSIS

- Atopic dermatitis
- Dandruff
- Acne rosacea
- Psoriasis
- Candidal infection
- Tinea capitis

DIAGNOSTIC STUDIES

- Usually none

NONPHARMACOLOGIC MANAGEMENT

- Exposure to sunlight
- Shampoo frequently (for scalp lesions)
- Apply warm peanut, olive, or mineral oil in PM to help remove thick scale, wash off in AM with shampoo (may use soft bristle brush to loosen scale)

PHARMACOLOGIC MANAGEMENT

- *Scalp*
  - ◊ OTC antiseborrheic shampoo containing selenium sulfide (Selsun Blue® shampoo), sulfur, salicylic acid, coal tar (leave in for 5-10 minutes, then rinse)
  - ◊ Topical steroid gel massaged into scalp 2-3 times per week (for scalp not responsive to OTC agents); taper steroid
- *Face*
  - ◊ 1% hydrocortisone cream (thin layer, short term)
- *Ears and scalp margin*
  - ◊ Fluorinated hydrocortisone cream (short term use only)
- *Eyelids*
  - ◊ Cleanse with dilute baby shampoo using a cotton swab
  - ◊ 1% ophthalmic hydrocortisone preparation
- *Other areas*
  - ◊ Antiseborrheic shampoo
  - ◊ Low potency hydrocortisone cream

CONSULTATION/REFERRAL

- Dermatologist for severe cases or cases which are unresponsive to therapy

FOLLOW-UP

- Individualize for patients

EXPECTED COURSE

- In infants, usually resolves by 8 months of age
- In adults, expect remissions and unpredictable exacerbations

POSSIBLE COMPLICATIONS

- Striae from use of fluorinated corticosteroids, especially if used on face
- Skin atrophy

PITYRIASIS ROSEA

DESCRIPTION

Idiopathic self-limiting skin disorder characterized by papulosquamous lesions distributed over the trunk and extremities

ETIOLOGY

- Unknown
-

INCIDENCE

- Common
- Males = Females
- Occurs in all age groups, but most common in ages 10-35 years

RISK FACTORS

- None known

ASSESSMENT FINDINGS

- "*Herald patch*" on trunk resembles tinea corporis and precedes the generalized rash
- *Salmon-colored oval plaques* 1-10 cm in diameter and with fine scales
- "*Collarette" of loose scales* along the border of the plaques
- Oval shaped lesions appear parallel to each other on the trunk, hence the term, "*Christmas tree*" pattern rash
- Mild pruritus; occasional reports of severe pruritus
- In children, lesions may be more papular and on face and distal extremities

DIFFERENTIAL DIAGNOSIS

- Tinea corporis, versicolor
- Viral exanthems
- Drug rash
- Secondary syphilis

DIAGNOSTIC STUDIES

- None usually needed
- Syphilis serology strongly suggested since secondary syphilis can present in this manner
- KOH if fungal infection suspected

NONPHARMACOLOGIC MANAGEMENT

- Lukewarm oatmeal bath to relieve itching
- Reassurance that condition is self-limiting
- Good hygiene to prevent bacterial secondary infections

PHARMACOLOGIC MANAGEMENT

- Antipruritics (topical or oral): Calamine lotion®, hydroxyzine (Atarax®)

CONSULTATION/REFERRAL

- Dermatologist if unresolved after 8-10 weeks

FOLLOW-UP

- Usually none needed
- Resolution usually 2-6 weeks

EXPECTED COURSE

- Benign course, resolution in 1-14 weeks

POSSIBLE COMPLICATIONS

- Secondary bacterial infection from scratching

BURNS

DESCRIPTION

Injury to skin and tissues caused by chemicals, thermal energy, radiation, or electricity

ETIOLOGY

- Excessive sun exposure
- Flames or hot water most common
- Electrical wires, lightning
- Chemical splashes: acids or bases

INCIDENCE

- Common
- Splashes and flames are most common causes
- Leading cause of death in children
- Hot water burns are common means of abuse

RISK FACTORS

- Occupational exposure to chemicals
- Carelessness
- Hot water heaters set too high, especially in the elderly
- Improper use of sunscreens
- Insensitivity (e.g., diabetes mellitus, paralysis)

ASSESSMENT FINDINGS

- *Partial thickness*: first and second degree burns
- *Full thickness*: third degree burns
- General distribution of burns may indicate source
- Straight burn lines may indicate child abuse (bilaterally symmetrical on extremities)
- Geriatric burns heal more slowly

Burns	Appearance
First-degree (superficial layers of epidermis)	Redness Tenderness No blisters
Second degree (epidermal injury with blister formation	Redness Tenderness Presence of blisters
Third degree (destruction of all skin elements)	Charred, leathery appearance of skin Skin may be white with red edges Very little tenderness

DIFFERENTIAL DIAGNOSIS

- Chemical vs. electrical vs. thermal vs. solar
- Scalded skin syndrome

DIAGNOSTIC STUDIES

- Usually none indicated for first- or second-degree burns of limited area
- Culture and sensitivity if infected
- EKG if electrical burn

PREVENTION

- Liberal sunscreen use
- In children, limit access to electrical cords, wires, chemicals, etc.
- Parental supervision
- Use of home smoke detectors and plan for evacuation of home in case of fire
- Knowledge of proper use of home fire extinguishers
- Set home water heaters 120-130°F

NONPHARMACOLOGIC MANAGEMENT

- Do not apply ice to burns. Apply cool water or saline only to clean. May use a mild soap.
- Remove clothing, jewelry, over and around burned areas

- Flush chemical burns with cool water for 30 minutes to 2 hours depending on substance and severity
- Remove blistered skin after rupturing blisters
- Clean and redress burn 1-2 times/day (frequency dependent on severity)
- Good nutrition during convalescence

PHARMACOLOGIC MANAGEMENT

- Apply antibacterial cream: bacitracin (around mucus membranes and face), silver sulfadiazine (Silvadene®)
- Consider biologic dressings (very expensive)
- Analgesics to relieve pain
- Tetanus prophylaxis if not within 10 years

CONSULTATION/REFERRAL

- Refer to specialist all burns not considered minor: second-degree burns >20% of body, all third-degree burns, burns of the eyes, hands, face, feet, or perineum, lightening burns, electrical burns, burns over joints
- Child/elderly protection for suspected abuse

FOLLOW-UP

- Most burns are minor and can be managed on an outpatient basis
- Depends on severity and age of patient, but follow-up 1-3 days and until resolved

EXPECTED COURSE

- First degree burns resolve without complications
- Second degree burns resolve in about 2 weeks

POSSIBLE COMPLICATIONS

- Bacterial secondary infection (usually Gram negative organisms)
- Scarring

SPIDER/INSECT BITES AND STINGS

DESCRIPTION

The injection of venom or another substance by a bee, wasp, ant, mosquito, flea, tick, or spider which can produce local or systemic hypersensitivity.

ETIOLOGY

- *Bees/wasps/ants*: local or systemic hypersensitivity reaction
- *Mosquitoes/fleas*: local or systemic hypersensitivity reaction
- *Ticks*: blood is sucked by the female tick and toxin may be injected which enables disease transmission
- *Spiders/scorpions/caterpillars*: venom injected can be necrotizing, hemolytic; reaction can be local, systemic, or both

INCIDENCE

- *Bees/wasps*: common
- *Mosquitoes/fleas*: most common insect bite; seasonal pattern of incidence
- *Ticks*: common in spring and early summer
- *Spiders/caterpillars*: common, bites from most spiders are harmless, but the brown recluse, black widow, and hobo spiders can cause local as well as systemic reactions

RISK FACTORS

- Contact with grasses, weeds, bushes, or dark, cool areas
- Residence in parts of the U.S. where certain insects or spiders are indigenous
- Previous bite by same insect or spider
- Wearing of bright-colored clothes or scented perfumes, cosmetics, lotions, soaps, etc.

- Improper protective clothing while exposed to insects or spiders

ASSESSMENT FINDINGS

- Bees/wasps
  - ◊ Local redness
  - ◊ Pruritus
  - ◊ Pain
  - ◊ Edema
  - ◊ Cellulitis
  - ◊ Anaphylaxis in susceptible individuals
- Mosquitoes/fleas
  - ◊ Urticarial wheal
  - ◊ Itching
  - ◊ Central punctum
  - ◊ Secondary bacterial infection (impetigo)
- Ticks
  - ◊ Presence of tick (which may go undetected for several days)
  - ◊ Erythematous halo
  - ◊ Pruritus if tick body parts remain under the skin
- Spiders/caterpillars
  - ◊ Punctate marks on the skin
  - ◊ Severe burning, stinging at site when bite occurs
  - ◊ Severe pain, swelling, burning, stinging for several hours after bite
  - ◊ Necrosis locally
  - ◊ Abdominal pain (black widow spider bite)
  - ◊ Local reaction can progress to systemic reaction in certain individuals; characterized by fever, chills, aches, rash, nausea, vomiting, diarrhea, cramps, shock

DIFFERENTIAL DIAGNOSIS

- Bites/stings from harmless insects/spiders vs. poisonous insects/spiders
- Contact dermatitis
- Cellulitis
- Allergic reaction
- Poison ivy/oak
- Acute abdomen

DIAGNOSTIC STUDIES

- Usually none indicated
- CBC
- Culture and sensitivity if secondarily infected

PREVENTION

- *See* Risk Factors
- Minimize contact with environments likely to harbor insects/spiders

NONPHARMACOLOGIC MANAGEMENT

- Cool compresses for itching/edema
- Elimination of fleas from home environment
- Firmly grasp tick with forceps or tweezers to remove (do not attempt to burn tick)
- Remove stinger
- Elevation of extremity for severe edema
- Application of ice to spider bites. **Avoid application of heat!**
- Examination of unprotected body parts after exposure to potential tick infested areas
- Possible debridement

PHARMACOLOGIC MANAGEMENT

- *Oral* antipruritics/antihistamines/analgesics/steroids
- *Topical* antipruritics/antihistamines/corticosteroids
- Application of insect repellents (may be absorbed systemically). Apply with caution in pediatric and elderly patients.
- Tetanus prophylaxis for spider bites
- Analgesics for spider bites
- Topical/systemic antibiotics for secondarily infected bites (*Refer to Furunculosis, Carbunculosis and Cellulitis antibiotic tables.*)
- Preloaded syringe of epinephrine for patients with potential for anaphylactic reaction
- Short course of steroids for severe local reactions which extend beyond two joints
- Anti-venoms

AGENT	ACTION	COMMENTS
Antihistamine/antipruritic (first generation) *Examples:* diphenhydramine (Benadryl®) hydroxyzine (Atarax®, Vistaril®)	Non-selectively block histamine binding sites centrally (in the brain) and peripherally	Common side effects are sedative and relief of itching. Don't use in symptomatic prostatic hypertrophy because of anti-cholinergic effects (inability to urinate). Monitor additive effects with EtOH, other sedative drugs. Cautious use in elderly where exaggerated effects may produce excessive sedation, dizziness, confusion, hypotension. Many available OTC.
Antihistamine/antipruritic (second generation) *Examples:* cetirizine (Zyrtec®) fexofenadine (Allegra®) loratadine (Claritin®)	Selectively block peripheral histamine binding and so sedation is not as common as with first generation agents	Advantage is lack of sedation (but not cetirizine). Once daily dosing. Generally well tolerated. Expensive compared to first generation agents.

CONSULTATION/REFERRAL

- **Don't delay treatment!** Reactions usually take place within 2-60 minutes.
- Emergency department for severe reactions
- Surgeon/dermatologist for severe local reactions
- Consider referral for severe reaction in the very young and very old

FOLLOW-UP

- Individualize by severity

EXPECTED COURSE

- Depends on type of bite, type of reaction, age of patient

POSSIBLE COMPLICATIONS

- Anaphylactic reactions possible
- Secondary bacterial infections
- Increased intensity of reactions with subsequent bites

SEBORRHEIC KERATOSIS

DESCRIPTION

Benign skin tumor

ETIOLOGY

- Unknown

INCIDENCE

- Common in middle-aged and older adults
- Appear on the trunk or temples

RISK FACTORS

- Unknown
- Perhaps sun exposure

ASSESSMENT FINDINGS

- Round or oval shaped
- Flesh colored or brown or black
- Waxy appearance, but may be scaling or crusted
- Appears "stuck on"
- Size varies from 0.25-3.0 cm

DIFFERENTIAL DIAGNOSIS

- Mole
- Malignant melanoma
- Basal cell carcinoma
- Squamous cell carcinoma

DIAGNOSTIC STUDIES

- None indicated when origin of lesion is obvious

References

Achar, S. (1996). Principles of skin biopsies for the family physician. *American Family Physician, 54*(8), 2411-2422.

American Academy of Pediatrics. (2003). *Red book: Report of the committee on infectious disease* (26th ed.). Elk Grove Village, IN: American Academy of Pediatrics.

Anderson, M.L. (2005). Atopic dermatitis: More than a simple skin disorder. *Journal of the American Academy of Nurse Practitioners, 17*, 249-255.

Bickley, L.S., & Szilagyi, P.G. (2003). *Bates' guide to physical examination and history taking* (8th ed.). Philadelphia: Lippincott Williams & Wilkins.

Branch, W.T. (2003). *Office practice of medicine* (4th ed.). Philadelphia: Saunders.

Burns, C.E., Brady, M.A., Blosser, C., Starr, N.B., & Dunn, A.M. (2004). *Pediatric primary care: A handbook for nurse practitioners* (3rd ed.). Philadelphia: W.B. Saunders.

Dambro, M.R. (2005). *Griffith's 5 minute clinical consult.* Philadelphia: Lippincott Williams & Wilkins.

Davis, R.E. (1997). Diagnosing neurofibromatosis type I in children. *The Nurse Practitioner, 22*(4), 73-81.

Diehl, K.B. (1996). Topical antifungal agents: An update. *American Family Physician, 54*, 1687-1692.

Elston, D.M. (2005). Bites and stings: Be prepared to respond quickly. *Clinical Advisor, 8(7)* 20-32.

Epstein, E. (2001). *Common Skin Disorders.* (5th ed.). Philadelphia: WB Saunders.

Goldstein, B.G. & Goldstein, A.O. (2001). Diagnosis and management of malignant melanoma. *American Family Physician 63*, 1359-1368, 1374.

Graber, M.A., & Lanternier, M.L. (Eds.) (2001). *The family practice handbook.* (4th ed.). St. Louis: Mosby.

Johnson, B.A. & Nunley, J.R. (2000). Treatment of seborrheic dermatitis. *American Family Physician, 61*, 2703-2710, 2713-2714.

Johnson, C.E., Stancin, T., Fattlar, D., Rowe, L.P., & Kumar, M.L. (1997). A long-term prospective study of varicella vaccine in healthy children. *Pediatrics, 100*, 761-766.

Kasper, D.L., Braunwald, E., Fauci, A.S., Hauser, S.L., Longo, D.L., Jameson, J.L., et al. (2004). *Harrison's principles of internal medicine* (16th ed.). New York: McGraw-Hill.

Kliegman, R.M., Greenbaum, L.A., & Lye, P.S. (2004). *Practical strategies in pediatric diagnosis and therapy* (2nd ed.). Philadelphia: W.B. Saunders.

Lobato, M.N., Vugia, D.J., & Friede, I.J. (1997). Tinea capitis in California children: A population-based study of a growing epidemic. *Pediatrics, 99*, 551-554.

Mangion, S. (2000). *Physical diagnosis secrets.* Philadelphia: Hanley and Belfus.

Mladenovic, J. (Ed.). (2003). *Primary care secrets.* (3rd Ed.). Philadelphia: Hanley and Belfus.

Nicol, N.H. (2000). Managing atopic dermatitis in children and adults. *The Nurse Practitioner, 25*(4), 58-76.

Noronha., P.A., & Zubkov, B. (1997). Nails and nail disorders in children and adults. *American Family Physician, 55*, 2129-2140.

Olson, A.L., Dietrich, A.J., Sox, C.H., Stevens, M.M., Winchell, C.W., & Ahles, T.A. (1997). Solar protection of children at the beach. *Pediatrics Electronic Pages.* [On-line serial]. Available: www.pediatrics.come1.

Rakel, R.E. (1998). *Essentials of family practice.* (2nd ed.). Philadelphia: WB Saunders.

Rager, E.L., Bridgeford, E.P., & Ollila, D.W (2005). Cutaneous melanoma: Update on prevention, screening, diagnosis, and treatment. *American Academy of Family Physicians, 72,* 269-276.

Reifsnider, E. (1997). Adult infectious skin conditions. *The Nurse Practitioner, 22*(11), 17-33.

Scheinfeld, N.S. (2005). Psoriasis: The "Nuts and bolts" of management. *Consultant, 45,* 798-807.

Schwartz, M.W. (Ed.). (2002). *The 5 minute pediatric consult.* (2nd ed.) Philadelphia: Lippincott Williams & Wilkins.

Singleton, J.K. (1997). Pediatric dermatoses: Three common skin disruptions in infancy. *The Nurse Practitioner, 22*(6), 32-50.

Stein, D.H. (1998). Tineas-superficial dermatophyte infections. *Pediatric Review, 19,* 368-372.

Supple, K. (2005). An overview of burn injury. *Advance for Nurse Practitioners, 13*(7), 24-29

Temple, M.E. (1999). Pharmacotherapy of tinea capitis. *Journal of the American Board of Family Practice, 12*(3), 236-242.

Treadwell, P.A. (1997). Dermatoses in newborns. *American Family Physician, 56,* 443-454.

Uphold, C.R., & Graham, M.V. (2003). *Clinical guidelines in family practice.* (4th ed.). Gainesville, FL: Barmarrae Books.

U.S. Preventive Services Task Force. (1996). *Guide to clinical preventive services.* (2nd ed.) Washington, D.C.: Office of Disease Prevention and Health Promotion, U.S. Government Printing Office.

Verdon, M.E., & Sigal, L.H. (1997). Recognition and management of Lyme disease. *American Family Physician, 56,* 427-438.

Ward, M. R. (1997). Reye's syndrome: An update. *The Nurse Practitioner, 22*(12*),* 45-53.

Zollo, A.J., Jr (Ed.). (2004). *Medical Secrets.* (4th ed.), St. Louis, MO: Mosby-Year Book.

Zoltan, T.B., Taylor, K.S., & Achar, S.A. (2005). Health issues for surfers. *American Academy of Family Physicians, 71,* 2313-2317.

3

DERMATOLOGIC DISORDERS: PEDIATRIC

Dermatologic Disorders: Pediatric

DIAPER DERMATITIS
(DIAPER RASH)

DESCRIPTION

Inflamed skin found in the diaper area

ETIOLOGY

- Irritant contact dermatitis
- Candidal infection
- Atopic dermatitis
- Seborrheic dermatitis

INCIDENCE

- Common
- Males = Females
- Common pediatric problem and in incontinent geriatric population

RISK FACTORS

- Prolonged contact with soiled/wet diaper
- Waterproof diapers
- Hot and humid climates
- Family history of dermatitis
- Diarrhea
- Recent treatment with oral antibiotics

ASSESSMENT FINDINGS

Irritant contact dermatitis	Chapped skin Rarely involves skin creases Dusky red rash
Candidal diaper rash	Bright beefy rash Satellite lesions visible Excoriated skin Often involves skin creases
Atopic diaper dermatitis	Excoriated skin Weeping, crusting lesions Not usually in skin creases
Seborrheic dermatitis	Patches or plaques may be present Dusky red appearance Other sites of seborrheic dermatitis often present (scalp, eyebrows) Usually found within skin creases

DIFFERENTIAL DIAGNOSIS

- Dermatitis: atopic vs. seborrheic vs. contact
- Candidiasis

DIAGNOSTIC STUDIES

- Usually none needed
- KOH preparation if possible fungal etiology

PREVENTION

- Change diapers frequently
- Avoid use of baby powder (retains moisture in creases)

NONPHARMACOLOGIC MANAGEMENT

- Leave dermatitis open to air as much as possible
- Change diapers frequently
- Treat at earliest sign of rash
- Cleanse skin with mild soap, pat dry, allow to air dry as long as possible after cleansing
- Avoid waterproof diapers, waterproof pants

PHARMACOLOGIC MANAGEMENT

- Zinc oxide to rash 3-4 times per day at first sign (serves as a moisture barrier)
- Antifungal cream for candidal diaper rash at each diaper change: clotrimazole cream, miconazole cream, econazole, others
- Low potency cortisone cream if moderate to severe inflammation present

CONSULTATION/REFERRAL

- Dermatologist for cases unresponsive to treatment
- Child protection if neglect is suspected

FOLLOW-UP

- Every 3-5 days until clear

EXPECTED COURSE

- Resolution with proper treatment in 4-7 days

POSSIBLE COMPLICATIONS

- Secondary bacterial or yeast infections
- Two or more types of dermatitis may exist concurrently

ROSEOLA, EXANTHEM SUBITUM

DESCRIPTION

A viral illness characterized by 3-5 days of high fever with a sudden disappearance of fever and the appearance of a blanching maculopapular rash lasting 1-2 days.

ETIOLOGY

- Human herpes virus 6B (HHV-6B)
- Roseola-like illnesses are associated with other types of viruses

INCIDENCE

- Very common in daycare attendees and preschoolers (usually prior to 3 years of age)

RISK FACTORS

- Contact with saliva/feces of a roseola patient during the fever phase (most contagious) or during the 7-17 day incubation period

ASSESSMENT FINDINGS

- Sudden onset of fever up to 104°F (40°C) for 3-5 days
- Child does not seem as ill as degree of fever would indicate
- Signs of mild upper respiratory infection may or may not be present
- Sudden disappearance of fever and appearance of maculopapular rash on trunk and spreading to extremities
- Nonpruritic rash
- Rash blanches with pressure

DIFFERENTIAL DIAGNOSIS

- Other viral illnesses
- Antibiotic rash
- Streptococcal rash

DIAGNOSTIC STUDIES

- Usually none needed

PREVENTION

- Avoid contact with respiratory secretions of infected persons

NONPHARMACOLOGIC MANAGEMENT

- Supportive care
- Cooling measures for elevated temperatures

PHARMACOLOGIC MANAGEMENT

- Analgesics/antipyretics
- Do not use aspirin due to risk of Reye's syndrome

CONSULTATION/REFERRAL

- Consult pediatrician if disease follows atypical course

FOLLOW-UP

- Usually none needed

EXPECTED COURSE

- Benign and self-limited
- Child may return to daycare as soon as afebrile

POSSIBLE COMPLICATIONS

- Seizures due to high fever (5-10% of children)
- Aseptic meningitis (rare)

FIFTH DISEASE
(Erythema Infectiosum, Slapped-Cheek Disease)

DESCRIPTION

A common viral infection characterized by an eruptive rash. Since it was the fifth disease described with an eruptive rash, it was named "Fifth Disease".

ETIOLOGY

- Parvovirus B19

INCIDENCE

- Most common in 5-15 year olds
- Also occurs in infants and adults
- Most common in early spring and late winter

RISK FACTORS

- Incubation period is 4-28 days (average = 16 days)
- Contact with a person before the rash erupts (communicable period ends when rash erupts)
- Nasal secretions and aerosolized respiratory droplets are means of transmission

ASSESSMENT FINDINGS

- Prodrome: low-grade fever, malaise, sore throat, lethargy (lasts 1-4 days)
- Rash
  - ◊ First phase often appears first on cheeks of face: intense red rash with circumoral pallor; hence the name "slapped-cheek disease"
  - ◊ Second phase of rash spreads to body and extremities over next few days: (macular and lacy appearing)
  - ◊ Final phase of rash may be pruritic and itch more intensely with exercise, sun exposure, or bathing (can last up to 21 days)
  - ◊ Palms and soles may be affected (lasts 7-20 days)
  - ◊ Children may return to school during the rash phase
  - ◊ Adults may have arthralgias and/or arthritis

DIFFERENTIAL DIAGNOSIS

- Rubella
- Enterovirus
- Lupus
- Drug rashes
- Other viral exanthems

DIAGNOSTIC STUDIES

- Usually none; diagnosis is made clinically
- B19 specific IgM (confirms acute infection)
- B19 specific IgG (confirms past infection)

PREVENTION

- Avoid exposure to persons with known infections
- Danger to fetus is primarily severe anemia due to RBC destruction and aplasia
- Pregnant women should avoid close contact with aplastic Parvo B19 patients because they are highly contagious

NONPHARMACOLOGIC MANAGEMENT

- Supportive care
- Rest

PHARMACOLOGIC MANAGEMENT

- No specific treatment
- Analgesics if needed

PREGNANCY/LACTATION CONSIDERATIONS

- Rash in pregnant women should be assessed for possible Parvo B19 infection
- Infection during pregnancy is associated with a 10% fetal death (greatest threat is before 14th week gestation)
- There is no indication for abortion or routine exclusion in the work place if known infected personnel are present
- Fetal ultrasound and α-fetoprotein testing can help assess fetal damage if documented infection and exposure has taken place

CONSULTATION/REFERRAL

- Obstetrician for known exposure
- Consider referral for immunocompromised patients

FOLLOW-UP

- Usually none needed

EXPECTED COURSE

- Rash may last up to 3 weeks
- Rash may fade, intensify depending on temperature, sunlight, exercise

POSSIBLE COMPLICATIONS

- Arthritis: adults more prone; may begin 2-3 weeks after onset of symptoms
- Aplastic crisis: may occur in patients with sickle cell or other types of anemias
- Fetal hydrops

RUBELLA

(German Measles, Three Day Measles, Third Disease)

DESCRIPTION

Acute viral infection of childhood (and adults) that may occur in two different forms:

- Acquired
- Congenital

ETIOLOGY

- Rubivirus, a member of the Togaviridae family of viruses

INCIDENCE

- <1000 cases annually are reported
- Congenital rubella syndrome occurs rarely
- Infection rates are highest for persons 5-9 years; but may affect any age
- Fetal infection if exposed during the first trimester is 50-80%
- Fetal infection if exposed during the second trimester is 10-20%
- Fetal infection if exposed during the third trimester is near zero

RISK FACTORS

- Lack of vaccination and subsequent exposure to viral particles by airborne transmission
- Incubation period is 14-21 days
- Most contagious when rash is erupting

ASSESSMENT FINDINGS

- *Acquired (postnatal)*
  - ◊ Mild catarrhal symptoms, conjunctivitis
  - ◊ Low-grade fever
  - ◊ Occipital lymph nodes are most commonly involved and are essentially diagnostic
  - ◊ Lymphadenopathy: postauricular, posterior cervical
  - ◊ Possible splenomegaly
  - ◊ Maculopapular rash (which starts on the face and spreads to chest) which usually lasts about 3 days
  - ◊ Possible desquamation
  - ◊ In adults and adolescents, arthralgia and arthritis common
- *Congenital*
  - ◊ Premature delivery
  - ◊ Fetal demise
  - ◊ Low birth weight
  - ◊ Eye defects: cataracts, glaucoma, retinopathy
  - ◊ Cardiac defects: patent ductus arteriosus, atrial and ventricular septal defects, coarctation of the aorta, pulmonic stenosis
  - ◊ Nervous system defects: mental retardation, psychomotor retardation, encephalitis, autism, deafness
  - ◊ Endocrine defects: thyroid disorders, diabetes mellitus, precocious puberty
  - ◊ Hematological defects: splenomegaly, thrombocytopenia, hepatitis

DIFFERENTIAL DIAGNOSIS

- Scarlet fever
- Roseola/Fifth disease
- Drug reactions
- Other viral exanthems

DIAGNOSTIC STUDIES

- Viral cultures from throat or urine (not usually needed)
- Rubella antibodies: titer of 1:10 or higher is considered immune

PREVENTION

- Routine immunization at 12-15 months, then age 4-6 years except during pregnancy
- Do not immunize patients during pregnancy
- Communicable in breast-milk

NONPHARMACOLOGIC MANAGEMENT

- Supportive care

PHARMACOLOGIC MANAGEMENT

- Usually none needed

PREGNANCY/LACTATION CONSIDERATIONS

- Pregnancy avoided for 1 month after vaccine
- Vaccine virus may be communicable through breast milk

CONSULTATION/REFERRAL

- Obstetrician for suspected exposure during pregnancy
- Refer for complications
- Report all cases to local public health authorities

FOLLOW-UP

- Individualize per patient

EXPECTED COURSE

- 50% of infections are asymptomatic
- Infection in early pregnancy has worse outcomes than those associated with infection after the 20th week

POSSIBLE COMPLICATIONS

- As described above for congenitally acquired infants
- Arthritis and arthralgia (common in adults)
- Encephalitis
- Bleeding (more common in children)

RUBEOLA
(Measles, Nine Day Measles, First Disease)

DESCRIPTION

Acute, highly contagious viral disease with a characteristic rash. Associated with a significant degree of morbidity and mortality worldwide.

ETIOLOGY

- Morbillivirus of the family Paramyxoviridae

INCIDENCE

- Outbreaks occurred in 1989-1990 (mortality and significant morbidity occurred)
- Since 1990, drastic decrease in incidence

RISK FACTORS

- Lack of immunization (MMR given at 12-15 months of age)
- Waiting rooms (up to 45% of known exposures have occurred here) with an infected patient (spread by microaerosolized respiratory droplets)
- Incubation period is 7-18 days, but usually about 10 days
- Patients are contagious from 1-2 days prior to onset of symptoms until 4 days after appearance of the rash

ASSESSMENT FINDINGS

- *Prodromal stage* (2-4 days)
  - ◊ Upper respiratory infection symptoms
  - ◊ Fever up to 104°F (40°C)
  - ◊ The 3-C's: cough, coryza, conjunctivitis
  - ◊ Presence of Koplik's spots (white spots on buccal mucosa) is pathognomonic
  - ◊ Malaise
- *Rash phase* (the more severe the rash, the more severe the illness)
  - ◊ Emergence of maculopapular rash and elevation of temperature up to 104.7°F (40.5°C) occur simultaneously,
  - ◊ Pharyngitis, cervical lymphadenopathy and splenomegaly often accompany rash
  - ◊ Rash appears behind forehead and ears initially
  - ◊ Over the first 24 hours, rash spreads to face, neck, and arms
  - ◊ Next 24 hours rash spreads to trunk and thighs
  - ◊ Rarely rash can become hemorrhagic leading to fatality
  - ◊ After 3-4 days, rash begins to clear and may leave a brownish discoloration and scaling

DIFFERENTIAL DIAGNOSIS

- Roseola
- Scarlet fever
- Other viral rashes
- Drug rashes
- Kawasaki Disease
- Steven-Johnson syndrome

DIAGNOSTIC STUDIES

- Measles specific IgM titers (must draw no sooner than 5 days after rash appears)
- Substantial rise in IgG titers between acute and convalescent phase
- Nasopharynx culture if done within 24 hours of onset of rash

PREVENTION

- Routine vaccination at 12-15 months, then age 4-6 years
- Respiratory isolation until 4 days after rash appears. Exception: Isolate immunocompromised patients for the entire illness
- Vaccination with live virus within 72 hours after exposure can provide protection
- Immunoglobulin if given within 6 days after exposure

NONPHARMACOLOGIC MANAGEMENT

- Antipyretic measures
- Oral fluids
- Antitussives
- Room humidification

PHARMACOLOGIC MANAGEMENT

- Water miscible vitamin A for children 6 months to 2 years in developing countries has been shown to decrease morbidity and mortality

PREGNANCY/LACTATION CONSIDERATIONS

- During pregnancy there is significant increase in fetal morbidity and mortality
- Immunoglobulin recommended for susceptible pregnant women who have been in contact with known rubeola patient

CONSULTATION/REFERRAL

- Report to local health department
- Consider referral for all severe cases, pregnant women, and immunocompromised patients

FOLLOW-UP

- Individualize for each patient

EXPECTED COURSE

- Mild to severe symptoms depending on age and immune status of patient

POSSIBLE COMPLICATIONS

- Otitis media (most common)
- Pneumonitis
- Diarrhea
- Encephalitis (rare)
- Laryngotracheitis

CHICKEN POX
(Varicella)

DESCRIPTION

A highly contagious viral illness characterized by the development of pruritic vesicles and papules on the skin, scalp and less commonly, on mucus membranes.

ETIOLOGY

- Varicella-zoster virus (VZV), a herpesvirus

INCIDENCE

- Common, but becoming less prevalent with the advent of the varicella vaccine
- Peak age is 5-9 years, but any age susceptible
- Outbreaks from January to May

RISK FACTORS

- Incubation period is about 2 weeks
- No prior history of varicella, no vaccination
- Immunocompromised status

ASSESSMENT FINDINGS

- Prodrome
  - ◊ Fever
  - ◊ Malaise
  - ◊ Anorexia, abdominal pain
  - ◊ Headache
- Rash Phase
  - ◊ Crops of lesions begin on trunk, become vesicles, then scabs in 6-10 hours
  - ◊ Successive crops appear over the next several days
  - ◊ Lesions may be found on any mucosal membrane: mouth, larynx, vagina

DIFFERENTIAL DIAGNOSIS

- Other viral illnesses
- Other herpetic illnesses
- Impetigo
- Contact dermatitis

DIAGNOSTIC STUDIES

- Usually none indicated except in pregnant women

PREVENTION

- Vaccination
  - ◊ 12 months to 12 years: given as single immunization (70-90% efficacy)
  - ◊ 13 years and older: two vaccinations 4-8 weeks apart (70% efficacy)
- Most contagious period is 2 days prior to appearance of rash and up to crusting of ALL lesions; therefore, keep infected individuals at home until lesions have crusted
- Passive immunization with VZIG (Varicella-zoster immune globulin) within 4 days of exposure for immunocompromised individuals
- If unable to administer VZIG within timeframe, consider acyclovir to decrease duration and time of viral shedding (recommended for high risk individuals)

NONPHARMACOLOGIC MANAGEMENT

- Supportive therapy
- Good hygiene to prevent bacterial secondary infections
- Cut fingernails short in young children to decrease incidence of bacterial infections from scratching
- Tepid baths for itching

PHARMACOLOGIC MANAGEMENT

- Antipruritics
- Antipyretics: **DO NOT GIVE ASPIRIN** due to increased risk of Reye's syndrome with varicella patients

PREGNANCY/LACTATION CONSIDERATIONS

- Do not vaccinate pregnant women
- In pregnant women who have never had chickenpox or immunization, avoid contact with recently vaccinated individuals for 6 weeks

- Fetal infection following maternal infection is 25%
- Increased incidence of pneumonia in women infected during pregnancy
- Congenital malformations seen in 5% of infants if mother was infected during the first or second trimester

CONSULTATION/REFERRAL

- Refer for newborns, immunocompromised, pregnant women, or severe cases

FOLLOW-UP

- Usually none needed if disease follows normal course
- If complications develop, individualize follow-up

EXPECTED COURSE

- Complete resolution in 2-3 weeks
- Lifelong immunity conferred after disease

POSSIBLE COMPLICATIONS

- Bacterial secondary infections
- Pneumonia (most common in adults and the elderly)
- Encephalitis (rare)
- Reye's syndrome (rare)
- Disseminated infection

SCARLET FEVER
(Scarlatina)

DESCRIPTION

Childhood disease characterized by sore throat, fever, and a scarlet "sandpaper" rash

ETIOLOGY

- Group A β-hemolytic *Streptococcus pyogenes* that produces an erythrogenic toxin

INCIDENCE

- Ages 6-12 years are most common
- Males = Females

RISK FACTORS

- Age 6-12 years
- Wound infection
- Burns

ASSESSMENT FINDINGS

- Sore throat
- Headache
- Fever and chills
- Vomiting
- Erythematous tonsils usually covered with an exudate; pharynx may have exudate as well
- Petechiae on palate
- White coating on tongue which sheds by day 2 or 3 and leaves a "strawberry" tongue with shiny red papillae
- Fine sandpaper rash begins on chest and axillae, then appears on abdomen and extremities; blanches with pressure
- Pastia's lines present (transverse red streaks in skin folds of antecubital space, abdomen, and axillae)
- Desquamation from face which proceeds over trunk and finally to hands and feet

DIFFERENTIAL DIAGNOSIS

- Pharyngitis: non scarlatina
- Measles
- Rubella
- Drug rash
- Viral exanthems
- Toxic shock syndrome
- Scalded skin syndrome

DIAGNOSTIC STUDIES

- Throat culture
- Rapid streptococcal test
- Antistreptolysin O (ASO) confirms infection but not helpful for diagnosis

PREVENTION

- Avoid contact with respiratory secretions of infected person
- Prophylactic penicillin NOT recommended after exposure to scarlet fever
- Antibiotic started within 10 days after onset effective in preventing rheumatic fever
- Antibiotic does not completely eliminate possibility of glomerulonephritis

NONPHARMACOLOGIC MANAGEMENT

- Supportive care
- Maintain hydration status

PHARMACOLOGIC MANAGEMENT

- Antipyretics for fever
- Penicillin is drug of choice
- Cephalosporins acceptable
- Erythromycin or advanced macrolides for penicillin allergic patients

CONSULTATION/REFERRAL

- Refer for severe cases

FOLLOW-UP

- Individualize per patient

EXPECTED COURSE

- Excellent prognosis after appropriate treatment

POSSIBLE COMPLICATIONS

- Sinusitis
- Otitis media
- Rheumatic fever
- Glomerulonephritis

COMMON, BENIGN PEDIATRIC SKIN LESIONS

(Mongolian Spots, Hemangiomas, Milia, Freckles)

DESCRIPTION

These skin lesions are variations from normal and are of no particular physical significance, but may be of cosmetic importance to parents.

ETIOLOGY

***Mongolian spots*: dermal pigmented cells**
***Hemangiomas*: dilation of capillaries**
***Milia*: superficial cysts filled with keratin**
***Freckles*: epidermal cells which contain an increased amount of pigment**

INCIDENCE

- Very common
- Patient education regarding permanency of lesion

RISK FACTORS

- Unknown for most lesions
- Maybe familial (Mongolian spots, freckles)
- Fair skinned, blue-eyed individuals (freckles)
- Ultraviolet (UV) light exposure (freckles)

ASSESSMENT FINDINGS

- *Mongolian spots*
  - ◊ Blue-black macular lesion (may be mistaken for bruising)
  - ◊ Prevalent in lumbosacral area of African-Americans, Native Americans, Hispanics, and Asians
  - ◊ Usually disappear by 3 years of age
- *Hemangiomas*
  - ◊ Raised
    - * Cavernous: appear bluish, located deep beneath the skin, not present at birth, appears within a few months of life and then disappears before the end of the first decade of life
    - * Capillary (strawberry hemangiomas): bright red vascular overgrowth, elevated, vary in size
  - ◊ *Flat*
    - * Port-wine stains: dark red to deep purple lesions present at birth,

frequently found on the face, do not fade with time

- *Milia*
  - ◊ White papules found on the forehead, face, chin, and cheeks of infants
  - ◊ 1-2 mm in size
  - ◊ Disappear a few weeks after birth
  - ◊ May appear on palate, referred to as Epstein's pearls
- *Freckles*
  - ◊ Light brown macules present in large numbers on skin exposed to UV light

DIFFERENTIAL DIAGNOSIS

- Mongolian spots: bruises, child abuse
- Hemangiomas: other types of vascular nevi
- Milia: molluscum contagiosum
- Freckles: measles

DIAGNOSTIC STUDIES

- Usually none indicated

PREVENTION

- *See* Risk Factors

NONPHARMACOLOGIC MANAGEMENT

- Reassure parents that these are benign lesions
- Laser treatment for port-wine stains

CONSULTATION/REFERRAL

- Dermatologist for questionable lesions

EXPECTED COURSE

- Benign lesions
- Course as described in assessment findings

CAFÉ AU LAIT SPOTS

DESCRIPTION

Brown, macular lesions which are almost always benign, but are also present in neurofibromatosis, a neurocutaneous syndrome.

ETIOLOGY

- An increase in the amount of melanin found within the melanocytes

INCIDENCE

- Common

RISK FACTORS

- Unknown
- Possible family history

ASSESSMENT FINDINGS

- Well marginated light brown macules usually <1.5 cm in diameter
- Usually less than 5 lesions present
- If >5 lesions are present which are >5 mm, suggests neurofibromatosis
- If 6 or more lesions are >15 mm in postpubertal child, strongly suggests neurofibromatosis
- Lesions may increase in size and number as person ages

DIFFERENTIAL DIAGNOSIS

- Freckles
- Neurofibromatosis

DIAGNOSTIC STUDIES

- Usually none indicated

NONPHARMACOLOGIC MANAGEMENT

- Patient education about regular examination of skin, reporting of changes to health care provider
- Measure and diagram location of lesions for identifying changes in lesions

CONSULTATION/REFERRAL

- Refer for suspected neurofibromatosis

FOLLOW-UP

- Annual visits to evaluate lesions

EXPECTED COURSE

- Benign course, no malignant changes expected
- Lesions may grow in size and number as patient ages

POSSIBLE COMPLICATIONS

- Neurofibromatosis

HERPANGINA

DESCRIPTION

Viral infection which causes fever and multiple vesicles and ulcerations on the posterior third of the mouth which involves the soft palate, uvula, tonsils, and pharynx.

ETIOLOGY

- Coxsackie A (most common) and B virus
- Rarely Echovirus

INCIDENCE

- Occurs in outbreaks during the summer and fall in children 3 months to 16 years

RISK FACTORS

- Contact with saliva of infected persons

ASSESSMENT FINDINGS

- High fever
- Severe throat pain which can cause impairment of fluid intake
- 1-2 mm grey-white vesicles on the posterior third of the mouth surrounded by an erythematous halo (before ulceration occurs)
- Drooling
- Coryza
- Anorexia
- Malaise
- Irritability
- GI symptoms

DIFFERENTIAL DIAGNOSIS

- Hand-foot-mouth disease
- Herpes simplex
- Gingivostomatitis
- Drug reaction

DIAGNOSTIC STUDIES

- Consider viral cultures of lesions (rarely performed)
- Consider quick streptococcal test

PREVENTION

- Avoid exposure to oral secretions of infected persons
- Good hygiene
- Good hand washing

NONPHARMACOLOGIC MANAGEMENT

- Maintain hydration and provide cool liquids frequently
- Avoid spicy foods
- Rest
- Teach parents to return to office with child if no improvement in 3-4 days
- Treatment is symptomatic

PHARMACOLOGIC MANAGEMENT

- Analgesics for fever and throat pain
- Consider topical anesthetic but cautious use in young children

CONSULTATION/REFERRAL

- None usually needed
- Refer for severe dehydration

FOLLOW-UP

- None usually needed

EXPECTED COURSE

- Ulcerations heal/resolve in 3-6 days
- Resolution usually by day 7

POSSIBLE COMPLICATIONS

- Unusual
- Dehydration (most frequent complication)

HAND-FOOT-AND-MOUTH DISEASE

DESCRIPTION

This is a highly contagious viral illness similar to herpangina, but the characteristic lesions appear on the buccal mucosa, palate, palms of the hands, soles of the feet and buttocks.

ETIOLOGY

- Coxsackie A 16 (most common)
- Other Coxsackie viruses
- Other enterovirus

INCIDENCE

- Common in children under 5 years
- Occurs in late summer and fall

RISK FACTORS

- Contact with oral, fecal, or respiratory secretions of infected persons (highly contagious)

ASSESSMENT FINDINGS

- Low-grade fever
- Malaise
- Abdominal pain
- 25% have enlarged anterior cervical nodes or submandibular nodes
- Oral manifestations may be small, red papules on the tongue and buccal mucosa which progress to ulcerative vesicles on an erythematous base which ulcerates
- Exanthem is rarely pruritic and may occur on the palms, soles, arms, legs, buttocks, fingers, and toes

DIFFERENTIAL DIAGNOSIS

- Herpangina
- Aphthous stomatitis
- Stevens-Johnson syndrome

DIAGNOSTIC STUDIES

- Usually none needed (diagnosis made from history and examination)

PREVENTION

- Avoid exposure to known infected persons
- Good hygiene
- Good hand washing

NONPHARMACOLOGIC MANAGEMENT

- Maintain hydration and provide cool liquids frequently
- Avoid spicy foods
- Rest
- Return to clinic if no improvement in 3-4 days
- Treatment is symptomatic

PHARMACOLOGIC MANAGEMENT

- Analgesics for pain and fever
- Topical antihistamine/anesthetic (aluminum hydroxide/magnesium hydroxide gel with diphenhydramine) applied to painful lesions (relief is short-lived)
- Topical lidocaine is NOT recommended because it can be absorbed from mucous membranes and may be toxic (adult & child fatalities reported)

CONSULTATION/REFERRAL

- Rarely needed because condition is self-limiting
- Refer for dehydration

FOLLOW-UP

- Usually none needed

EXPECTED COURSE

- Resolution within 7 days of onset

POSSIBLE COMPLICATIONS

- Myocarditis (extremely rare)
- Meningitis, encephalitis

References

Achar, S. (1996). Principles of skin biopsies for the family physician. *American Family Physician, 54*, 2411-2422.

American Academy of Pediatrics. (2003). *Red book: Report of the committee on infectious disease* (26th ed.). Elk Grove Village, IN: American Academy of Pediatrics.

Bickley, L.S., & Szilagyi, P.G. (2003). *Bates' guide to physical examination and history taking* (8th ed.). Philadelphia: Lippincott Williams & Wilkins.

Branch, W.T. (2003). *Office practice of medicine* (4th ed.). Philadelphia: Saunders.

Burns, C.E., Brady, M.A., Blosser, C., Starr, N.B., & Dunn, A.M. (2004). *Pediatric primary care: A handbook for nurse practitioners* (3rd ed.). Philadelphia: W.B. Saunders.

Dambro, M.R. (2005). *Griffith's 5 minute clinical consult.* Philadelphia: Lippincott Williams & Wilkins.

Davis, R.E. (1997). Diagnosing neurofibromatosis type I in children. *The Nurse Practitioner, 22*(4), 73-81.

Diehl, K.B. (1996). Topical antifungal agents: An update. *American Family Physician, 54*, 1687-1692.

Epstein, E. (2001). *Common Skin Disorders.* (5th ed.). Philadelphia: WB Saunders.

Gilber, D.N., Moellering, R.C., Eliopoulos, G.M., & Sande, M.A. (Eds.). (2004). *Sanford Guide to Antimicrobial Therapy* (34th ed.). Hyde Park, VT: Antimicrobial Therapy.

Goldstein, B.G. & Goldstein, A.O. (2001). Diagnosis and management of malignant melanoma. *American Family Physician, 63*, 1359-1368, 1374.

Graber, M.A., & Lanternier, M.L. (2001). *The family practice handbook.* (4th Ed.). St. Louis: Mosby.

Hahn, R.G., Knox, L.M., & Forman, T.A. (2005). Evaluation of poststreptococcal illness. *American Family Physician, 71*, 1949-1954.

Johnson, B.A. & Nunley, J.R. (2000). Treatment of seborrheic dermatitis. *American Family Physician, 61*, 2703-2710, 2713-2714.

Johnson, C.E., Stancin, T., Fattlar, D., Rowe, L.P., & Kumar, M.L. (1997). A long-term prospective study of varicella vaccine in healthy children. *Pediatrics, 100*, 761-766.

Kasper, D.L., Braunwald, E., Fauci, A.S., Hauser, S.L., Longo, D.L., Jameson, J.L., et al. (2004). *Harrison's principles of internal medicine* (16th ed.). New York: McGraw-Hill.

Kliegman, R.M., Greenbaum, L.A., & Lye, P.S. (2004). *Practical strategies in pediatric diagnosis and therapy* (2nd ed.). Philadelphia: W.B. Saunders.

Lobato, M.N., Vugia, D.J., & Friede, I.J. (1997). Tinea capitis in California children: A population-based study of a growing epidemic. *Pediatrics, 99*, 551-554.

Mangion, S. (2000). *Physical diagnosis secrets.* Philadelphia: Hanley and Belfus.

Mladenovic, J. (Ed.). (2003). *Primary care secrets.* (3rd Ed.). Philadelphia: Hanley and Belfus.

Nicol, N.H. (2000). Managing atopic dermatitis in children and adults. *The Nurse Practitioner, 25*(4): 58-76.

Noronha., P.A., & Zubkov, B. (1997). Nails and nail disorders in children and adults. *American Family Physician, 55*, 2129-2140.

Olson, A.L., Dietrich, A.J., Sox, C.H., Stevens, M.M., Winchell, C.W., & Ahles, T.A. (1997). Solar protection of children at the beach. *Pediatrics Electronic Pages.* [On-line serial]. Available: www.pediatrics.come1.

Rakel, R.E. (1998). *Essentials of family practice.* (2nd ed.). Philadelphia: WB Saunders.

Reifsnider, E. (1997). Adult infectious skin conditions. *The Nurse Practitioner, 22*(11), 17-33.

Schwartz, M.W. (Ed.). (2002). *The 5 minute pediatric consult.* (2nd ed.) Philadelphia: Lippincott Williams & Wilkins.

Singleton, J.K. (1997). Pediatric dermatoses: Three common skin disruptions in infancy. *The Nurse Practitioner, 22*(6), 32-50.

Stein, D.H. (1998). Tineas-superficial dermatophyte infections. *Pediatric Review, 19*, 368-372.

Temple, M.E. (1999). Pharmacotherapy of tinea capitis. *Journal of the American Board of Family Practice*; *12*, 236-242.

Treadwell, P.A. (1997). Dermatoses in newborns. *American Family Physician, 56*, 443-454.

Uphold, C.R., & Graham, M.V. (2003). *Clinical guidelines in family practice.* (4th ed.). Gainesville, FL: Barmarrae Books.

U.S. Preventive Services Task Force. (1996). *Guide to clinical preventive services.* (2nd ed.) Washington, D.C.: Office of Disease Prevention and Health Promotion, U.S. Government Printing Office.

Verdon, M.E., & Sigal, L.H. (1997). Recognition and management of Lyme disease. *American Family Physician, 56*, 427-438.

Ward, M. R. (1997). Reye's syndrome: An update. *The Nurse Practitioner, 22*(12*)*, 45-53.

Zollo, A.J., Jr (Ed.). (2004). *Medical Secrets.* (4th ed.), St. Louis, MO: Mosby-Year Book.

4

EAR, NOSE, AND THROAT DISORDERS

Ear, Nose, and Throat Disorders

COMMON COLD
(Nasopharyngitis, URI)

DESCRIPTION

An infection of the upper respiratory tract caused by a virus. The symptoms may last for 3-10 days and are usually self-limiting.

ETIOLOGY

- Rhinoviruses are the most common cause
- Influenza viruses
- Parainfluenza viruses
- Adenoviruses
- Coronaviruses

INCIDENCE

- Adults: 2-4 annually
- Children: 6-10 annually

RISK FACTORS

- Exposure to infected individuals
- Psychological stress
- Touching of contaminated surfaces and subsequent touching of nose or conjunctiva

ASSESSMENT FINDINGS

- Most common symptoms: Nasal stuffiness, sneezing, scratchy, irritated throat/hoarseness
- Red/irritated nasal mucosa with mucus discharge
- Malaise, headache
- Cough
- Occasionally fever

DIFFERENTIAL DIAGNOSIS

- Allergic rhinitis
- Influenza
- Sinusitis
- Mumps
- Rubeola

DIAGNOSTIC STUDIES

- Usually none indicated
- CBC if symptoms persist: elevated WBC indicates bacterial infection
- Culture of nasal washings (usually not helpful)

PREVENTION

- Good hand washing
- Avoid exposure to infected individuals
- Adequate rest
- Stress management
- Zinc lozenges (thought to prevent viral replication) and vitamin C have failed to demonstrate clinical benefit

NONPHARMACOLOGIC MANAGEMENT

- Increased rest
- Fluids
- Humidify inspired air
- Discontinue tobacco products
- Hard candy or lozenges for scratchy throat
- Saline nose drops and bulb syringe for infants
- Avoid tobacco products and alcohol
- Teach patients that hand washing is the single most effective preventive measure

PHARMACOLOGIC MANAGEMENT

- Decongestants for nasal congestion to promote drainage (oral route is preferred over topicals because prolonged topical use, >4-5 days, can lead to dependence and rebound stuffiness also called *rhinitis medicamentosa*)
- Cough suppressants helpful for cough due to nocturnal post nasal drip and/or tracheobronchial irritation

Antihistamines have NOT been shown to alleviate symptoms; however, OTCs are widely used.

- Acetaminophen/NSAIDs for fever and/or aches and pains
- Cough expectorants not shown to be effective for the common cold

Avoid aspirin in children to reduce risk of Reye's Syndrome.

PREGNANCY/LACTATION CONSIDERATIONS

- Medications ONLY if absolutely needed
- Most mild decongestants considered safe for short term use

FOLLOW-UP

- None usually needed

EXPECTED COURSE

- Complete resolution by 10 days

POSSIBLE COMPLICATIONS

- Sinusitis
- Pneumonia
- Otitis media
- Asthma in individuals who have asthma triggered by viral infections

INFLUENZA
(Grip, Grippe, Flu)

DESCRIPTION

A highly contagious, acute viral illness of the respiratory tract which involves the nasal mucosa, pharynx, respiratory tract and the conjunctiva. Most frequent time of occurrence is during winter months.

ETIOLOGY

- Influenza virus types A and B

INCIDENCE

- Occurs world-wide
- Virus undergoes phenomenon of *antigenic variation* (minor genetic alterations which account for human inability to develop lasting immunity and thus an unending need for vaccination)
- Prevalence is highest in school age population
- Severe disease occurs more frequently in the elderly, pregnant women in the 3rd trimester, infants, and patients with chronic diseases

RISK FACTORS

- Closed or crowded conditions (e.g., schools, prisons, nursing homes)
- Presence of chronic disease, especially respiratory

ASSESSMENT FINDINGS

- High fever of sudden onset
- Cough
- Rhinorrhea
- Pharyngitis
- Headache
- Malaise, myalgias, and arthralgias
- Irritated mucous membranes
- Cervical lymphadenopathy
- GI complaints in children

DIFFERENTIAL DIAGNOSIS

- Common cold
- RSV and other viral illnesses
- Pneumonia
- Tonsillitis

DIAGNOSTIC STUDIES

- Usually none are needed to make diagnosis during an epidemic
- Nasal swab for typing (A or B)
- CBC: leukocytosis
- Chest x-ray if pneumonia is suspected

PREVENTION

Immunization	
Persons at high risk for complications	**Especially cardiac and pulmonary patients, and others with chronic diseases**
6-23 month olds	
Groups at high risk to transmit disease	**Health care workers**
Medications	
Rimantadine	Effective against Influenza A virus if administered within 48 hours after exposure Only approved for prophylaxis Preferred over amantadine
Amantadine	Effective against Influenza A virus if administered within 48 hours after exposure May shorten duration and severity of disease

- Vaccination is >70% effective against preventing the disease
- Must vaccinate *annually* with new vaccine

Do NOT administer if patient has had an anaphylactic reaction to eggs.

NONPHARMACOLOGIC MANAGEMENT

- Minimize contact with others (i.e. home from work of school)
- Saline nose drops/spray
- Decongestants (oral route preferred over topical)
- Increased fluids
- Rest
- Good hand washing
- Cessation of tobacco products and alcohol
- Humidify air to prevent drying of respiratory secretions
- Patient education regarding disease, treatment, comfort measures, etc.

PHARMACOLOGIC MANAGEMENT

Influenza Type A	Influenza Type B
Zanamivir Oseltamivir Amantadine Rimantadine*	Zanamivir Oseltamivir

**Preferred because of fewer side effects*

- Must start medications as soon as possible but within 48 hours
- Acetaminophen/ibuprofen for fever, aches, and pains
- Cough suppressant for nocturnal, nonproductive cough

PREGNANCY/LACTATION CONSIDERATIONS

- Safe to immunize during pregnancy
- Amantadine is contraindicated during pregnancy

FOLLOW-UP

- None needed if disease is uneventful and no symptoms linger
- Follow-up for complications is dependent on severity of disease and medical status of patient
- Follow-up needed if symptoms persist longer than 10 days

EXPECTED COURSE

- Favorable outcome

POSSIBLE COMPLICATIONS

- Pneumonia
- Otitis media
- Acute sinusitis
- Croup
- Bronchitis
- Death

SINUSITIS

DESCRIPTION

Inflammation of the paranasal sinuses due to bacterial, viral, or fungal infection; or allergic reaction.

ETIOLOGY

Acute sinusitis	**Bacterial** *Streptococcus* sp. (most common) *Haemophilus influenza* (common in smokers) *Staphylococcus* sp. **Viral** Rhinovirus Coronavirus Influenza A & B Parainfluenza virus RSV
Chronic sinusitis	Gram negative more likely Anaerobic organisms

INCIDENCE

- Common in all ages
- Males = Females

RISK FACTORS

- Allergies
- Tooth abscess (25% of chronic sinusitis is due to tooth abscess)
- Swimming in contaminated water
- Any condition which results in swollen nasal mucous membranes
- Anatomical abnormalities which prevent normal mucosal drainage

ASSESSMENT FINDINGS

- Fever
- Nasal congestion and/or discharge (may be purulent and/or bloody)
- Headache
- Sore throat from persistent postnasal discharge
- Pain over cheeks and upper teeth (maxillary sinuses)
- Pain and tenderness over eyebrows (frontal sinuses)
- Pain and tenderness behind and between eyes (ethmoid sinuses)
- Cough
- Postnasal discharge
- Periorbital edema

DIFFERENTIAL DIAGNOSIS

- Viral, bacterial, or allergic rhinitis
- Dental abscess
- Headaches
- Wegener's granulomatosis

DIAGNOSTIC STUDIES

- CBC: elevated WBC count if bacterial infection
- Sinus x-rays: opaque areas seen on radiographs; air-fluid levels seen
- CT scan: most useful tool to evaluate recurrent sinusitis
- Transillumination: opacification with air-fluid levels if sinus cavity is infected

PREVENTION

- Promote drainage by avoiding irritants which increase swelling in mucous membranes and cause retention of sinus exudate
- Good hand washing to prevent upper respiratory infections
- Management of allergic rhinitis

NONPHARMACOLOGIC MANAGEMENT

- Avoid environmental irritants (cigarette smoke)
- Manage allergic rhinitis appropriately
- Humidified air can improve mucus clearance
- Irrigation of sinuses or normal saline nose drops
- Increase fluid intake

- Patient education regarding disease, treatment options, etc.

PHARMACOLOGIC MANAGEMENT

- Antibiotics: for acute infections and patients with moderate to severe infection
- May switch to antibiotic with β-lactamase coverage if first course of antibiotics ineffective
- Decongestants: oral route preferred over topical
- Pretreat with decongestants prior to air travel
- Analgesics for headache

AGENT	ACTION	COMMENTS
Antibiotics ***PCN*** *Examples:* amoxicillin (Amoxil®)	Inhibit cell wall synthesis of Gram positive (Staph, Strep) bacteria and are most effective against organisms with rapidly dividing cell walls	Penicillin contains a beta lactam ring in its chemical structure. Therefore, PCN is rendered ineffective if the organism produces the enzyme, beta lactamase. Generally well tolerated; watch for hypersensitivity reactions.
Extended spectrum PCN *Examples:* amoxicillin/clavulanate	Exactly as for PCN, but addition of clavulanate extends antimicrobial spectrum (covers many Gram negative organisms too) and protects PCN molecule if the organism produces beta lactamase	Monitor for PCN hypersensitivity. Clavulanate associated with diarrhea.
Cephalosporins ***Second generation*** *Examples:* cefprozil (Cefzil®) cefuroxime (Ceftin®) cefaclor (Ceclor®)	Inhibit cell wall synthesis of bacteria Contains beta lactam ring like PCN Provides coverage of many Gram positive and Gram negative bacteria but NOT those organisms that produce beta lactamase	Well tolerated Cross sensitivity (≈2-10%) with the PCN. Do NOT administer if patient has had anaphylactic response to PCN.
Third generation *Examples:* cefdinir (Omnicef®) cefixime (Suprax®) ceftibuten (Cedax®) cefpodoxime (Vantin®)	Exactly as for second generation cephalosporins but covers many more Gram negative organisms; and if organism produces beta-lactamase the antibiotic remains effective.	Same as for second generation cephalosporins. Good choice if patient is PCN allergic and needs beta lactamase coverage.
Oral decongestants *Examples:* pseudoephedrine (Sudafed®) phenylephrine (Endal®)	Act on adrenergic receptors affecting sympathetic tone of the blood vessels and causing vasoconstriction This results in mucous membrane shrinkage and improved ventilation	Do not use in patients with hypertension. Cautious use in patients with thyroid disease, CAD, PAD, arrhythmias, prostate disease, and glaucoma.
Topical decongestants *Examples:* Oxymetazoline (Afrin®) Phenylephrine (Neo-Synephrine®)	Same mechanism of action as oral agents, but effect is local or minimally systemic	Topical agents work faster but are more likely to bring about rhinitis medicamentosa if used > 4 days. May produce burning, stinging especially when sprayed on irritated mucous membranes.

PREGNANCY/LACTATION CONSIDERATIONS

- Sinusitis may be aggravated by physiologic nasal congestion due to pregnancy
- Mild decongestant use considered safe for short-term use
- Avoid antibiotics unless absolutely necessary
- Avoid tetracyclines, quinolones, sulfa during pregnancy or lactation

CONSULTATION/REFERRAL

- Refer to ENT for infection which will not clear
- Consider immediate referral for periorbital cellulitis
- Stiff neck may indicate meningitis

FOLLOW-UP

- Indicated until clinically free of infection

EXPECTED COURSE

- Good prognosis for acute sinusitis
- Chronic sinusitis frequently recurs unless causative factor is treated (e.g., allergic rhinitis, drainage problems) or eliminated (e.g., mechanical obstruction)

POSSIBLE COMPLICATIONS

- Abscess
- Meningitis
- Periorbital cellulitis

PHARYNGITIS/TONSILLITIS

DESCRIPTION

An acute inflammation of the pharynx/tonsils

ETIOLOGY

Causes	
Viral*	**Bacterial**
Rhinovirus Adenovirus Parainfluenza Epstein-Barr virus (mononucleosis)	Group A β-hemolytic *Streptococcus*** Haemophilus influenzae *Mycoplasma pneumonia* *Chlamydia pneumoniae* *Neisseria gonorrhoeae* No pathogen can be isolated in many cases

**Most common pathogen*
** *Common depending on time of year*

INCIDENCE

- Prevalent in school age population, but occurs in all age groups (5-18 years most common age group)
- More common during winter months

RISK FACTORS

- Exposure during Group A β-hemolytic *Streptococcus* (GABHS) infection outbreaks
- Family history of rheumatic fever places higher risk if GABHS is untreated
- Crowded conditions
- Daycare attendance
- Chronic illness (e.g., diabetes mellitus)
- Oral sex

ASSESSMENT FINDINGS

- Sore throat and pharyngeal edema
- Tonsillar exudate and/or enlarged tonsils
- Malaise
- Clinical findings are not specific for diagnosis of bacterial or viral illness
- Suggestive of streptococcal infection:
  - ◊ Cervical adenopathy
  - ◊ Fever >102°F (38.8°C)
  - ◊ Foul or sweet odor on breath
  - ◊ Absence of other upper respiratory
  - ◊ findings (cough, nasal congestion, etc.)
  - ◊ Petechiae on soft palate (> 6 suggestive of streptococcal infection)

- Suggestive of viral infection:
  - ◊ Conjunctivitis

DIFFERENTIAL DIAGNOSIS

- Upper respiratory illness
- Tonsillitis
- Mononucleosis
- Peritonsillar abscess
- Epiglottitis

DIAGNOSTIC STUDIES

- Quick streptococcal test (75-80% sensitivity): must get good swab of tonsillar pillars and posterior pharynx
- A negative result should be confirmed by throat culture (gold standard)
- CBC: shift to the left
- Monospot if infectious mononucleosis suspected

PREVENTION

- Avoid contact with infected persons during outbreaks
- Good hand washing, especially during cold weather months
- Teach patients not to share drinking glasses, eating utensils, etc.
- Prompt treatment of individuals with family history of rheumatic fever

NONPHARMACOLOGIC MANAGEMENT

- Gargling with warm salt water
- Increase amount of fluids consumed
- Patient education regarding disease, course, and treatment

PHARMACOLOGIC MANAGEMENT

- Antipyretics/analgesics (acetaminophen, ibuprofen) for fever and throat pain

Antibiotic treatment used to prevent sequelae of rheumatic fever secondary to Strep pharyngitis.

Medication	Treatment
Penicillin G	One IM injection
Penicillin V *Amoxicillin* *Erythromycin*	Requires 10 days of treatment
First generation cephalosporin	Requires 10 days of treatment
Second generation cephalosporin	5 days of treatment
Azithromycin	Requires 5 days of treatment

CONSULTATION/REFERRAL

- Evidence of acute renal failure and reddish, tea-colored urine (2-3 weeks post infection) may indicate acute poststreptococcal glomerulonephritis
- Tonsillar edema and upper airway obstruction

FOLLOW-UP

- None usually needed

EXPECTED COURSE

- Peak fever and pain on days 2 and 3
- Lasts 4-10 days

POSSIBLE COMPLICATIONS

- Upper airway obstruction
- Acute poststreptococcal glomerulonephritis after streptococcal infection
- Splenic rupture in infectious mononucleosis infection (rare)
- Rheumatic fever after streptococcal infections
- Peritonsillar abscess

Do not use tetracycline or sulfonamides for Strep eradication because of resistance.

PERITONSILLAR ABSCESS
(Quinsy)

DESCRIPTION

Complication of pharyngitis or tonsillitis which manifests itself initially as a cellulitis and develops into an infection between the anterior and posterior tonsillar pillars.

ETIOLOGY

- *Streptococcus sp.*
- *Staphylococcus aureus*
- *Haemophilus influenzae*
- Anaerobic bacteria

INCIDENCE

- Rare in young children, but more common in young adults/adolescents

RISK FACTORS

- Concurrent or previous pharyngitis/tonsillitis/supraglottitis
- Penetrating trauma in the nasopharyngeal area

ASSESSMENT FINDINGS

- Fever
- Severe sore throat
- Dysphagia
- Trismus: pain on opening of mouth
- Erythematous, swollen, soft palate
- Displaced uvula
- Medially displaced tonsil
- Unilateral neck and/or ear pain
- Torticollis toward side of abscess
- Cervical adenopathy

DIFFERENTIAL DIAGNOSIS

- Epiglottitis
- Severe tonsillitis/pharyngitis
- Peritonsillar cellulitis
- Retropharyngeal abscess

DIAGNOSTIC STUDIES

- Ultrasound or CT with contrast will show abscess
- Quick streptococcal test
- CBC: shift to the left
- Lateral neck X-rays if retropharyngeal abscess or epiglottitis is part of differential
- Diagnosis can be made after physical exam usually

PREVENTION

- Early, appropriate treatment of pharyngitis/tonsillitis
- Tonsillectomy after severe or recurrent peritonsillar abscess

NONPHARMACOLOGIC MANAGEMENT

- Inpatient admission
- Maintain patent airway until referral to emergency department or ENT

PHARMACOLOGIC MANAGEMENT

- Intravenous penicillin for *Streptococcus* infections
- Intravenous cephalosporins for staphylococcal or anaerobic bacterial infections

CONSULTATION/REFERRAL

- Referral to ENT for likely incision and drainage (I&D)

FOLLOW-UP

- Peritonsillar abscesses tend to recur; teach patients early signs and symptoms
- Oral course of antibiotics for 10-14 days after incision and drainage
- Tonsillectomy may be indicated 6 weeks after acute event

EXPECTED COURSE

- Complete recovery

POSSIBLE COMPLICATIONS

- Airway obstruction
- Recurrence if abscess is not incised and drained

EPIGLOTTITIS
(Supraglottitis)

DESCRIPTION

A life-threatening infection of the epiglottis and surrounding tissues which can cause sudden and critical narrowing of the airway; a medical emergency.

ETIOLOGY

- *Haemophilus influenza* (incidence has decreased since Hib vaccine in use)
- *Streptococcus sp.*
- *Staphylococcus*
- Viral pathogens

INCIDENCE

- Uncommon in children <2 years
- Most common in 2-5 year olds
- May occur at any age including adults

RISK FACTORS

- Foreign body aspiration

ASSESSMENT FINDINGS

- Abrupt onset of high fever and sore throat
- Beefy red pharynx
- Drooling or spitting out of saliva because too painful to swallow
- Muffled voice
- Dyspnea, tachypnea, and inspiratory stridor if respiratory compromise occurs
- "Sniffing posture" (child leans forward and hyperextends neck to maintain patent airway)

Do not attempt to visualize the pharynx if epiglottitis is suspected!

DIFFERENTIAL DIAGNOSIS

- Croup: has characteristic brassy cough not usually found in epiglottitis
- Bacterial tracheitis
- Foreign body aspiration
- Peritonsillar abscess

DIAGNOSTIC STUDIES

- Diagnosis made usually with history and appearance of child
- Do NOT use tongue depressor in examination until airway is secured
- Lateral neck x-ray: characteristic "thumbprint" but contraindicated unless airway secured
- CBC: elevated WBC

PREVENTION

- Hib immunization for toddlers & young children

Airway management is priority intervention!

NONPHARMACOLOGIC MANAGEMENT

- **Maintain patent airway!**
- Arrange for transfer to quickest medical facility which can intubate/manage airway
- Keep patient calm, quiet
- Have supplemental oxygen available until transfer

PHARMACOLOGIC MANAGEMENT

- Intravenous antibiotics to cover gram positive organisms, β-lactamase- producing organisms, and *H. influenza* type b

CONSULTATION/REFERRAL

- Refer to nearest medical facility which can provide intubation/airway management

FOLLOW-UP

- After hospitalization is dependent on patient's condition

EXPECTED COURSE

- Approximately 8% mortality
- Good prognosis if airway management and appropriate antibiotic therapy are initiated in a timely manner

POSSIBLE COMPLICATIONS

- Sudden closure of airway resulting in hypoxia, arrest, and death
- Pneumonia

INFECTIOUS MONONUCLEOSIS (IM)

(Mono, Kissing Disease)

DESCRIPTION

Viral illness characterized by malaise and fatigue

ETIOLOGY

- Epstein-Barr virus (EBV) of the herpes family of viruses (almost entirely)

Incubation period is 30-50 days.

INCIDENCE

- About 50/100,000 people; up to 5% in susceptible college students
- By young adulthood, about 90% are seropositive
- Most common age is teens and early twenties

RISK FACTORS

- Contact with oral or fecal secretions of an infected person

ASSESSMENT FINDINGS

- Malaise and fatigue
- Tetrad:
    - ◊ Fatigue can last days to weeks
    - ◊ Fever
    - ◊ Pharyngitis can be painful, severe, and exudative
    - ◊ Lymphadenopathy: anterior and posterior cervical nodes most common
- Splenomegaly (found in 50% of patients)
- Headache
- Tonsillitis
- Mild hepatomegaly
- Palatal petechiae

DIFFERENTIAL DIAGNOSIS

- Group A β-hemolytic streptococcal infection (detection does not rule out IM and IM does not rule out co-infection with Strep)
- Cytomegalovirus (CMV)
- Adenovirus
- Herpes simplex
- Lymphoma/Leukemia
- Rubella
- Viral hepatitis
- Viral tonsillitis

DIAGNOSTIC STUDIES

- Monospot used for screening of heterophil antibodies: most likely time to be positive is 2nd or 3rd week of illness. This is less diagnostic in younger children (<5 years), but is diagnostic about 90% of the time in adolescents and adults.
- EBV titers (positive in 100% of patients)
- Atypical monocytosis
- Liver function tests: may see elevated liver enzymes

- CBC: lymphocytosis

PREVENTION

- Avoid contact with secretions of infected persons
- Good handwashing
- Isolation NOT necessary
- No blood donation for at least 6 months

NONPHARMACOLOGIC MANAGEMENT

- Rest
- No vigorous exercise, contact sports, or heavy lifting for about 2 months because of potential for splenic rupture (may resume activities sooner if spleen returns to prior non-enlarged state)
- Warm, salt water gargles
- Teach that convalescence may take weeks
- Avoid stress
- Eat well balanced diet with extra fluids

PHARMACOLOGIC MANAGEMENT

- Acetaminophen for fever, aches, pain /other analgesics (aspirin should be avoided because of risk of Reye's syndrome)
- Antiviral medications have not been shown to decrease length or severity of infection

Avoid ampicillin in patients with IM due to increased susceptibility to reactions (i.e., characteristic "ampicillin rash").

- Avoid steroids unless severe pharyngeal erythema (use may prolong illness)

CONSULTATION/REFERRAL

- For marked pharyngeal swelling that may threaten airway (consider steroids)
- Symptoms persisting longer than 2 weeks
- Immunocompromised individuals

FOLLOW-UP

- In 1-2 weeks and more often if patient's condition dictates

EXPECTED COURSE

- Duration is variable
- Acute phase lasts about 2 weeks
- Complete resolution may take several weeks

POSSIBLE COMPLICATIONS

- Chronic EBV infection (chronic fatigue syndrome)
- Splenic rupture (rare)
- Encephalitis
- Airway obstruction
- Blood dyscrasias
- Other complications effecting nearly every body system

EPISTAXIS
(Nosebleed)

DESCRIPTION

Severe bleeding which occurs from the nose, nasal cavity, or part of the nasopharynx.

This is a symptom, not a disease.

ETIOLOGY

- Idiopathic (most common)
- Epistaxis digitorum (nose picking)
- Bleeding tendency (associated with aplastic anemias, leukemias, hereditary coagulopathies, decreased platelet and clotting functions)
- Infection of the sinuses or upper respiratory tract
- Hypertension
- Liver disease
- Trauma

Kiesselbach's plexus is part of the anterior portion of the septum and is particularly subject to injury and, thus, is a frequent site of anterior hemorrhages.

INCIDENCE

- Most common ages are under 10 years and over 50 years

RISK FACTORS

- Idiopathic (most common)
- Epistaxis digitorum (nose picking)
- Blood dyscrasias/coagulopathy
- Chronic/acute sinus infections
- Uncontrolled hypertension
- Hepatitis or other liver diseases
- Blunt nose trauma
- Cocaine use

ASSESSMENT FINDINGS

- Nostril hemorrhage
- Dried blood in naris from prior bleeds
- Hemoptysis
- Nausea from swallowing blood
- Hematemesis

DIFFERENTIAL DIAGNOSIS

- Because epistaxis is a symptom, not a disease, the underlying cause must be identified (*see* Etiology)

DIAGNOSTIC STUDIES

- Usually none
- CBC if bleeding severe
- Hemoglobin to evaluate for anemia, platelet count
- Clotting studies as indicated
- Liver function tests (may be elevated)

PREVENTION

- Avoid placing objects in nose
- Keep fingernails short
- Management of hypertension, upper respiratory infections
- Lubricate nares during upper respiratory infections if tendency to have nosebleeds
- Humidification at night to prevent drying of mucous membranes
- General measures to stop nosebleeds if they occur

NONPHARMACOLOGIC MANAGEMENT

- Analgesics if needed
- Ice packs over nose
- Upright posture
- Teach patient proper technique to apply pressure to nose during times of bleeding
- Nasal endoscopy for cauterization
- Nasal packing
- Surgical cauterization/arterial ligation for intractable bleeds

PHARMACOLOGIC MANAGEMENT

- Phenylephrine spray (Neo-Synephrine®)
- Vasoconstrictor-impregnated cotton pledget (0.25% phenylephrine or 1:1000 epinephrine)
- Silver nitrate sticks to bleeding area (Painful!)

CONSULTATION/REFERRAL

- Physician (ENT) for severe anterior bleeds, posterior nasal bleeds, recurrent bleeds
- Consider referral in the elderly (can be severe)

FOLLOW-UP

- Depends on etiology and severity of hemorrhage

EXPECTED COURSE

- Prognosis depends on underlying cause
- For idiopathic epistaxis, prognosis is excellent with proper treatment

POSSIBLE COMPLICATIONS

- Hemorrhage
- Sinusitis
- Abscess
- Tachycardia, hypertension, arrhythmias from systemic effects of topical vasoconstrictors

ALLERGIC RHINITIS

DESCRIPTION

Inflammation of the mucous membranes of the nasal tract with subsequent mucosal edema, clear discharge, sneezing, and nasal stuffiness

ETIOLOGY

- Any substance or condition which causes an IgE mediated response characterized by rupture of mast cells and release of histamines, leukotrienes, prostaglandins, and other substances
- Most common seasonal allergens are pollens from grass, trees, and weeds
- Most common perennial allergens are mold, animal dander, dust mites

INCIDENCE

- Up to 20% of children
- Up to 30% of adolescents
- Usually diminishes with age
- Most common age of onset is 10-20 years

RISK FACTORS

- Family history
- Other atopic diseases (e.g., asthma, eczema)
- Repeated exposure to the allergic substance
- Noncompliance with treatment

ASSESSMENT FINDINGS

- "*Allergic shiners*": dark discolored areas beneath the lower eyelids as a result of impeded lymphatic and venous drainage
- Conjunctival injection
- Pale, boggy turbinates with clear nasal secretions
- "*Allergic salute*": transverse crease on tip of nose due to long-term wiping of nose in an upward direction
- Nasal polyps may be present
- Mouth breathing
- Palpable lymph nodes
- Enlarged tonsils and adenoids

DIFFERENTIAL DIAGNOSIS

- Vasomotor rhinitis
- Rhinitis medicamentosa
- Infection
- Tumors
- Nasal foreign body

DIAGNOSTIC STUDIES

- CBC: eosinophilia if acute reaction
- Consider cultures if infection is suspected
- Allergy testing
- Sinus films if indicated

PREVENTION

- Minimize continuous exposure to commonly known allergens
- Remove offending allergens/avoid exposure
- Adherence to pharmacological regimen

NONPHARMACOLOGIC MANAGEMENT

- Avoidance/elimination of offending allergen (e.g., frequent vacuuming, dusting, remove feather pillows from bedroom, change air conditioner filter frequently, removal of house plants, pet control, removal carpentry, stuffed animals)
- Surgical removal of polyps
- Surgical reduction of turbinates to relieve obstruction

PHARMACOLOGIC MANAGEMENT

- Saline nasal spray helps to "wash" offending particles which are trapped in airways
- Antihistamines (nonsedating and sedating available)
- Nasal steroids (preferred agent for most cases)
- Systemic steroids (avoid if possible & use only short-term)
- Topical cromolyn (mast cell stabilizer)
- Decongestants, oral or topical

AGENT	ACTION	COMMENTS
Antihistamine ***First Generation*** *Examples:* diphenhydramine (Benadryl®) hydroxyzine (Atarax®, Vistaril®)	Non-selectively block histamine binding sites in the brain (centrally) and peripherally	Don't use in symptomatic prostatic hypertrophy because of anti-cholinergic effects (inability to urinate). Monitor additive effects with EtOH, other sedative drugs. Cautious use in elderly where exaggerated effects may produce excessive sedation, dizziness, confusion, hypotension. Many available OTC.
Antihistamine ***Second Generation*** *Examples:* cetirizine (Zyrtec®) fexofenadine (Allegra®) loratadine (Claritin®)	Selectively block peripheral histamine binding	Advantage is lack of sedation for all but cetirizine. Once daily dosing improves compliance. Generally well tolerated. Expensive compared to first generation agents.
Topical nasal steroids *Examples:* budesonide (Rhinocort ®) fluticasone (Flonase ®) mometasone (Nasonex ®) triamcinolone (Nasacort ®)	Exert glucocorticoid activity on the nasal mucosa and thus have local anti-inflammatory effects	Considered "gold standard" in treatment of allergic rhinitis. Minimal systemic absorption. Can produce drying of nasal mucosa and bleeding can result. Can contribute to fungal nasal infections (rare).

CONSULTATION/REFERRAL

- Allergist for testing when persistent symptoms occur despite treatment
- ENT for sinus related etiologies
- Emergency department for severe allergic response to allergens

FOLLOW-UP

- 2-4 weeks after initial evaluation and then every 3-6 months depending on patient and severity of symptoms

EXPECTED COURSE

- Allergies tend to diminish in severity as individuals age
- Allergic response is heightened each time allergen is contacted

POSSIBLE COMPLICATIONS

- Otitis media
- Secondary infections of sinuses, tonsils, pharynx
- Sinusitis
- Epistaxis
- Facial changes (e.g., allergic salute, allergic shiners)

HEARING LOSS

DESCRIPTION

Partial or complete hearing loss. Three types:

- *Conductive*: involving the external auditory canal or the middle ear
- *Sensorineural*: involving the inner ear or the 8th cranial nerve
- Components of both conductive and sensorineural

ETIOLOGY

Conductive:

- Anything that can occlude or mechanically block sound from traveling through the external auditory canal or the middle ear

Sensorineural:

- Anything that prevents sound from traveling through the inner ear or prevents the 8th cranial nerve from functioning

Type	Cause
Conductive	Cerumen impaction Tympanic membrane perforation Fluid (serous otitis media) Tympanosclerosis
Sensorineural	Acoustic neuroma Ménière's Disease Ototoxic drugs (ASA, gentamicin) Injury due to noise Viral (especially after mumps) Presbycusis (related to aging)

INCIDENCE

- >20 times more common in adults than children
- More common in the elderly

RISK FACTORS

- Chronic allergic conditions
- Conditions which cause eustachian tube obstruction
- Heredity
- Use of ototoxic drugs
- Aging (presbycusis)
- Exposure to loud noise
- Syphilis
- Congenital rubella infection

ASSESSMENT FINDINGS

- Hard of hearing
- Tinnitus
- Dizziness
- Withdrawal from group discussions and social activities

DIFFERENTIAL DIAGNOSIS

- Conductive hearing loss
- Sensorineural hearing loss
- Conductive and sensorineural hearing losses

DIAGNOSTIC STUDIES

- Audiometry: used to quantify hearing loss
- Tuning fork tests: tuning forks with frequencies of 256, 512, 1024, and 2048 Hz are used
- Whisper test: evaluates patient's gross hearing ability

WEBER TEST **Confirms result of Rinne and tests for lateralization of sound**	**RINNE TEST** **Normal is AC > BC**	**RESULTS**
Tone heard louder in affected ear	Tone heard louder in affected ear BC > AC	Conductive hearing loss
Tone heard louder in unaffected ear	AC > BC	Sensorineural hearing loss

AC = air conduction *BC = bone conduction*

PREVENTION

- Avoid loud noise exposure (e.g., guns, loud music, occupational exposure)
- Use of earplugs when exposed to loud noises
- Treat upper respiratory infections and monitor for ear problems
- Minimize exposure to ototoxic medications ("mycin" are famous for ototoxicity)
- Avoid flying or diving if upper respiratory infection is present to prevent rupture of tympanic membrane

NONPHARMACOLOGIC MANAGEMENT

- Removal of cerumen with warm water
- Development of lip reading skills for untreatable forms of hearing loss
- Hearing aid when appropriate

PHARMACOLOGIC MANAGEMENT

- Agents used to soften ear wax if cerumen impaction
- Consider antibiotics to treat otitis media

CONSULTATION/REFERRAL

- ENT for any conductive problem which does not respond after initial treatment
- ENT for any sensorineural hearing loss

FOLLOW-UP

- Depends on etiology, but for conductive hearing loss problems, follow up needed to insure resolution of problem

EXPECTED COURSE

- Sensorineural hearing loss usually unresponsive to treatment
- Conductive hearing losses usually improve with treatment, or, no progression of loss

POSSIBLE COMPLICATIONS

- Depends on etiology of problem
- Middle ear problems may progress to chronic problems
- Permanent hearing loss from loud noise exposure
- Delayed speech in young children

OTITIS EXTERNA
(Swimmer's Ear)

DESCRIPTION

An infection of the external auditory canal producing much inflammation, itching, and/or pain

ETIOLOGY

Bacterial	Fungal
Pseudomonas (most common pathogen) *Staphylococcus* *Streptococcus*	*Aspergillus* (most common fungal pathogen) *Candida albicans*

INCIDENCE

- More common in summer months

RISK FACTORS

- Swimming
- Hearing aid use
- Diabetes
- Hot, humid climates
- Trauma to external canal (cotton swab use, foreign objects)
- Not drying ears after showering or profuse perspiration

ASSESSMENT FINDINGS

- Otalgia/conductive hearing loss
- Edema and redness in the external auditory canal
- Itching in the external auditory canal
- Purulent discharge
- Tragal and/or pinna pain
- Normal tympanic membrane

DIFFERENTIAL DIAGNOSIS

- Wisdom tooth eruption
- Temporomandibular joint disease
- Tympanic membrane rupture
- Foreign body
- Hearing loss

DIAGNOSTIC STUDIES

- Culture of discharge (usually not necessary)

PREVENTION

- Avoid prolonged ear exposure to hot, humid conditions
- Dry ears after showering and swimming
- Do not place objects in the ear which may cause trauma to the external auditory canal (cotton swab, paper clips, matches, toothpicks)
- Treat ear infections aggressively
- 2% acetic acid (50:50 solution with water) drops after swimming (helps restore acidic pH of ear)
- Treat eczema before it effects the external auditory canal
- Teach methods of prevention

NONPHARMACOLOGIC MANAGEMENT

- Thorough cleansing of the external auditory canal
- Use of cotton ear wick to facilitate passage of medication into an edematous, painful ear canal

PHARMACOLOGIC MANAGEMENT

- Otic antibiotic/corticosteroid drops for 5-10 days (Cortisporin®, Cipro® otic)
- 2% Acetic acid drops/antifungal agent if fungal infection present
- Analgesics for ear pain

CONSULTATION/REFERRAL

- Refer to ENT if evidence of systemic involvement (fever)
- Poor response to therapy

FOLLOW-UP

- Usually none

EXPECTED COURSE

- Improvement in 24-48 hours with treatment
- Resolution in a few days

POSSIBLE COMPLICATIONS

- Cellulitis/chondritis
- Infection at contiguous bone

OTITIS MEDIA

DESCRIPTION

Two types:

- *Acute otitis media* (AOM) is a sudden onset of middle ear effusion and signs or symptoms of local or systemic illness
- *Otitis media with effusion* (OME) is fluid accumulation in the middle ear without evidence of infection; also called a middle ear effusion (MEE)

ETIOLOGY

Acute otitis media:

- Bacteria/viruses

Age Group	Agent for Acute Otitis Media
< 14 years	*Streptococcus pneumoniae* *H. influenzae* *Moraxella catarrhalis* Group A β-hemolytic *Streptococcus* *S. aureus*
> 14 years	*Streptococcus pneumoniae* *H. influenza* *S. aureus* Viral: RSV, Influenza

Agent	Incidence
Streptococcus pneumoniae	About 33% incidence
H. influenzae	About 33% incidence Nearly half produce beta lactamase Most prevalent organism in children who have received Prevnar®; no longer Strep
Moraxella catarrhalis	About 12% incidence About 90% produce beta lactamase

Otitis media with effusion:
- Probably due to incomplete resolution of AOM or eustachian tube obstruction

INCIDENCE

- More common in winter months
- Most common in 6 months to 3 years
- Lowest incidence in breast fed babies

RISK FACTORS

- Daycare attendance
- Familial disposition (common in siblings)
- Craniofacial abnormalities
- Upper respiratory infection
- Allergic rhinitis
- Second hand cigarette smoke
- First episode of AOM <12 months old
- Bottle feeding while in supine position

ASSESSMENT FINDINGS

Acute otitis media:
- Ear pain and irritability
- Decreased tympanic membrane (TM) mobility (observed using pneumatic otoscopy)
- Distorted landmarks
- Displaced light reflex
- Dull, opaque TM
- Possible bulging TM
- Fever
- GI symptoms (nausea, vomiting, diarrhea)
- Diminished hearing
- Pulling on ear
- Dizziness

Otitis media with effusion:
- Usually asymptomatic
- Dull TM
- Decreased mobility
- Visible air-fluid interface
- Visible air bubbles
- Diminished hearing

DIFFERENTIAL DIAGNOSIS

- Otitis externa may present like AOM with TM rupture
- Tumors (cholesteatoma)
- Crying may cause the TM to appear red on examination
- Referred pain from jaw or teeth

DIAGNOSTIC STUDIES

- Pneumatic otoscopy
- Consider referral for tympanocentesis to obtain culture (rarely performed)
- Tympanometry to measure TM compliance

PREVENTION

- Breastfeeding
- Avoid cigarette smoke exposure
- Do not put baby to sleep in horizontal position with bottle
- Antibiotic prophylaxis for recurrent AOM (controversial)

NONPHARMACOLOGIC MANAGEMENT

- Local heat
- Myringotomy
- Swallowing to help the eustachian tube ventilate
- Patient and family education regarding treatment, disease, comfort measures, etc.

PHARMACOLOGIC MANAGEMENT

Antibiotics do NOT relieve pain in the first 24 hours!

- Analgesics (i.e. acetaminophen, ibuprofen, otalgic drops) for 2-3 days if no symptoms of systemic illness (80% of patients resolve with analgesics)
- **Exception**: If child is < 6 months old, amoxicillin (80-90 mg/kg/d) is first choice

unless PCN allergic, β-lactamase-producer suspected, severe illness (39°C or severe otalgia), or recent antibiotic exposure

- Second line: Amoxicillin/clavulanate for β-lactamase coverage, newer generation macrolides, 2nd, 3rd generation cephalosporins, clindamycin

ACUTE OTITIS MEDIA		
AGENT	**ACTION**	**COMMENTS**
PCN *Examples:* amoxicillin (80-90 mg/kg/d) (Amoxil®)	Inhibit cell wall synthesis Not stable in the presence of beta lactamase producer	Give in divided doses. Considered first line agent in most cases. Consider amoxicillin/clavulanate if failure after 48-72 hrs.
amoxicillin/clavulanate (80-90 mg/kg/d amox and 6.4 mg/kg/d clavulanate) (Augmentin ES®)	Inhibit cell wall synthesis Clavulanate broadens spectrum of coverage	Give in divided doses. Use first line if patient has severe illness, has had recent antibiotic exposure.
Second generation Cephalosporin *Examples:* cefuroxime (Ceftin®)	Inhibit cell wall synthesis and is more stable in presence of beta lactamase producers than other 2nd generation agents	Consider first line if patient is PCN allergic (non-Type I allergic reaction). Consider ceftriaxone (Rocephin®) if failure after 48-72 hours.
Third generation Cephalosporin *Examples:* cefpodoxime (Vantin®) cefdinir (Omnicef®)	Inhibit cell wall synthesis Stable in the presence of beta lactamase producers	First line agent for PCN allergic (non-type I allergic reaction). Consider ceftriaxone (Rocephin®) if failure after 48-72 hours.
Extended Spectrum Macrolides *Examples:* azithromycin (Zithromax®) clarithromycin (Biaxin®)	Inhibit protein synthesis by binding to the 50S ribosomal subunit	First line for PCN allergic (Type I allergic reaction) Consider clindamycin, if failure after 48-72 hours.

CONSULTATION/REFERRAL

- ENT referral for recurrent (3 occurrences in 6 months or 4 in one year)
- ENT consultation for headache (may signal meningitis, epidural abscess)
- ENT referral for mastoiditis
- Refer if language delay detected
- Refer/consult for neonates

FOLLOW-UP

- Recheck ears in 4 weeks and follow until resolution or referral
- Re-evaluate sooner if symptoms persist

EXPECTED COURSE

- Improvement in 48-72 hours
- At 4 weeks approximately 50% will still have middle ear effusion (MEE)
- At 3 months about 10% will still have MEE

POSSIBLE COMPLICATIONS

- TM perforation
- Conductive and/or sensorineural hearing loss
- Acute mastoiditis
- Meningitis
- Epidural abscess
- Language delay from hearing loss

MASTOIDITIS

DESCRIPTION

A bacterial infection of the mastoid antrum and cells that can be asymptomatic or life-threatening. Usually is a result of untreated or under treated acute otitis media.

ETIOLOGY

- *Streptococcus pneumoniae*
- Group A β-hemolytic *Streptococcus*
- *H. influenza*
- *S. aureus*
- *Pseudomonas aeruginosa*

RISK FACTORS

- Age < 2 years
- Cholesteatoma (from chronic mastoiditis)
- Recurrent or persistent otitis media
- Immunocompromised state
- Untreated/undertreated otitis media

ASSESSMENT FINDINGS

- Persistent, throbbing otalgia
- Fever
- Postauricular swelling and tenderness
- Auricular protrusion (pinna displaced laterally and inferiorly)
- Possible creamy, profuse otorrhea since TM perforation often precedes mastoiditis
- Possible hearing loss

DIFFERENTIAL DIAGNOSIS

- Severe otitis externa
- Neoplasm of the mastoid bone
- Parotitis or mumps (swelling is over the parotid vs. preauricular area)
- Cellulitis

DIAGNOSTIC STUDIES

- Middle ear aspirate
- Mastoid radiographs: demonstrates clouding of air cells
- Myringotomy
- CBC: demonstrates shift to left

PREVENTION

- Early treatment of otitis media
- Early identification of cholesteatoma

NONPHARMACOLOGIC MANAGEMENT

- Keep ear dry
- Water precautions
- Myringotomy to drain middle ear (refer)

PHARMACOLOGIC MANAGEMENT

- Antibiotics (usually intravenous) on basis of most likely organisms until cultures are known
- Topical antibiotics
- Analgesics for pain
- Antipyretics for fever

CONSULTATION/REFERRAL

- ENT referral for myringotomy, hospitalization, intravenous antibiotic management
- Neurologist or ENT for suspected meningitis

FOLLOW-UP

- Depends on patient condition and age, but weekly follow-up after discharge
- Postinfection follow-up needed with audiograms to assess hearing loss

EXPECTED COURSE

- Depends on severity of infection, but prognosis is good if proper therapy initiated early

POSSIBLE COMPLICATIONS

- Meningitis
- Intracranial abscess
- Facial nerve paralysis

VERTIGO
(Dizziness)

DESCRIPTION

The sensation or impression that an individual is moving, or that objects around him are moving, when actually no movement is occurring.

ETIOLOGY

- A disturbance in the equilibratory apparatus with either peripheral or central causes

Peripheral Etiologies:
- Otogenic
  - ◊ Ménière's disease
  - ◊ Myringitis
  - ◊ Infections of inner ear
  - ◊ Otitis media
  - ◊ Labyrinthitis
  - ◊ Obstructed eustachian tubes
  - ◊ Benign positional vertigo
- Toxic
  - ◊ Excessive alcohol ingestion
  - ◊ Salicylates
  - ◊ Potent diuretics
  - ◊ Ototoxic drugs (especially aminoglycosides)
- Environmental
- Motion sickness
- Neurological
- 8th cranial nerve tumors (acoustic neuroma)

Central Etiologies:
- Circulatory
  - ◊ Transient ischemic attacks (TIA)
  - ◊ Postural hypotension
- Neurologic
  - ◊ Multiple sclerosis
  - ◊ Temporal lobe seizures
  - ◊ Cervical vertebra disorders
  - ◊ Syphilis
- Other
  - ◊ Hypothyroidism
  - ◊ Psychiatric illness

INCIDENCE

- Unknown
- Usually in 20-60 year olds

RISK FACTORS

- Depends on etiology

ASSESSMENT FINDINGS

All findings listed below are possible depending on the etiology:
- Asymptomatic except vertigo
- Nystagmus when extraocular movements are tested (peripheral or central)
- Tinnitus (peripheral or central)
- Hearing loss, (peripheral) ear pain
- Paroxysmal, episodic attacks of vertigo (peripheral)
- Carotid bruit (central)
- Persistent vertigo (central)
- Headache, diplopia, slurred speech (central)
- Hypotension (central)

ASSESSMENT FINDINGS IN MOST COMMON CAUSES OF VERTIGO

Benign positional vertigo:
- Vertigo
- Nystagmus with shifts in head position
- No hearing loss or tinnitus
- Nausea, vomiting

Vestibulopathy:
- Vertigo with position changes
- No hearing loss
- No tinnitus
- Nausea, vomiting
- Often follows gastrointestinal or upper respiratory infections

Ménière's Disease:
- Sudden vertigo
- Tinnitus

- Hearing loss
- Ear fullness
- Nausea
- Vomiting

DIFFERENTIAL DIAGNOSIS

- Vestibular disease
- Neuromas, other tumors
- Cardiac and vascular pathologies
- Sensory deficits
- Psychiatric illnesses
- Metabolic disorders

DIAGNOSTIC STUDIES

- Audiometry to discern hearing loss
- Rinne and Weber tests
- Test cranial nerve and cerebellar function
- Syphilis serology to rule out syphilis
- Consider TSH to rule out thyroid disease
- Consider hematocrit/hemoglobin to rule out anemia
- Consider fasting blood sugar levels to rule out diabetes and hypoglycemia
- Blood pressure checks in 3 positions to rule out hypotension
- Auditory Brainstem Response to rule out acoustic neuroma
- Consider CT/MRI to rule out central lesions
- Consider in selected patients the Nylen-Barany maneuver or Hallpike maneuver
- Electronystagmography (ENG) to help differentiate central and peripheral lesions

PREVENTION

- Teach safety measures to patients who have vertigo

NONPHARMACOLOGIC MANAGEMENT

- Depends on etiology
- Rest in bed with eyes closed during acute attack
- Handrails at home for chronic multisensory deficits
- Good lighting
- Use of a cane or walker

PHARMACOLOGIC MANAGEMENT

- Depends on etiology
- Antihistamines: meclizine (Antivert®), promethazine (Phenergan®), dimenhydrinate (Dramamine®), transdermal scopolamine

CONSULTATION/REFERRAL

- Refer if any neurological symptoms exist
- Refer any problems that are disabling and/or progressive

FOLLOW-UP

- Dependent on etiology

EXPECTED COURSE

- Dependent on etiology, but generally, peripheral causes have better prognosis than central causes

References

Berman, S., Byrns, P.J., Bondy, J., Smith, P.J., & Lezotte, D. (1997). Ootitis media-related antibiotic prescribing patterns, outcomes, and expenditures in a pediatric medicaid population. *Pediatrics, 100*(4), 585-592.

Bickley, L.S., & Szilagyi, P.G. (2003). *Bates' guide to physical examination and history taking* (8th ed.). Philadelphia: Lippincott Williams & Wilkins.

Branch, W.T. (2003). *Office practice of medicine* (4th ed.). Philadelphia: Saunders.

Brown, C.S., Parker, N.G., & Stegbauer, C.C. (1999). Managing allergic rhinitis. *The Nurse Practitioner*, 24(6): 107-120.

Burns, C.E., Brady, M.A., Blosser, C., Starr, N.B., & Dunn, A.M. (2004). *Pediatric primary care: A handbook for nurse practitioners* (3rd ed.). Philadelphia: W.B. Saunders.

Conboy-Ellis, K. (2005). Management of seasonal allergic rhinitis: Comparative efficacy of the new-generation prescription antihistamines. *Journal of the American Academy of Nurse Practitioners, 17*(8), 295-301.

Cozad, J. (1996). Infectious mononucleosis. *The Nurse Practitioner, 21*(3), 14-28.

Daly, K.A., Selvius, R.E., & Lindgren, B. (1997). Knowledge and attitudes about otitis media risk: Implications for prevention. *Pediatrics 100*(6), 931-936.

Dambro, M.R. (2005). *Griffith's 5 minute clinical consult.* Philadelphia: Lippincott Williams & Wilkins.

Fell, E. (2000). An update on lyme disease and other tick-borne illnesses. *The Nurse Practitioner*, 25(10): 38-55.

Gilber, D.N., Moellering, R.C., Eliopoulos, G.M., & Sande, M.A. (Eds.). (2004). *Sanford Guide to Antimicrobial Therapy* (34th ed.). Hyde Park, VT: Antimicrobial Therapy.

Graber, M.A., & Lanternier, M.L. (Eds.) (2001). *The family practice handbook.* (4th ed.). St. Louis: Mosby.

Hanson, M.J. (1996). Acute otitis media in children. *The Nurse Practitioner, 21*(5), 72-81.

Hahn, R.G., Knox, L.M., & Forman, T.A. (2005). Evaluation of poststreptococcal illness. *American Family Physician, 71,* 1949-1954.

Hara, J.H. (1996). The red eye: Diagnosis and treatment. *American Family Physician, 54*(8), 2423-2436.

Kasper, D.L., Braunwald, E., Fauci, A.S., Hauser, S.L., Longo, D.L., Jameson, J.L., et al. (2004). *Harrison's principles of internal medicine* (16th ed.). New York: McGraw-Hill.

Kliegman, R.M., Greenbaum, L.A., & Lye, P.S. (2004). *Practical strategies in pediatric diagnosis and therapy* (2nd ed.). Philadelphia: W.B. Saunders.

Lucente, F. & Grady, H.E. (1999). Essentials of Otolaryngology. (4th ed.). Philadelphia: Lippincott Williams & Wilkins.

Mangion, S. (2000). *Physical diagnosis secrets.* Philadelphia: Hanley and Belfus.

Mladenovic, J. (Ed.). (2003). *Primary care secrets.* (3rd Ed.). Philadelphia: Hanley and Belfus.

Morrow, G.L., & Abbott, R.L. (1998). Conjunctivitis. *American Family Physician, 57*, 735-746.

Osguthorpe, J.D. (2001). Adult rhinosinusitis: diagnosis and management. *American Family Physician, 63,* 69-76.

Perkins, A. (1997). An approach to diagnosing the acute sore throat. *American Family Physician, 55*, 131-140.

Pryor, M.P. (1997). Noisy breathing in children. *Postgraduate Medicine 101*(2), 103-112.

Rabinowitz, P.M. (2000). Noise-induced hearing loss. *American Family Physician, 61,* 2749-2756, 2759-2760.

Rakel, R.E. (Ed.). (1998). *Essentials of family practice.* (2nd ed.). Philadelphia: WB Saunders.

Ruppert, S.D. (1996). Differential diagnosis of common causes of pediatric pharyngitis. *The Nurse Practitioner, 21*(4), 38-49.

Ruppert, S.D. (1996). Differential diagnosis of pediatric conjunctivitis. *The Nurse Practitioner, 21*(7), 12-26.

Schwartz, M.W. (Ed.). (2002). *The 5 minute pediatric consult.* (2nd ed.) Philadelphia: Lippincott Williams & Wilkins.

Scott, P.T., Clark, J.B., & Miser, W.F. (1997). Pertussis: An update on primary prevention and outbreak control. *American Family Physician, 56,* 1121-1130.

Shaw, L. (1997). Protocol for detection and follow-up of hearing loss. *Clinical Nurse Specialist: The Journal for Advanced Nursing Practice, 11*(6), 240-245.

Tasman, W., & Jaeger, E.A. (2005). *Duane's Clinical Ophthalmology on CD-ROM.* Philadelphia: J.B. Lippincott Co.

Uphold, C.R., & Graham, M.V. (2003). *Clinical guidelines in family practice.* (4th ed.). Gainesville, FL: Barmarrae Books.

U.S. Preventive Services Task Force. (1996). *Guide to clinical preventive services.* (2nd ed.) Washington, D.C.: Office of Disease Prevention and Health Promotion, U.S. Government Printing Office.

Ward, M. R. (1997). Reye's syndrome: An update. *The Nurse Practitioner, 22*(12), 45-53.

Wingate, S. (1999). Treating corneal abrasions. *The Nurse Practitioner*, *24*(6): 53-68.

Zollo, A.J., Jr (Ed.). (2004). *Medical Secrets.* (4th ed.), St. Louis, MO: Mosby-Year Book.

5

ENDOCRINE DISORDERS

Endocrine Disorders

**Denotes pediatric diagnosis*

DIABETES MELLITUS
Type I

DESCRIPTION

A leading serious chronic illness of children and young adults characterized by insulin deficiency, hyperglycemia, and glucosuria.

ETIOLOGY

- Insulin deficiency and hyperglycemia result from destruction of β-cells of the pancreas
- β-cell destruction may be a result of genetic predisposition in combination with environmental triggers

INCIDENCE

- Peak age at onset is 8 to 12 years; peaking in adolescence
- Approximately 10% of all diabetics
- Highest incidence is in Caucasian Americans
- Male = female

RISK FACTORS

- Diabetes mellitus Type I or 2 in a first-degree relative
- Presence of HLA DR3, DR4, B8, B15 genes on Chromosome 6

ASSESSMENT FINDINGS

- Acute onset of polydipsia, polyphagia, polyuria ("the 3 P's"), weight loss, fatigue
- Dehydration
- Decreased energy level
- Confusion
- Fruity odor to breath if diagnosed during diabetic ketoacidosis
- Failure to grow and gain weight in small children and infants

DIFFERENTIAL DIAGNOSIS

- Diabetes mellitus Type II
- Pancreatic disease
- Salicylate poisoning

DIAGNOSTIC STUDIES

- Fasting plasma glucose $\geq$ 126 mg/dL *(on 2 occasions)* *OR*
  Random glucose level $\geq$ 200 mg/dL
  OR
  2 hour plasma glucose $\geq$ 200 mg/dl *(during an oral GTT)*
- Impaired fasting glucose (IFG) $\geq$ 100 mg/dl *(pre-diabetes)*
- Glucosuria
- Ketonuria
- Glycosylated hemoglobin increased in patient with symptoms longer than 1 month **(not used for diagnosis)**
- Electrolytes
- C-peptide insulin level
- Urinalysis for presence of glucose or ketones

PREVENTION OF COMPLICATIONS

- Normoglycemia by "tight control": maintenance of HgbA1C near nondiabetic range (5.5 – 6.5%)
- Smoking avoidance or cessation
- Exercise daily
- Maintenance of ideal body weight
- Education about insensate foot care
- Limit dietary fat intake

MANAGEMENT

- Multidisciplinary treatment: integration of insulin therapy (cornerstone of therapy), nutrition management, exercise

Assessments:
- Physical examinations every three months focused on growth, development and sexual development (poor glucose control affects growth)
- Blood pressure and cardiac examination
- Funduscopic and vision examination at time of diagnosis, then, annual dilated eye exam and if having visual problems
- Oral examination

- Palpation of thyroid
- Abdominal examination
- Skin examination
- Neurological examination
- Examine feet for pulses, cleanliness, odor, swelling, mobility, nail thickness, bruises, pressure points; include sensory evaluation

Insulin therapy:

- Changes in insulin dose:
  Based on several day trends of CBG and are done by increments of 1-2 units
- Insulin
  - ◊ *AM regular insulin* affects glucose pre-lunch
  - ◊ *AM NPH/Lente* affects glucose post lunch/pre-supper
  - ◊ *PM rapid acting* affects glucose post-supper
  - ◊ *PM regular* affects glucose at bedtime
  - ◊ *PM NPH/Lente* affects glucose early AM

Summary of Insulin Therapy	
Rapid acting	Lispro/Aspart – works almost immediately with injection (may be used in lieu of regular insulin)
Short acting	Regular
Intermediate acting	NPH Lente
Long acting	Ultralente
Peak less	Lantus
Pre-mixed	70/30 50/50
Calculation of Daily Insulin Requirements	
Adults	0.8 to 1 u/kg/day divided into 2 doses, $^2/_3$ dose in morning and $^1/_3$ in evening
Children	0.25 u/kg/day
Adolescents	1.25-1.5 u/kg/day due to accelerated growth and metabolic rate
Insulin pump delivers individualized basal metabolic rate with bolus at meal times	

Type I Diabetes Mellitus by Injection		
2 Dose Regimen (usually inadequate to maintain normal glycemic control) Calculate total daily requirements as above then 2/3 in am, 1/3 in pm		
AM	1:2 ratio regular/rapid acting for NPH/Lente	
PM	1:1 ratio regular/rapid acting to NPA/Lente	
3 Dose Regimen		
	NPH/Lente	Regular/Rapid Acting
AM	20-30%	25%
PM		25%
HS	20-30%	
Glargine OR regular/rapid acting		
AM		20-30%
PM		20-30%
HS	50%	
4 Dose Regimen		
	NPH/Lente	Regular/Rapid Acting
Breakfast		√
Lunch		√
Dinner		√
Bedtime	√√	
√ = based on amount eaten √√ = basal rate		

Nutrition therapy:

- Goal is a well balanced diet providing consistency in timing and intake
- Formula to determine caloric intake:
  - ◊ 100 calories x age in years + 1000 = total calories
  - ◊ 20% protein
  - ◊ 30% fat (<7% saturated fat)
  - ◊ 50% carbohydrate

Exercise:

- Regular aerobic exercise is preferred

- Recommended daily to increase the number of insulin receptors, and insulin secretion; allows more efficient glucose utilization

General:

- Formulate sick day plan
- Develop contingency plan for management of hypoglycemia
- Medic alert bracelet
- School personnel/co-workers should be aware

PREGNANCY/LACTATION CONSIDERATIONS

- Goal is maintenance of fasting plasma glucose (FPG) from 60-105 mg/dL and postprandial level <120 mg/dL
- Dietary management:
  - ◊ Well-balanced meals with a limited intake of concentrated sweets
  - ◊ Refer to registered dietitian and diabetes educator
- Self-monitoring of glucose 4 or more times a day
- Oral antihyperglycemic agents contraindicated in pregnancy
- Breastfeeding is encouraged because of its positive effect on HDL
- 28 weeks: maternal assessment of fetal activity should begin, with daily kick counts
- 32 weeks: twice weekly nonstress testing
- Increased risk of maternal and fetal complications:
  - ◊ Accelerates development of retinopathy and pregnancy-induced hypertension
  - ◊ Spontaneous abortion and congenital anomalies
  - ◊ Macrosomia, shoulder dystocia, hypoglycemia, hypokalemia, stillbirth

CONSULTATION/ REFERRAL

- Endocrinologist
- Diabetic educator
- Registered dietitian
- Obstetrician during pregnancy

FOLLOW-UP

- Frequency of visits dependent on course of illness
- Hemoglobin A_1C every 3 months
- Screen for microalbuminuria annually
- Annual total urinary protein once positive for microalbuminuria
- Annual serum creatinine in adults and in children if proteinuria is present
- Lipid profile, if >2 years of age, at diagnosis, then annually once control is established
- Annual ECG in adults
- Thyroid function tests every 2-3 years

EXPECTED COURSE

- Lifelong illness with course dependent on glucose control
- Use of insulin pump shown to decrease complications, but requires intensive management and training

POSSIBLE COMPLICATIONS

- Ketoacidosis
- Hypoglycemia
- Chronic microvascular disease: retinopathy, renal failure, peripheral neuropathy
- Skin ulcerations, gangrene of lower extremities
- Macrovascular disease, premature atherosclerosis

DIABETES MELLITUS
Type II

DESCRIPTION

Abnormal insulin secretion, resistance to insulin in target tissues, and/or decrease in insulin receptors

ETIOLOGY

- Influenced by genetics as well as environmental factors

- High body mass with central obesity is strongest environmental factor
- Inactivity

INCIDENCE

- 90% of diabetes mellitus cases in the U.S. are Type II with usual age of onset >30 years
- Incidence is rising in all age groups
- Increased in African-Americans, American Indians, Latino-Americans, Pacific Islanders, Mexican-Americans

RISK FACTORS

- Obesity
- History of gestational diabetes
- History of delivery of macrosomic infant
- Family history of Type II diabetes

ASSESSMENT FINDINGS

- Usually discovered on routine examination chemistry panel and urinalysis: glucosuria, proteinuria, and hyperglycemia
- Obesity
- Polydipsia, polyuria, polyphagia, fatigue
- Blurred vision
- Chronic skin infections
- Balanitis sometimes seen in elderly males
- Chronic candidal vulvovaginitis in women
- May present with hyperosmolar state or coma

Long Term Effects Of Hyperglycemia
Hypertension Renal failure CAD, MI Peripheral neuropathy CVA Severe peripheral vascular insufficiency

DIFFERENTIAL DIAGNOSIS

- Diabetes mellitus Type I
- Cushing's syndrome
- Pheochromocytoma
- Corticosteroid use

DIAGNOSTIC STUDIES

American Diabetes Association Diagnostic Criteria	
Fasting Plasma Glucose	≥ 126 mg/dL on 2 occasions
Random Plasma Glucose	≥ 200 mg/dL *OR* 2 hour plasma glucose ≥ 200 mg/dl during an oral GTT
Pre-diabetes	fasting glucose between 100 mg/dl and 125 mg/dl

- To differentiate Type I from Type II diabetes mellitus: C peptide levels will be below normal in Type I diabetes mellitus and normal or above normal in Type II diabetes mellitus

PREVENTION

- ADA recommends adults over age 45 years be screened every 3 years, more often with fasting plasma glucose close to 126 mg/dL
- Focus on education regarding: obesity, diet, exercise, sequelae, treatments
- Avoidance of obesity

NONPHARMACOLOGIC MANAGEMENT

- Weight loss: primary goal of obese patient; even modest weight loss of 5-10 lbs is helpful in increasing insulin sensitivity
- Nutrition plan:
  - ◊ 3 visits with registered dietitian at diagnosis and ongoing follow-up visits semi-annually to annually
  - ◊ ≈ 50% carbohydrates
  - ◊ ≈ 30% protein
  - ◊ ≈ 20% fat (limit cholesterol to 300 mg/day)
- Avoid alcohol
- Avoid smoking
- Exercise
  - ◊ To increase insulin secretion, glucose utilization, and HDL
  - ◊ Endurance exercise is optimal (e.g., walking)

- ◊ Perform stress test first if older than age 35 years and diabetic
- Periodic physical examinations:
  - ◊ Blood pressure and cardiac examination
  - ◊ Funduscopic and vision examination at time of diagnosis, then if diabetic for 5 years or more, or if having visual problems
  - ◊ Oral examination
  - ◊ Thyroid palpation
  - ◊ Skin examination
  - ◊ Neurological examination
  - ◊ Abdominal examination
  - ◊ Examine feet for pulses, cleanliness, odor, swelling, mobility, nail thickness, bruises, pressure points; include sensory evaluation

PHARMACOLOGIC MANAGEMENT

- Should begin if not normoglycemic after 3 months of nonpharmacologic therapy or immediately if symptomatic

AGENT	ACTION	COMMENTS
Sulfonylurea agents *Examples:* chlorpropamide (Diabinese®) glyburide (Micronase®, DiaBeta®) glipizide (Glucotrol®) glimepiride (Amaryl®)	Potentiate insulin secretin from the pancreas (long-acting secretagogue)	May cause hypoglycemia. Tend to cause weight gain. Ideal use in insulinopenic patients, non-obese patients. Elderly are particularly sensitive to these agents. Monitoring glucose carefully in patients with renal or hepatic impairment because inability to metabolize and/or eliminate these agents can produce profound hypoglycemia. May be given as monotherapy or in combination with metformin or TZD or insulin.
Biguanides *Example:* metformin (Glucophage®)	Decrease production of glucose in the liver; decrease absorption of glucose in the intestine, and improve insulin sensitivity by increasing peripheral glucose uptake and utilization	Does not produce hypoglycemia; may produce weight loss, improvement of lipid profiles. Avoid in binge drinkers. Careful use in patients with CHF, renal and hepatic dysfunction. May be used as monotherapy or in combination with TZD, insulin, sulfonylureas. Diarrhea, flatulence are common initial side effects. Ideal use: obese, insulin resistant patient
Thiazolidinediones (TZD) *Examples:* Rosiglitazone (Avandia®) Pioglitazone (Actos®)	Inhibit gluconeogenesis in the liver, improve insulin liver sensitivity in the skeletal muscle and adipose tissue, (and consequently reduce circulating insulin levels in hyperinsulinemic patients)	Monitor ALT/AST at initiation, then at least every 2 months for one year, then periodically. Monitor for fluid retention which may exacerbate CHF. May be used as monotherapy or in combination with metformin, insulin, sulfonylureas. Ideal use: obese, hyperinsulinemic patient, renal dysfunction.
Meglitinides *Examples:* repaglinide (Prandin®) nateglinide (Starlix®)	Potentiates insulin secretion from pancreas (short-acting secretagogue)	Pre-prandial dosing only. Should not be used with sulfonylureas. Use with caution in hepatic patients and the elderly. May be used as monotherapy or with metformin. Ideal use: patients with post-prandial glucose elevation, renal dysfunction patients.

AGENT	ACTION	COMMENTS
Alpha glucosidase inhibitors *Examples:* Miglitol (Glyset®) Acarbose (Precose®)	Delay absorption of carbohydrates following a meal resulting in a smaller rise in glucose elevation. These agents do NOT enhance action of insulin	Contraindicated in patients with inflammatory bowel disorders; If hypoglycemia results, do not administer sucrose (absorption will be delayed) instead, administer dextrose. Flatulence and diarrhea are common side effects. May be used as monotherapy or with a sulfonylurea. Ideal patient: mild clinical presentation; post-prandial hyperglycemia.
Combination agents: *Examples:* Avandia® plus metformin (Avandamet®) metformin plus glipizide (Metaglip®) glyburide plus metformin (Glucovance®) Others		

- Insulin
  - ◊ Used if oral therapy fails
  - ◊ Initial therapy is usually *BIDS*: *B*edtime *I*nsulin, *D*aytime *S*ulfonylurea
  - ◊ Usually begins at 0.1 to 0.2 u/kg of NPH at night
  - ◊ Eventually insulin may be added during the day

Type II Diabetes Mellitus by Injection		
2 Dose Regimen (usually inadequate to maintain normal glycemic control) Calculate total daily requirements as above then 2/3 in am, 1/3 in pm		
AM	1:2 ratio regular/rapid acting for NPH/Lente	
PM	1:1 ratio regular/rapid acting to NPA/Lente	
3 Dose Regimen		
	NPH/Lente	Regular/Rapid Acting
AM	20-30%	25%
PM		25%
HS	20-30%	
Glargine OR regular/rapid acting		
AM		20-30%
PM		20-30%
HS	50%	
4 Dose Regimen		
	NPH/Lente	Regular/Rapid Acting
Breakfast		√
Lunch		√
Dinner		√
Bedtime	√√	
√ = based on amount enter √√ = basal rate		

- Antihypertensive treatment for blood pressure >130/80 mm Hg, preferably with ACE inhibitors
- Early aggressive therapy for hyperlipidemia-statins preferred

PREGNANCY/LACTATION CONSIDERATIONS

- Goal is fasting glucose from 60-105 mg/dL and postprandial level <120 mg/dL
- Universal screening at 24 to 28 weeks gestation for detection of gestational diabetes. If glucose >140 mg/dL one hour

after 50 grams oral glucose load, 3-hour GTT is recommended.

- Initial management is dietary: well-balanced meals with decreased intake of concentrated sweets
- Refer to registered dietitian and diabetes educator
- Addition of insulin if glucose >105 mg/dL fasting or 120 mg/dL 2 hours postprandial
- Self-monitoring of glucose four times a day or more
- Women with gestational diabetes have an increased risk of developing Type II diabetes mellitus later, thus follow-up is warranted
- Increased risk of maternal and fetal complications:
  - ◊ Pregnancy accelerates development of retinopathy and pregnancy-induced hypertension
  - ◊ Increased risk of spontaneous abortion, stillbirth, and congenital anomalies
  - ◊ Increased risk of macrosomia resulting in shoulder dystocia
- 28 weeks: maternal assessment of fetal activity should begin, with daily kick counts
- 32 weeks: twice weekly nonstress testing
- Breastfeeding is encouraged as it helps increase HDL

CONSULTATION/REFERRAL

- Endocrinologist
- Registered dietitian
- Diabetic educator
- Ophthalmologist
- Early referral to foot specialist when needed

FOLLOW-UP

- Success is measured by glycemic control and avoidance of tissue organ damage
- Annual total urinary protein once microalbuminuria present; then total urinary protein
- Annual lipid profile
- Annual serum creatinine
- Annual ECG
- Thyroid function tests if indicated
- If treated with diet, fasting glucose $\leq$ 126 mg/dL
- If treated with medication, hemoglobin A_1C every 3 months; goal is < 6.5%
- Annual dilated eye and visual examination at time of diagnosis, then annually, or if complaints of visual problems
- Foot inspection at each visit
- Education at each visit

EXPECTED COURSE

- Dependent on glucose control
- Usually complications develop 10-15 years after onset but can present earlier, if undetected for years before diagnosis

POSSIBLE COMPLICATIONS

- Nephropathy, renal failure
- Peripheral neuropathy
- Retinopathy
- Cardiovascular and peripheral vascular disease
- Glaucoma, cataracts, blindness
- Skin ulcerations, gangrene of lower extremities; limb amputations
- Charcot foot

HYPOGLYCEMIA

DESCRIPTION

Excessive secretion of epinephrine along with dysfunction of the central nervous system as a reaction to insufficient plasma glucose

ETIOLOGY

- Reactive
  - ◊ Alimentary hyperinsulinism due to gastrectomy, gastrojejunostomy, pyloroplasty, or vagotomy

- ◊ Ingestion of fructose or galactose by a child with fructose intolerance or galactosemia
- ◊ Leucine sensitivity in infants
- Idiopathic
- Insulinoma
- Imbalance between production of glucose by the liver and its utilization in peripheral tissue
- Post-GI surgery associated with dumping syndrome

INCIDENCE

- Most prevalent in older adults

RISK FACTORS

- Hormone deficiencies
- Enzyme defects
- Severe malnutrition with muscle wasting and fat depletion
- Third trimester of pregnancy
- Liver disease
- Alcoholism
- Salicylates
- Insulinoma (Islet cell tumor)
- Exogenous insulin, sulfonylurea, quinine, disopyramide, pentamidine
- Endotoxic shock

ASSESSMENT FINDINGS

CNS dysfunction (if glucose dropping gradually):

- Headache
- Visual disturbance
- Confusion, elderly with recurrent hypoglycemia may have dementia-like presentation
- Hunger
- Clumsiness
- Convulsions
- Loss of consciousness

Excessive epinephrine secretion (if sudden decrease in glucose):

- Diaphoresis
- Tremor
- Nervousness
- Dizziness
- Anxiety

DIFFERENTIAL DIAGNOSIS

- CNS disorders
- Emotional disorders
- Factitious disease: self-induction by injection of insulin or ingestion of oral hypoglycemic agents

DIAGNOSTIC STUDIES

- Best to perform when patient is symptomatic: simultaneous plasma glucose, plasma insulin, and C peptide levels
- Diagnostic is:
  - ◊ Plasma insulin level: elevated (values vary in laboratories)
  - ◊ C peptide level: increased
  - ◊ Plasma glucose: decreased
  - ◊ Reversal of symptoms with ingestion of glucose
- Cortisol level
- Drug assay, including sulfonylurea and alcohol
- Liver function studies
- CT scan or abdominal ultrasound to assess for tumors
- If postprandial hypoglycemia suspected, 5-hour oral glucose tolerance test

NONPHARMACOLOGIC MANAGEMENT

- Avoidance of fasting is all that is usually required
- Oral carbohydrate for alert patient (oral fruit juice)
- Surgery is treatment of choice for insulinoma
- High protein diet with restricted carbohydrates, frequent small meals
- Avoid causative agents
- Counseling if hypoglycemia is self-induced

PHARMACOLOGIC MANAGEMENT

- If there is confusion or coma: initially, intravenous bolus of 25-50 gram glucose as 50% concentrate, followed by constant glucose infusion, until able to eat a meal
- GlucaGen IM
- Hormone replacement in pituitary or adrenal insufficiency

CONSULTATION/REFERRAL

- Hormone deficiencies: endocrinologist
- Insulinoma: endocrinologist to confirm diagnosis, then surgeon

FOLLOW-UP

- Variable, dependent on etiology and treatment

EXPECTED COURSE

- With recognition of cause and appropriate treatment, prognosis is favorable

POSSIBLE COMPLICATIONS

- Risk associated with surgery for insulinoma
- Tissue damage or death if glucose deficit is prolonged

HYPERTHYROIDISM
(Thyrotoxicosis)

DESCRIPTION

Clinical state that results when the body's tissues are exposed to an increased level of circulating thyroid hormone. Manifestations are related to excessive metabolic activities in body tissues.

ETIOLOGY

- Most common cause is Graves' disease, an autoimmune disorder with a genetic component.
- Other causes include thyroid nodules, ingestion of thyroid hormones, pituitary gland dysfunction, and thyroiditis (Hashimoto's).

INCIDENCE

- Common, affects 0.1% of women and 0.3% of men
- Typical patient is aged mid-20-40 years old at diagnosis

RISK FACTORS

- Family history of thyroid disease
- Thyroid replacement hormone ingestion
- Other autoimmune disorders

ASSESSMENT FINDINGS

- Weight loss incongruent with daily dietary intake and exercise level
- Most common symptoms are nervousness, dyspnea, intolerance to heat and perspiring, palpitations and tachycardia
- Thyroid enlargement (2 to 6 times) may be accompanied by vascular thrill or bruit
- Atrial fibrillation, systolic murmur, cardiac failure (common presentation in the elderly)
- Fatigue, weakness, diminished quadriceps strength
- Bowel movements frequent and soft
- Skin changes, warm, moist, hyperpigmented, smooth, flushes easily
- Hair and nails soft and thin
- Labile emotions
- Tremors, rapid deep tendon reflexes
- Oligomenorrhea
- Vision changes, blurred, double, photophobia, tearing
- Exophthalmos, eyelid retraction and lag
- Accelerated growth in children

DIFFERENTIAL DIAGNOSIS

- Anxiety
- Arrhythmias
- Diabetes
- Malignancy
- Menopause
- Normal aging
- Pheochromocytoma
- Pregnancy

DIAGNOSTIC STUDIES

- T_3 - ↑
- T_4 - ↑
- Free thyroxine index - ↑
- TSH: low or not detectable

PREVENTION

- Periodically monitor TSH and T_4 of patient on thyroid replacement therapy

NONPHARMACOLOGIC MANAGEMENT

- Surgery: thyroidectomy, although not the preferred method of treatment, may be offered if remission does not occur after use of antithyroid drugs; hypothyroidism is frequent long-term outcome

PHARMACOLOGIC MANAGEMENT

Antithyroid drugs *Examples:* propylthiouracil (PTU) methimazole (MMI, Tapazole®)	Block synthesis of thyroid hormone Expect improvement in 2 to 3 weeks and euthyroid state in 4 to 6 weeks Remission may occur Remain on drug 1 to 2 years, then gradual trial withdrawal *Most children are treated with antithyroid drugs, neonates for 2 to 3 months*
Radioactive Iodine (RAI)	Taken orally in 1 or 2 doses, causes atrophy of thyroid gland Results in permanent hypothyroidism
Supportive management	Propranolol may be given initially to relieve catecholamine effects (e.g., tachycardia, tremors, lid lag, and anxiety) Discontinue once antithyroid drugs take effect Multivitamin supplements with calcium and vitamin D (thyrotoxicosis is a causative factor in development of osteoporosis) Anticoagulation with warfarin (Coumadin®) for atrial fibrillation

PREGNANCY/LACTATION CONSIDERATIONS

- PTU is used at lowest dose that keeps serum T_4 at upper limit of normal
- PTU does not cross the placenta
- Pregnancy is an absolute contraindication to the use of RAI

CONSULTATION/REFERRAL

- Surgeon if thyroidectomy is chosen as form of management
- Emergency department for thyroid storm, an extreme form of hyperthyroidism
- Endocrinologist for management during pregnancy and in children
- Ophthalmologist for patient with infiltrative ophthalmopathy

FOLLOW-UP

- Long term evaluation for recurrence of hyperthyroidism or development of hypothyroidism is necessary, regardless of treatment choice
- TSH and T_4 every 4 weeks until euthyroid, then every 3 to 6 months on antithyroid drugs
- TSH at 6 weeks, 12 weeks, 6 months, and annually if RIA therapy used
- Baseline CBC to be repeated if agranulocytosis is suspected
- Liver function tests (LFT): rare hepatic abnormality effect of antithyroid drugs

EXPECTED COURSE

- With antithyroid drug therapy there is a 25-90% chance of permanent remission
- With RIA or surgery, great majority of patients eventually become hypothyroid

POSSIBLE COMPLICATIONS

- An episode of major depression commonly follows treatment of hyperthyroidism, possibly due to unmasking of depression, or damaged relationships due to behavior changes or illness' effect on neurotransmitters

- Thyroid storm: an extreme form of hyperthyroidism with severe anxiety, fever, nausea, vomiting, abdominal pain and cardiac failure
- Visual disturbance due to ophthalmopathy
- Myxedema
- Cardiac failure in patients with underlying heart disease

HYPOTHYROIDISM

DESCRIPTION

Clinical state that results from either a reduction in the amount of circulating free thyroid hormone, or from resistance to the action of thyroid hormone

ETIOLOGY

- Majority of cases are due to primary thyroid gland failure from autoimmune destruction (Hashimoto's thyroiditis)
- Ablative therapy for hyperthyroidism
- Other causes are congenital, and secondary or tertiary, due to pituitary or hypothalamic disease

INCIDENCE

- Predominant age is >40 years
- Females > Males

RISK FACTORS

- Elderly
- Family history
- Postpartum
- Pituitary disease
- Hypothalamic disease
- Autoimmune diseases
- Treatment of hyperthyroidism

ASSESSMENT FINDINGS

- Severity of clinical symptoms range from asymptomatic to myxedema coma
- Lethargy, delayed deep tendon reflexes
- Mild weight gain, swelling of hands and feet, macroglossia, periorbital edema
- Intolerance to cold
- Constipation
- Menstrual irregularities, decreased libido, infertility
- Memory loss, dull facial expression, depression
- Muscle cramps, arthralgias, paresthesias
- Coarse dry skin, hair loss from body and scalp, brittle nails
- Bradycardia, enlarged heart
- Reduced systolic and increased diastolic blood pressure
- Anemia
- Hyponatremia
- Atrophic or enlarged thyroid

DIFFERENTIAL DIAGNOSIS

- Depression
- Dementia
- Chronic heart failure
- Kidney failure

DIAGNOSTIC STUDIES

- Serum TSH is increased in thyroprivic and goitrous hypothyroidism (often > 20 μu/ml); normal or undetectable in pituitary or hypothalamic hypothyroidism
- T_3 and T_4 decreased
- Free T_4 index ↓ = T_3 resin uptake x total serum T_4

PREVENTION

- Periodic monitoring of thyroid hormone levels for those patients being treated for hyperthyroidism
- Newborn screening with TSH and/or T_4 at 2-6 days of age

NONPHARMACOLOGIC MANAGEMENT

- Educate parents that children may manifest behavioral problems at the beginning of treatment
- Assess growth and development in children

- High fiber diet to prevent constipation
- Diet for weight loss/fat reduction if obese
- Educate regarding need for lifelong compliance with thyroid replacement medication and need to report signs of toxicity, infection, or cardiac symptoms
- Subclinical hypothyroidism: slightly elevated TSH and nonspecific symptoms; reasonable to treat and periodically monitor TSH
- Congenital hypothyroidism: educate parents about etiology, importance of treatment with L-thyroxine to prevent mental retardation, and need for follow-up care
- Annual lipid level assessment

PHARMACOLOGIC MANAGEMENT

- L-thyroxine daily, beginning at lower dose in elderly or in presence of cardiac disease

PREGNANCY/LACTATION CONSIDERATIONS

- L-thyroxine dose requirements rise by 25-50% beginning in first trimester
- TSH should be assessed at 8 weeks gestation and at 20 to 24 weeks gestation
- Reduce L-thyroxine to prepregnancy dose immediately after delivery
- Breastfeeding is not a contraindication to L-thyroxine therapy

CONSULTATION/REFERRAL

- Refer to pediatric endocrinologist: congenital hypothyroidism
- Refer to physician: myxedema coma

FOLLOW-UP

- Measure TSH after patient has been on L-thyroxine for 6 weeks, and every 6-8 weeks until within normal limits, then annually, unless symptomatic
- In secondary or tertiary hypothyroidism, monitor T_4 rather than TSH
- Examine periodically for signs of thyrotoxicity (e.g., tremor or tachycardia)
- Congenital hypothyroidism: monitor T_4 and TSH periodically
- Acquired hypothyroidism: monitor initial response to medication at 4 to 6 weeks with TSH and by symptoms, then monitor TSH annually

EXPECTED COURSE

- Improvement is expected 2 weeks after initiation of medication
- Signs and symptoms should resolve in 3 to 6 months
- Lifelong therapy is needed

POSSIBLE COMPLICATIONS

- Myxedema coma: life-threatening, severe hypothyroidism; may require intravenous L-thyroxine and cardiorespiratory assistance
- Thyrotoxicity
- Treatment induced CHF in elderly or patient with CAD
- Bone demineralization due to over-treatment over a long period
- Mental retardation associated with congenital hypothyroidism if not treated
- Growth and development delays in children

THYROID NODULE

DESCRIPTION

Thyroid mass that is discrete and functions without influence from the pituitary gland

ETIOLOGY

- Unknown

INCIDENCE

- Most common in elderly and women
- Uncommon in children, but if present, >60% are malignant
- <5% are malignant in adults
- Common in iodine deficient areas

RISK FACTORS

- Iodine deficiency
- Exposure to ionizing radiation: history of irradiation to head, neck, or chest
- Family history

ASSESSMENT FINDINGS

- Both benign and malignant nodules often asymptomatic
- May have symptoms of either hypothyroidism or hyperthyroidism
- Fixed, firm, nontender, large nodules not accompanied by symptoms of thyroid dysfunction more likely to be malignant
- Multiple nodules occur in Hashimoto's thyroiditis
- Hoarseness, dysphagia
- Cervical lymphadenopathy

DIFFERENTIAL DIAGNOSIS

- Benign nodules
- Malignant nodules
- Cysts

DIAGNOSTIC STUDIES

- Thyroid function tests: serum thyroid stimulating hormone (TSH) and free-thyroxine index (FTI) often normal
  If thyrotoxic, malignancy is less likely
- Thyroid imaging: radionuclide scan should be performed on all nonpregnant patients who present with a thyroid nodule. 90% of "cold" (decreased amount of radionuclide uptake) nodules are not malignant
- High resolution ultrasound helpful in distinguishing cysts from solid lesions
- Fine needle aspiration biopsy: best method to determine malignancy

NONPHARMACOLOGIC MANAGEMENT

- Adequate iodine intake
- Surgery if needle biopsy indicates thyroid cancer

PHARMACOLOGIC MANAGEMENT

- Follow guidelines for hypothyroidism or hyperthyroidism if thyroid function affected

PREGNANCY/LACTATION CONSIDERATIONS

- Avoid radionuclide scan

CONSULTATION/REFERRAL

- Endocrinologist if unresponsive to treatment
- Surgeon for malignant or disfiguring nodules

FOLLOW-UP

- Annual evaluation of benign nodules for size and thyroid function if euthyroid
- Follow guidelines for hypothyroid and hyperthyroid if thyroid function is abnormal
- Malignant nodules will require thyroid replacement postoperatively to suppress serum TSH level; thyroid scan and chest x-ray at 6 months, then annually thereafter

EXPECTED COURSE

- Malignant nodules: good survival rate, require annual evaluation
- Benign nodules require long-term management of thyroid dysfunction

POSSIBLE COMPLICATIONS

- Recurrence of tumor
- Complications of hyperthyroidism or hypothyroidism or pharmacologic therapy

CUSHING'S SYNDROME

DESCRIPTION

Hyperfunctioning of the adrenal cortex resulting in excessive exposure of the tissues to cortisol and/or other corticosteroids

ETIOLOGY

- The most common cause is exogenous use of glucocorticoids
- ACTH-dependent etiologies: pituitary adenoma, non pituitary ACTH-producing tumors
- ACTH-independent etiology: autonomous cortisol production from adrenal tissue

INCIDENCE

- Females > males 3:1
- Rare in infancy and childhood

RISK FACTORS

- Long term use of corticosteroids
- Adrenal tumor
- Pituitary tumor

ASSESSMENT FINDINGS

- Truncal obesity, dorsal cervical fat pad ("buffalo hump")
- Amenorrhea, clitoral hypertrophy
- Central weight gain
- Edema, moon face
- Abdominal striae, thin skin with poor wound healing, ecchymosis
- Hirsutism
- Hypertension
- Weakness and fatigue
- Glucosuria, polyuria, polydipsia
- Osteoporosis
- Personality changes, mood changes
- Slow growth in children
- Hyperpigmentation

DIFFERENTIAL DIAGNOSIS

- Obesity
- Diabetes mellitus
- Syndrome X
- Alcoholism
- Depression

DIAGNOSTIC STUDIES

- Initial screening: overnight dexamethasone suppression test
- Definitive diagnosis: failure to suppress urinary cortisol to <30 μg/dL or plasma cortisol to <5 μg/dL or 17-hydroxysteroid excretion to <3 mg/dL after a low dose dexamethasone suppression test (0.5 mg dexamethasone every 6 hours for 48 hours)
- 24 hour urinary cortisol
- AM and PM plasma cortisol
- CT abdomen to visualize adrenals
- Pituitary MRI with gadolinium contrast to detect pituitary source
- X-ray of lumbar spine: osteoporosis common

PREVENTION

- Limit corticosteroid use

NONPHARMACOLOGIC MANAGEMENT

- Surgery is treatment of choice if tumor is present
- High protein diet, potassium supplements
- Educate: early treatment of infection, daily weights, emotional lability
- Reduce pituitary ACTH production:
    - ◊ Transsphenoidal resection
    - ◊ Radiation
- Reduce adrenocortical cortisol secretion:
    - ◊ Bilateral adrenalectomy

PHARMACOLOGIC MANAGEMENT

- Medical therapy alone is not usually appropriate
- Medication should be prescribed and managed by an endocrinologist:
    - ◊ Ketoconazole (Nizoral®) to suppress cortisol production

CONSULTATION/REFERRAL

- Endocrinologist
- Surgeon

FOLLOW-UP

- Replacement glucocorticoid therapy may be needed for up to 1 year after surgery (lifelong if bilateral adrenalectomy is performed)
- Stress need for gradual glucocorticoid withdrawal
- Patient should wear identification bracelet stating need for glucocorticoid replacement
- Patients exhibiting signs of recurrence should undergo measurement of urine free cortisol

EXPECTED COURSE

- Normal hypothalamic-pituitary-adrenal activity is expected within 3 to 24 months of surgery if at least one adrenal gland remains.
- Recurrence occurs in a minority of patients
- If surgery is not feasible, lifelong medical therapy is required
- Pregnancy can cause exacerbation

POSSIBLE COMPLICATIONS

- Osteoporosis
- Metastasis of malignant tumors

ADDISON DISEASE

DESCRIPTION

Hypofunction of the adrenal gland which results in inadequate release of glucocorticoids and mineralocorticoids. Also called hypoadrenocorticism

ETIOLOGY

- 80% of cases due to autoimmune process which causes adrenal destruction
- AIDS is an increasing etiological factor
- Tuberculosis
- Acute withdrawal after long-term corticosteroid therapy

INCIDENCE

- All ages affected; predominantly 30-50 year olds
- Females > Males

RISK FACTORS

- Family history of adrenal insufficiency
- CMV
- AIDS
- Prolonged use of steroids followed by a stressor like infection, trauma, or surgery
- Medications which potentiate adrenal failure:
  - ◊ Rifampin
  - ◊ Phenytoin (Dilantin®)
  - ◊ Ketoconazole (Nizoral®)
  - ◊ Opiates
- Other immune disorders

ASSESSMENT FINDINGS

- Slowly progressive
- Fatigue, weakness, anorexia, nausea and vomiting, weight loss, amenorrhea
- Hypotension
- Depression
- Cutaneous and mucosal pigmentation (e.g., tanning, freckles, blue-black areolas and mucous membranes)
- Cold intolerance

DIAGNOSTIC STUDIES

- Early stages of disease:
  - ◊ Subnormal rise in cortisol levels after adrenal stimulation with ACTH
- Later stages:
  - ◊ Serum sodium, chloride, and bicarbonate: decreased
  - ◊ Serum potassium: increased
  - ◊ ECG: nonspecific ST segment changes

- ◊ EEG: generalized slowing
- ◊ Serum calcium: increased
- ◊ BUN, creatinine: increased
- ◊ CBC: normocytic anemia, lymphocytosis, eosinophilia
- ◊ Low cortisol levels 8-9 AM
- Abdominal CT scan: small adrenals
- Chest x-ray: decreased heart size

DIFFERENTIAL DIAGNOSIS

- Hyperparathyroidism
- Secondary or tertiary adrenocortical insufficiency
- Depression
- Myopathies
- Heavy metal poisoning
- Anemia

NONPHARMACOLOGIC MANAGEMENT

- Correct precipitating factors
- Diet with adequate sodium, chloride, and potassium replacement

PHARMACOLOGIC MANAGEMENT

- Synthetic hydro cortisol and cortisone
- Intravenous NaCl to treat dehydration
- 5 S's: salt, sugar, steroids, support, search for precipitating illness

CONSULTATION/REFERRAL

- Endocrinologist

FOLLOW-UP

- Periodic assessment of:
  - ◊ Blood pressure
  - ◊ Electrolytes/blood sugar
  - ◊ Strength
  - ◊ Appetite
  - ◊ Plasma renin
  - ◊ Heart size

EXPECTED COURSE

- Excellent prognosis
- Requires lifelong replacement therapy with monitoring for adequacy and avoidance of overdose
- 100% lethal without treatment

POSSIBLE COMPLICATIONS

- Acute adrenal crisis (more likely in elderly)
- Psychosis
- Hyperkalemia
- Hyperpyrexia
- Osteoporosis
- Complications of steroid therapy

GYNECOMASTIA

DESCRIPTION

Occurrence of mammary tissue hypertrophy in males causing enlargement of one or both breasts

ETIOLOGY

- Estrogen-androgen imbalance related to effects of puberty, aging, or drugs
- In newborns, from stimulation by maternal hormones
- Estrogen secreting tumor

INCIDENCE

- Occurs in 1/3 of normal males during early puberty
- Occurs in 40-60% of men over age 50 years

RISK FACTORS

- Adrenal hyperplasia
- Klinefelter's syndrome
- Bronchogenic carcinoma
- Drugs:
  - ◊ Tricyclic antidepressants, phenothiazine, diazepam
  - ◊ Ketoconazole (Nizoral®)
  - ◊ Nonsteroidal agents

- ◊ Spironolactone, methyldopa, digitalis
- ◊ Phenytoin (Dilantin®)
- ◊ Cimetidine (Tagamet®)

- Heavy marijuana smoking
- Alcoholism
- Carcinoma of the liver
- Family history
- Obesity
- Thyroid disease: hypo/hyperthyroidism

ASSESSMENT FINDINGS

- Firm, solitary irregular lumps of fat may be attached to underlying skin
- May be unilateral, usually bilateral
- Often tender
- No nipple retraction, increase in pigmentation, ulceration, or nipple discharge
- Testicular size and mass normal considering Tanner stage
- No thyromegaly, tachycardia, or diaphoresis
- No axillary lymphadenopathy
- No abdominal organomegaly or masses

DIFFERENTIAL DIAGNOSIS

- Pseudogynecomastia: fatty tissue around breast, no glandular tissue
- Breast cancer
- Obesity
- Cyst
- Neurofibroma

DIAGNOSTIC STUDIES

- None needed unless accompanied by abnormalities which demand further evaluation
- Mammography and/or sonography helpful in differentiating physiological from pathological
- Chest x-ray

PREVENTION

- Education about avoidance of precipitating drugs
- Include breast examination for adolescent males; discuss in matter of fact manner; boys may not raise questions independently

MANAGEMENT

- Reassure adolescents of transient nature (< 2 years duration)
- Reassure postpubertal males of negative evaluation and lack of pathology
- Seek exogenous source of estrogen if there is increased nipple pigmentation

CONSULTATION/REFERRAL

- Physician/endocrinologist if accompanied by abnormal exam findings or if persists >2 years, or if >4 cm in diameter
- Surgeon for abnormal findings or for aesthetic reasons

FOLLOW-UP

- Evaluate pubertal boys every 3-6 months

EXPECTED COURSE

- Pubertal males: should normalize in 2 years or less

POSSIBLE COMPLICATIONS

- Negative impact on self-image or lifestyle may justify surgical removal

PRECOCIOUS PUBERTY

DESCRIPTION

Premature physical maturation resulting in the appearance of secondary sexual characteristics, accelerated growth, and onset of puberty (before age 7 years in Caucasian girls, 6 years in African American girls, and before age 9 years in boys). Normal mean age of sexual development in girls is 10 to 13 years, and in boys 11 to 16 years.

ETIOLOGY

- 90% of girls have no underlying pathology
- Boys are often found to have central nervous system disorders (e.g., hamartomas, astrocytomas, or gliomas)
- 50% of male cases are idiopathic
- Exogenous source of estrogen (e.g., child's ingestion of mother's oral contraceptives)

INCIDENCE

- Females > Males
- Some cases are familial
- 5000-6000 children in U.S. affected

RISK FACTORS

- CNS trauma or inflammation
- Hypothalamic hamartoma
- CNS tumors and space-occupying lesions
- Congenital adrenal hyperplasia
- Gonadal tumors
- Hypothyroidism

ASSESSMENT FINDINGS

- Progression of sexual development is normal but early development of:
  - ◊ Pubic hair
  - ◊ Axillary hair
  - ◊ Breasts
  - ◊ Testicular enlargement
  - ◊ Rapid onset acne
  - ◊ Body odor
- Sperm and ova are mature resulting in fertility
- Advanced bone age
- Advanced linear growth: child is initially tall for age, then epiphyses close, resulting in eventual short stature
- Increased appetite
- Emotional lability
- Genital maturation
- Leukorrhea
- Vaginal bleeding, menarche

DIFFERENTIAL DIAGNOSIS

- Adrenarche: presence of pubic hair, typically in girls aged 5-8 years of age
- Premature thelarche: isolated precocious development of breast tissue
- Pseudoprecocious puberty due to testicular or ovarian tumor
- Premature pubarche: isolated appearance of pubic hair

DIAGNOSTIC STUDIES

- Tanner staging
- Chart growth
- Luteinizing hormone (LH) and follicle stimulating hormone (FSH): present (detectable) in precocious puberty
- Blood testosterone level (boys): elevated
- Blood estradiol level (girls): may be low in early stages, then elevated
- Dehydroepiandrosterone sulfate (DHEA-S): elevated
- TSH to rule out hypothyroidism as etiology
- X-ray of hand and wrist to determine bone age
- Skeletal age: advanced osseous maturation
- MRI, CT, pelvic ultrasound, testicular ultrasound to rule out tumors or cysts of ovaries, testicles, or adrenals: enlarged ovaries and uterus and enlarged pituitary gland in precocious puberty

NONPHARMACOLOGIC MANAGEMENT

- Educate:
  - ◊ Greater risk for sexual abuse
  - ◊ Safe storage of oral contraceptives
  - ◊ Effect on peer relationships, body image and sexuality

PHARMACOLOGIC MANAGEMENT

- Administration of gonadotropin-releasing hormone, in consultation with pediatric endocrinologist
  - ◊ Leuprolide acetate for depot suspension (Lupron Depot-PED®) (intramuscular)
  - ◊ Histrelin acetate (Supprelin®) (subcutaneous)
  - ◊ Nafarelin acetate (Synarel®) (subcutaneous or intranasal)
  - ◊ Medroxyprogesterone acetate (Depo-Provera®)

CONSULTATION/REFERRAL

- Referral to pediatric endocrinologist for elimination of cause, or if idiopathic, for administration of gonadotropin-releasing hormone
- Early referral is important to avoid early epiphyseal closure and short stature
- Early referral is also important, especially for boys, because they are more likely to have CNS or other tumors

FOLLOW-UP

- Evaluate every 3 to 6 months
- Drug therapy is discontinued once adequate height is achieved
- Mother's menstrual history is considered when deciding when to let menstruation commence

EXPECTED COURSE

- Sex hormone levels remain suppressed as long as therapy is continued
- Once therapy is discontinued, puberty resumes. Menarche and ovulation appear within a few months.
- Drug therapy does not reverse changes that have already occurred:
    - ◊ Breast size will not be reduced
    - ◊ Height will not diminish

POSSIBLE COMPLICATIONS

- Sexual abuse, pregnancy
- Social and psychological ramifications
- Short stature

References

American Diabetes Association. (2002). Report of the expert committee on the diagnosis and classification of diabetes mellitus. [Electronic version]. *Diabetes Care 25,* S5-S20.

Appel, S. (2005). Calculating insuling resistance in the primary care setting: Why should we worry about insulin levels in euglycemic patients. *Journal of the American Academy of Nurse Practitioners, 17(8),* 331-336.

Aring, A.M., Jones, D.E., & Falko, J.M. Yates, J. (2005). Evaluation and Prevention of diabetic neuropathy. *American Family Physician, 71,* 2123-2128.

Behrman, R.E., Kliegman, R.M., Arvin, A.M., & Nelson, W.E. (Eds.). (1996). *Nelson textbook of pediatrics* (15th ed.). Philadelphia: Saunders.

Bickley, L.S., & Szilagyi, P.G. (2003). *Bates' guide to physical examination and history taking* (8th ed.). Philadelphia: Lippincott Williams & Wilkins.

Bradshaw, K. (1997). Diagnosing and treating precocious puberty. *Hospital Medicine, 33*(9), 40-49.

Branch, W.T. (2003). *Office practice of medicine* (4th ed.). Philadelphia: Saunders.

Burns, C.E., Brady, M.A., Blosser, C., Starr, N.B., & Dunn, A.M. (2004). *Pediatric primary care: A handbook for nurse practitioners* (3rd ed.). Philadelphia: W.B. Saunders.

Dambro, M.R. (2005). *Griffith's 5 minute clinical consult.* Philadelphia: Lippincott Williams & Wilkins.

Desai, S.P. (2004). *Clinician's guide to laboratory diagnosis* (3rd ed.). Hudson, OH:Lexi-Comp.

Douaihy, K. (2005). Prediabetes and atherosclerosis: What's the connection? *The Nurse Practitioners, 30*(6), 24-35.

Erick, L. (1997). Partners in prevention. *Advance for Nurse Practitioners, 5*(9), 28-33, 72.

Fischbach, F.T., & Dunning, M.B. (2003). *A manual of laboratory & diagnostic tests* (7th ed.). Philadelphia: Lippincott Williams & Wilkins.

Flick, M., & Schumann, L. (1997). Noninsulin-dependent diabetes mellitus. *Journal of the American Academy of Nurse Practitioners, 9*(7), 337-343.

Graber, M.A., & Lanternier, M.L. (Eds.) (2001). *The family practice handbook.* (4th ed.). St. Louis: Mosby.

Greenspan, F.S., & Gardner, D.G. (2003). *Basic and clinical endocrinology* (7th ed.). New York:McGraw-Hill.

Gutowski, C. (1999). Understanding the new pharmacologic therapy for Type II diabetics. *The Nurse Practitioner, 24*(6), 15-25.

Kasper, D.L., Braunwald, E., Fauci, A.S., Hauser, S.L., Longo, D.L., Jameson, J.L., et al. (2004). *Harrison's principles of internal medicine* (16th ed.). New York: McGraw-Hill.

Lecesse, C. (1997). A promising horizon. *Advance for Nurse Practitioners, 5*(10), 60-62.

Mangion, S. (2000). *Physical diagnosis secrets.* Philadelphia: Hanley and Belfus.

Mladenovic, J. (Ed.). (2003). *Primary care secrets.* (3rd Ed.). Philadelphia: Hanley an

Pasuli, K., & McFarland, K. (1997). Management of diabetes in pregnancy. *American Family Physician, 55,* 2731-2738.

Peters, S. (1996). Precocious puberty. *Advance for Nurse Practitioners, 4*(10), 26-29.

Rakel, R.E. (Ed.). (1998). *Essentials of family practice.* (2nd ed.). Philadelphia: WB Saunders.

Seller, R. (2000). *Differential diagnosis of common complaints* (4th ed.). Philadelphia: W.B. Saunders.

Stoner, G.D. (2005). Hyperosmolar hyperglycemic state. *American Family Physician, 71*, 1723-1730.

Schwartz, M.W. (Ed.). (2002). *The 5 minute pediatric consult.* (2nd ed.) Philadelphia: Lippincott Williams & Wilkins.

Thorp, M.L. (2005) Diabetic nephropathy: Common questions. *American Family Physician, 72*, 96-99.

Trachtenbarg, D.E. (2005). Diabetic Ketoacidosis. *American Family Physician, 71*, 1705-1714.

Umeh, L. Wallagen, M., Nicoloff, N. (1999). Identifying diabetic patients at high risk for amputation. *The Nurse Practitioner*, *24*(8), 56-70.

Uphold, C.R., & Graham, M.V. (2003). *Clinical guidelines in family practice.* (4th ed.). Gainesville, FL: Barmarrae Books.

Woeber, K.A. (2000). Update on the management of hyperthyroidism and hypothyroidism. *Archives of Family Medicine*, *9*, 743-747.

Zollo, A.J., Jr (Ed.). (2004). *Medical Secrets*. (4th ed.), St. Louis, MO: Mosby-Year Book.

6

GASTROINTESTINAL DISORDERS

Gastrointestinal Disorders

* *Denotes pediatric diagnosis*

GASTROESOPHAGEAL REFLUX DISEASE
(GERD)

DESCRIPTION

Movement of gastrointestinal contents up the esophagus or larynx facilitated by decreased lower esophageal sphincter (LES) tone

INCIDENCE

- Affects up to 1/3 of Americans at some time in their lives
- Affects 81% of patients 60 years of age or older
- Common in pregnant women

RISK FACTORS

- Factors which may reduce LES tone:
  - ◊ Alcohol
  - ◊ Anticholinergics
  - ◊ Calcium channel blockers
  - ◊ Chocolate, peppermint
  - ◊ Fatty foods
  - ◊ Hormones: estrogen, progesterone, glucagon, secretin
  - ◊ Pregnancy
  - ◊ Meperidine
  - ◊ Nicotine
  - ◊ Theophylline
- Aging
- Zenker's diverticulum
- Irritation of esophageal mucosa by:
  - ◊ NSAIDs
  - ◊ Tetracycline
  - ◊ Quinidine
  - ◊ Caffeine
- Increased gastric acid secretion: acidic foods
- Delay in gastric emptying: fatty foods
- Zollinger-Ellison syndrome
- Obesity
- Diabetes mellitus, diabetic gastroparesis

ASSESSMENT FINDINGS

- Pyrosis (heartburn) is cardinal symptom, burning beneath sternum, typically postprandial and nocturnal
- Regurgitation, ("sour, hot"): 60%
- Chest pain: 33%
- Dysphagia, odynophagia: 15-20%
- Esophageal pain referred to neck, mid-back, and upper abdomen
- Chronic cough
- Chronic sore throat/Hoarseness
- Erosion of teeth by acid
- Ulceration: hemoptysis, hematemesis, fatigue, anemia
- Barrett's esophagitis (small number of patients): replacement of the squamous epithelium of the esophagus by columnar epithelium, which may be further complicated by adenocarcinoma in 2-5% of cases

DIFFERENTIAL DIAGNOSIS

- Cardiac disease
- Esophageal spasm or infection
- Cholelithiasis
- Peptic ulcer disease
- Lower respiratory infection: bronchitis, pneumonia
- Asthma
- Pulmonary edema

DIAGNOSTIC STUDIES

- Patient with one episode of heartburn that responds well to nonpharmacologic and acid suppressant therapy may require no further investigation
- Manometry followed by pH testing: motility test to determine LES and esophageal function
- Esophageal pH testing to detect pathologic reflux
- Endoscopy to observe effects of esophagitis and obtain biopsy for histology

- 50% of symptomatic patients have NERD (nonerosive reflux disease)

NONPHARMACOLOGIC MANAGEMENT

- Education: physical causes of GERD, common aggravating and ameliorating factors, and lifestyle changes to control GERD:
    - ◊ Avoid recumbence until 2 hours after meals
    - ◊ Elevate head of bed, including entire chest
    - ◊ Reduce size of meals and amount of fat, acid, spices, caffeine, and sweets
    - ◊ Smoking cessation
    - ◊ Reduce alcohol consumption
    - ◊ Lose weight if indicated
    - ◊ Avoid stooping, bending after meals and tight fitting garments
- Surgical interventions, crural tightening or fundoplication, reserved for patient with stricture, hemorrhage, Barrett's esophagitis, chronic aspiration or intractable symptoms

PHARMACOLOGIC MANAGEMENT

AGENT	ACTION	COMMENTS
Antacids *Examples:* calcium carbonate (Mylanta®, Tums®) aluminum hydroxide (ALternaGEL®)	Neutralize hydrochloric acid in the stomach to rapidly cause pH to rise	Produces rapid relief of heartburn symptoms. Use with caution in patients with CHF, renal failure, edema, cirrhosis. Decreases absorption of many drugs: tetracyclines, digoxin, benzodiazepines, iron, and many others.
H_2 antagonists *Examples:* cimetidine (Tagamet®) ranitidine (Zantac®) famotidine (Pepcid®) nizatidine (Axid®)	Inhibit gastric acid secretion by inhibiting H_2 receptors of the gastric parietal cells	Cimetidine associated with many drug interactions. Long term therapy may be associated with B_{12} deficiency. May take several days for relief to occur. Allow one hour between H_2 blocker and antacid consumption.
Proton Pump Inhibitors (PPIs) *Examples:* omeprazole (Prilosec®) lansoprazole (Prevacid®) rabeprazole (Aciphex®) esomeprazole (Nexium®) pantoprazole (Protonix ®)	Potently suppress gastric acid secretion by inhibiting the hydrogen/potassium pump in gastric parietal cells	Therapy > 3 years may lead to B_{12} malabsorption. Take at same time each day. Best if taken before a meal when hydrogen/potassium pumps are most active.

CONSULTATION/REFERRAL

- Cardiologist: severe chest pain, radiating pain
- Gastroenterologist:
    - ◊ Dysphagia
    - ◊ Unexplained weight loss
    - ◊ Vomiting
    - ◊ GI bleeding
    - ◊ Anemia
    - ◊ Palpable abdominal mass
    - ◊ Recurrent or refractory symptoms
    - ◊ Long history of alcohol and/or nicotine abuse
    - ◊ Regular NSAID use

FOLLOW-UP

- CBC
- Screen for B12 deficiency after long-term PPI use
- Barrett's esophagitis: endoscopy and biopsy every 1 to 2 years

EXPECTED COURSE

- Most patients respond well to combined nonpharmacologic and pharmacologic therapies, but symptoms return once medication is withdrawn

POSSIBLE COMPLICATIONS

- Ulceration
- Stricture
- Barrett's esophagitis
- High-grade dysplasia
- Esophageal adenocarcinoma
- Aspiration pneumonia

PEPTIC ULCER DISEASE (PUD)

DESCRIPTION

A chronic ulceration involving the stomach or the duodenum.

ETIOLOGY

- *Helicobacter pylori* infection: bacteria attach to gastric epithelial cells and secrete enzymes which break down the mucous layer
- NSAID-related ulcers: NSAID use results in the inhibition of prostaglandin synthesis
- Zollinger-Ellison syndrome: tumors in the walls of the pancreas or intestines secrete high levels of gastrin

INCIDENCE

- Uncommon before puberty; incidence increases with age
- 1-2% of U.S. population
- Duodenal ulcer 4 times more common than gastric ulcer

RISK FACTORS

- NSAID use, especially multiple NSAIDs at high doses
- Concomitant use of NSAIDs and systemic corticosteroids
- Cigarette smoking
- Stress
- Previous ulcer disease
- *H. pylori* infection
- Age >60 years

ASSESSMENT FINDINGS

- Duodenal ulcer:
    - ◊ Burning epigastric pain awakens patient early morning and is relieved by food and antacids
- Gastric ulcer:
    - ◊ Nausea and vomiting
    - ◊ Pain exacerbated by eating
    - ◊ Early satiety
- Acute GI hemorrhage:
    - ◊ Coffee ground emesis
    - ◊ Tarry, black, or bloody stools
- Iron deficiency anemia due to occult blood loss
- Epigastric tenderness
- Perforation: board-like abdomen with rebound tenderness

DIFFERENTIAL DIAGNOSIS

- Gastroesophageal reflux disease (GERD)
- Myocardial infarction, cardiac disease
- Esophageal spasm
- Cholelithiasis
- Lower respiratory infection
- Pancreatitis

DIAGNOSTIC STUDIES

- Endoscopy for direct visualization
- Double contrast barium radiography of the upper gastrointestinal system: ulcer appears as discrete crater
- *H. pylori* serologic antibody measurement
- Urea breath test, biopsy for *H. pylori*
- Serum gastrin: elevated in Zollinger-Ellison syndrome

PREVENTION

- Eradicate *H. pylori*

- Attempt alternative therapeutics to avoid long-term NSAID use
- Use lowest dose of NSAID that is effective
- Concomitant use of NSAID and misoprostol (Cytotec®) or proton pump inhibitor

NONPHARMACOLOGIC MANAGEMENT

- Avoid cigarette smoking, caffeine, and any foods that exacerbate symptoms
- Lifestyle modifications
- Surgery (vagotomy or gastroduodenal anastomosis) reserved for ulcers resistant to medical treatment

PHARMACOLOGIC MANAGEMENT

- Based on etiology

NSAID-related ulcers:
- Misoprostol (Cytotec®) or PPI use along with NSAID: preventive for both duodenal and gastric NSAID-related ulcer complications (e.g., perforation)
- Treat NSAID-related duodenal ulcers for 4-12 weeks with proton pump inhibitor (PPI)
- Discontinue NSAID if possible
- Consider COX-2 inhibitor

H. pylori-related ulcer:
- Quadruple therapy for 2 weeks
  - ◊ 98% eradication rate
  - ◊ PPI plus 2 antibiotics; clarithromycin and amoxicillin (alternatives are tetracycline, metronidazole, rifampin)
- Single antibiotic regimens discouraged

Zollinger-Ellison syndrome:
- Proton pump inhibitors
- Surgical correction if pharmacologic therapy fails
  - ◊ Definitive therapy is removal of gastrinoma
  - ◊ Vagotomy to reduce acid secretion
  - ◊ Parathyroidectomy if Zollinger-Ellison syndrome is associated with multiple endocrine neoplasia type 1 (MEN1)

CONSULTATION/REFERRAL

- Refer patients with Zollinger-Ellison syndrome to gastroenterologist
- Refer patients who have failed treatment to gastroenterologist

FOLLOW-UP

- Monitor clinical response of duodenal ulcer
- Confirmation of eradication of *H. pylori* is by CLO test biopsy, or urea breath test (serology is limited in usefulness due to the persistence of antibodies for years after successful treatment)
- Gastric ulcer: endoscopy with cytology and biopsy to confirm healing at 6 to 12 weeks
- Symptom improvement does not imply absence of malignancy

EXPECTED COURSE

- Recurrence of *H. pylori* infection is rare (<1%), but possible with a positive response to *H. pylori* therapy
- NSAID-related gastric ulcers may require months of therapy
- Zollinger-Ellison syndrome: complete surgical removal of gastrinoma cures 25% of patients

POSSIBLE COMPLICATIONS

- Hemorrhage
- Perforation
- Gastric outlet obstruction

ACUTE GASTROENTERITIS (AGE)

DESCRIPTION

Acute infection causing inflammation of the stomach and intestinal lining resulting in vomiting, diarrhea, and fever

ETIOLOGY

- Infection is by the fecal-oral route, and possibly by the respiratory route

- Pathogens invade the intestinal mucosa, resulting in a decreased area available for fluid absorption
- Viruses, bacteria, and parasites are responsible
- Most infections in healthy hosts in the U.S. are viral
    - ◊ Rotavirus is most common pathogen in age <1 year
    - ◊ Norwalk-like viruses also common
    - ◊ Adenovirus, astrovirus, coxsackievirus, echovirus less common
- Bacterial infections are less common, but usually more severe
    - ◊ *Campylobacter jejuni* most common bacterial pathogen in children
    - ◊ *Salmonella* most common cause of food-borne illness in the U.S.
    - ◊ Other common pathogens: *Shigella, Escherichia coli, Yersinia enterocolitica, Clostridium difficile*
- Parasitic
    - ◊ *Giardia lamblia* most common parasitic agent in U.S.

INCIDENCE

- Common in all ages
- Incidence is decreasing in U.S.

RISK FACTORS

- Improper handwashing and food preparation
- Day care center attendance
- Recent use of antibiotics (*C. difficile* common)
- Lack of sanitation
- Immunocompromised status
- Recent travel to developing countries

ASSESSMENT FINDINGS

- Hyperactive bowel sounds
- Diarrhea (3 or more loose stools in 24 hours)
- Blood in stool
- White cells in the stool (common with *Salmonella, Shigella, Campylobacter*)
- Nausea, vomiting, usually precede diarrhea
- Anorexia
- Fever
- Tenesmus (a strong urge to defecate caused by an anal sphincter spasm)
- Abdominal cramps
- Dehydration
    - ◊ Poor skin turgor
    - ◊ Dry mucous membranes
    - ◊ Flattened or sunken fontanels
    - ◊ Tachycardia, tachypnea
    - ◊ Oliguria
- Lethargy
- Pale skin color

DIFFERENTIAL DIAGNOSIS

- Viral, bacterial, or parasitic infection
- Anatomical abnormalities
- Medication
- Food intolerances
- Appendicitis
- Irritable bowel syndrome
- Fecal impaction

AGENT	ONSET	SIGNS/SYMPTOMS	COMMENTS
S. aureus	30 min to 6 hrs	Nausea, vomiting, cramps, soft stool	Creamy food is common source (egg salad, cream filled pastries), undercooked poultry
Salmonella	6-72 hrs	Nausea, vomiting, cramps, bloody stool, WBCs in stool	Undercooked poultry, red meats Contaminated pets, turtles Reportable
Shigella	Usually 2-4 days	Abdominal pain, fever, watery diarrhea, WBCs in stool	Fecal-oral route; homosexual transmission Reportable
E. coli	10 hrs to 6 days	Cramps, no fever, watery diarrhea	Causative agent of Traveler's diarrhea Contaminated water/food are common sources
Campylobacter	1-7 days	Nausea, vomiting, fever, abdominal pain, watery, bloody diarrhea, WBCs in stool	Causative agent is undercooked poultry Unpasteurized milk, contaminated H_2O
Giardia (Protozoan)	1-4 weeks	Foul smelling stools abdominal pain, flatulence	Spread by fecal-oral route Contaminated H_2O is a common source
C. difficile	Observed after antibiotic usage, commonly fluoroquinolones	Fever, bloody, watery diarrhea, cramps WBCs in stool	Discontinue antibiotics if possible Rehydrate aggressively; tissue culture most sensitive for diagnosis

DIAGNOSTIC STUDIES

- Usually none necessary unless symptoms are severe and last >48 hours
- Stool for WBC: rare scattered leukocytes are normal; may suggest Crohn's disease, ulcerative colitis, ischemic colitis, *Shigella, Salmonella, Campylobacter*
- Stool cultures: Shigella, Salmonella, Campylobacter, E. coli commonly identified
- Blood or mucus present in stool
- Stool for ova and parasites
- Urinalysis, culture, and sensitivity
- In infants and elderly consider assessment for dehydration: BUN, specific gravity, electrolytes

PREVENTION

- Hygiene
- Avoidance of risk factors
- Shigella: culture all symptomatic contacts and treat those with positive stool cultures; report to local health department

NONPHARMACOLOGIC MANAGEMENT

- Correct dehydration, orally if possible
- Rehydrating with soft drinks, gelatin, and apple juice is not advisable due to the high carbohydrate, low electrolyte composition; commercially prepared rehydration products help avoid this problem: Pedialyte®, CeraLyte®, Infalyte®
- Age appropriate diet as soon as possible
- Reintroduce solid foods within 24 hours of onset of diarrhea
- *BRAT* diet no longer recommended because it provides inadequate protein, fat, and calories
- May develop temporary lactose intolerance
- Monitor oral intake, urine output, and bowel movements; count wet diapers

PHARMACOLOGIC MANAGEMENT

Use of antidiarrheal agents is discouraged; the offending agent must be excreted.

Organism	Treatment
S. aureus	Antibiotics not recommended
Salmonella	Antibiotics not recommended because it prolongs carrier state by slowing excretion of organisms. Treatment recommended (Bactrim® or ciprofloxacin) for patients with valvular heart disease, immunocompromised states.
Shigella	Bactrim® bid x 3-5 days If acquired outside US, ciprofloxacin x 10 days
E. coli	Bactrim® bid x 3 days May use ciprofloxacin (Cipro®) in adults
Campylobacter	Erythromycin qid x 5 days, or Cipro® bid x 7 days
Giardia (Protozoan)	Metronidazole TID x 5 days
C. difficile	Metronidazole 3-4 daily x 10-14 days, Questran® for diarrhea

PREGNANCY/LACTATION CONSIDERATIONS

- Antibiotics indicated when there is a bacterial pathogen identified
- Refer if there is dehydration, intractable symptoms, or bloody diarrhea

CONSULTATION/REFERRAL

- Parenteral rehydration for intractable symptoms, extremes in age, or shock
- Neurologic symptoms
- Severe abdominal pain

FOLLOW-UP

- Telephone contact within 3 days

EXPECTED COURSE

- Both viral and bacterial gastroenteritis is usually self-limiting and resolves without medication in 5 days unless patient is at age extremes or immunocompromised
- Salmonella infection: diarrhea may continue for up to 2 weeks

POSSIBLE COMPLICATIONS

- Cardiovascular collapse from dehydration and acidosis
- Colonic perforation/septicemia
- Carrier state

CHOLECYSTITIS

DESCRIPTION

Inflammation of the gallbladder; can be acute or chronic

ETIOLOGY

- Gallstone obstruction of the gallbladder-cystic duct junction results in inflammation (90-95%) and acute pain
- In a small number of cases, gallbladder inflammation occurs without stone formation
- Obstruction of common bile duct can cause jaundice, light colored stools, and biliary colic
- Obstruction of pancreatic duct can produce pancreatitis, pain over the upper abdomen, nausea and vomiting
- Gallbladder sludge

Test	Classic	with Bile Duct Obstruction	with Pancreatitis
CBC	Mild leukocytosis	Leukocytosis	Leukocytosis
Bilirubin	Mild elevation	Elevated	Elevated
Amylase	Normal		Elevated
LFTs	Slightly elevated	Normal	Elevated
ALP	Normal	Elevated	Normal
GGT	Normal	Elevated	Normal

INCIDENCE

- Increases with age and BMI; most common in ages 50 to 70 years
- Females > Males (2:1)
- Very common in Native Americans

RISK FACTORS

- Pregnancy
- Rapid weight loss
- Obesity
- Gallstones
- Surgery or trauma
- Sickle cell anemia
- Parenteral alimentation over prolonged period

ASSESSMENT FINDINGS

- Murphy's sign: inspiratory arrest with deep palpation of right upper quadrant (RUQ) (classic sign)
- RUQ pain, may be unremitting, with or without rebound pain, may radiate to right shoulder or subscapular area
- Nausea and vomiting/anorexia
- Attack follows meal (especially high in fat) by 1-6 hours
- Low grade fever
- Palpable RUQ mass

DIFFERENTIAL DIAGNOSIS

- Peptic ulcer disease
- Cardiac disease
- Pancreatitis
- Hepatitis
- Bowel obstruction
- Appendicitis

DIAGNOSTIC STUDIES

- Ultrasound is most sensitive and specific test to diagnose cholecystitis
- Ultrasound demonstrates presence of gallstones, thickening of wall of gallbladder, fluid, and enlargement
- Endoscopic retrograde cholangiopancreatography (ERCP) used to see biliary and pancreatic ducts to detect common bile duct stones

PREVENTION

- Avoid risk factors
- During parenteral feeding, administer cholestyramine (Questran®) daily

NONPHARMACOLOGIC MANAGEMENT

- Severe attacks: nothing by mouth
- Mild attacks: avoid fatty meals
- Nasogastric tube for persistent nausea or abdominal distention
- Laparoscopic or open cholecystectomy within 72 hours of diagnosis

PHARMACOLOGIC MANAGEMENT

- Prevention of gallstones post bariatric procedures, during rapid weight loss periods or during mild acute attack with functioning gallbladder: ursodeoxycholic acid (Ursodiol®, Actigall®)
- Prevention of stones while patient on TPN: cholecystokinin
- Broad spectrum antibiotics (e.g., third-generation cephalosporin) should be started preoperatively and maintained into immediate postoperative period
- Analgesia
- Antiemetic

CONSULTATION/REFERRAL

- Outpatient if symptoms mild
- Surgeon if biliary colic > 6 hours, toxic appearing, or intractable pain

FOLLOW-UP

- Throughout postoperative period

EXPECTED COURSE

- Stones may recur in bile ducts after cholecystectomy
- Gallstones usually recur in 3 to 6 months if cholecystectomy is not performed

POSSIBLE COMPLICATIONS

- Empyema of the gallbladder: bacterial invasion of the gallbladder

- Emphysematous cholecystitis: infection with a gas-forming bacteria
- Perforation: requires aggressive fluid replacement, antibiotics and emergency surgical exploration
- Cholecystenteric fistula: gallbladder perforates into duodenum or colon; should be treated as a bowel obstruction with fluid replacement, nasogastric suction, and surgical exploration

VIRAL HEPATITIS

DESCRIPTION

Viral infection affecting the liver. Five viral agents with different antigenic properties are known to be responsible, all causing illnesses that are clinically similar, with various degrees of severity. Hepatitis B, C, and D can cause chronic infections.

ETIOLOGY

Hepatitis Type	Etiology	Mode of Transmission
A	HAV	Contaminated food-H_2O, fecal-oral route
B	HBV	Blood borne/body fluids
C	HCV	Blood borne
D	HDV	Body fluids, blood borne
E	HEV	Fecal-oral

Hepatitis D virus (HDV) is transmitted only after infection with HBV.

Hepatitis Type	Incubation Period
A	2-7 weeks
B	6-23 weeks
C	2-26 weeks
D	2-8 weeks
E	2-9 weeks

INCIDENCE

HAV:

- Occurrence increases with age; rare in infants due to maternal antibodies
- More common in temperate climates; occurs most often in late fall and early winter
- 33% of Americans have antibodies

HBV:

- Endemic areas are Alaska, Southeast Asia, Pacific Islands, Africa
- Perinatal transmission to newborns is 80%

HCV:

- Most common cause of both acute and chronic viral hepatitis
- Accounts for 43% of cases of new hepatitis in the U.S.

HDV:

- 5% of those infected with HBV are also infected with HDV

HEV:

- Sporadic incidence in Asia, Africa, and Central America

RISK FACTORS

HAV and HEV:

- Travel to endemic areas
- Ingestion of contaminated food, water, milk, or shellfish
- Poor personal hygiene
- Crowded living conditions
- Lower socioeconomic status

HBV:

- Injecting drug use
- Homosexual activity
- Engaging in sexual activity with multiple partners
- Health care workers
- Renal dialysis patients
- Body piercing
- Tattoo recipients (not likely but possible)
- All adolescents are considered high risk

HCV:

- Low socioeconomic status, homelessness
- Sharing toothbrushes, razors
- Homosexual activity
- HIV positive status increases risk of HCV if exposed

- Injecting drug use
- Tattoos and body piercing
- Transfusions, renal dialysis

HDV:
- Infection with HBV

ASSESSMENT FINDINGS

- Children often asymptomatic
- Vast majority of adults are asymptomatic or minimally symptomatic
- Illness is often more severe in the elderly
- Malaise, fever, jaundice, dark urine are most common symptoms
- Nausea, vomiting, anorexia, abdominal pain (RUQ), liver enlargement
- Clay-colored stools
- Markedly elevated serum alanine aminotransferase (ALT), aspartate aminotransferase (AST)
- Bilirubin, alkaline phosphatase may elevated
- Transient neutropenia and lymphopenia followed by lymphocytosis
- Measure PT, PTT, albumin, glucose, electrolytes (for severe hepatitis)

In all types of hepatitis, ALT levels are higher than AST.

DIFFERENTIAL DIAGNOSIS

Children and adolescents:
- Hemolytic-uremic syndrome
- Reye's syndrome
- Chronic hemolytic diseases
- Wilson's disease
- Cystic fibrosis
- Infectious mononucleosis
- CMV
- Coxsackievirus
- Toxoplasmosis
- Acute cholangitis (infection of the bile duct)
- Drug toxicity and poisonings

Adults:
- All differential diagnoses for adolescents and children
- Hepatic malignancy
- Autoimmune, alcoholic, or ischemic hepatitis
- Acute cholecystitis
- Disseminated sepsis

DIAGNOSTIC STUDIES

Consider testing for co-infection with HDV in sexually active, gay men who have HBV.

Hepatitis Type	Markers of Acute Disease	Markers of Chronic Disease/Infectivity	Markers of Recovery
A	IgM anti-HAV	None	IgG anti-HAV
B	IgM anti-HBc (the core) HBsAg *(can also indicate chronic infection)*	HBsAg, HBeAg *(high infectivity)*	Anti-HBs *(surface antibody)*
C	PCR HCV-RNA *(sensitive within 10 days of exposure)* Anti-HCV *(may be negative early)*	Anti-HCV	Undetectable HCV-RNA
D	Anti-HDV	Total anti-HDV	None
E	IgM anti-HEV	None	None

Hepatitis B Lab Interpretation		
Markers	**Results**	**Interpretation**
HBsAg Anti-HBc Anti-HBs	Negative Negative Negative	No infection No immunity
HBsAg Anti-HBc Anti-HBs	Negative Positive Positive	Immune due to natural infection
HBsAg Anti-HBc Anti-HBs	Negative Negative Positive	Immune due to immunization
HBsAg Anti-HBc IgM anti-HBc Anti-HBs	Positive Positive Positive Negative	Acutely infected
HBsAg Anti-HBc IgM anti-HBc Anti-HBs	Positive Positive Negative Negative	Chronically infected

From: Guidelines for Viral Hepatitis Surveillance and Case Management. (July 14, 2005). Atlanta, GA: Center for Disease Control.

PREVENTION

Hepatitis A
- Sanitation and hygiene
- Hepatitis A vaccine: three-dose vaccine schedule for use in persons over age 2 years who are at risk of contracting hepatitis A
- Exposure: Passive immunization with human gamma globulin (IG) for persons who are immunodeficient, nonimmunized or under immunized

Hepatitis B
- Avoidance of risk behaviors and universal precautions
- Hepatitis B vaccine for all newborns and those at risk
- Exposure: Hepatitis B immunoglobulin (HBIG) along with Hepatitis B vaccine to unimmunized or anti-HBs-negative persons
- Infants born to HBsAg-positive women should receive Hepatitis B vaccine within 12 hours of birth along with HBIG
- Screen all pregnant women for Hepatitis B

Hepatitis C
- Universal precautions
- No immunization available

Hepatitis D
- Universal precautions
- Prevention of HBV with immunization (since HDV cannot be transmitted in the absence of HBV)

Hepatitis E
- Sanitation and hygiene

NONPHARMACOLOGIC MANAGEMENT

- Measurement of PT, PTT, albumin, electrolytes, glucose, and CBC
- Education regarding illness, transmission, and cost and side effects of treatment
- Liver biopsy is done to determine extent of liver involvement (especially HBV, HCV)
- High calorie diet, best tolerated in morning
- Abstain from alcohol
- Avoid large doses of acetaminophen, iron and drugs metabolized by the liver
- Blood precautions for patients with Hepatitis B and C
- Maintain fluid balance

PHARMACOLOGIC MANAGEMENT

General:
- Cholestyramine (Questran®) alleviates pruritus
- Avoid steroids, glucocorticoids

Hepatitis B (chronic):
- No treatment recommended for acute HBV
- Interferon-alpha (IFN-a®)
- Lamivudine (Epivir®)

Hepatitis C:
- Pegylated interferon + ribavirin
- Interferon alfa (for acute episode)
- Pegylated Interferon alfa 2a
- Pegylated Interferon alfa 2b

CONSULTATION/REFERRAL

- Gastroenterologist for Hepatitis B, C, D
- For liver biopsy if disease persists

FOLLOW-UP

- 6 to 12 months after acute illness, measure ALT, AST, bilirubin and globulin levels

- 6 months after acute illness measure HBsAg or HBeAg to determine whether there is chronic infection
- Surveillance for hepatocellular carcinoma

EXPECTED COURSE

HAV:

- Excellent prognosis; once acute infection resolves, expect liver functions to return to normal

HBV:

- Chronic hepatitis develops in 2% of immunocompetent adults
- Chronic hepatitis develops in >90% of infants infected perinatally
- 40% of chronic hepatitis cases result in cirrhosis
- Hepatocellular carcinoma may occur, although this usually happens several decades after primary infection

HCV:

- 95% of acute infections become chronic, some of which progress to cirrhosis and hepatocellular carcinoma

POSSIBLE COMPLICATIONS

- Chronic active infection
- Hepatocellular carcinoma
- Cirrhosis
- Glomerulonephritis
- Fulminant hepatitis and hepatic necrosis
- Pancreatitis

DIVERTICULITIS

DESCRIPTION

Diverticula, outpouchings that can occur along the wall of the large intestine, become infected, with resultant inflammation.

ETIOLOGY

- Aerobic and anaerobic bacteria invade diverticula

INCIDENCE

- Diverticulosis, the presence of diverticula, is common; especially in Western cultures where low fiber diets predominate
- Diverticulitis is uncommon, increases with age
- 2200-3000/100,000 in U.S.

RISK FACTORS

- Low fiber, low residue diet
- Diverticulosis
- Age >50 years

ASSESSMENT FINDINGS

- Abdominal pain (due to tension in the wall of the colon), typically left lower quadrant, with or without palpable mass
- Rebound tenderness, board like rigidity
- Anorexia
- Nausea and vomiting
- Diarrhea, constipation
- Abdominal distention
- Fever

DIFFERENTIAL DIAGNOSIS

- Gynecologic disorders
- Urologic disorders
- Appendicitis
- Ulcerative colitis
- Lactose intolerance
- Crohn's disease
- Irritable bowel syndrome
- Colon cancer
- Infective colitis
- Ischemic colitis

DIAGNOSTIC STUDIES

- Computed tomography (CT) scan, with or without contrast, is least invasive and provides the most information about presence, location, and extent of inflammation but cannot detect presence of bleeding
- Barium enema used to diagnose diverticulosis
- CBC: leukocytosis
- SED rate elevated
- Colonoscopy/flexible sigmoidoscopy to rule out malignancy, ulcerative colitis, or ischemic colitis

PREVENTION

- High fiber diet

NONPHARMACOLOGIC MANAGEMENT

- Rest
- NPO during acute episode; advance to clear liquids in small volume at frequent intervals, advance to high fiber diet
- Surgery may be indicated if patient experiences frequent recurrences
- Recommend high fiber diet

PHARMACOLOGIC MANAGEMENT

- Antibiotics effective against pericolitis
  - ◊ Oral antibiotics for mild cases:
    - * Ciprofloxacin and metronidazole (Flagyl®) for 1 week
    - * Sulfamethoxazole-trimethoprim (Bactrim®)
  - ◊ Intravenous antibiotics for severe cases: triple therapy: ampicillin, gentamicin (Garamycin®), and metronidazole (Flagyl®)
- Treat pain with antispasmodics such as hyoscyamine (Levsin®)

CONSULTATION/REFERRAL

- Gastroenterologist if moderate or severe symptoms exist
- Indications for surgical consult:
  - ◊ Severe, repeated, or extensive disease
  - ◊ Carcinoma suspected
  - ◊ Abdominal drainage, colostomy, or colon resection indicated

EXPECTED COURSE

- Symptoms completely resolve in 1 to 2 weeks
- >2/3 of patients fully recover without recurrence
- Colon resection is almost always curative

POSSIBLE COMPLICATIONS

- Perforation
- Abscess formation
- Sepsis
- Enteroenteric or enterovesical fistula
- Peritonitis

APPENDICITIS

DESCRIPTION

Inflammation of the vermiform appendix, which is a projection from the apex of the cecum

ETIOLOGY

Obstruction of the appendix secondary to stool, inflammation, stricture, foreign body, or neoplasm. The obstructed lumen prevents drainage. The resultant increased pressure decreases mucosal blood flow, and the appendix becomes hypoxic.

INCIDENCE

- Most common between ages 5 and 50 years
- Males > Females

RISK FACTORS

- Family history
- Abdominal neoplasm

ASSESSMENT FINDINGS

- Abdominal pain, usually severe and initially throughout the abdomen, or periumbilical area, later becomes localized to the right lower quadrant (RLQ)
- Anorexia, abdominal pain, nausea and vomiting are most common symptoms (in this order)
- Constipation and diarrhea occur after the pain
- Maximum abdominal tenderness and rigidity occurs over the right rectus muscle (McBurney's point)
- Psoas sign: pain with right thigh extension
- Obturator sign: pain with internal rotation of flexed right thigh
- Fever, usually 99-101° F (37.2-38.3°C)
- Patients frequently flex the right lower extremity when supine to relieve muscle tension
- May have urinary frequency, urgency, and dysuria
- Decreased bowel sounds
- Elderly may present with weakness, anorexia, tachycardia, and abdominal distention

DIFFERENTIAL DIAGNOSIS

- Mittelschmerz
- Ruptured ectopic pregnancy
- Pelvic inflammatory disease
- Gastroenteritis
- Gastric ulcer, duodenal ulcer
- Cholecystitis
- Urinary tract infection
- Inflammatory bowel disease
- Recurrent abdominal pain
- Renal calculi

- Urinalysis: may be positive for red blood cells and leukocytes
- Urine pregnancy test: negative
- KUB: may show gas filled appendix
- CT scan: diagnostic test of choice

NONPHARMACOLOGIC MANAGEMENT

- Keep NPO
- Instruct to refrain from using laxatives, enemas, or from applying heat to the abdomen
- Prompt surgery is the treatment of choice: appendectomy

PHARMACOLOGIC MANAGEMENT

- Preoperative antibiotics may be prescribed by surgeon (e.g., cefoxitin)

CONSULTATION/REFERRAL

- Prompt surgical referral

FOLLOW-UP

- Routine postoperative assessment is at 2 weeks and 6 weeks
- May require postoperative antibiotics if perforation has occurred

EXPECTED COURSE

- Quick recovery usually follows surgery
- Activity should be restricted for 2-6 weeks

POSSIBLE COMPLICATIONS

- Ruptured appendix, often manifested by cessation of pain
- Abscess
- Peritonitis

IRRITABLE BOWEL SYNDROME (IBS)

DESCRIPTION

Common intestinal disorder manifested by cramping, abdominal pain, bloating, and changes in bowel habits (e.g., constipation and/or diarrhea)

ETIOLOGY

- Unknown
- Stress is believed to be a factor

INCIDENCE

- Common: affects 15% of population of U.S.
- Rare in children and adolescents
- Predominant age: late 20's
- Female > Male

RISK FACTORS

- Family history

ASSESSMENT FINDINGS

- Crampy abdominal pain in lower quadrant
- Constipation and/or diarrhea
- Mucus in stools
- Abdominal distention
- No significant weight loss
- No bleeding, persistent severe pain, or fever

DIFFERENTIAL DIAGNOSIS

- Inflammatory bowel disorders
- Gastroenteritis
- Ingestion of antacids containing magnesium
- Lactose intolerance
- Celiac sprue
- Thyroid disorders

DIAGNOSTIC STUDIES

- Sigmoidoscopy to rule out other disorders: may show spasm or increased mucosal folds
- Barium enema to rule out other disorders: normal
- Sedimentation rate: normal
- CBC: normal
- Stool for ova, parasites, occult blood: negative

NONPHARMACOLOGIC MANAGEMENT

- Stress management
- Heat to abdomen
- Education about illness
- Avoid stimulants known to cause difficulty

PHARMACOLOGIC MANAGEMENT

- Bulk-producing agents (may make some patients worse): psyllium (Metamucil®)
- Antidiarrheal agents if diarrhea is present: loperamide (Imodium®)
- Antispasmodic agents: dicyclomine (Bentyl®), hyoscyamine sulfate (Levsin®)
- Anticholinergics: phenobarbital-hyoscyamine-atropine-scopolamine (Donnatal®)
- Antiflatulents: simethicone (Mylicon®)
- 5-HT receptor agonists: tegaserod (Zelnorm®)
- Low dose SSRIs (off label use)

CONSULTATION/REFERRAL

- Gastroenterologist for treatment failure

FOLLOW-UP

- Variable, dependent on symptoms

EXPECTED COURSE

- Recurrence with stress to be expected
- Does not increase risk of inflammatory bowel disease or colon cancer

INFLAMMATORY BOWEL DISEASE (IBD)

DESCRIPTION

Inflammatory bowel diseases (IBD) are chronic disorders of the GI tract distinguished by the recurrent inflammatory involvement of intestinal segments. Two main types are Crohn's disease and ulcerative colitis.

CROHN'S DISEASE

DESCRIPTION

Chronic, slowly progressive inflammation of the small intestine (most common), and/or large intestine, often involving the terminal ileum; disease ranges from mild to refractory in severity. Typically several locations of the intestines with sections in between are unaffected.

ETIOLOGY

- Idiopathic

INCIDENCE

- Females > Males
- 15% have family history
- Caucasians > African-Americans or Asians
- Peak age at onset is 15 to 25 years, then smaller peak at 55 to 65 years
- Three- to sixfold increased incidence in Jewish population

RISK FACTORS

- Family history
- Cigarette smoking

ASSESSMENT FINDINGS

- Diarrhea, including nocturnal
- Fever
- Abdominal pain and tenderness
- Weight loss
- Abdominal mass
- Fistulas
- Intestinal obstruction (uncommon)
- Hematochezia
- Megacolon
- Extracolonic disease: uveitis, arthritis, dermatitis, sclerosing cholangitis (< 10%)
- Bone age in children usually delayed by 2 years

DIFFERENTIAL DIAGNOSIS

- Ulcerative colitis, ischemic colitis
- NSAID adverse effects
- Enteritis
- Intestinal pathogenic bacteria
- Malignancy
- Irritable bowel syndrome
- Appendicitis
- Peptic ulcer disease
- Renal colic

DIAGNOSTIC STUDIES

- Colonoscopy with biopsy: submucosal inflammation with pseudopolyps, edema, and strictures; biopsy often reveals granulomatous inflammation
- Anti glycan antibody: elevated in 75% of cases
- Barium X rays
- Sedimentation rate: elevated
- CBC: anemia
- Albumin: below normal if severe disease
- Electrolytes: imbalances
- B_{12}, folate: deficient
- Stool for leukocytes, culture and sensitivity to rule out other causes for symptoms

NONPHARMACOLOGIC MANAGEMENT

- Maintain nutrition and weight:
  - ◊ May be helpful to decrease fat and increase fiber to treat diarrhea
  - ◊ Low lactose diet for small intestine involvement
  - ◊ Low fiber diet if strictures present
- Sitz baths helpful if perirectal disease present
- Drainage of perirectal abscess if present
- Manage extracolonic manifestations
- Refer to Crohn's and Colitis Foundation of America for information and support
- Surgery when indicated:
  - ◊ Abscess
  - ◊ Intestinal obstruction
  - ◊ For ostomy placement

PHARMACOLOGIC MANAGEMENT

Maintenance:

- Mesalamine (Asacol®, Pentasa®, Rowasa®)

- Antibiotics (if perirectal involvement): metronidazole (Flagyl®) reduces bacteria, granuloma formation
- Folate supplement while taking sulfasalazine, which inhibits folate absorption
- Antispasmodics and antidiarrheals may be helpful

Acute exacerbation:
- Corticosteroids initiated with poor response to first-line therapy
- Sulfasalazine (Azulfidine®)

If poor response to other treatments: Immunomodulating therapy
- Azathioprine (Imuran®)
- 6-mercaptopurine (Purinethol®)
- Cyclosporine (Sandimmune®)
- Methotrexate
- Infliximab (Remicade®): good patient response

PREGNANCY/LACTATION CONSIDERATIONS

- Pregnancy not contraindicated
- Long-term sulfasalazine therapy is associated with reversible sterility in males

CONSULTATION/REFERRAL

- Gastroenterologist

FOLLOW-UP

- Frequency dependent on severity
- Monitor weight, symptoms, CBC, sedimentation rate, Vitamin B_{12}, folate levels
- Changes in weight are helpful in determining need to increase or decrease medications
- Endoscopy indicated if symptoms change
- Annual liver function tests

EXPECTED COURSE

- Chronic illness with recurrences and exacerbations
- Surgery usually needed every 4-7 years for the average patient
- Full activities and normal, but often shortened life can be expected

POSSIBLE COMPLICATIONS

- Fistulae
- Colon perforation
- Toxic megacolon
- Adenocarcinoma
- Malnutrition

ULCERATIVE COLITIS

DESCRIPTION

Chronic inflammation of the colonic mucosa and submucosa; the inflammation is continuous, widespread and superficial, almost always involves the rectum, and may spread throughout the colon.

ETIOLOGY

- Unknown

INCIDENCE

- More common in developed countries
- Peak occurrence ages 15-40 years, and again at 50-70 years
- Increased frequency of occurrence in Jewish population
- Male = Female

RISK FACTORS

- Positive family history

ASSESSMENT FINDINGS

- Fecal incontinence, bloody diarrhea, rectal bleeding
- Tenesmus (cramping pain of the anal or vesical sphincter), abdominal pain

- Weight loss (possibly from malignancy)
- Fever, tachycardia, anemia

DIFFERENTIAL DIAGNOSIS

- Infectious colitis
- Ischemic colitis
- Crohn's disease
- Irritable bowel syndrome
- Diarrhea associated with antibiotic use
- Hemorrhoids
- Diverticulitis
- Lactose intolerance
- Arthralgia/arthritis

DIAGNOSTIC STUDIES

- Sigmoidoscopy with biopsy: establishes whether inflammation is present
- Plain abdominal films: identifies toxic megacolon and should be used in UC patients who present with fever, abdominal pain, leukocytosis
- Colonoscopy with biopsy to define extent of involvement
- Air contrast barium enema: often normal in early disease
- CBC to detect anemia and leukocytosis
- Sedimentation rate: elevated
- pANCA (perinuclear antineutrophil cytoplasmic antibody): elevated in 85% of patients
- Serum electrolytes: hypokalemia

NONPHARMACOLOGIC MANAGEMENT

- Complete bowel rest indicated in acute fulminant disease only
- Surgery is curative and should be considered in cases of disease that is unresponsive to 2-3 weeks of medical therapy
- Referral to National Foundation for Ileitis and Colitis

PHARMACOLOGIC MANAGEMENT

Aminosalicylates:

- Sulfasalazine (Azulfidine®) (drug of choice)
- Mesalamine (Asacol®, Pentasa®): if disease limited to left side of colon and rectum
- Olsalazine (Dipentum®)

Corticosteroids:

- Prednisone
- Steroid enemas/suppositories
- Prednisolone
- Methylprednisolone

Immuno modulators (used in patients who fail to respond to other therapies):

- Methotrexate
- Azathioprine (Imuran®)
- 6-mercaptopurine (Purinethol®)
- Cyclosporine (Sandimmune®)

Anticholinergic agents:

- Dicyclomine (Bentyl®)
- Hyoscyamine (Levsin®)

Antidiarrheal agents:

- Contraindicated in severe active disease
- May be useful in mild, stable disease with caution (could precipitate toxic megacolon)

PREGNANCY/LACTATION CONSIDERATIONS

- Sulfasalazine, topical and oral 5-ASA, and corticosteroids have not been associated with birth defects and can be used in pregnancy and lactation
- Congenital abnormalities have been associated with the use of azathioprine

CONSULTATION/REFERRAL

- Gastroenterologist
- Severe colitis requires prompt hospitalization

FOLLOW-UP

- Regular, close practitioner/patient relationship is important for the detection of exacerbations, complications, and for emotional support
- Patients with extensive or long-standing disease require surveillance for colorectal cancer (every 1-2 years after disease

present for 7-8 years) with annual colonoscopy with biopsies

EXPECTED COURSE

- Variable, dependent on extent of disease
- Chronic illness with remissions and exacerbations

POSSIBLE COMPLICATIONS

- Toxic megacolon
- Perforation
- Colon cancer
- Fluid and electrolyte imbalances
- Liver disease
- Stricture formation

CONSTIPATION

DESCRIPTION

Painful, difficult passage of small amounts of hard, dry stool, usually fewer than three times a week

ETIOLOGY

- Slow, sluggish colonic contractions cause excessive absorption of water by the colon; hard, dry stools move through the colon slowly

INCIDENCE

- Reported most often at age extremes
- The most common GI complaint in the U.S.

RISK FACTORS

- Age extremes
- Lack of dietary fiber
- Inadequate fluid intake
- Sedentary lifestyle
- Ignoring the urge to defecate
- Change in routine
- Medications
  - ◊ Antidepressants
  - ◊ Anticholinergics
  - ◊ Antihypertensives
  - ◊ Antihistamines
  - ◊ Calcium supplements
  - ◊ Iron supplements
  - ◊ Narcotics
  - ◊ Antacids containing aluminum
  - ◊ Diuretics
  - ◊ Anticonvulsants
- Irritable bowel syndrome
- Laxative abuse
- Neurologic, metabolic, and endocrine disorders
- Diverticulosis
- Hirschsprung's disease
- Intestinal obstruction

ASSESSMENT FINDINGS

- Decrease in number of bowel movements compared to patient's "usual" ("usual" is 3-5 times weekly)
- Hard, dry stools
- Pain and difficulty with defecation
- Abdominal distention

DIFFERENTIAL DIAGNOSIS

- Encopresis secondary to constipation
- Irritable bowel syndrome
- Colorectal cancer
- Obstipation (fecal impaction)
- Hirschsprung's disease
- Anorectal stenosis
- Anal fissure
- Hemorrhoids
- Hypothyroidism
- Depression

DIAGNOSTIC STUDIES

- Abdominal x-ray if structural abnormalities: suspected accumulation of stool in the sigmoid colon
- Barium enema if obstruction or Hirschsprung's disease is suspected
- Sigmoidoscopy or colonoscopy for visualization and biopsy

- Colorectal transit study used for chronic constipation; demonstrates how quickly food moves through the colon
- Anorectal manometry to evaluate anal sphincter muscle function
- Stool for occult blood: negative
  - ◊ Should be repeated on at least 3 different stool specimens before being considered negative
- Thyroid studies: normal

PREVENTION

- Establish regular toileting routine; respond to the urge to have a bowel movement
- High fiber diet (20 to 35 grams/day): beans, whole grains, bran, fruit, vegetables
- Adequate intake of water and juice (1.5 to 2 liters/day) and elimination of caffeine, which has a dehydrating effect
- Adequate exercise
- Avoidance of medications that contribute to constipation
- Limit use of laxatives, enemas, and stool softeners

NONPHARMACOLOGIC MANAGEMENT

- Dietary and lifestyle changes (*see* Prevention)

PHARMACOLOGIC MANAGEMENT

AGENT	ACTION	COMMENTS
Bulk producing laxatives *Examples:* methylcellulose (Citrucel®) psyllium (Metamucil®) polycarbophil (Fibercon®)	Hold water in stool to soften it, increase bulk and stimulate peristalsis	Take with plenty of water. Well tolerated. Minimal side effects. OK to use daily and long-term. Useful in patients with irritable bowel syndrome or diverticular disease.
Stool softeners *Examples:* Docusate (Colace®, Doxidan®, Surfak®)	Cause stool to absorb more fat and water	Take with plenty of water. Helpful for painful anorectal conditions like hemorrhoids. Short-term use only.
Osmotic Agents *Examples:* Corn syrup (especially useful in pediatric patients) Lactulose (Chronulac®)	Osmotic effect causes fluid to be retained in colon, increasing peristalsis	Works in 24-48 hours. Can be used long-term (lactulose only). May cause significant distention with flatulence.
Stimulants *Examples:* bisacodyl (Dulcolax®) cascara (Cascara®) senna (Senokot®, Ex-Lax®)	Act on the intestinal mucosa and alter secretion of H_2O and electrolytes	Chronic use leads to dependency. May discolor urine (senna, cascara).
Lubricants/Emollients *Example:* Mineral oil	Prevent colon from absorbing water from the stool	Potentially decreases absorption of fat-soluble vitamins (A, D, E, & K). May cause anal seepage.
Saline laxatives *Examples:* Magnesium sulfate (Epsom salt®) Magnesium hydroxide (Milk of Magnesia®)	Cause fluid retention in the colon which increases peristaltic activity	Use cautiously or avoid in patients on sodium restricted diets, CHF, renal dysfunction (up to 20% of magnesium can be absorbed).

PREGNANCY/LACTATION CONSIDERATIONS

- Stress dietary management
- Bulk-forming agents and occasional stool softeners may be used
- Category B: lactulose, magnesium sulfate

CONSULTATION/REFERRAL

- Gastroenterologist for treatment failure or ongoing constipation
- Surgeon for complications of hemorrhoids, fissures, rectal prolapse

FOLLOW-UP

- Regular follow-up evaluation needed until resumption of regular bowel function
- Monitor electrolytes, BUN, and creatinine of chronic laxative user

EXPECTED COURSE

- Brief, occasional constipation responds well to treatment
- Can become chronic and lifelong

POSSIBLE COMPLICATIONS

- Hemorrhoids
- Anal fissures
- Rectal prolapse
- Laxative abuse syndrome (LAS)
- Fecal impaction
- Fluid and electrolyte imbalances due to laxative use
- Acquired megacolon

HEMORRHOIDS

DESCRIPTION

Varicose veins of the hemorrhoidal venous plexus

- *Internal hemorrhoids*: those that occur above the dentate line
- *External hemorrhoids*: folds of perianal skin resulting from prior perianal swelling; symptomatic only when becoming thrombosed

ETIOLOGY

- Veins of the hemorrhoidal plexus become engorged as a result of:
    - ◊ Passage of stool: shearing force, straining
    - ◊ Increased venous pressure (e.g., pregnancy, CHF)

INCIDENCE

- Common in adults
- Males = Females

RISK FACTORS

- Constipation, straining with defecation
- Chronic diarrhea
- Pregnancy: due to constipation and direct effect of gravid uterus
- Hypertension, congestive heart failure
- Prolonged sitting
- Obesity
- Colon malignancy

ASSESSMENT FINDINGS

Internal hemorrhoids:

- Painless bleeding with defecation
- Feeling of incomplete evacuation after bowel movements

External hemorrhoids:

- Anal itching
- Pain with defecation
- Anal protrusion of blue, shiny mass
- Can be acutely painful

DIFFERENTIAL DIAGNOSIS

- Rectal prolapse
- Rectal neoplasm
- Condyloma

DIAGNOSTIC STUDIES

- Stool for occult blood: if positive, refer for colonoscopy. Do **not** assume bleeding is due to hemorrhoids. Should be repeated on at least 3 different stool specimens before being considered negative.
- Anoscopy: visualization of bright red or purple masses
- Sigmoidoscopy

PREVENTION

- Avoid constipation
- Refrain from prolonged sitting and straining with bowel movements

NONPHARMACOLOGIC MANAGEMENT

- Sitz baths alleviate pain
- Education about prevention
- High fiber diet and liberal water intake
- Cold packs
- Rubber band ligation (for internal hemorrhoids only)
- Infrared coagulation (external hemorrhoids)
- Sclerotherapy
- Hemorrhoidectomy for severe cases

PHARMACOLOGIC MANAGEMENT

- See *Constipation*
- Fiber supplements
- Stool softeners
- Analgesic ointment: benzocaine (Hurricaine®), dibucaine (Nupercainal®)
- Corticosteroid preparations (for itching and shrinking swollen hemorrhoids): hydrocortisone (Anusol-HC®)

PREGNANCY/LACTATION CONSIDERATIONS

- Hemorrhoids that occur with pregnancy usually resolve without treatment after delivery

CONSULTATION/REFERRAL

- Surgeon if conservative management is ineffective

FOLLOW-UP

- None needed unless symptoms persist

EXPECTED COURSE

- May resolve spontaneously or as a result of treatment
- May be recurrent and chronic

POSSIBLE COMPLICATIONS

- Thrombosis
- Rectal prolapse
- Infection
- Incontinence

PYLORIC STENOSIS

DESCRIPTION

Narrowing of the pyloric sphincter that occurs in infancy due to hypertrophy of the pyloric muscle which leads to obstruction

ETIOLOGY

- Probably familial
- More common in first born males

INCIDENCE

- Caucasians
- Males > Females (5:1)
- Usual onset is 3-4 weeks to 5 months of age

RISK FACTORS

- Family history

ASSESSMENT FINDINGS

- Projectile nonbilious vomiting, progressive in severity and frequency
- Usually begins after 2 weeks of age

- Olive-shaped mass palpable in right upper quadrant of abdomen (hypertrophied pylorus)
- Peristaltic waves visible across abdomen after feeding
- Insatiable hunger with weight loss and dehydration

DIFFERENTIAL DIAGNOSIS

- Gastroesophageal reflux
- Inappropriate feeding
- Gastritis
- Congenital adrenal hyperplasia

DIAGNOSTIC STUDIES

- Upper gastrointestinal series: thin, elongated pyloric canal ("string sign")
- Ultrasound is replacing contrast x-ray: clearly shows hypertrophied pyloric muscles and narrowed pyloric channel

MANAGEMENT

- Correction of fluid and electrolyte imbalances
- Surgical correction

CONSULTATION/REFERRAL

- For surgical pyloromyotomy

FOLLOW-UP

- Educate to introduce feedings gradually after surgery
- Routine pediatric care

EXPECTED COURSE

- Surgery remedies disorder

HIRSCHSPRUNG'S DISEASE
(Congenital Aganglionic Megacolon)

DESCRIPTION

Congenital absence of ganglion cells in a section of the wall of the large intestine resulting in lack of motility in that region, accumulation of feces, and dilation of the colon

ETIOLOGY

- Familial
- Often associated with trisomy 21

INCIDENCE

- Occurs 1 in 2 - 5000 births in the U.S.
- Males > Females

RISK FACTORS

- Family history
- Down syndrome

ASSESSMENT FINDINGS

- Failure to pass meconium within 48 hours of birth
- Constipation, obstipation
- Distended abdomen with palpable mass of feces
- Poor feeding, failure to thrive
- Vomiting
- Explosive diarrhea or flatus after finger rectal exams
- Anemia secondary to chronic blood loss from colon

DIFFERENTIAL DIAGNOSIS

- Acquired megacolon
- Idiopathic constipation, obstipation
- Ileal atresia
- Meconium plug, meconium ileus

DIAGNOSTIC STUDIES

- CBC: anemia, leukocytosis

- Abdominal x-rays: dilated loops of bowel
- Biopsy: absence of ganglion cells

MANAGEMENT

- Removal of accumulated feces
- Correction of fluid and electrolyte imbalances
- Education: diet after surgery, signs of dehydration, colostomy care if needed

CONSULTATION/REFERRAL

- Surgeon for resection of affected bowel and possible colostomy

FOLLOW-UP

- Throughout recuperative period

EXPECTED COURSE

- Favorable prognosis if corrected before complications occur

POSSIBLE COMPLICATIONS

- Toxic enterocolitis
- Perforated bowel

INTUSSUSCEPTION

DESCRIPTION

An emergent condition in which one bowel segment becomes invaginated into another

ETIOLOGY

- Idiopathic in infants age 5-9 months (90% of cases)
- Associated with predisposing conditions in neonates, older children, and adults (10% of cases)
- *See* Risk Factors

INCIDENCE

- Peak age is 5-9 months
- Can occur at any age but most common 6-12 months of age
- Up to 4/1000 live births in the U.S.
- Males > Females: 3:2

RISK FACTORS

- Hypertrophy of Peyer's patches (mucous membrane of the small intestine)
- Neoplasm
- Lead paint (in adults)
- Meckel's diverticulum
- Foreign body
- Henoch-Schönlein purpura
- Appendicitis
- Recent viral upper respiratory or gastrointestinal infection (21%)

ASSESSMENT FINDINGS

- Classic triad (frequently late findings):
  - ◊ Abdominal pain, often colicky
  - ◊ Vomiting (almost always occurs)
  - ◊ Bloody stools resembling "currant jelly"
- Lethargy
- Irritability
- May present with right upper quadrant mass
- May present with fever

DIFFERENTIAL DIAGNOSIS

- Intestinal perforation
- Gastroenteritis
- Enterocolitis
- Parasitic infection
- Tumors

DIAGNOSTIC STUDIES

- Stool for occult blood: often positive
- Gold standard for diagnosis is barium enema:
  - ◊ "Coiled spring" appearance
  - ◊ Often therapeutic, may reduce intussusception

- Plain abdominal x-ray to exclude intestinal perforation before barium enema
- Abdominal ultrasound can sometimes identify other etiologies of pain (e.g., appendicitis, ovarian sources, urinary tract source)

MANAGEMENT

- Rehydration
- Emergency nonsurgical or surgical reduction

CONSULTATION/REFERRAL

- Radiologist
- Surgeon

FOLLOW-UP

- Throughout postoperative period

EXPECTED COURSE

- Spontaneous reduction while awaiting surgery is known to occur
- Recurrence rate after barium enema reduction is 10%
- Recurrence rate after surgery is <4%

POSSIBLE COMPLICATIONS

- Can be fatal without prompt treatment
- Bowel ischemia
- Bowel perforation
- Sepsis

COLIC

DESCRIPTION

A symptom complex, in an otherwise healthy infant, that is characterized by episodes of inconsolable crying, accompanied by apparent abdominal pain. Tends to occur at predictable times of the day, often in the evening, and may last for several hours.

ETIOLOGY

- Unknown
- Possibly due to immaturity of the gastrointestinal tract

INCIDENCE

- Usually begins at age 3 weeks and resolves by age 3 to 4 months

RISK FACTORS

- Family tension
- First-time parents

ASSESSMENT FINDINGS

- Parent describes infant as:
  - ◊ Rigid
  - ◊ Fists clenched
  - ◊ Legs flexed upon abdomen
  - ◊ Irritable
  - ◊ Frequent flatus
- Normal growth
- Abdomen may be distended due to ingestion of air with crying
- Normal stools
- Normal physical exam

DIFFERENTIAL DIAGNOSIS

- Gastroesophageal reflux
- Infection
- Injury
- Incarcerated hernia
- Food intolerance

NONPHARMACOLOGIC MANAGEMENT

- Educate parents about comfort measures and feeding techniques
  - ◊ Rhythmic rocking in a swing or car
  - ◊ Continuous monotonous noise (e.g., fan, hairdryer, or clothes dryer)
  - ◊ Slow feeding with frequent burping
  - ◊ Pacifier
- Parental reassurance and encouragement with emphasis on infant's healthy status, and normal growth and development

- Formula changes are usually ineffective
- Breastfeeding mothers may be able to identify foods in their diet that contribute

PHARMACOLOGIC MANAGEMENT

- Treatment is controversial
- Simethicone (Mylicon®)

CONSULTATION/REFERRAL

- Breastfeeding consultant as indicated

FOLLOW-UP

- Close telephone contact and more frequent visits for education and support

EXPECTED COURSE

- Usually resolves by itself by age 3 months

PINWORMS
(Enterobiasis)

DESCRIPTION

Intestinal infestation with *Enterobius vermicularis*, a white, thread-like parasite one centimeter in length

ETIOLOGY

- The eggs of *Enterobius vermicularis* are ingested from contaminated fingers and fomites
- After hatching, become larvae in the intestines, and travel to the rectum

INCIDENCE

- The most common parasitic infestation in children in the U.S.
- Predominant age is preschool to 14 years

RISK FACTORS

- Family contact
- Day care center attendance, institutional residence
- Poor hygiene
- Crowded living conditions
- Warm climate

ASSESSMENT FINDINGS

- Perianal itching, vulvovaginitis
- Enuresis
- Abdominal pain
- Irritability, restlessness
- Anorexia
- Parent may directly visualize female worm at night or early in the morning by shining a flashlight on the perianal area

DIFFERENTIAL DIAGNOSIS

- Idiopathic pruritus ani
- Dermatitis
- Lichen planus
- Scabies
- Vaginitis

DIAGNOSTIC STUDIES

- Transparent adhesive tape test ("Scotch" tape test): identification of ova on low power microscopy after touching tape to perianal area

PREVENTION

- Avoidance of risk factors
- Hygiene

NONPHARMACOLOGIC MANAGEMENT

Educate parent and child:

- Careful handwashing, hygiene
- Wash clothing and bedding in hot water at time of treatment
- Ova remain viable for 3 weeks in a moist environment
- Discourage scratching
- Keep hands away from face and mouth

PHARMACOLOGIC MANAGEMENT

- Treat all family members simultaneously with anthelminthics:
  - ◊ Mebendazole (Vermox®)
  - ◊ Pyrantel pamoate (Antiminth®)
- Topical antipruritic cream may relieve itching

PREGNANCY/LACTATION CONSIDERATIONS

- Anthelminthics contraindicated in pregnancy

CONSULTATION/REFERRAL

- Usually none needed

FOLLOW-UP

- Anthelminthics to be repeated in 2 weeks

EXPECTED COURSE

- Easily resolved, but re infestation is common

POSSIBLE COMPLICATIONS

- Excoriation and impetigo from scratching
- Urinary tract infection, urethritis
- Endometritis, salpingitis

ENCOPRESIS

DESCRIPTION

Incontinence of stool after age 4 years

- Primary encopresis: child has never been toilet trained successfully
- Secondary encopresis: child previously trained begins to soil

ETIOLOGY

- Unclear
- Appears to be associated with emotional as well as physiologic factors, such as constipation
- Often associated with anger

INCIDENCE:

- Males > Females
- Affects >1% of children 4 years and older
- More common in low socioeconomic backgrounds

RISK FACTORS

- Dehydration or inadequate fluid intake
- Inappropriate use of laxatives
- Major life or family stress
- Inappropriate toilet training
- Physical or sexual abuse
- Painful bowel movements
- Changes in diet

ASSESSMENT FINDINGS

- Constipation present > 80% of time
- Painful bowel movements
- Fecal/foul odor surrounds child
- Hiding during play
- Attempting to retain stool
- Large amount of stool noted on abdominal exam
- Stool often of large volume

DIFFERENTIAL DIAGNOSIS

- Developmental delay
- Cerebral palsy
- Hirschsprung's disease
- Anal fissure
- Anorectal stenosis
- Hypothyroidism
- Hypercalcemia

DIAGNOSTIC STUDIES

- If associated with constipation, abdominal x-ray is indicated: may show accumulation of stool

PREVENTION

- Educate parents regarding appropriate toilet training and bowel habits
- Assist with stress management
- Early detection of abuse

NONPHARMACOLOGIC MANAGEMENT

Encopresis without constipation:

- Assist with development of appropriate bowel routine; instruct to use the bathroom at specific times
- Reinforce appropriate bowel habits with rewards

Encopresis with constipation:

- High fiber diet
- Increase fluid intake
- Limit milk intake in child >1 year of age
- Encourage child to take responsibility for toileting
- Sit on toilet 10 minutes twice a day after meals
- Administer enemas to evacuate colon if impacted
- Educate parents not to punish child for soiling
- Biofeedback may be helpful

PHARMACOLOGIC MANAGEMENT

Encopresis without constipation:

- Avoid use of laxatives

Encopresis with constipation:

- Administer stool softeners or laxatives if not impacted
- Mineral oil for children >age 5 years (prevents absorption of fat soluble vitamins; **cautious use**!)

CONSULTATION/REFERRAL

- Psychological counseling may be needed

FOLLOW-UP

- Evaluate in 1 week to determine if colon successfully evacuated
- Repeat enemas if necessary
- Teach parent to use laxatives/enemas if stool is retained for >48 hours, or if soiling resumes
- Recheck monthly for 6 months
- Continue stool softeners until child has not soiled for 1 month

EXPECTED COURSE

- Condition can be managed successfully in 80-90% of cases with aggressive treatment and adequate parental education

POSSIBLE COMPLICATIONS

- High-risk of difficulty with social and family relations
- Psychogenic megacolon
- Recurrent UTI
- Anal fissures

RECURRENT ABDOMINAL PAIN
(Functional Abdominal Pain)

DESCRIPTION

Childhood condition in which there are three or more episodes of functional abdominal pain occurring over a 3 month period

ETIOLOGY

- Unknown

INCIDENCE:

- Affects 10% of school age children
- Peak age is 9 years
- Females > Males

RISK FACTORS

- Emotional stress
- Maternal depression, overprotection, or rigidity
- Defective family coping skills
- Family history

ASSESSMENT FINDINGS

- Abdominal pain
  - ◊ Often periumbilical, may be generalized
  - ◊ May be sharp or dull
  - ◊ Constant, or intermittent
  - ◊ Rarely nocturnal
  - ◊ Accompanied by dramatic response and complicated rituals
- School absenteeism
- May include low grade fever, nausea, and vomiting
- Usually no change in bowel habits, sometimes constipation reported
- Pain medication reported as ineffective

DIFFERENTIAL DIAGNOSIS

- Urinary tract infection
- Gastroenteritis
- Lactose intolerance
- Depression
- Irritable bowel syndrome
- Acute abdomen (e.g., appendicitis)

DIAGNOSTIC STUDIES

- CBC with differential: normal
- Urinalysis: normal
- Urine pregnancy test: negative
- Flat and erect x-ray of abdomen: negative
- Breath hydrogen test: no evidence of lactose intolerance

NONPHARMACOLOGIC MANAGEMENT

- Support patient and family, ensuring that pain is taken seriously
- Introduce the possibility that the pain is functional (inorganic)
- Discuss relationship between stress and pain
- Encourage normal activities, including regular school attendance
- Increase dietary fiber if there is constipation

PHARMACOLOGIC MANAGEMENT

- Pain medication is generally not helpful

CONSULTATION/REFERRAL

- Mental health professional if there is family or behavioral dysfunction

FOLLOW-UP

- Provide ongoing support with emphasis on lack of organic cause and lack of physical danger
- Teach signs and symptoms of emergent pain, acute abdomen

EXPECTED COURSE

- Resolves gradually
- Course variable

References

Ament, P., & Childers, S. (1997). Prophylaxis and treatment of NSAID-induced gastropathy. *American Family Physician, 55*(11), 51-61.

Beers, M.H., & Berkow, R (Eds.). (1999). *The Merck manual of diagnosis and therapy* (17th ed.). Rahway, NJ: Merck.

Behrman, R.E., Kliegman, R.M., Arvin, A.M., & Nelson, W.E. (Eds.). (1995). *Nelson textbook of pediatrics* (15th ed.). Philadelphia: W.B. Saunders.

Bickley, L.S., & Szilagyi, P.G. (2003). *Bates' guide to physical examination and history taking* (8th ed.). Philadelphia: Lippincott Williams & Wilkins.

Branch, W.T. (2003). *Office practice of medicine* (4th ed.). Philadelphia: Saunders.

Burns, C.E., Brady, M.A., Blosser, C., Starr, N.B., & Dunn, A.M. (2004). *Pediatric primary care: A handbook for nurse practitioners* (3rd ed.). Philadelphia: W.B. Saunders.

Castell, D., Richter, J., & Spichler, S. (1996). Achieving better outcomes for patients with GERD. *Patient Care, 30*(8), 20-42.

Center for Disease Control and Prevention (2004). Acute Hepatitis B Among Children and Adolescents. *MMWR 53,* (43).

Dambro, M.R. (2005). *Griffith's 5 minute clinical consult.* Philadelphia: Lippincott Williams & Wilkins.

Damianos, A., & McGarrity T. (1997). Treatment strategies for *Helicobacter pylori* infection. *American Family Physician, 55*, 265-284.

Desai, S.P. (2004). *Clinician's guide to laboratory diagnosis* (3rd ed.). Hudson, OH:Lexi-Comp. Added to sections??????

Fischbach, F.T., & Dunning, M.B. (2003). *A manual of laboratory & diagnostic tests* (7th ed.). Philadelphia: Lippincott Williams & Wilkins.

Gilber, D.N., Moellering, R.C., Eliopoulos, G.M., & Sande, M.A. (Eds.). (2004). *Sanford Guide to Antimicrobial Therapy* (34th ed.). Hyde Park, VT: Antimicrobial Therapy.

Graber, M.A., & Lanternier, M.L. (Eds.) (2001). *The family practice handbook.* (4th ed.). St. Louis: Mosby.

Kasper, D.L., Braunwald, E., Fauci, A.S., Hauser, S.L., Longo, D.L., Jameson, J.L., et al. (2004). *Harrison's principles of internal medicine* (16th ed.). New York: McGraw-Hill.

Kong, A.P., & Stamos, M.J. (2005). Anorectal complaints: Office diagnosis and treatment. *Consultant, 45,* 731-738.

Lindsey, T., Watts-Tate, N., Southwood, E., Routhieaux, J., Beatty, J., Calamaras, D., et al.(2005). Rural health alert: *Helicobacter pylori* in well water. *Journal of the American Academy of Nurse Practitioners, 17*, 283-289.

Mangion, S. (2000). *Physical diagnosis secrets.* Philadelphia: Hanley and Belfus.

McManus, T.J. (2000). Helicobacter pylori: An emerging infectious disease. *The Nurse Practitioner, 25*(8), 40-50.

Middlemiss, C. (1997). Gastroesophageal reflux disease: A common condition in the elderly, *The Nurse Practitioner, 22* (11), 51-61.

Mladenovic, J. (Ed.). (2003). *Primary care secrets.* (3rd Ed.). Philadelphia: Hanley and Belfus.

National Institute of Health. (1995). *Constipation.* (DHHS Publication No. 97-2754). Washington, D.C.: U.S. Department of Health & Human Services.

National Digestive Diseases Information Clearinghouse. (n.d.) *Constipation.* Retrieved August 1, 2005, from http://www.digestive.niddk.nih.gov/ddiseases/pubs/constipation/.

Pisarra, V.H. (1999). Recognizing the various presentation of appendicitis. *The Nurse Practitioner*, *24*(8): 42-53.

Rakel, R.E. (Ed.). (1998). *Essentials of family practice.* (2nd ed.). Philadelphia: WB Saunders.

Schwartz, M.W. (Ed.). (2002). *The 5 minute pediatric consult.* (2nd ed.) Philadelphia: Lippincott Williams & Wilkins.

Shapira, S.C. (2005). Hepatitis B: Latest treatment guidelines. *Consultant, 45*, 605-610.

Tierney, L.M.,Jr., McPhee, S.J., Papadahis, M.A. (2004) *Current medical diagnosis and treatment.* (44th ed.). New York: McGraw-Hill Professional Publishing.

Uphold, C.R., & Graham, M.V. (2003). *Clinical guidelines in family practice.* (4th ed.). Gainesville, FL: Barmarrae Books.

U.S. Preventive Services Task Force. (1996). *Guide to clinical preventive services.* (2nd ed.) Washington, D.C.: Office of Disease Prevention and Health Promotion, U.S. Government Printing Office.

Wilson, T.R. (2005). The ABCs of Hepatitis. *The Nurse Practitioners, 30*(6), 12-21.

Winslow, B., & Westfall, J. (1996). Intussusception. *American Family Physician, 54,* 213-217.

Yates, J. (2005). Traveler's diarrhea. *American Family Physician, 71,* 2095-2100.

Zollo, A.J., Jr (Ed.). (2004). *Medical Secrets.* (4th ed.), St. Louis, MO: Mosby-Year Book.

7

HEALTH PROMOTION: ADULT

Health Promotion: Adult

PRIMARY, SECONDARY, TERTIARY PREVENTION

The US Preventive Services Task Force's Guide to Preventive Services (2nd edition, 1996) defines ***primary preventive measures*** as "those provided to individuals to prevent the onset of a targeted condition." (pp. xli).

Example: Routine MMR administration to a healthy, 12 month old

The US Preventive Services Task Force's Guide to Preventive Services (2nd edition, 1996) defines ***secondary preventive measures*** as those which "identify and treat asymptomatic persons who have already developed risk factors or preclinical disease, but in whom the disease has not become clinically apparent." (pp. xli).

Example 1: Screening mammogram in a 50 year old female

Example 2: Screening for elevated cholesterol levels

Tertiary preventive measures are used in patients with established clinical disease. The purpose of the measures is to minimize complications associated with the disease, prevent progression of the disease, and/or to restore the patient to his highest possible level of functioning.

Example 1: Use of cholesterol lowering medications in a patient with coronary artery disease

Example 2: Use of an oral anti-hyperglycemic medication in a diabetic patient to achieve normal blood sugar values

Some recommendations for adults by the U.S. Preventive Services Task Force's (USPSTF) Guide to Clinical Preventive Services 2005

ASPRIN FOR PRIMARY PREVENTION OF CARDIOVASCULAR EVENTS

- Adults at risk for coronary heart disease because of age, gender, hypertension, hyperlipidemia, family history, or smoking may benefit from daily dose of aspirin
- Benefit: prevention of MI
- Risk: possible gastrointestinal or cerebral bleed (risk may be greater in older adults)
- Optimal dose is not known but 75 mg – 325 mg daily is reasonable

SCREENING:

BREAST CANCER SCREENING

- There is insufficient evidence to recommend teaching or performing self-breast exam to help decrease mortality from breast cancer
- Screening with mammography for women aged 40 and older should be done every 1-2 years depending on risk for breast cancer
- There is no recommendation as to the age to discontinue screening with mammography

CERVICAL CANCER SCREENING

- Screening should begin after a woman has been sexually active for 3 years or age 21; whichever comes first
- It is unclear as to the optimal age to discontinue screening, but, screening after age 65 yielded low results in previously screened women
- There were no differences in outcomes in patients who were screened annually compared to those screened every 3 years

- Discontinuation of cervical screening after total hysterectomy (for benign reasons) is appropriate

CHLAMYDIA INFECTION SCREENING

- Sexually active women aged 25 and younger, even if asymptomatic, are at increased risk for infection and therefore, should be screened
- There is insufficient evidence to recommend a screening interval but consideration should be given to risk factors for infection, change in partners, pregnancy status
- Risk factors include age, unmarried status, African-American race, history of an STD, having new or multiple sexual partners, inconsistent use of contraceptive barrier products, and cervical ectopy
- Women at increased risk, even if asymptomatic, should be screened
- Benefit is unknown for screening high risk men

COLORECTAL CANCER SCREENING

- Beginning at age 50 years, men and women of average risk should be screened using fecal occult blood (FOBT), flexible sigmoidoscopy, colonoscopy, **OR** double-contrast barium enema (BE)
- Annual FOBT has a high rate of false positives
- Colonoscopy can be performed at 10 year intervals; flexible sigmoidoscopy, BE at 5 year intervals
- Persons at increased risk should consider screening at an earlier age. Examples of increased risk are history of colon cancer in a first degree relative before age 60 years, familiar polyposis, ulcerative colitis, personal history of colorectal cancer
- Colonoscopy has the highest degree of sensitivity and specificity of all screening tests available but is more expensive and associated with higher risks

DIABETES MELLITUS

- There is insufficient evidence to recommend routine screening for elevated glucose levels in asymptomatic adults
- Screening is recommended for adults who have hypertension, hyperlipidemia, polyuria, or polydipsia

HYPERTENSION SCREENING

- All persons $\geq$18 years of age should be periodically screened for hypertension with blood pressure measurement (no recommendation is made as to the intervals between measurements)
- 2 abnormal measurements should be made on at least 2 different visits over a period of 1 to several weeks before a diagnosis of hypertension should be considered

LIPID DISORDERS

- Men aged $\geq$ 35 and women aged $\geq$ 45 years should be screened for lipid disorders and treated if found to be at high risk for development of coronary artery disease (CAD)
- Men aged 20-35 and women aged 20-45 should be screened if they have other risk factors for coronary artery disease
- Risk factors include: personal history of diabetes, family history of CAD or hyperlipidemia, HTN, or tobacco use
- Screening should include measurement of total cholesterol and HDL only (these can be measured in a non-fasting state). Abnormal results should be confirmed.
- Optimal intervals for screening, and age to stop screening, are uncertain

OBESITY

- All adult patients should be screened for obesity
- Counseling and behavioral interventions should be offered to promote weight loss in adults who are obese

SCREENING FOR OSTEOPOROSIS

- Women aged 65 and older should be screened for osteoporosis
- Women at increased risk of fractures should be screened starting at age 60

EDUCATION AND COUNSELING

NUTRITION

- Whole grains: at least half of daily consumption should be whole grains
- Veggies: several daily servings with emphasis on dark green and orange ones
- Fruits: several daily servings of fresh, canned, frozen, or dried
- Milk should be low fat or no fat
- Meat/Beans: lean meats, more fish, nuts, beans
- Oils: minimize use but avoid solid fats
- Women should consume adequate calcium:
  - ◊ Adults age <25 years: 1200-1500 mg/day
  - ◊ Adults age 25-50 years: 1200 mg/day
  - ◊ Postmenopausal women: 1200-1500 mg/day
  - ◊ Pregnant and nursing women: 1200-1500 mg/day
- Individuals who follow a vegetarian diet should be instructed to consume a wide variety of legumes, grains, nuts, seeds, and vegetables to ensure appropriate protein intake

EXERCISE

- Regular physical activity for all adults (most days of the week) because of its proven efficacy in reducing risk of CHD, hypertension, and obesity, and its positive effect on general well-being
- Progressive activity over several months toward achievement of cardiovascular fitness
- Development and maintenance of muscular strength and joint flexibility
- Inclusion of regular weight-bearing exercise to promote bone density
- Discourage sporadic vigorous exercise in favor of consistently performed, moderate-level activities

SMOKING CESSATION

- Promote smoking cessation for all adults on a regular basis
- Pregnant women should be counseled on the effect of smoking on fetal health
- Parents should be counseled on the effect of smoking on child health
- 87% of cancers of the lung, bronchus, and trachea are associated with smoking
- Smoking significantly increases the risk for many cancers, stroke, CAD, peripheral vascular disease
- Discourage exposure to second hand smoke (environmental tobacco smoke) increases the risk lung cancer, heart disease, lower respiratory tract infections in children and infants, increases risk of SIDS, aggravates symptoms of asthma, etc.

SAFETY

- Lap/shoulder belt use
- Bicycle and motorcycle helmets
- Smoke detectors
- Firearm safety
- Avoidance of alcohol/drug use while driving, boating, swimming

ALCOHOL ABUSE

- Patients with evidence of alcohol dependence should be offered advice and counseling regarding reduction of consumption, and the role of alcohol in current medical or psychosocial problems
- A decreased risk of coronary artery disease is associated with low to moderate alcohol consumption in adults aged $\geq$ 65 years (2 drinks/day for men; 1 drink or less per day for women)

DENTAL HEALTH

- Daily flossing and brushing with fluoride toothpaste
- Regular preventive dental care
- Avoidance of tobacco

SEXUALLY TRANSMITTED DISEASES

- Sexual behavior counseling should be based on individual risk factors and local epidemiology
  - ◊ Abstinence

- ◊ Maintenance of a mutually monogamous sexual relationship
- ◊ Latex condom use for those with multiple partners, casual partners
- ◊ Female condom for women whose male partner uses no condom
- ◊ Diaphragm and spermicide helpful in reducing risk of gonorrhea and chlamydia, but not as effective as male condoms and not proven effective against HIV and other STDs
- ◊ Pregnant women at risk of STDs should be educated regarding potential fetal risk
- ◊ Alcohol and drug use is associated with high-risk sexual behavior

CONTRACEPTION

- Contraceptive counseling should be based on information obtained though direct questioning about sexual activity, contraceptive use, and concern about pregnancy

TESTICULAR CANCER

- Patients at high risk for the development of testicular cancer (e.g., those with a history of cryptorchidism or atrophic testes) should be informed of their increased risk and instructed on testicular self-examination and to seek appropriate medical attention if an abnormality is noted

SOLAR DAMAGE

- All adults should receive counseling to avoid excess sun and use protective clothing to prevent solar damage and associated risk of skin cancer
- Basal cell and squamous cell carcinoma are in epidemic proportions in the U.S.

VACCINE SCHEDULE FOR ADULTS

Latest vaccine information: *www.cdc.gov/nip*

- **Tetanus-diphtheria (Td):** 0, 2, and 8-14 months
  - ◊ Standard regimen is Td booster every 10 years
  - ◊ Primary series if not completed is 3 doses: first 2 doses are 4 weeks apart, third dose is 6-12 months after the second dose
  - ◊ International travelers should receive a booster every 10 years
  - ◊ Precaution: first trimester of pregnancy

- **Influenza vaccine:** annual vaccination with current vaccine at or around October
  - ◊ Inactivated influenza vaccination is indicated for the following adults:
    - * Residents of chronic care facilities
    - * Chronic cardiopulmonary disorders
    - * Chronic metabolic diseases
    - * Hemoglobinopathies
    - * Immunosuppression
    - * Renal dysfunction
    - * Health care providers
    - * Pregnancy is a not a contraindication to receiving the inactivated influenza vaccine; do not use FluMist®
    - * For healthy persons aged 5-49 who do not have contact with high risk persons, FluMist® may be administered

- **Pneumococcal vaccine:** 1 dose recommended for the following adults:
  - ◊ All immunocompetent individuals age 65 years or older
  - ◊ High-risk groups:
    - * Institutionalized persons age 50 years or older
    - * Most chronic diseases
    - * Chronic cardiac or pulmonary disease (excluding asthma)
    - * Diabetes mellitus
    - * Anatomic asplenia
    - * Native American and Alaska Native populations living in an area identified as high risk
  - ◊ *Revaccination* recommended after 5 years for individuals at highest risk for

morbidity and mortality from pneumococcal infection:
  * Persons ≥ 65 years of age for whom ≥ 5 years has passed and were ≤ 65 years at the initial vaccination
  * Persons with severe chronic disease
- ◊ Safety in pregnancy is unknown

- **Measles-mumps-rubella (MMR) vaccine** should be administered to all persons born after 1956 who lack evidence of immunity
  - ◊ In adults, administer one dose; a second dose should be administered to young adults in settings where there is risk of infection (schools) or exposure, work in healthcare facilities, plan to travel internationally
  - ◊ Not recommended after age 50 years
  - ◊ Contraindicated in pregnancy
  - ◊ After immunization, counsel to avoid pregnancy for 4 weeks

- **Hepatitis B vaccine** recommended for all young adults and for susceptible adults in high-risk groups; first 2 doses 1 month apart, then a third dose 6 months later. High risk groups include:
  - ◊ Men who have sex with men
  - ◊ Injecting drug users and their sex partners
  - ◊ History of sexual activity with multiple partners in the last 6 months
  - ◊ History of recently acquired sexually transmitted disease
  - ◊ International travelers to countries where HBV is endemic
  - ◊ Recipients of blood products, hemodialysis patients
  - ◊ Persons in jobs with frequent exposure to blood products
  - ◊ Pregnancy is not a contraindication in a high risk person

- **Hepatitis A vaccine** is recommended for all adults at high risk, 2 doses, 6-12 months apart:
  - ◊ Persons with clotting factor disorders or chronic liver disease
  - ◊ Persons living in or traveling to endemic areas
  - ◊ Men who have sex with men
  - ◊ Users of injection or street drugs
  - ◊ Military personnel
  - ◊ Certain hospital and laboratory workers
  - ◊ Institutionalized persons and workers in institutions

- **Varicella vaccine**, 2 doses given 4-8 weeks apart
  - ◊ Recommended for healthy adults with no history of varicella infection who might be at high risk
  - ◊ Do not administer during pregnancy; counsel to avoid pregnancy for 4 weeks after vaccine

CHEMOPROPHYLAXIS

NEURAL TUBE DEFECTS

- Daily multivitamins containing 0.4 mg folic acid are recommended for all fertile women in case of unplanned or planned pregnancy to reduce the risk of neural tube defects
- Daily multivitamin containing folic acid supplementation of 0.4-1.0 mg is recommended for all women planning pregnancy beginning at least 1 month prior to conception and continuing through the first trimester
- Women with a history of a previous pregnancy affected by a neural tube defect who are planning pregnancy are advised to supplement their folic acid intake with 4 mg/day beginning 1-3 months prior to conception and continuing through the first trimester of pregnancy

HEPATITIS B EXPOSURE

- *Postexposure recommendations*
  Initiate Hepatitis B immunization and give hepatitis B immune globulin (HBIG) in the following circumstances:

- ◊ Birth of an infant to a hepatitis B surface antigen (HBsAg)-positive mother
- ◊ Household exposure of an infant <1 year of age to a primary caregiver with acute HBV
- ◊ Percutaneous or permucosal exposure to HBsAg-positive blood
- ◊ Sexual exposure to a HBsAg-positive person

HEPATITIS A EXPOSURE

- *Postexposure recommendations*
  Initiate Hepatitis A immunization and administer immune globulin as soon as possible within 2 weeks after exposure to:
  - ◊ Sexual contacts
  - ◊ Close household contacts
  - ◊ Staff and children at day care centers where a case is recognized
  - ◊ Staff and patients at custodial institutions where HAV transmission has occurred
  - ◊ Food handlers in establishments where a food handler is diagnosed with HAV

MENINGITIS

- *Postexposure prophylaxis*
  Rifampin/ciprofloxacin for meningococcal meningitis:
  - ◊ Casual contacts do not need prophylaxis
  - ◊ Household contacts of persons with meningococcal infection
  - ◊ Daycare contacts of persons with meningococcal infection
  - ◊ Individuals with direct exposure to oral secretions of a person with meningococcal infection (e.g., kissing)
  - ◊ The meningococcal vaccine is also recommended for persons age 3 months or older in all outbreaks caused by serogroup A strains, and for persons at least 2 years of age in all outbreaks caused by serogroup C, Y, and W-135 strains

Rifampin is contraindicated during pregnancy.

TETANUS

- *Postexposure prophylaxis*
  - ◊ Initiate tetanus toxoid (Td) if an individual presents with a minor, clean wound, and >10 years has elapsed since the last dose
  - ◊ If an individual presents with a serious, contaminated wound, tetanus toxoid is recommended if >5 years have elapsed since the last dose

RABIES

- Individuals at high risk of contact with the rabies virus should receive pre-exposure prophylaxis against rabies:
  - ◊ Animal handlers
  - ◊ Rabies laboratory workers
  - ◊ Persons planning to spend >1 month in an endemic area
- Persons with frequent exposure should have antibody level checked every 6 months and should receive a booster injection as their titers drop below protective levels
- Indications for postexposure prophylaxis with human rabies immune globulin (HRIG) against rabies:
  - ◊ Dependent on type of animal and circumstances of attack (consult local health department)
    - * Carnivorous wild animal, bat
    - * Unprovoked attack

SPECIAL CONSIDERATIONS: ELDERLY ADULTS

SCREENING:

CAROTID ARTERY STENOSIS

- Patients >age 60 years at high risk for vascular disease are likely to benefit from screening with auscultation for bruits and follow-up carotid ultrasound
- The most effective intervention to prevent brain attack is still smoking cessation and treatment of hypertension

ABDOMINAL AORTIC ANEURYSM

- Men >age 60 years with risk factors (e.g., vascular disease, family history of abdominal aortic aneurysm (AAA), hypertension, and smoking) are at highest risk for AAA and would benefit most from abdominal palpation or abdominal ultrasound to screen for AAA

PROSTATE CANCER

- Screening for prostate cancer is controversial and should be limited to individuals with a life expectancy >10 years, using digital rectal exam (DRE) and prostatic specific antigen (PSA), and performed only after the patient has been given information regarding the potential benefit and harm of early detection and treatment
- PSA of 4.0 ng/ml detects the majority of prostate cancers; however, PSA may not detect early prostate cancer

GLAUCOMA

- Caucasian patients with diabetes, severe myopia, family history of glaucoma, and/or >age 65 years of age are at greatest risk of developing glaucoma and may benefit from screening for increased intraocular pressure. Effective screening is best performed by an eye specialist with the benefit of proper equipment

HEARING IMPAIRMENT

- Older adults are at risk for hearing impairment, particularly presbycusis (progressive loss of hearing and sound discrimination characterized by inability to hear the consonants *s*, *sh*, and *f*, which are high-frequency sounds)
- Screening for hearing impairment by questioning regarding hearing is recommended
- Audiometric testing is appropriate follow-up if questioning reveals the possibility of hearing difficulty

ACTIVITIES OF DAILY LIVING

- Information regarding ability to perform activities of daily living should be solicited from patients and from family members. Direct questioning may be accompanied by brief standardized questionnaires, but questionnaires are not a reliable substitute for interview. If dementia is suspected, further assessment to exclude primary causes (e.g., depression, physical illness, and medication effect) is important.

DEPRESSION

- Clinicians should maintain a high index of suspicion for depressive symptoms in elderly patients who have suffered recent losses, or those with chronic illness

ABUSE

- Elderly dependent adults who present with multiple injuries, or with an unsatisfactory explanation for injuries, should be assessed for abuse and followed accordingly

CERVICAL CANCER

- Women >age 65 years do not appear to benefit from Pap testing if previous Pap smears have been repeatedly normal; however, many women in this age group have not been previously tested consistently and may still benefit from the screening

POLYPHARMACY

- Older adults tend to be on multiple medications
- "Brown Bag Test": encourage elderly patient to bring all medications for each clinic visit so prescriber may assess medications for drug interactions, contraindications, duplications, etc.

DISEASE PREVENTION FOR THE INTERNATIONAL TRAVELER

For Latest Information: *www.cdc.gov*

MALARIA

- Malaria is transmitted through the bite of an infected female *Anopheles* mosquito, by blood transfusion, and congenitally
  - ◊ Endemic in Central America, South America, Sub-Saharan Africa, India, Southeast Asia, Middle East, and Oceania
  - ◊ Stay in well screened area, use mosquito nets, clothing to cover body
  - ◊ High-risk hours are between dusk and dawn
  - ◊ Adherence to specific antimalarial drug regimen

TRAVELERS' DIARRHEA

- Risk is associated with travel to developing countries: Latin America, Middle East, Asia, parts of the Caribbean, and southern Europe
- Transmitted through ingestion of fecally contaminated food and fluids
- Educate regarding food and beverage intake
- Avoid raw and undercooked meat and fish, fresh fruit, drinks with ice, local tap water, ground-grown vegetables, foods sold by street venders, and dairy products
- Fluids safe to ingest are bottled carbonated beverages, canned fruit juices, beer, wine, drinks with boiled water (e.g., tea, coffee)
- Non antimicrobial medications: bismuth subsalicylate (Pepto-Bismol®), loperamide (Imodium®)
- Antimicrobial agents:
  - ◊ Trimethoprim sulfamethoxazole (Bactrim®, Septra®)
  - ◊ Doxycycline (Vibramycin®)
  - ◊ Norfloxacin (Noroxin®)
  - ◊ Ciprofloxacin (Cipro®)
- Rehydration regimen recommended by World Health Organization (WHO):
  - ◊ Dissolve $^1/_2$ teaspoon table salt, $^1/_2$ teaspoon baking soda, $^1/_4$ teaspoon KCl, and $2^1/_2$ tablespoons sucrose in 1 L drinkable water
  - ◊ Drink 2-5 L/day

SCHISTOSOMIASIS

- Avoid swimming in fresh water in endemic areas
- Adequately chlorinated and salt water are safe

HEPATITIS A AND B

Immunizations are recommended before travel to areas where these diseases may be endemic

TETANUS

Up to date immunization is recommended before travel outside the US

OBESITY

DESCRIPTION

Condition of increased body weight that leads to increased morbidity and mortality. Defined as weight 20% greater than an individual's ideal body weight. Abdominal (android) obesity carries increased risk for long-term health problems.

ETIOLOGY

- Multifactorial: genetic, social, developmental, psychological, metabolic
- Imbalance between food intake and energy expenditure
- Insulinoma
- Diabetes mellitus
- Glucocorticosteroid drug therapy
- Cushing's syndrome
- Hypothyroidism
- Hypothalamic disorders

INCIDENCE

- On increase in the U.S.
- Prevalence of obesity
  - ◊ 20-30% in adult males
  - ◊ 30-40% in adult females
  - ◊ 11-15% in adolescents

RISK FACTORS

- Decreased socioeconomic status
- High fat diet
- Parental obesity
- Sedentary life-style
- Increased television viewing, especially among children

ASSESSMENT FINDINGS

- Weight >20% over ideal body weight
- Weight for height >95th percentile in infants and children
- Can also be expressed as body mass index (BMI)
  - ◊ BMI = body weight (kg) ÷ body height^2 (m)
  - ◊ A BMI of >28.5 is considered obese in men, and >27.5 in women
- A simpler way is to determine ideal body weight:
  - ◊ Men: 106 lbs + 6 lbs/inch over 5 feet
  - ◊ Women: 100 lbs + 5 lbs/inch over 5 feet
- Abdominal (android) obesity: waist: hip ratio >0.85 in women and >0.95 in men. (To obtain, divide waist measurement by hip measurement)
- Use food diaries and self-assessments to determine eating habits

DIAGNOSTIC STUDIES

- Not needed for diagnosis, but can assist with identification of underlying problem and development of treatment plan
- Thyroid function studies
- Lipid profile
- Blood glucose

PREVENTION

- Well-balanced diet following USDA Food Guide Pyramid
- Regular exercise

NONPHARMACOLOGIC MANAGEMENT

- Severely restrictive diets are not recommended
- Counseling regarding life-long behavior changes
- Well-balanced diet following USDA Food Guide Pyramid
- Behavior modification
- Determine caloric requirement for body weight and activity level

PREGNANCY/LACTATION CONSIDERATIONS

- Well-balanced diet should be maintained in pregnancy
- Restrictive caloric intake is not recommended in pregnancy
- Common time of onset or worsening of obesity

CONSULTATION/REFERRAL

- Refer to community organizations for weight loss and maintenance programs (e.g., Weight Watchers)
- Refer for nutritional counseling

FOLLOW-UP

- Long-term frequent follow-up

EXPECTED COURSE

- Chronic condition that is rarely cured
- Long-term maintenance of weight loss difficult
- Dependent on sustained patient motivation

POSSIBLE COMPLICATIONS

- Increased mortality
- Cardiovascular disease
- Diabetes mellitus
- Hypertension
- Hyperlipidemia
- Cholelithiasis especially with rapid weight loss
- Osteoarthritis
- Hypoventilation
- Gout
- Thromboembolism
- Sleep apnea
- Low self-esteem
- Decreased mobility
- Decreased exercise tolerance

References

Alder, M., & Chisholm, B. (1991). Health promotion and disease prevention for the international traveler. *Nurse Practitioner*, *16*(5), 10-25.

Bickley, L.S., & Szilagyi, P.G. (2003). *Bates' guide to physical examination and history taking* (8th ed.). Philadelphia: Lippincott Williams & Wilkins.

Branch, W.T. (2003). *Office practice of medicine* (4th ed.). Philadelphia: Saunders.

Centers for Disease Control and Prevention. (2002). Recommended adult immunization schedule. *MMWR,* vol. 53 no. 45, Q1-Q4.

Centers for Disease Control and Prevention. (2005). Prevention and control of influenza: Recommendations of the Advisory Committee on Immunization Practices (ACIP). *MMWR,* vol. 54, RR-8.

Gates, T.J. (2001). Screening for cancer: evaluating the evidence. *American Family Physician*, *63*, 513-22.

Graber, M.A., & Lanternier, M.L. (Eds.). (2001). *The family practice handbook* (4th ed.). St. Louis: Mosby.

Houde, S. C. & Melillo, K. D. (2000). Physical activity and exercise counseling in primary care. *The Nurse Practitioner*, *25*(8), 9-37.

Huntzinger, A. (2005). CDC releases guidelines for improving vaccination rates among high-risk adults. *American Academy of Family Physicians, 72,* 338-339.

Kemp, C. & Potyk, D. (2005). Cancer screening principles and controversies. *The Nurse Practitioner, 30*(8), 46-50.

Mladenovic, J. (Ed.). (2003). *Primary care secrets.* (3rd ed.). Philadelphia: Hanley and Belfus.

Murray, R.B., & Zentner, J.P. (1997). *Nursing assessment and health promotion strategies through the lifespan.* (6th ed.). Norwalk, CT: Appleton & Lange.

Tierney, Jr., L., McPhee, S.J., & Papadakis, M.A. (2004). *Current Medical Diagnosis & Treatment* (44th ed.). New York: McGraw Hill.

Uphold, C.R., & Graham, M.V. (2003). *Clinical guidelines in family practice.* (4th ed.). Gainesville, FL: Barmarrae Books.

U.S. Preventive Services Task Force. (1996). *Guide to clinical preventive services.* (2nd ed.) Washington, D.C.: Office of Disease Prevention and Health Promotion, U.S. Government Printing Office.

Yates, J. (2005). Traveler's diarrhea. *American Family Physician, 71,* 2095-2100.

Zoorob, R., Anderson, R., & Cafala, C. (2001). Cancer screening guidelines. *American Family Physician*, 63, 1101-1112.

Zuber T. J. (2001). Flexible sigmoidoscopy. *American Family Physician*, 63: 1375-80, 1383-1384, 1385-1388.

8

HEALTH PROMOTION: PEDIATRIC

Health Promotion: Pediatric

PRIMARY, SECONDARY, TERTIARY PREVENTION

The US Preventive Services Task Force's Guide to Preventive Services (2nd edition, 1996) defines ***primary preventive measures*** as "those provided to individuals to prevent the onset of a targeted condition." (pp. xli).

Example: Routine MMR administration to a healthy, 12 month old

The US Preventive Services Task Force's Guide to Preventive Services (2nd edition, 1996) defines ***secondary preventive measures*** as those which "identify and treat asymptomatic persons who have already developed risk factors or preclinical disease, but in whom the disease has not become clinically apparent." (pp. xli).

Example 1: Screening mammogram in a 50 year old female

Example 2: Screening for elevated cholesterol levels

Tertiary preventive measures are used in patients with established clinical disease. The purpose of the measures is to minimize complications associated with the disease, prevent progression of the disease, and/or to restore the patient to his highest possible level of functioning.

Example 1: Use of cholesterol lowering medications in a patient with coronary artery disease

Example 2: Use of an oral anti-hyperglycemic medication in a diabetic patient to achieve normal blood sugar values

TANNER STAGES OF PHYSICAL DEVELOPMENT

FEMALE BREASTS

- **STAGE 1**
  - ◊ Prepubertal: papilla elevated above chest wall
- **STAGE 2**
  - ◊ Breast bud stage: breast and papilla form small mound, areola increases in diameter
- **STAGE 3**
  - ◊ Breast and areola enlarge, no separation in contours
- **STAGE 4**
  - ◊ Secondary mound formed by areola and papilla about at level of breast
- **STAGE 5**
  - ◊ Adult breast: nipple projects, areola becomes part of contour of breast

MALE GENITALIA

- **STAGE 1**
  - ◊ Testes one centimeter, scrotum and penis are size seen in early childhood
- **STAGE 2**
  - ◊ Slight enlargement of testes (2-3 centimeters), scrotum becomes reddened and textured
- **STAGE 3**
  - ◊ Further testicular growth (3-4 centimeters), slight enlargement of penis
- **STAGE 4**
  - ◊ Penis increases in length and diameter, testes enlarge (4-5 centimeters)
- **STAGE 5**
  - ◊ Adult genitalia, (testes 5 centimeters)

PUBIC HAIR

- **STAGE 1**
  - ◊ No pubic hair present
- **STAGE 2**
  - ◊ Sparse, lightly pigmented, straight along border of labia/base of penis

- **STAGE 3**
  - ◊ Hair becomes more pigmented, coarse, curled, and more abundant
- **STAGE 4**
  - ◊ Pubic hair is abundant but covers smaller area than found in adult (in females, not found on medial surface of thigh)
- **STAGE 5**
  - ◊ Adult hair distribution, female distributed as reverse triangle
- **STAGE 6**
  - ◊ Hair grows up linea alba

NEWBORN
(Birth to One Month)

TERMS

- Preterm: gestational age less than 37 weeks
- AGA (appropriate for gestational age): preterm or term babies whose measurements are between the 10th and 90th percentiles
- SGA (small for gestational age): refers to babies whose measurements fall below the 10th percentile
- LGA (large for gestational age): refers to babies whose lengths and weights are above 90th percentile regardless of age

NEWBORN ASSESSMENT/SCREENING:

- Charts for male and female infants and children can be found: www.cdc.gov/growthcharts

Growth should always be plotted on growth charts.

NORMAL ASSESSMENT/SCREENING

- **LENGTH**
  - ◊ Average is 20 inches
- **WEIGHT**
  - ◊ Always compare weight with gestational age
  - ◊ Average is 7.5 lbs
  - ◊ Weight between 6-12 lbs
  - ◊ Babies lose 10% of birth weight in first 3 or 4 days of life
- **HEAD**
  - ◊ Circumference measured at largest circumference above the ears
  - ◊ Average is 13 to 14 inches (33.0-35.6 cm)

***Hydrocephalus*: an excess amount of CSF which accumulates in the ventricles.**
***Microcephalus*: a skull that is abnormally small and is usually associated with mental retardation.**

  - ◊ Cranial molding: occurs with vertex delivery due to overriding of cranial bones at the sutures
  - ◊ Breech delivery: swelling and ecchymosis to presenting part, absence of cranial molding

***Caput succedaneum*: swelling and/or ecchymosis of the scalp over the presenting part, resolves within a few days**
***Cephalhematoma*: accumulation of blood which produces swelling that does not cross suture lines, disappears over several weeks to months**

  - ◊ Fontanels
    - * Posterior (1 cm in diameter) rarely palpable at birth, closes by 2 months of age, slight depression is normal
    - * Anterior (2-3 cm in diameter) remains palpable until 9-18 months, slightly depressed is normal

The anterior fontanel should always be open at birth and about the size of your thumbnail.

- **EYES**
  - ◊ Red reflex should be present bilaterally
  - ◊ Absent red reflex may indicate congenital cataracts, retinoblastoma
  - ◊ PERRL
  - ◊ Chemical conjunctivitis due to silver nitrate or erythromycin ointment may be seen
  - ◊ Purulent eye discharge usually associated with gonococcus, chlamydia, or herpes

- ◊ Eyes should open symmetrically but may appear puffy (normal)
- ◊ Disconjugate gaze is normal in the newborn
- ◊ Retinopathy of prematurity (formerly called retrolental fibroplasia): develops in premature infants presumably related to use of high oxygen concentrations, apnea, and sepsis. Resulting blindness is irreversible.
- ◊ Hypertelorism (wide set eyes): present in Down syndrome

Newborns see best at about 12 inches.

- **EARS**
  - ◊ Assess risk factors for hearing problems: NICU admission for ≥ 2 days, congenital CMV, herpes, or rubella infections, bilirubin ≥20 mg/dL, family history of hearing problems, abnormalities of the pinna and ear canal
  - ◊ Inspect ears for positioning
    - * Low set ears: may indicate renal or genetic abnormality, multisystem syndrome
  - ◊ Assess gross hearing by observing for startle response to loud noise
  - ◊ Auditory evoked response testing for high risk patients

- **NARES**
  - ◊ Patency assessed by closing mouth and each naris separately or passing small catheter into nasopharynx

No nasal flaring should be present.

- **MOUTH**
  - ◊ Palate: intact
  - ◊ Cleft palate: a fissure in the mid palate usually associated with the clef lip
  - ◊ Access frenulum length

Short frenulum makes tongue movement difficult and impedes speech.

- ◊ Short frenulum makes tongue movement difficult and impedes speech
- ◊ Epstein's pearls: small, white, cysts on the palate and gums; common
- ◊ Natal teeth sometimes present: possible risk of aspiration if very loose

- **NECK**
  - ◊ Webbing: excessive amounts of skin seen in Turner's and Noonan's syndromes
  - ◊ Masses: thyroglossal cysts, hematoma in the sternocleidomastoid muscle
  - ◊ Torticollis: turning of head to one side due to shortening of the sternocleidomastoid muscle

- **CLAVICLE**
  - ◊ May be fractured in LGA babies delivered vaginally, usually resolves without treatment
  - ◊ Crepitus sometimes present if clavicle fractured
  - ◊ Decreased movement of arm on affected side, if clavicle fractured
  - ◊ Ecchymosis visible from injury

- **HEART**
  - ◊ Normal rate is 120-160 beats per minute
  - ◊ Murmurs common (only 10% are significant)
  - ◊ Marked sinus arrhythmia (normal)
  - ◊ Femoral pulses equal and strong

Coarctation of the aorta should be suspected when femoral pulses are unequal or weak.

- ◊ Dextrocardia, situs inversus: assess PMI location to rule out
- ◊ Cardiac murmurs may present with cyanosis or heart failure

- **SKIN**
  - ◊ No jaundice should be present at birth
  - ◊ Lanugo: fine, dark, hair over the trunk and shoulders; seen in prematurity
  - ◊ Vernix: white, greasy, thick material found on infant's skin; seen in prematurity
  - ◊ Milia: multiple, tiny (1 mm) papules on the forehead, cheeks, and nose; common
  - ◊ Acrocyanosis: bluish skin changes to feet and hands normal during first few days of life due to heat loss

Observe for peripheral cyanosis which usually indicates cardiac or respiratory problems.

- ◊ Meconium staining may occur if first stool is passed in utero. Infant's skin and fingernails may be stained

- ◊ "Stork bite" on nape of neck, eyelids; common
- ◊ Mongolian spot (hyperpigmented nevi): usually in sacral and gluteal area; common

- **ABDOMEN**
  - ◊ No masses or distention should be present
  - ◊ Palpate kidneys to assess for agenesis or hypoplasia
  - ◊ Umbilical hernia should be easily reducible if present; common
  - ◊ Umbilical stump should fall off by the 14th day
  - ◊ Failure to pass meconium stool within 24 hours of birth is abnormal

- **GENITALIA (MALE)**
  - ◊ Urethral opening should be at the tip of penis (*see* Hypospadias)

Circumcision is delayed for hypospadias because foreskin may be used during repair.

  - ◊ Palpate scrotum for presence of testes (*see* Cryptorchidism)
  - ◊ Testes descended into scrotum or able to be retrieved to scrotum. Must be monitored. If unable to palpate, refer to urologist.
  - ◊ Hydrocele is common (identify by transillumination of scrotum)
  - ◊ Assess for inguinal hernia

- **GENITALIA (FEMALE)**
  - ◊ Labia and vagina should be patent
  - ◊ White discharge may be present (normal), small amount blood tinged discharge may be present (normal for the first few days)

Ambiguous genitalia always abnormal.

- **PATENT ANUS AND RECTUM**

- **HIP DYSPLASIA** (*see* Orthopedic Disorders)

- **FOOT ABNORMALITIES**
  - ◊ Foot curvatures often due to intrauterine molding (in-toeing and out-toeing)
  - ◊ Tibial curvatures (seldom pathologic)
    - * *genu varum*: bowleg
    - * *genu valgum*: knock-knee
  - ◊ Club foot (talipes): talipes equinovarus most common, foot is plantar flexed, inverted, and significantly adducted (may require casting in the nursery if severe)
  - ◊ Metatarsus adductus: adduction of the forefoot (no treatment needed usually)

- **NEUROLOGICAL**
  - ◊ Muscle tone: observe tone, symmetry, and movement
  - ◊ Assess spine for spinal bifida, pilonidal dimple
  - ◊ Reflexes
    - * Moro
    - * Palmar grip
    - * Rooting
    - * Sucking
    - * Stepping/placing response
  - ◊ Cranial Nerves (CN)
    - * CN II (optic): assessed by checking response to bright light (squinting)
    - * CN III (oculomotor), IV (trochlear), VI (abducens): tested by observing infant's ability to gaze in all directions
    - * CN V (trigeminal), IX (glossopharyngeal), X (vagus), and XII (hypoglossal): tested by observing sucking and swallowing
    - * CN VII (facial): tested by observing symmetrical facial movements during crying
    - * CN VIII (acoustic): tested by observing startle reaction to loud noise

- **SCREENING**
  - ◊ Phenylketonuria (PKU)
  - ◊ Congenital hypothyroidism
  - ◊ Hemoglobinopathy
  - ◊ Ideal time for screening of PKU is 24 hours after birth because metabolites may not have been produced before this time

- **NEWBORN DEVELOPMENT**
  - ◊ Observe interaction of parent(s) with infant for feeding, holding, and caring for baby
  - ◊ Observe baby's suck reflex and/or attachment
  - ◊ Observe response to sound, blinking, crying, parents' voice, and face
  - ◊ Posture should be flexed

- **ANTICIPATORY GUIDANCE**
  - ◊ Newborn infant will feed every 2-3 hours. Awaken to feed if 4 hours have elapsed without feeding.
  - ◊ Breastfed and formula fed infants usually do not require vitamin D supplementation. Supplementation is needed if the lactating woman's diet is lacking in vitamin D or if formula is not vitamin D fortified and the infant does not have adequate exposure to sunlight.

NEVER place infants < 6 months of age in direct sunlight.

  - ◊ Discuss car seat use (rear facing in the back seat; center placed is safest until 20 pounds *and* 1 year of age)
  - ◊ Place infant on back or side for sleeping

Do not place pillows in infant's crib and always place sides of crib in "up" position.

  - ◊ Never leave unattended while changing diaper. Do not use baby powder.
  - ◊ Discuss importance of smoke free environment with caregiver
  - ◊ Review signs and symptoms of illness and course of action: fever, dehydration, vomiting, jaundice, etc.
  - ◊ Discuss cord care
  - ◊ Discuss circumcision if applicable
  - ◊ Discuss frequency of bowel movements/wet diapers
  - ◊ Use clothing/blanket to maintain body temperature

TWO MONTHS

- **NORMAL GROWTH/ASSESSMENT SCREENING**
  - ◊ Length: one inch per month
  - ◊ Weight: about one ounce per day
  - ◊ Head circumference: 0.5 inches per month
  - ◊ Plot all on growth chart

- **EYES**
  - ◊ Red reflex bilaterally
  - ◊ Dacryostenosis (*see* Ophthalmic Disorders)
  - ◊ Dacryocystitis; common
  - ◊ Assess for strabismus
  - ◊ Assess ability to visually track object

- **EARS**
  - ◊ Assess gross hearing

- **MOUTH**
  - ◊ Assess suck reflex
  - ◊ Check for oral candidiasis

- **HEART**
  - ◊ Evaluate for presence of cardiac murmurs
  - ◊ Evaluate femoral pulses bilaterally for coarctation of the aorta

- **SKIN**
  - ◊ Assess for cradle cap
  - ◊ Assess for diaper rash
  - ◊ Assess for atopic dermatitis if family history
  - ◊ Assess for signs of abuse

- **ABDOMEN**
  - ◊ Assess for abdominal masses
  - ◊ Assess for umbilical hernia

- **GENITALIA (MALE)**
  - ◊ Assess for bilaterally descended testes
  - ◊ Identify hydrocele by transillumination
  - ◊ Assess for inguinal hernia

- **GENITALIA (FEMALE)**
  - ◊ Assess for labial adhesions

- **MUSCULOSKELETAL**
  - ◊ Assess for hip dysplasia
  - ◊ Assess for torticollis
  - ◊ Assess for metatarsus adductus

- **NEUROLOGICAL**
  - ◊ Check palmar grasp
  - ◊ Check plantar grasp

- ◊ Check Moro reflex
- ◊ Check stepping response
- ◊ Assess rooting reflex
- ◊ Check for tonic neck ("fencing" reflex appears at 2-3 months)
- ◊ Assess Babinski reflex

- **SCREENING**
  - ◊ Assess gross hearing
  - ◊ Assess lead risk
  - ◊ Developmental screening (e.g., Denver Developmental Screening Tool)

- **DEVELOPMENT**
  - ◊ Infant should focus on face
  - ◊ Grasps rattle if placed in hand
  - ◊ Smiles, coos
  - ◊ Able to lift head 45° and has some control when torso held upright

- **ANTICIPATORY GUIDANCE**
  - ◊ Discuss car seat use
  - ◊ Place infant on back/side for sleeping
  - ◊ Review signs and symptoms of illness/course of action
  - ◊ Encourage infant-parent interactions
  - ◊ Encourage parents to take brief periods of time away from baby
  - ◊ No solid foods, do not place cereal in bottle
  - ◊ Do not give honey or plain water in bottle

Honey may expose infant to spores of *Clostridium botulinum*.

  - ◊ Discuss infant care, colic, immunizations and possible side effects

FOUR MONTHS

- **NORMAL GROWTH/ASSESSMENT SCREENING**
  - ◊ Length: one inch per month
  - ◊ Weight: about one ounce per day
  - ◊ Head circumference: 0.5 inches per month
  - ◊ Plot all on growth chart

- **EYES**
  - ◊ Red reflex should be present bilaterally
  - ◊ Dacryostenosis (*see* Ophthalmic Disorders)
  - ◊ Dacryocystitis; common
  - ◊ Assess for strabismus
  - ◊ Assess ability to visually track object

- **EARS**
  - ◊ Assess gross hearing

- **MOUTH**
  - ◊ Assess suck reflex
  - ◊ Assess for presence of oral candidiasis

- **HEART**
  - ◊ Evaluate for presence of cardiac murmurs

- **SKIN**
  - ◊ Assess for cradle cap
  - ◊ Assess for diaper rash
  - ◊ Assess for atopic dermatitis, especially if family history
  - ◊ Assess for signs of abuse

- **ABDOMEN**
  - ◊ Assess for abdominal masses
  - ◊ Assess for umbilical hernia

- **GENITALIA (MALE)**
  - ◊ Assess for bilaterally descended testes
  - ◊ Identify hydrocele by transillumination
  - ◊ Assess for inguinal hernia

- **GENITALIA (FEMALE)**
  - ◊ Assess for labial adhesions

- **MUSCULOSKELETAL**
  - ◊ Assess for hip dysplasia
  - ◊ Assess for metatarsus adductus

- **NEUROLOGICAL**
  - ◊ Check plantar grasp
  - ◊ Assess Moro reflex
  - ◊ Assess stepping response

- ◊ Rooting reflex (disappears by 4 months except during sleep)
- ◊ Check for tonic neck ("fencing" reflex appears at 2-3 months)
- ◊ Assess Babinski reflex

- **SCREENING**
  - ◊ Gross hearing
  - ◊ Assess lead risk
  - ◊ Developmental screening (e.g., Denver Developmental Screening Tool)

- **DEVELOPMENT**
  - ◊ Infant should focus on face
  - ◊ Grasps rattle if placed in hand
  - ◊ Smiles, coos, recognizes caregivers' voice and touch
  - ◊ Able to hold and control head when held upright
  - ◊ No head lag when pulled upright
  - ◊ Raises body on hands
  - ◊ Rolls prone to supine
  - ◊ Follows light 180°

- **ANTICIPATORY GUIDANCE**
  - ◊ Discuss car seat use
  - ◊ Discuss infant care
  - ◊ Discuss teething and measures to soothe painful gums
  - ◊ Avoid bottle propped in bed or held in bed
  - ◊ No vitamin mineral supplement is needed at this time if formula fed or well-nourished Mom who breastfeeds (otherwise, infant may be at risk)
  - ◊ Discuss childproofing home (small, sharp, or dangerous objects, poisons, medications)
  - ◊ Discuss introduction of solid foods: cereal first, then pureed fruit and vegetables
  - ◊ Development of bedtime ritual
  - ◊ Provide age appropriate toys
  - ◊ Play peek-a-boo and pat-a-cake
  - ◊ Have Poison Control Center number in case of accidental ingestion (syrup of ipecac should ONLY be administered when specifically directed by Poison Control Center)

Syrup of ipecac should not be administered:
- * **If ingestion of acids, alkalis, hydrocarbons, sharp objects, or seizure-inducing drugs has occurred**
- * **To children <6 months of age**
- * **In cases of diminished gag reflexes or coma**

SIX MONTHS

- **NORMAL GROWTH ASSESSMENT SCREENING**
  - ◊ Length: grows $^{1}/_{2}$ inch per month
  - ◊ Weight: gains about 3-4 ounces per week; doubled birth weight at this age
  - ◊ Head circumference: 0.25 inches per month
  - ◊ Plot all on growth chart

- **EYES**
  - ◊ Red reflex should be present bilaterally
  - ◊ Dacryostenosis (*see* Ophthalmic Disorders)
  - ◊ Dacryocystitis; common
  - ◊ Assess for strabismus
  - ◊ Assess ability to visually track object

- **EARS**
  - ◊ Assess gross hearing

- **MOUTH**
  - ◊ Assess for tooth eruption
    - * Lower central incisors (6 months)
    - * Lower lateral incisors (7 months)
    - * Upper central incisors (7.5 months)

- **HEART**
  - ◊ Evaluate for presence of cardiac murmurs

- **SKIN**
  - ◊ Assess for cradle cap
  - ◊ Assess for diaper rash
  - ◊ Assess for atopic dermatitis if family history
  - ◊ Assess for signs of abuse

- **ABDOMEN**
  - ◊ Assess for abdominal masses
  - ◊ Assess for umbilical hernia

- **GENITALIA (Male)**
  - ◊ Assess for bilaterally descended testes
  - ◊ Identify hydrocele by transillumination
  - ◊ Assess for inguinal hernia

- **GENITALIA (FEMALE)**
  - ◊ Assess for labial adhesions

- **MUSCULOSKELETAL**
  - ◊ Assess for hip dysplasia
  - ◊ Assess for metatarsus adductus
  - ◊ Assess for flat feet
  - ◊ Assess muscle tone

- **NEUROLOGICAL**
  - ◊ Check plantar grasp
  - ◊ Moro reflex disappearance at about 6 months
  - ◊ Stepping response still present
  - ◊ Rooting (disappears by 4 months except during sleep)
  - ◊ Tonic neck ("fencing" reflex disappears at about 6 months)
  - ◊ Assess Babinski reflex

- **SCREENING**
  - ◊ Gross hearing
  - ◊ Assess for anemia in the following situations
    - * Low socioeconomic status
    - * Birthweight <1500 grams
    - * Low iron formula used (not recommended)
    - * Whole milk prior to 1 year of age (not recommended)
  - ◊ Developmental screening (e.g., Denver Developmental Screening Tool)

- **DEVELOPMENT**
  - ◊ Bears weight and stands when placed
  - ◊ Sits with support/maybe unassisted
  - ◊ Rolls supine to prone
  - ◊ No head lag when pulled upright
  - ◊ Able to place object in opposite hand and in mouth
  - ◊ Recognizes parents
  - ◊ Says "dada" or "baba"
  - ◊ Babbles
  - ◊ Smiles, squeals, laughs, imitates some sounds

- **ANTICIPATORY GUIDANCE**
  - ◊ Discuss childproofing home (small, sharp, or dangerous objects, poisons, medications)
  - ◊ Be aware of hazards at child's level: buckets, electric sockets, etc.
  - ◊ Discuss introduction of solid foods 2-3 times per day. If solid foods have not been introduced, initiate at this age.
  - ◊ Needs iron fortified cereal at least twice daily if breast fed
  - ◊ Needs iron fortified cereal even if infant consumes iron fortified formula
  - ◊ Discuss foods that are a choking hazard (e.g., nuts, hot dogs, whole grapes, hard candy)
  - ◊ Introduce a cup for liquids
  - ◊ Dental care: clean teeth with soft brush and plain water
  - ◊ Fluoride supplements if not sufficient amounts in drinking water www.ada.org/public/topics/fluoride/facts/tables for fluoride supplementation
  - ◊ Use distraction, schedules, and routines as discipline; be consistent
  - ◊ Put baby in bed to sleep while still awake

Baby will learn how to console self when awakens at nighttime.

  - ◊ Play peek-a-boo and pat-a-cake
  - ◊ Provide opportunities for exploring
  - ◊ Do not use baby walkers

NINE MONTHS

- **NORMAL GROWTH/ASSESSMENT SCREENING**
  - ◊ Length: grows $^1/_2$ inch per month
  - ◊ Weight: about 3-4 ounces per week
  - ◊ Head circumference: 0.25 inches per month
  - ◊ Plot all on growth chart

- **EYES**
  - ◊ Red reflex should be present bilaterally
  - ◊ Dacryostenosis (*see* Ophthalmic Disorders)
  - ◊ Dacryocystitis; common
  - ◊ Assess for strabismus
  - ◊ Assess ability to visually track object

- **EARS**
  - ◊ Assess gross hearing

- **MOUTH**
  - ◊ Assess for tooth eruption
    - * Upper lateral incisors

- **HEART**
  - ◊ Evaluate for presence of cardiac murmurs

- **SKIN**
  - ◊ Assess for cradle cap
  - ◊ Assess for diaper rash
  - ◊ Assess for atopic dermatitis if family history
  - ◊ Assess for signs of abuse

- **ABDOMEN**
  - ◊ Assess for abdominal masses
  - ◊ Assess for umbilical hernia

- **GENITALIA (Male)**
  - ◊ Assess for bilaterally descended testes
  - ◊ Identify hydrocele by transillumination
  - ◊ Assess for inguinal hernia

- **GENITALIA (FEMALE)**
  - ◊ Assess for labial adhesions

- **MUSCULOSKELETAL**
  - ◊ Assess for hip dysplasia
  - ◊ Assess for metatarsus adductus
  - ◊ Assess for flat feet
  - ◊ Assess muscle tone

- **NEUROLOGICAL**
  - ◊ Check plantar grasp
  - ◊ Stepping reflex disappears at 9 months
  - ◊ Babinski reflex still intact

- **SCREENING**
  - ◊ Assess gross hearing
  - ◊ Assess lead risk
  - ◊ Assess for anemia: Hemoglobin and/or hematocrit
  - ◊ Developmental screening (e.g., Denver Developmental Screening Tool)

- **DEVELOPMENT**
  - ◊ Crawls, creeps, and scoots
  - ◊ Sits independently
  - ◊ Pulls to stand
  - ◊ Bangs, shakes, drops, and throws objects
  - ◊ Able to feed self with finger foods
  - ◊ Responds to own name and understands a few words
  - ◊ Stranger anxiety develops

- **ANTICIPATORY GUIDANCE**
  - ◊ Discuss childproofing home (small, sharp, or dangerous objects, poisons, medications, etc.)
  - ◊ Be aware of hazards at child's level: buckets, electric sockets, bath tub, check hot water thermostat (setting should be $<$ 120°)
  - ◊ Discuss introduction of mashed foods and finger foods, start table foods
  - ◊ Discuss weaning from bottle
  - ◊ Discuss nuts, hot dogs, whole grapes, hard candy, tough meat, etc. as choking hazards
  - ◊ Fluoride supplements if not sufficient amounts in drinking water
  - ◊ Brush teeth daily and at bedtime
  - ◊ Use distraction as discipline
  - ◊ Limit rules, but enforce consistently
  - ◊ Put baby to bed awake
  - ◊ Play peek-a-boo and pat-a-cake
  - ◊ Provide opportunities for exploring
  - ◊ Do not use baby walkers

TWELVE MONTHS (Toddler)

- **NORMAL GROWTH/ASSESSMENT SCREENING**
  - ◊ Length: grows three inches annually
  - ◊ Weight: gains about 4½ to 6½ lbs annually; should have tripled weight by this time
  - ◊ Head circumference: one inch annually
  - ◊ Plot all on growth chart
  - ◊ Initial dental screening 12-36 months of age (when cooperative)

- **EYES**
  - ◊ Red reflex should be present bilaterally
  - ◊ If dacryostenosis present refer to ophthalmologist
  - ◊ Dacryocystitis; common
  - ◊ Assess for strabismus
  - ◊ Assess ability to visually track object

- **EARS**
  - ◊ Assess gross hearing

- **MOUTH**
  - ◊ Assess teeth for decay and eruption
    - * Lower first molars

- **HEART**
  - ◊ Evaluate for presence of cardiac murmurs
  - ◊ Normal heart rate: 80-160 beats per minute

- **SKIN**
  - ◊ Assess for diaper rash
  - ◊ Assess for atopic dermatitis if family history
  - ◊ "Stork bites" usually disappear by this age
  - ◊ Assess for signs of abuse

- **ABDOMEN**
  - ◊ Assess for abdominal masses
  - ◊ Assess for umbilical hernia

- **GENITALIA (MALE)**
  - ◊ Descended testes (if not descended bilaterally, refer to urologist)
  - ◊ Identify hydrocele by transillumination (if hydrocele still present at this time, refer to urologist)
  - ◊ Assess for inguinal hernia

- **GENITALIA (FEMALE)**
  - ◊ Assess for labial adhesions

- **MUSCULOSKELETAL**
  - ◊ Assess for hip dysplasia
  - ◊ Assess for metatarsus adductus
  - ◊ Assess feet
  - ◊ Assess gait

- **NEUROLOGICAL**
  - ◊ Rooting (may be present up to 12 months during sleep)

- **SCREENING**
  - ◊ Gross hearing
  - ◊ Assess lead risk
  - ◊ Assess for anemia if high risk

Annual PPD recommended if:
*** Low socioeconomic status**
*** Prior exposure to tuberculosis**
*** Foreign birth**

  - ◊ Mantoux skin using purified protein derivative test considered most reliable for tuberculosis screening
  - ◊ Developmental screening (e.g., Denver Developmental Screening Tool)

- **DEVELOPMENT**
  - ◊ Pulls to stand, may take a few steps
  - ◊ Bangs blocks together
  - ◊ Uses pincer grasp and able to point
  - ◊ Says 2-4 words
  - ◊ Looks for dropped or hidden objects
  - ◊ Responds to own name and understands a few words
  - ◊ Feeds self and drinks from cup
  - ◊ Waves and says "bye-bye", "dada", and "mama"
  - ◊ Imitates vocalizations

- **ANTICIPATORY GUIDANCE**
  - ◊ Child car seat can face forward if child weighs at least 20 pounds (seat must remain in car's rear seat)

- ◊ Re-examine home for dangerous objects, poisons
- ◊ Home safety around lawnmowers, moving cars in driveway, animals, streets, pool, bathtub, etc.
- ◊ Provide healthy food choices and 2-3 nutritious snacks daily (expect decrease in appetite)
- ◊ Start on whole milk rather than 2%, fat is needed for adequate brain development

Begin weaning from bottle.

- ◊ Avoid nuts, hot dogs, whole grapes, hard candy, tough meat, etc.
- ◊ Allow toddler to feed self (wash hands often; especially before eating)
- ◊ Fluoride supplements if not sufficient amounts in drinking water
- ◊ Brush teeth daily and at bedtime
- ◊ Do not allow child to bite or hit
- ◊ Limit rules, but enforce consistently
- ◊ Praise, talk, show affection to child
- ◊ Provide opportunities for exploring environment
- ◊ Expect curiosity about genitals

FIFTEEN MONTHS
(Toddler)

- **NORMAL GROWTH/ASSESSMENT SCREENING**
  - ◊ Length: three inches annually
  - ◊ Weight: about 4½ to 6½ lbs annually
  - ◊ Head circumference: one inch annually
  - ◊ Plot all on growth chart
- **EYES**
  - ◊ Red reflex should be present bilaterally
  - ◊ Assess for strabismus
  - ◊ Assess ability to visually track object
- **EARS**
  - ◊ Assess gross hearing
- **MOUTH**
  - ◊ Assess teeth for decay and eruption
    - * Upper first molars (14 months)
    - * Lower cuspids (16 months)
- **HEART**
  - ◊ Evaluate for presence of cardiac murmurs
- **SKIN**
  - ◊ Assess for diaper rash
  - ◊ Assess for nevi, *café au lait* spots, and birth marks which have not disappeared
  - ◊ Assess for signs of abuse
- **ABDOMEN**
  - ◊ Assess for abdominal masses
  - ◊ Assess for umbilical hernia
- **GENITALIA (MALE)**
  - ◊ Assess for bilaterally descended testes
  - ◊ Assess for inguinal hernia
- **GENITALIA (FEMALE)**
  - ◊ Assess for labial adhesions
- **MUSCULOSKELETAL**
  - ◊ Assess for hip dysplasia
  - ◊ Assess for metatarsus adductus
  - ◊ Assess feet
  - ◊ Assess gait
- **SCREENING**
  - ◊ Assess gross hearing
  - ◊ Assess lead risk
  - ◊ Consider PPD if at high risk
  - ◊ Developmental screening (e.g., Denver Developmental Screening Tool)
- **DEVELOPMENT**
  - ◊ Walks well and is able to stoop
  - ◊ Can point to a body part
  - ◊ Says 3-10 words
  - ◊ Stacks two blocks
  - ◊ Follows simple commands
  - ◊ Feeds self and drinks from cup
  - ◊ Points, grunts, pulls to show what he wants
  - ◊ Listens to a story

- **ANTICIPATORY GUIDANCE**
  - ◊ Use toddler car seat in car's rear seat
  - ◊ Re-examine home for dangerous objects, poisons
  - ◊ Recheck home safety
  - ◊ Supervise around lawnmowers, moving cars in driveway, animals, streets, pools, and bathtubs
  - ◊ Provide healthy food choices. Do not force to eat.
  - ◊ Discuss nuts, hot dogs, whole grapes, hard candy, tough meat, etc. as choking hazards
  - ◊ Allow toddler to feed self. Fluoride supplements if not sufficient amounts in drinking water
  - ◊ Brush teeth daily and at bedtime
  - ◊ Do not allow child to bite or hit
  - ◊ Limit rules, but enforce consistently
  - ◊ Praise, talk, show affection to child. Give individual attention.
  - ◊ Provide opportunities for exploring environment
  - ◊ Expect curiosity about genitals

EIGHTEEN MONTHS
(Toddler)

- **NORMAL GROWTH/ASSESSMENT SCREENING**
  - ◊ Length: grows three inches annually
  - ◊ Weight: about 4½ to 6½ lbs annually
  - ◊ Head circumference: one inch annually
  - ◊ Plot all on growth chart

- **EYES**
  - ◊ Red reflex should be present bilaterally
  - ◊ Assess for strabismus
  - ◊ Assess ability to visually track object

- **EARS**
  - ◊ Assess gross hearing

- **MOUTH**
  - ◊ Assess teeth for decay and eruption
    - * Upper cuspids (18 months)
    - * Lower 2nd molars (20 months)

- **HEART**
  - ◊ Evaluate for presence of cardiac murmurs

- **SKIN**
  - ◊ Assess for diaper rash
  - ◊ Assess for nevi, *café au lait* spots, and birth marks which have not disappeared
  - ◊ Assess for signs of abuse

- **ABDOMEN**
  - ◊ Assess for abdominal masses
  - ◊ Assess for umbilical hernia

- **GENITALIA (MALE)**
  - ◊ Assess for inguinal hernia

- **GENITALIA (FEMALE)**
  - ◊ Assess for labial adhesions

- **MUSCULOSKELETAL**
  - ◊ Assess for hip dysplasia
  - ◊ Assess for metatarsus adductus
  - ◊ Assess feet
  - ◊ Assess gait

- **SCREENING**
  - ◊ Assess gross hearing
  - ◊ Assess lead risk
  - ◊ Consider PPD if at high risk
  - ◊ Developmental screening (e.g., Denver Developmental Screening Tool)

- **DEVELOPMENT**
  - ◊ Able to walk backwards
  - ◊ Can throw a ball
  - ◊ Says 15-20 words
  - ◊ Imitates words, uses two word phrases
  - ◊ Points to multiple body parts
  - ◊ Shows affection, kisses
  - ◊ Able to voice 1 or 2 wants
  - ◊ Listens to a story, points and names objects in book
  - ◊ Begins to scribble spontaneously
  - ◊ Stacks 3-4 blocks

- **ANTICIPATORY GUIDANCE**
  - ◊ Use toddler car seat in car's rear seat
  - ◊ Do not place child in front seat of car if airbag is present
  - ◊ Re-examine home for dangerous objects, poisons
  - ◊ Recheck home safety
  - ◊ Supervise around lawnmowers, moving cars in driveway, animals, streets, pools, and bathtubs
  - ◊ Provide healthy food choices. Do not force to eat.
  - ◊ Discuss nuts, hot dogs, whole grapes, hard candy, tough meat, etc. as choking hazards
  - ◊ Allow toddler to feed self with spoon and hands
  - ◊ Should no longer use bottles
  - ◊ Fluoride supplements if not sufficient amounts in drinking water
  - ◊ Brush teeth daily and at bedtime
  - ◊ Do not allow child to bite or hit
  - ◊ Limit rules, but enforce consistently. Reassure child once negative behavior has stopped.
  - ◊ Praise, talk, show affection to child. Give individual attention.
  - ◊ Expect curiosity about genitals
  - ◊ Assess child's readiness for toilet training

TWO YEARS
(Toddler)

- **NORMAL GROWTH/ASSESSMENT SCREENING**
  - ◊ Length: grows three inches annually
  - ◊ Weight: about 4½ to 6½ lbs annually
  - ◊ Head circumference: one inch annually
  - ◊ Plot all on growth chart
  - ◊ Consider initial dental screening (12-36 months of age)

- **EYES**
  - ◊ Red reflex should be present bilaterally
  - ◊ Assess for strabismus
  - ◊ Assess ability to visually track object

- **EARS**
  - ◊ Assess gross hearing

- **MOUTH**
  - ◊ Assess teeth for decay and eruption
    - * Upper 2nd molars (24 months)

- **HEART**
  - ◊ Evaluate for presence of cardiac murmurs

- **SKIN**
  - ◊ Assess for signs of abuse

- **ABDOMEN**
  - ◊ Assess for abdominal masses
  - ◊ Assess for umbilical hernia

- **GENITALIA (MALE)**
  - ◊ Assess for inguinal hernia

- **GENITALIA (FEMALE)**
  - ◊ Assess for labial adhesions

- **MUSCULOSKELETAL**
  - ◊ Assess feet
  - ◊ Assess gait

- **SCREENING**
  - ◊ Assess lead risk
  - ◊ Consider PPD if at high risk
  - ◊ Developmental screening (e.g., Denver Developmental Screening Tool)

- **DEVELOPMENT**
  - ◊ Able to walk up and down stairs one step at a time
  - ◊ Can kick a ball
  - ◊ Says at least 20 words
  - ◊ Imitates words, uses two word phrases
  - ◊ Imitates adults
  - ◊ Follows two step commands
  - ◊ Stacks 5 blocks

- **ANTICIPATORY GUIDANCE**
  - ◊ Use toddler car seat
  - ◊ Re-examine home for dangerous objects, poisons

- ◊ Recheck home safety
- ◊ Supervise closely
- ◊ Provide healthy food choices. Do not force to eat.
- ◊ Fluoride supplements if not sufficient amounts in drinking water
- ◊ Brush teeth daily and at bedtime
- ◊ Begin to encourage self care
- ◊ Limit rules, but enforce consistently. Use time-out for behavior: one minute for each year of age.
- ◊ Toilet train when child is ready
- ◊ Expect curiosity about genitals
- ◊ Limit television viewing time to one hour per day of age appropriate programming

THREE YEARS
(Toddler)

- **NORMAL GROWTH/ASSESSMENT SCREENING**
  - ◊ Length: grows three inches annually
  - ◊ Weight: about 4½ to 6½ lbs annually
  - ◊ Head circumference: one inch annually
  - ◊ Plot all on growth chart
  - ◊ Initial dental screening if not taken place yet

- **EYES**
  - ◊ Red reflex should be present bilaterally
  - ◊ Assess for strabismus
  - ◊ Assess ability to visually track object
  - ◊ Normal vision is 20/50

- **EARS**
  - ◊ Assess gross hearing

- **MOUTH**
  - ◊ Assess teeth for decay and eruption

- **HEART**
  - ◊ Evaluate for presence of cardiac murmurs
  - ◊ Normal heart rate is 80-120 beats per minute

- **SKIN**
  - ◊ Assess for signs of abuse

- **ABDOMEN**
  - ◊ Assess for abdominal masses
  - ◊ Assess for umbilical hernia

- **GENITALIA (MALE)**
  - ◊ Assess for inguinal hernia

- **GENITALIA (FEMALE)**
  - ◊ Assess for labial adhesions

- **MUSCULOSKELETAL**
  - ◊ Assess gait

- **SCREENING**
  - ◊ Vision and hearing if cooperative
  - ◊ Blood pressure screen; taller and heavier children will have higher blood pressure (consult a pediatric BP table)
  - ◊ Assess lead risk if not done previously
  - ◊ Consider PPD if at high risk
  - ◊ Developmental screening (e.g., Denver Developmental Screening Tool)

- **DEVELOPMENT**
  - ◊ Able to jump
  - ◊ Can stand on one foot
  - ◊ Can kick a ball
  - ◊ Able to ride a tricycle
  - ◊ Says name, age, and gender
  - ◊ Knows gender of others
  - ◊ Able to copy a circle, cross
  - ◊ Able to recognize colors

- **ANTICIPATORY GUIDANCE**
  - ◊ Use toddler car seat in car's rear seat
  - ◊ Re-examine home for dangerous objects, poisons
  - ◊ Supervise closely
  - ◊ Provide healthy food choices. Do not force to eat.
  - ◊ Fluoride supplements if not sufficient amounts in drinking water
  - ◊ Brush teeth daily and at bedtime
  - ◊ Encourage self care

- ◊ Limit rules, but enforce consistently. Use time-out for unacceptable behavior: 1 minute for each year of age.
- ◊ Expect curiosity about genitals. Use correct terms when referring to genitals.
- ◊ Limit television viewing time to one hour daily of age appropriate programming
- ◊ Help with fears

FOUR YEARS
(Preschool)

- **NORMAL GROWTH/ASSESSMENT SCREENING**
  - ◊ Length: grows three inches annually
  - ◊ Weight: about 4½ to 6½ lbs annually
  - ◊ Head circumference: one inch annually
  - ◊ Plot all on growth chart

- **EYES**
  - ◊ Red reflex should be present bilaterally
  - ◊ Assess for strabismus
  - ◊ Assess ability to visually track object
  - ◊ Normal vision is 20/40

- **EARS**
  - ◊ Assess gross hearing

- **MOUTH**
  - ◊ Assess teeth for decay and eruption

- **HEART**
  - ◊ Evaluate for presence of cardiac murmurs

- **SKIN**
  - ◊ Assess for signs of abuse

- **ABDOMEN**
  - ◊ Assess for abdominal masses
  - ◊ Assess for umbilical hernia

- **GENITALIA (MALE)**
  - ◊ Assess for inguinal hernia

- **GENITALIA (FEMALE)**
  - ◊ Assess for labial adhesions

- **MUSCULOSKELETAL**
  - ◊ Assess gait

- **SCREENING**
  - ◊ Vision and hearing (should be cooperative)
  - ◊ Blood pressure screen (consult a pediatric BP table)
  - ◊ Assess lead risk if not done previously
  - ◊ Consider PPD if at high risk
  - ◊ Developmental screening (e.g., Denver Developmental Screening Tool)

- **DEVELOPMENT**
  - ◊ Able to sing a song
  - ◊ Can hop on one foot
  - ◊ Able to throw a ball overhand
  - ◊ Able to draw a person with three parts
  - ◊ Able to cut and paste
  - ◊ Able to build a tower with 10 blocks
  - ◊ Says first and last name, age, and gender
  - ◊ Counts to 5
  - ◊ Able to copy a square
  - ◊ Able to dress self with supervision

- **ANTICIPATORY GUIDANCE**
  - ◊ Uses car seat/seat belt depending on size and weight
  - ◊ Teach about stranger safety, neighborhood safety, and teach to swim if around any type of water activities
  - ◊ Re-examine home for dangerous objects, poisons
  - ◊ Continue to supervise closely
  - ◊ Provide healthy food choices. Do not force to eat.
  - ◊ Fluoride supplements if not sufficient amounts in drinking water
  - ◊ Educate about preventive and emergency dental care
  - ◊ Encourage assertiveness, not aggression
  - ◊ Limit rules, but enforce consistently. Use time-out for unacceptable behavior: 1 minute for each year of age.
  - ◊ Expect curiosity about genitals. Use correct terms.

◊ Limit television viewing to one hour per day of age appropriate screening

◊ Enroll in school or some specific learning environment

FIVE YEARS
(Preschool)

- **NORMAL GROWTH/ASSESSMENT SCREENING**
  - ◊ Length: grows 2½ inches annually
  - ◊ Weight: about 5-7 lbs annually
  - ◊ Head circumference: negligible growth
  - ◊ Plot all on growth chart

- **EYES**
  - ◊ Red reflex should be present bilaterally
  - ◊ Assess ability to visually track object
  - ◊ Normal vision is 20/30

- **EARS**
  - ◊ Assess gross hearing

- **MOUTH**
  - ◊ Assess teeth for decay and eruption

- **HEART**
  - ◊ Evaluate for presence of cardiac murmurs

- **SKIN**
  - ◊ Assess for signs of abuse

- **ABDOMEN**
  - ◊ Assess for abdominal masses
  - ◊ Assess for umbilical hernia

- **GENITALIA (MALE)**
  - ◊ Assess for inguinal hernia

- **MUSCULOSKELETAL**
  - ◊ Assess gait

- **SCREENING**
  - ◊ Vision and hearing
  - ◊ Blood pressure (consult pediatric BP table)
  - ◊ Assess lead risk if not done previously
  - ◊ Consider PPD if at high risk
  - ◊ Developmental screening (e.g., Denver Developmental Screening Tool)

- **DEVELOPMENT**
  - ◊ Able to draw a person with body, head, arms, legs
  - ◊ Able to recognize most letters and can print some
  - ◊ Plays make believe
  - ◊ Learns address and phone number
  - ◊ Can define at least one word
  - ◊ Counts on fingers
  - ◊ Able to copy a triangle; knows colors
  - ◊ Able to dress self without help
  - ◊ Able to skip, tiptoe
  - ◊ Begins to understand right and wrong
  - ◊ Plays cooperatively and enjoys playmate's company

- **ANTICIPATORY GUIDANCE**
  - ◊ Uses seatbelt in car's back seat (if weighs 60 pounds or head is higher than back of seat) or booster car seat if doesn't meet weight and height requirements
  - ◊ Teach about personal hygiene
  - ◊ Teach about stranger safety, playground safety, pedestrian safety
  - ◊ Needs after school supervision
  - ◊ Continue to supervise closely
  - ◊ Provide healthy food choices
  - ◊ Fluoride supplements if not sufficient amounts in drinking water
  - ◊ Educate about preventive and emergency dental care
  - ◊ Encourage assertiveness, not aggression
  - ◊ Limit rules, but enforce consistently. Use time-out for unacceptable behavior: 1 minute per year of age.
  - ◊ Encourage self-discipline
  - ◊ Limit television viewing to one hour per day of age appropriate programming
  - ◊ Teach how to resolve conflict and deal with anger appropriately
  - ◊ Household chores

SIX YEARS
(School Age)

- **NORMAL GROWTH/ASSESSMENT SCREENING**
  - ◊ Length: grows 2½ inches annually
  - ◊ Weight: about 5-7 lbs annually
  - ◊ Head circumference: negligible growth
  - ◊ Plot all on growth chart

- **EYES**
  - ◊ Red reflex should be present bilaterally
  - ◊ Assess ability to visually track object
  - ◊ Normal vision is 20/20

- **EARS**
  - ◊ Assess gross hearing

- **MOUTH**
  - ◊ Assess teeth for decay and eruption
    - * Assess for upper and lower first molars
    - * Assess for lower central incisors

- **HEART**
  - ◊ Evaluate for presence of cardiac murmurs
  - ◊ Normal heart rate is 70-110 beats per minute

- **SKIN**
  - ◊ Assess for signs of abuse

- **ABDOMEN**
  - ◊ Assess for abdominal masses
  - ◊ Assess for umbilical hernia

- **GENITALIA (MALE)**
  - ◊ Assess for inguinal hernia

- **MUSCULOSKELETAL**
  - ◊ Assess gait

- **SCREENING**
  - ◊ Vision and hearing
  - ◊ Blood pressure (consult pediatric BP table)
  - ◊ Assess lead risk if not done previously
  - ◊ Consider PPD if at high risk
  - ◊ Developmental screening (e.g., Denver Developmental Screening Tool)

- **SCHOOL PERFORMANCE**
  - ◊ Interview child: Does he like school? What subject does he like the best? Like the least?
  - ◊ Interview parent: Does child keep up with other children at school? Does he follow school rules?

- **ANTICIPATORY GUIDANCE**
  - ◊ Review immunization status
  - ◊ Use seatbelt in back seat of car
  - ◊ Reinforce personal hygiene
  - ◊ Teach about stranger safety, playground safety, pedestrian safety
  - ◊ Needs after school supervision
  - ◊ Continue to supervise closely
  - ◊ Provide healthy food choices. Teach about what constitutes healthy choices.
  - ◊ Fluoride supplements if not sufficient amounts in drinking water
  - ◊ Educate about preventive and emergency dental care
  - ◊ Enforce rules consistently. Have firm rules for acceptable behavior.
  - ◊ Encourage self-discipline
  - ◊ Limit TV watching to one hour per day
  - ◊ Teach how to resolve conflict and deal with anger appropriately
  - ◊ Household chores
  - ◊ Encourage reading
  - ◊ Patient should ask questions daily about school and give individual attention
  - ◊ Answer questions regarding sexuality. Provide age-appropriate books.

EIGHT YEARS
(School Age)

- **NORMAL GROWTH/ASSESSMENT SCREENING**
  - ◊ Use drape for exam
  - ◊ Length: 2½ inches annually
  - ◊ Weight: about 5-7 lbs annually
  - ◊ Head circumference: negligible growth
  - ◊ Plot height/weight on growth chart

- **EYES**
  - ◊ Red reflex should be present bilaterally
  - ◊ Assess ability to visually track object

- **EARS**
  - ◊ Assess gross hearing

- **MOUTH**
  - ◊ Assess teeth for decay and eruption
    - * Assess for upper central incisors (7-8 years)
    - * Assess for lower lateral incisors (7-8 years)
    - * Assess for upper lateral incisors (8-9 years)

- **HEART**
  - ◊ Evaluate for cardiac murmurs

- **SKIN**
  - ◊ Assess for signs of abuse

- **ABDOMEN**
  - ◊ Assess for abdominal masses
  - ◊ Assess for umbilical hernia

- **GENITALIA (MALE)**
  - ◊ Assess for inguinal hernia
  - ◊ Assess Tanner stage

- **GENITALIA (FEMALE)**
  - ◊ Assess for early puberty
  - ◊ Assess Tanner stage

- **MUSCULOSKELETAL**
  - ◊ Assess for scoliosis

- **SCREENING**
  - ◊ Vision and hearing
  - ◊ Blood pressure (consult pediatric table)
  - ◊ Assess lead risk
  - ◊ Consider PPD is at high risk

- **SCHOOL PERFORMANCE**
  - ◊ Interview child: Does he like school? What subject does he like the best? Like the least? How are grades?
  - ◊ Interview parent: Any particular concerns? Reading/doing math at grade level?

- **ANTICIPATORY GUIDANCE**
  - ◊ Uses seatbelt
  - ◊ Reinforce pedestrian, neighborhood, stranger, sports safety
  - ◊ Reinforce personal hygiene
  - ◊ Needs after school supervision and supervision with friends
  - ◊ Provide healthy food choices. Teach about what constitutes healthy choices.
  - ◊ Fluoride supplements if not sufficient amounts in drinking water
  - ◊ Educate about preventive and emergency dental care
  - ◊ Enforce rules consistently. Have firm rules for acceptable behavior. Provide consequences.
  - ◊ Encourage self-discipline
  - ◊ Limit TV watching to one hour per day
  - ◊ Teach how to resolve conflict and deal with anger appropriately
  - ◊ Household chores
  - ◊ Needs personal space
  - ◊ Encourage reading
  - ◊ Parent should ask questions daily about school and give individual attention
  - ◊ Answer questions regarding sexuality. Provide age-appropriate books.

TEN YEARS
(School Age)

- **NORMAL GROWTH/ASSESSMENT SCREENING**
  - ◊ Use drape for exam
  - ◊ Length: grows 2½ inches annually
  - ◊ Weight: about 5-7 lbs annually
  - ◊ Head circumference: negligible growth
  - ◊ Body mass index

- **EYES**
  - ◊ Red reflex should be present bilaterally
  - ◊ Assess ability to visually track object

- **EARS**
  - ◊ Assess gross hearing

- **MOUTH**
  - ◊ Assess teeth for decay and eruption
    - * Assess for lower cuspids (9-10 years)
    - * Assess for first bicuspids (10-11 years)

- **HEART**
  - ◊ Evaluate for presence of cardiac murmurs
  - ◊ Heart rate: 70-110 beats per minute

- **SKIN**
  - ◊ Assess for signs of abuse

- **ABDOMEN**
  - ◊ Assess for abdominal masses
  - ◊ Assess for umbilical hernia

- **GENITALIA (MALE)**
  - ◊ Assess for inguinal hernia
  - ◊ Assess for early puberty
  - ◊ Assess Tanner stage

- **GENITALIA (FEMALE)**
  - ◊ Assess for early puberty
  - ◊ Assess Tanner stage

- **MUSCULOSKELETAL**
  - ◊ Assess for scoliosis

- **SCREENING**
  - ◊ Vision and hearing
  - ◊ Blood pressure (consult pediatric table)
  - ◊ Assess lead risk
  - ◊ Consider PPD if at high risk

- **SCHOOL PERFORMANCE**
  - ◊ Interview child: Does he like school? What subject does he like the best? Like the least? How are grades? Does he participate in extracurricular activities?
  - ◊ Interview parent: Any particular concerns? Reading/doing math at grade level?

- **ANTICIPATORY GUIDANCE**
  - ◊ Uses seatbelt
  - ◊ Reinforce sports safety
  - ◊ Counsel regarding tobacco, alcohol, and drugs
  - ◊ Reinforce personal hygiene
  - ◊ Needs after school supervision and supervision with friends
  - ◊ Provide healthy food choices. Teach about what constitutes healthy choices.
  - ◊ Fluoride supplements if not sufficient amounts in drinking water
  - ◊ Teach about preventive and emergency dental care
  - ◊ Enforce rules consistently. Have firm rules for acceptable behavior. Provide consequences.
  - ◊ Encourage self-discipline
  - ◊ Prepare for sexual development and puberty; encourage abstinence and answer questions
  - ◊ Teach how to resolve conflict and deal with anger appropriately
  - ◊ Household chores
  - ◊ Needs personal space
  - ◊ Encourage reading; parent should ask questions daily about school; give individual attention
  - ◊ Encourage child to pursue talents and likes

EARLY ADOLESCENCE
(11, 12, 13, and 14 years)

- **HISTORY/ASSESSMENT**
  - ◊ Use drape for exam
  - ◊ Allow adolescent to be primary historian
  - ◊ Consider interview and examination alone

- **GROWTH SPURT**
  - ◊ Females: about 11 years of age
  - ◊ Males: about 13 years of age

- **EYES**
  - ◊ Red reflex should be present bilaterally
  - ◊ Assess ability to visually track object

- **EARS**
  - ◊ Assess gross hearing

- **MOUTH**
  - ◊ Assess teeth for decay and tooth eruption
    - * Assess for upper cuspids, lower second bicuspids (11-12 years)
    - * Assess for lower second molars (11-13 years)
    - * Assess for upper second molars (12-13 years)

- **HEART**
  - ◊ Evaluate for presence of cardiac murmurs

- **SKIN**
  - ◊ Assess for signs of abuse, tattoos, acne

- **ABDOMEN**
  - ◊ Assess for umbilical hernia

- **GENITALIA (MALE)**
  - ◊ Assess for inguinal hernia
  - ◊ Assess Tanner stage
  - ◊ Ask about whether "wet dreams" are occurring. Educate regarding same.
  - ◊ Discuss/teach testicular self exam, especially if history of undescended testicles or single testicle
  - ◊ Ask about whether sexually active and about use of birth control, condoms
  - ◊ Gynecomastia, common

- **GENITALIA (FEMALE)**
  - ◊ Assess Tanner stage
  - ◊ Ask about whether periods have started and if regular
  - ◊ Assess for condyloma or lesions
  - ◊ Instruct regarding self breast exam
  - ◊ Ask about whether sexually active and about use of birth control and condoms
  - ◊ Pregnancy history
  - ◊ Annual pelvic exam if sexually active for 3 years or more
    - * Assess for condyloma or other lesions

- **MUSCULOSKELETAL**
  - ◊ Assess for scoliosis

- **SCREENING**
  - ◊ Vision and hearing
  - ◊ Blood pressure
  - ◊ Consider PPD if at high risk
  - ◊ If sexually active: test for sexually transmitted diseases

- **SCHOOL PERFORMANCE**
  - ◊ How are grades? How much school is missed? For what reasons?
  - ◊ Does student participate in extracurricular activities?
  - ◊ Interview parent: Any particular concerns?

- **ANTICIPATORY GUIDANCE**
  - ◊ Counsel regarding adequate sleep, exercise, healthy habits
  - ◊ Encourage healthy food choices
  - ◊ Maintain appropriate weight
  - ◊ Counsel regarding tobacco, alcohol, and drugs. Discuss prevention of substance abuse.
  - ◊ Reinforce personal hygiene
  - ◊ Counsel regarding body changes during puberty, sexual feelings, sexually transmitted diseases
  - ◊ Fluoride supplements if not sufficient amounts in drinking water
  - ◊ Educate about preventive and emergency dental care

- ◊ Enforce rules consistently. Have firm rules for acceptable behavior. Provide consequences.
- ◊ Encourage self-discipline
- ◊ Teach how to resolve conflict and deal with anger appropriately
- ◊ Household chores
- ◊ Needs personal space
- ◊ Parent should ask questions daily about school and after school activities
- ◊ Give individual attention
- ◊ Encourage child to pursue talents and likes. Discuss college, vocational training, military, and careers.
- ◊ Take on responsibilities, learn new skills

MIDDLE ADOLESCENCE
(15, 16, and 17 years)

- **HISTORY/ASSESSMENT**
  - ◊ Use drape for exam
  - ◊ Allow adolescent to be primary historian
  - ◊ Interview and examination alone
  - ◊ Interview parents separately

- **EYES**
  - ◊ Red reflex should be present bilaterally
  - ◊ Assess ability to visually track object

- **EARS**
  - ◊ Assess gross hearing

- **MOUTH**
  - ◊ Assess teeth for decay and tooth eruption
  - ◊ Assess for upper and lower third molars (17-21 years)

- **HEART**
  - ◊ Evaluate for presence of cardiac murmurs

- **SKIN**
  - ◊ Assess for signs of abuse, tattoos, acne

- **GENITALIA (MALE)**
  - ◊ Assess for inguinal hernia
  - ◊ Assess Tanner stage
  - ◊ Gynecomastia common
  - ◊ Reinforce importance of testicular self exam, especially if history of undescended testicles and/or single testicle
  - ◊ Ask about whether sexually active and about use of birth control and condoms

- **GENITALIA (FEMALE)**
  - ◊ Assess Tanner stage
  - ◊ Ask about whether periods are regular and any associated problems
  - ◊ Pregnancy history
  - ◊ Reinforce importance of self-breast exam
  - ◊ Ask about whether sexually active and about use of birth control and condoms
  - ◊ Annual pelvic exam if sexually active for 3 years or more
    - * Assess for condyloma or lesions if sexually active

- **MUSCULOSKELETAL**
  - ◊ Assess for scoliosis

- **SCREENING**
  - ◊ Vision and hearing
  - ◊ Blood pressure
  - ◊ Consider PPD if at high risk
  - ◊ If sexually active: test for sexually transmitted diseases

- **SCHOOL PERFORMANCE**
  - ◊ How are grades? How much school is missed? For what reasons?
  - ◊ Does he participate in extracurricular activities?
  - ◊ Interview parent: Any particular concerns?

- **ANTICIPATORY GUIDANCE**
  - ◊ Counsel regarding adequate sleep, exercise, healthy habits
  - ◊ Car safety: speed limits, seat belt use, abstinence from alcohol, drugs while driving
  - ◊ Encourage healthy food choices. Maintain appropriate weight.

- ◊ Counsel regarding tobacco, alcohol, and drugs. Discuss prevention of substance abuse.
- ◊ Reinforce personal hygiene if appropriate
- ◊ Counsel regarding sexually transmitted diseases, pregnancy, safe sex
- ◊ Fluoride supplements if not sufficient amounts in drinking water (up to age 16 years)
- ◊ Educate about preventive and emergency dental care
- ◊ Enforce rules consistently. Have firm rules for acceptable behavior. Provide consequences.
- ◊ Encourage self-discipline
- ◊ Teach how to resolve conflict and deal with anger appropriately
- ◊ Household chores
- ◊ Needs personal space
- ◊ Parent should ask questions daily about school and after school activities
- ◊ Give individual attention
- ◊ Encourage adolescent to pursue talents and interests; discuss college, vocational training, military, careers
- ◊ Take on responsibilities, learn new skills

LATE ADOLESCENCE
(18, 19, 20, and 21 years)

- **HISTORY/ASSESSMENT**
  - ◊ Use drape for exam
  - ◊ Adolescent is primary historian
  - ◊ Interview and examination alone
  - ◊ Interview parents separately

- **EYES**
  - ◊ Red reflex should be present bilaterally
  - ◊ Assess ability to visually track object

- **EARS**
  - ◊ Assess gross hearing

- **MOUTH**
  - ◊ Assess teeth for decay and eruption
  - ◊ Assess for upper and lower third molars (17-21 years)

- **HEART**
  - ◊ Evaluate for presence of cardiac murmurs

- **SKIN**
  - ◊ Assess for signs of abuse, tattoos, acne

- **GENITALIA (MALE)**
  - ◊ Assess for inguinal hernia
  - ◊ Assess Tanner stage
  - ◊ Gynecomastia (less common than in early adolescence; may be due to drug use)
  - ◊ Reinforce importance of testicular self exam, especially if history of undescended testicles and/or single testicle
  - ◊ Ask about whether sexually active and about use of birth control and condoms

- **GENITALIA (FEMALE)**
  - ◊ Tanner stage
  - ◊ Ask if periods are regular and about any associated problems
  - ◊ Pregnancy history
  - ◊ Reinforce importance of self breast exam
  - ◊ Ask about whether sexually active and about use of birth control and condoms
  - ◊ Annual pelvic exam if sexually active for 3 years or more or at age 21 years
    - * Assess for condyloma or lesions if sexually active

- **MUSCULOSKELETAL**
  - ◊ Assess for scoliosis

- **SCREENING**
  - ◊ Vision and hearing
  - ◊ Blood pressure
  - ◊ Consider PPD if at high risk
  - ◊ If sexually active: test for gonorrhea, chlamydia, HIV, syphilis other sexually transmitted diseases

- **SCHOOL/JOB PERFORMANCE**
  - ◊ How are grades? How much school is missed? For what reasons?
  - ◊ Does he participate in extracurricular activities?
  - ◊ How is job going?

- **ANTICIPATORY GUIDANCE**
  - ◊ Counsel regarding adequate sleep, exercise, healthy habits
  - ◊ Car safety: speed limits, seat belt use, abstinence from alcohol, drugs while driving
  - ◊ Encourage healthy food choices. Maintain appropriate weight.
  - ◊ Counsel regarding tobacco, alcohol, and drugs. Discuss prevention of substance abuse.
  - ◊ Reinforce personal hygiene if appropriate
  - ◊ Counsel regarding sexually transmitted diseases, pregnancy, safe sex
  - ◊ Brush teeth and encourage regular dental care
  - ◊ Enforce rules consistently. Have firm rules for acceptable behavior. Provide consequences.
  - ◊ Encourage self-discipline
  - ◊ Needs personal space
  - ◊ Encourage adolescent to pursue talents and interests
  - ◊ Discuss college, vocational training, military, careers
  - ◊ Take on responsibilities, learn new skills

IMMUNIZATIONS

Recommended Childhood and Adolescent Immunization Schedule

Retrieved from http://www.cdc.gov/nip

FIGURE. Recommended childhood and adolescent immunization schedule,[1] by vaccine and age — United States, 2005

Vaccine	Birth	1 mo	2 mos	4 mos	6 mos	12 mos	15 mos	18 mos	24 mos	4–6 yrs	11–12 yrs	13–18 yrs
Hepatitis B[2]	HepB #1	only if mother HBsAg (-)										
		HepB #2			HepB #3				HepB series			
Diphtheria, tetanus, pertussis[3]			DTaP	DTaP	DTaP		DTaP			DTaP	Td	Td
Haemophilus influenzae type b[4]			Hib	Hib	Hib[4]	Hib						
Inactivated poliovirus			IPV	IPV	IPV					IPV		
Measles, mumps, rubella[5]						MMR #1				MMR #2	MMR #2	
Varicella[6]						Varicella			Varicella			
Pneumococcal[7]			PCV	PCV	PCV	PCV			PCV		PPV	
Influenza[8]					Influenza (yearly)				Influenza (yearly)			
- - - - - - - Vaccines below red line are for selected populations - - - - - - -												
Hepatitis A[9]									Hepatitis A series			

Range of recommended ages | Catch-up immunization | Preadolescent assessment

1. This schedule indicates the recommended ages for routine administration of currently licensed childhood vaccines, as of December 1, 2004, for children aged ≥18 years. Any dose not administered at the recommended age should be administered at any subsequent visit when indicated and feasible. The Catch-up immunization indicates age groups that warrant special effort to administer those vaccines not previously administered. Additional vaccines might be licensed and recommended during the year. Licensed combination vaccines may be used whenever any components of the combination are indicated and other components of the vaccine are not contraindicated. Providers should consult package inserts for detailed recommendations. Clinically significant adverse events that follow immunization should be reported to the vaccine adverse Event Reporting System; guidance is available at http://www.vaers.org or by telephone, 800-822-7967.

2. Hepatitis B (HepB) vaccine. All infants should receive the first dose of HepB vaccine soon after birth and before hospital discharge; the first dose may also be administered by age 2 months if the mother is hepatitis B surface antigen (HBsAg) negative. Only monovalent HepB may be used for the birth dose. Monovalent or combination vaccine containing HepB may be used to complete the series. Four doses of vaccine may be administered when a birth dose is administered. The second dose should be administered at least 4 weeks after the first dose, except for combination vaccines, which cannot be administered before age 6 weeks. The third dose should be administered at least 16 weeks after the first dose and at least 8 weeks after the second dose. The final dose in the vaccination series (third or fourth dose should not be administered before age 24 weeks. **Infants born to HBsAg positive mothers** should receive HepB and 0.5 ml of hepatitis B immune globulin (HBIG) at separate sites within 12 hours of birth. The second dose is recommended at age 1-2 months. The final dose in the immunization series should not be administered before age 24 weeks. These infants should be tested for HBsAg and antibody to HBsAg at age 9-15 months. **Infants born to mothers whose HBsAg status is unknown** should receive the first dose of the HepB series within 12 hours of birth. Maternal blood should be drawn as soon as possible to determine the mother's HBsAg status; if the HBsAg test is positive, the infant should receive HBIG as soon as possible (no later than age 1 week). The second dose is recommended at age 1-2 months. The last dose in the immunization series should not be administered before age 24 weeks.

3. Diphtheria and tetanus toxoids and acellular pertussis (DTaP) vaccine. The fourth dose of DTaP may be administered as early as age 12 months, provided 6 months have elapsed since the 3rd dose and the child is unlikely to return at age 15-18 months. The final dose in the series should be administered at age ≥4 years. Tetanus and diphtheria toxoids (Td) is recommended at age 11-12 years if at least 5 years have elapsed since the last dose of tetanus and diphtheria toxoid-containing vaccine. Subsequent routine Td boosters are recommended every 10 years.

4. Haemophilus influenzae type b (Hib) conjugate vaccine. Three Hib conjugate vaccines are licensed for infant use. If PRP_OMP (PedvaxHIB® or ComVax® (Merck) is administered at ages 2-4 months, a dose at age 6 month is not required. DTaP/Hib combination products should not be used for primary immunization in infants at ages 2, 4, or 6 months but can be used as boosters after any Hib vaccine. The final dose in the series should be administered at age ≥12 months.

5. Measles, mumps, and rubella (MMR) vaccine. The second dose of MMR is recommended routinely at age 4-6 years but may be administered during any visit, provided at least 4 weeks have elapsed since the first dose and both doses are administered beginning at or after age 12 months. Those who have not previously received the second dose should complete the schedule by age 11-12 years.

6. Varicella vaccine. Varicella vaccine is recommended at any visit at or after age 12 months for susceptible children (i.e., those who lack a reliable history of chickenpox). ≥13 years should receive 2 doses administered at least 4 weeks apart.

7. Pneumococcal vaccine. The heptavalent pneumococcal conjugate vaccine (PCV) is recommended for all children aged 2-23 months and for certain children ages 24-59 months. The final dose in the series should be administered at age ≥12 months. Pneumococcal polysaccharide vaccine (PPV) is recommended in addition to PCV for certain groups at high risk. See MMWR 2000;49(No. RR-9).

8. Influenza vaccine. Influenza vaccine is recommended annually for children aged >6 months with certain risk factors (including, but not limited to asthma, cardiac disease, sickle cell disease, human immunodeficiency virus (HIV), and diabetes), health-care workers, and other persons (including household members) in close contact with persons in groups at high risk (see MMWR 2004;53(No. RR-6)). In addition, healthy children aged 6-23 months and close contacts of healthy children aged 0-23 months are recommended to receive influenza vaccine because children in this age group are at substantially increased risk for influenza-related hospitalizaions. For health persons aged 5-49 years, the intranasaly administered, live, attenuated influenza vaccine (LAIV) is an acceptable alternative to the intramuscular trivalent inactivated influenze vaccine (TIV). See MMWR 2004;53(No. RR-6). Children receiving TIV should be administered a dosage appropriate for their age (0.25mL if aged 6-35 months or 0.5 mL if aged ≥3 years). Children aged ≤8 years who are receiving influenza vaccine for the first time should receive 2 doses (separately by at least 4 weeks for TIV and at least 6 weeks for LAIV).

9. Hepatitis A vaccine. Hepatitis A vaccine is recommended for children and adolescents in selected states and regions and for certain groups at high risk; consult your local public health authority. Children and adolescents in these states, regions, and groups who have not been immunized against hepatitis A can begin the hepatitis A immunization series during any visit. The 2 doses in the series should be administered at least 6 months apart. See MMWR 1999;48(No. RR12).

Immunization schedules are updated in January of each year. Refer to www.cdc.gov/nip for the latest schedules.

References

American Academy of Pediatrics. (2003). *Red book: Report of the committee on infectious disease* (26th ed.). Elk Grove Village, IN: American Academy of Pediatrics.

Behrman, R.E., Kliegman, R.M., Arvin, A.M., & Nelson, W.E. (Eds.). (1995). *Nelson textbook of pediatrics* (15th ed.). Philadelphia: W.B. Saunders.

Biagilli, F. (2005). Child safety seat counseling: Three keys to safety. *American Family Physician, 72*, 473-478.

Bickley, L.S., & Szilagyi, P.G. (2003). *Bates' guide to physical examination and history taking* (8th ed.). Philadelphia: Lippincott Williams & Wilkins.

Branch, W.T. (2003). *Office practice of medicine* (4th ed.). Philadelphia: Saunders.

Burns, C.E., Brady, M.A., Blosser, C., Starr, N.B., & Dunn, A.M. (2004). *Pediatric primary care: A handbook for nurse practitioners* (3rd ed.). Philadelphia: W.B. Saunders.

Centers for Disease Control and Prevention. (2005). Recommended childhood and adolescent immunization schedule. *MMWR*, vol. 53, no. 51 & 52.

Graber, M.A., & Lanternier, M.L. (Eds.). (2001). *The family practice handbook.* (4th Ed.). St. Louis: Mosby.

Houde, S. C. & Melillo, K. D. (2000). Physical activity and exercise counseling in primary care. *The Nurse Practitioner*, *25*(8), 9-37.

Kliegman, R.M. (1996). *Practical strategies in pediatric diagnosis and therapy*. Philadelphia: W.B. Saunders .

Mathur, A., & Kamat, D. (2005). Travel risks: How to help parents protect infants and young children. *Consultant, 45(8)*, 900-904.

Mladenovic, J. (Ed.). (2003). *Primary care secrets.* (3rd Ed.). Philadelphia: Hanley and Belfus.

Murray, R.B., & Zentner, J.P. (1997). *Nursing assessment and health promotion strategies through the lifespan.* (6th ed.). Norwalk, CT: Appleton & Lange.

Schwartz, M.W. (Ed.). (2002). *The 5 minute pediatric consult.* (2nd ed.) Philadelphia: Lippincott Williams & Wilkins.

U.S. Public Health Service, Bureau of Maternal and Child Health. (1994). *Bright futures: Guidelines for health supervision of infants, children, and adolescents.* Washington, D.C.: Author.

Uphold, C.R., & Graham, M.V. (2003). *Clinical guidelines in family practice.* (4th ed.). Gainesville, FL: Barmarrae Books.

9

HEMATOLOGIC PROBLEMS

Hematologic Problems

**Denotes pediatric diagnosis*

IRON DEFICIENCY ANEMIA

DESCRIPTION

Microcytic, hypochromic anemia which occurs when iron loss exceeds intake of iron and subsequently, iron stores become depleted. Associated with chronic blood loss.

> **Microcytosis: red blood cell is smaller than average (<80fL)**
> **Hypochromia: describes a decreased amount of hemoglobin found in red blood cells**

ETIOLOGY

Common causes:

- Heavy menses
- GI bleeding
- Decreased iron intake; especially vegetarians
- Gastrointestinal cancer
- Increased iron requirements
- Pregnancy
- Lactation
- Poor iron absorption

INCIDENCE

- 7-10% of adult population
- Females > Males
- Most common type of anemia in U.S.
- Most common anemia in infancy and childhood, especially at 9-24 months of age (10-20%)

RISK FACTORS

- *See* Etiology
- Infants and toddlers
- Adolescents
- Pregnancy
- Low birthweight infant
- Chronic ASA, NSAID use

ASSESSMENT FINDINGS

- Asymptomatic
- Tinnitus
- Headache
- Dyspnea on exertion
- Fatigue
- Tachycardia
- Palpitations
- Inability to concentrate
- Irritability in young children
- Pallor (best seen in conjunctivae)
- Koilonychia (spoon-shaped, brittle nails)
- Cold intolerance
- Frequent infections
- Pica (craving for ice, starch, clay, or other unusual substance)

DIFFERENTIAL DIAGNOSIS

- α- and β- thalassemia trait
- Sideroblastic anemia
- Gastric carcinoma (especially in the elderly)
- Anemia of chronic disease
- Hypothyroidism
- Renal failure
- Lead toxicity

DIAGNOSTIC STUDIES

- Hemoglobin: decreased for age, <12 g/dL in adults
- RBC: decreased
- Mean corpuscular volume (MCV): decreased (<80 fl)
- Red cell distribution width (RDW): increased

> **MCV: describes the size of the average RBC**
> **Anisocytosis: describes the variability of RBC size**
> **RDW: measure of the variability of the RBC size**

- Serum ferritin: decreased (best non-invasive test in adults)
- Serum iron: decreased
- Total iron-binding capacity (TIBC): increased
- Reticulocyte count: increased

> **TIBC: ability of the RBC to bind circulating iron**
> **Reticulocyte count: measure of the ability of the bone marrow to produce RBCs**

- Peripheral smear: hypochromic, microcytic red blood cells, anisocytosis, poikilocytosis
- Bone marrow aspiration is gold standard for diagnosis, but rarely needed
- As indicated to diagnose underlying problem

Poikilocytosis: describes different RBC shapes

PREVENTION

- Screening recommended for pregnant women and high-risk infants
- Adequate intake of iron in diet
- Infant diet should include iron-fortified formula and cereal
- Breastfed infants should receive iron supplementation from age 4 months of age
- Smoking cessation or avoidance

NONPHARMACOLOGIC MANAGEMENT

- Diet rich in foods containing protein and iron (e.g., meat, dried beans, dark green, leafy vegetables)
- Increase fiber in diet to counteract constipating effect of iron replacement therapy

Patient education about Iron Replacement

Teach patients about iron replacement therapy:

Take 1-2 hours before meals on empty stomach for greatest absorption

Take with meals if GI upset occurs, but be aware that this decreases iron absorption

Do not take concomitantly with antacids, tetracycline, dairy products

Bowel movements will be very dark in color

Iron is highly toxic, keep out of children's reach

Place iron drops in back of mouth to reduce staining of teeth in infants and young children

Administration of iron with vitamin C enhances absorption

- Transfusion of packed red blood cells indicated if anemia severe and patient symptomatic
- Energy conservation with frequent rest periods
- Attempt to identify hidden source of bleeding

Food may reduce absorption of iron by 50%.

PHARMACOLOGIC MANAGEMENT

AGENT	ACTION	COMMENTS
Iron *Examples:* ferrous sulfate (≈ 20% iron) Feosol® ferrous gluconate (≈ 12% iron) Fergon® ferrous fumarate (≈ 33% iron) Femiron®, Feostat®	Iron is poorly absorbed but incorporated into RBCs in hemoglobin, myoglobin, and many enzymes	Approximately 10% of iron intake is absorbed. During anemic states, the body absorbs 2-3 times more. Generally, 4-6 months of iron replacement are needed to correct iron deficiency anemia.

Adults need about 180 mg of elemental iron daily during anemic states.
Children need about 3 mg/kg/d during anemic states.

PREGNANCY/LACTATION CONSIDERATIONS

- Common during pregnancy
- Iron supplementation almost always needed

CONSULTATION/REFERRAL

- If hemoglobin not increased after one month of iron replacement therapy, referral dependent on underlying cause

FOLLOW-UP

- Repeat hemoglobin one month after therapy initiated
- Dependent on underlying cause

EXPECTED COURSE

- Rapid hematological response is typical
- Curable with iron therapy, but recurrence common unless underlying cause successfully managed

POSSIBLE COMPLICATIONS

- Congestive heart failure
- Tissue hypoxia
- Neurological and intelligence deficits in children

ANEMIA OF CHRONIC DISEASE

DESCRIPTION

Mild to moderate normochromic, normocytic (usually, but can be microcytic) anemia associated with chronic disease. Red blood cell life span is shortened from the normal 120 days to 60-90 days.

Normocytic: describes an average size of RBC
Normochromia: describes the average amount of hemoglobin found in red blood cells

ETIOLOGY

- Unknown

INCIDENCE

- Most common in elderly with chronic illness
- Also seen in children with chronic illness

RISK FACTORS

- Presence of chronic infectious, inflammatory, and/or malignant disease

ASSESSMENT FINDINGS

- Dependent on underlying disease
- Asymptomatic
- Dyspnea on exertion
- Fatigue
- Headache
- Anorexia
- Weight loss
- Lightheadedness after mild exercise

DIFFERENTIAL DIAGNOSIS

- Iron deficiency anemia
- Thalassemia
- Sideroblastic anemia

DIAGNOSTIC STUDIES

- CBC with peripheral smear: normocytic, normochromic red blood cells; leukocytosis common
- Hemoglobin: 7-11 g/dL range
- Serum iron: decreased
- Total iron-binding capacity (TIBC): normal to slightly decreased
- Transferrin saturation: usually decreased
- Serum ferritin: normal or increased
- Red cell distribution width (RDW): normal (11.5-14.5%)
- Mean corpuscular volume (MCV): normal or slightly decreased
- Reticulocyte count: normal or decreased

MANAGEMENT

- Treatment aimed at control of underlying disease process
- Administration of iron is not indicated
- Transfusion of packed red blood cells (PRBC) indicated if patient becomes very symptomatic
- Energy conservation with frequent rest periods

CONSULTATION/REFERRAL

- As needed for management of underlying chronic condition

FOLLOW-UP

- As needed for evaluation and management of underlying chronic condition

EXPECTED COURSE

- Dependent on underlying chronic condition

POSSIBLE COMPLICATIONS

- Worsening of underlying chronic condition

GLUCOSE-6-PHOSPHATE DEHYDROGENASE DEFICIENCY
(G-6-PD Deficiency)

DESCRIPTION

Normocytic anemia caused by absence of glucose-6-phosphate dehydrogenase (G-6-PD). Congenital sex-linked red blood cell enzyme deficiency which leaves the patient susceptible to hemolysis after ingestion of substances with oxidant properties.

ETIOLOGY

- X-linked recessive disorder

INCIDENCE

- Most prevalent in persons of Mediterranean and African descent
- 16% of African-American males are affected and 1-2% of females
- Affects >200 million people

RISK FACTORS

- Mediterranean or African descent
- Family history of G-6-PD deficiency

ASSESSMENT FINDINGS

- Symptoms develop 24-48 hours after ingestion of substances that have oxidant properties
- Pallor
- Jaundice
- Dark urine

DIFFERENTIAL DIAGNOSIS

- α- and β-thalassemia trait
- Sideroblastic anemia
- Anemia of chronic disease
- Hypothyroidism
- Lead toxicity

DIAGNOSTIC STUDIES

- Hemoglobin/hematocrit: decreased during acute episode
- Mean corpuscular volume: normal
- G-6-PD level: decreased
- Peripheral smear: Heinz bodies

PREVENTION

- Screening of persons with risk factors

MANAGEMENT

- Teach patients to avoid the following substances
  - ◊ Antimalarials (primaquine, chloroquine)
  - ◊ Sulfonamides
  - ◊ Phenacetin
  - ◊ Aspirin
  - ◊ Chloramphenicol
  - ◊ Nitrofurantoin

- ◊ Furazolidone
- ◊ Trimethoprim-sulfamethoxazole (Bactrim®)
- ◊ Fava beans
- Packed red cell transfusion may be necessary

CONSULTATION/REFERRAL

- Refer to hematologist

EXPECTED COURSE

- Excellent prognosis if diagnosed early and person avoids substances that cause hemolysis

POSSIBLE COMPLICATIONS

- Severe anemia

LEAD TOXICITY
(Plumbism, Lead Poisoning)

DESCRIPTION

Occurs as a result of exposure to lead, characterized by sideroblastic anemia

Sideroblastic anemia occurs when iron is not able to be incorporated into the heme molecule.

ETIOLOGY

- Exposure to lead either by ingestion or inhalation

INCIDENCE

- Most common in children under 5 years of age
- May occur in adults

RISK FACTORS

- Residing or frequent visitation to home built before 1960
- Sibling or playmate with lead toxicity
- Child of adult with occupational exposure
- Living near busy highway or hazardous waste dump
- Ingestion of soil containing lead (pica)
- Member of occupation associated with lead over exposure (plumbers, pipe fitters, welders, firing range workers, painters)

ASSESSMENT FINDINGS

Mild:
- Intermittent abdominal pain
- Irritability
- Lethargy
- Mild fatigue
- Myalgias
- Paresthesias
- Learning disorders in children

Moderate:
- Constipation
- Diffuse abdominal pain
- General fatigue
- Headache
- Loss of libido
- Tremor
- Vomiting
- Weight loss

Severe:
- Abdominal colic due to abdominal muscle spasm
- Metallic taste in mouth
- Coma
- Encephalopathy
- Lead lines
- Motor neuropathy (wrist drop)
- Oliguria
- Renal failure
- Seizures

DIFFERENTIAL DIAGNOSIS

- Iron deficiency anemia
- Mental retardation
- Seizure disorder
- Colic
- Acute abdominal pain

- Encephalopathy

DIAGNOSTIC STUDIES

- Lead level >10 mg/dL is considered abnormal (screen is a finger stick)
- Abnormal finger stick screening values should be confirmed by venipuncture test
- Hemoglobin and hematocrit: slightly decreased
- Serum creatinine: elevated
- Erythrocyte protoporphyrin: elevated
- Urinalysis

PREVENTION

- Screening of children at risk for lead exposure at 10-14 months of age & then again at 2 years
- Primary prevention in workplace:
    - ◊ Engineering controls: substitution of less hazardous material, isolation via containment structure, appropriate ventilation
    - ◊ Personal protective equipment: respirator
    - ◊ Work practices: removal of lead accumulation, personal hygiene practices, periodic inspection/maintenance of control equipment

LEAD LEVEL INTERPRETATION	
Level	**Interpretation**
≤9 μg/dL	Unexposed or normal
10-40 μg/dL	Acceptable levels for long-term exposure, retest in 6 months
40-50 μg/dL	Close observation and follow-up indicated, retest in 2 months
≥50 μg/dL *on average of last three levels or* ≥60 μg/dL	Removal from exposure, retest within 1 month

NONPHARMACOLOGIC MANAGEMENT

- Increased iron and Vitamin C intake in diet
- Remove source of lead exposure
- Removal of worker from exposure if level ≥60 μg/dL
- Reportable to local health department

PHARMACOLOGIC MANAGEMENT

- Lead chelation agent as indicated by lead levels and clinical manifestations (oral or parenteral)
- Oral agent approved for chelation in children: succimer (Chemet®)
- Iron supplementation

CONSULTATION/REFERRAL

- If lead chelation therapy required

EXPECTED COURSE

- If detected early, excellent prognosis

POSSIBLE COMPLICATIONS

- Lead encephalopathy

In children:

- Decreased IQ scores
- Poor muscle coordination
- Shortened attention span
- Increased incidence of behavior problems

SICKLE CELL ANEMIA

DESCRIPTION

A group of genetic disorders characterized by chronic severe hemolytic anemia resulting from destruction of brittle erythrocytes; associated with intermittent episodic events (crises). Sickle cell trait is usually asymptomatic without anemia.

Sickle shaped red blood cells are inflexible, very fragile, and increase the blood's viscosity. Patients should always be well hydrated to help prevent crises.

ETIOLOGY

- Inherited autosomal recessive disorder

INCIDENCE

- Most common of the clinically significant hemoglobinopathies
- Affects more than 50,000 Americans
- 1 in 500 African-Americans have sickle cell disease
- 1 in 1000 Hispanics have sickle cell disease
- 1 in 10 African-Americans carry sickle cell trait
- Also seen to lesser degree in persons from Mediterranean area

RISK FACTORS FOR CRISIS

- Hypoxemia
- Infection
- Dehydration
- Fever

ASSESSMENT FINDINGS

- Asymptomatic in early months of life
- Pallor
- Hand-foot syndrome (symmetric, painful swelling of the hands and feet in infants and young children)
- Failure to thrive
- Acute painful vaso-occlusive episodes, especially of bones, joints, abdomen, and back
- Delayed maturation (physical and sexual); Males > Females
- Increased incidence of streptococcal infections
- Frequency of complications and secondary damage increases with age

DIFFERENTIAL DIAGNOSIS

- Other hemoglobinopathies (e.g., thalassemia)
- Other causes of acute pain in bones, joints, and abdomen (e.g., rheumatic fever, rheumatoid arthritis, osteomyelitis, acute abdomen, leukemia)

DIAGNOSTIC STUDIES

- Sickledex is the screening test; if positive then Hemoglobin electrophoresis
- Sickle cell disease: Hb S predominates and Hb A absent
- Sickle cell trait: Hb S and A are present
- Peripheral smear: few irreversibly sickled RBCs, polynucleated RBCs

PREVENTION

- *See* Risk Factors
- Screening of all high-risk infants for sickle cell disease
- Screening of couples preconceptually

NONPHARMACOLOGIC MANAGEMENT

- Regular dental care
- Regular developmental assessment
- Keep immunizations up to date
- Good hydration at all times
- Family should have a "sick day plan" (includes early identification of infection and immediate treatment)
- Usual childhood activities
- Hospitalization for crises
- Maintenance of good nutrition and adequate hydration
- Avoid smoking/alcohol
- Patient/family education about importance of prompt, aggressive treatment of infections
- Teach early recognition of complications

PHARMACOLOGIC MANAGEMENT

- Prophylactic penicillin BID from 2 months until at least 5 - 6 years of age (may consider continuing until puberty)
- Folic acid supplementation
- NSAIDs for pain management in milder crises
- Narcotic analgesics may be needed for pain control during severe crises
- Polyvalent pneumococcal vaccine
- Routine childhood immunizations

PREGNANCY/LACTATION CONSIDERATIONS

- Highest risk during third trimester and delivery
- Fetal mortality: 35-40%
- Complications during pregnancy: increased number and severity of crises, eclampsia, infections, pulmonary infarction, phlebitis
- Increased risk of prematurity, intrauterine growth restriction, and fetal death
- Best managed by perinatal team in tertiary care center

CONSULTATION/REFERRAL

- Refer to hematologist
- Refer for genetic counseling

FOLLOW-UP

- Dependent on frequency/severity of crises and complications

EXPECTED COURSE

- Anemia is chronic and lifelong
- Frequent complications occur during adolescence and twenties
- Most common causes of death: infections, embolic events
- Life expectancy of persons with sickle cell trait is not affected

POSSIBLE COMPLICATIONS

- Body image and sexual identity problems

- Low self-esteem
- Priapism
- Aseptic necrosis of femoral head
- Skin ulcerations
- Cardiomegaly
- Abnormal hepatic function
- Infarcts: splenic, cerebral, pulmonary, bone
- Hematuria
- Retinopathy
- Chronic pulmonary disease
- Pneumonia
- Meningitis
- Pyelonephritis
- Sepsis

THALASSEMIA

DESCRIPTION

A group of hereditary disorders that causes an overproduction of specific chains in the hemoglobin molecule. These chains tend to aggregate and precipitate in red blood cells causing premature red blood cell hemolysis. These anemias are characterized by hypochromia and microcytosis.

There are two main types and multiple variants:

- *β*-thalassemia: deficient synthesis of *β*-globin chains causing severe anemia, classified by severity and clinical type:
  - ◊ Major (Cooley's anemia, homozygous *β*-thalassemia): very severe disease; rarely live to adulthood
  - ◊ Intermedia: less severe disease; normal lifespan but delayed puberty
  - ◊ Minor (trait, heterozygous β-thalassemia): the least severe disease and most common form; normal lifespan
- *α*-thalassemia: deficient synthesis of *α*-globin chains causing mild anemia with variable degrees of clinical disease

ETIOLOGY

- Autosomal recessive

INCIDENCE

- Occurs throughout the U.S.
- Prevalent in the Mediterranean region, Middle East, India, African, and Southeast Asia
- Thalassemia trait affects 3-5% of above ethnic groups

RISK FACTORS

- Family history

ASSESSMENT FINDINGS

β-thalassemia major:

- Usually becomes symptomatic about 3 months after birth
- Pallor
- Failure to thrive
- Increased respiratory rate
- Fatigue
- Splenomegaly/hepatomegaly
- Pathological fractures

α- and β-thalassemia minor: (trait)

- Asymptomatic
- Mild pallor
- Mild splenomegaly

DIFFERENTIAL DIAGNOSIS

- Iron deficiency anemia
- Other microcytic, hypochromic anemias

DIAGNOSTIC STUDIES

β-thalassemia major:

- Red blood cells (RBC): decreased
- Hemoglobin: <5 g/dL
- Hematocrit: may be as low as <10%
- Peripheral smear: microcytosis, hypochromia, target cells

> **Target cell: a red blood cell with a "bull's eye" or "target" in the center of the cell. Normal red blood cells are biconcave discs.**

- Red cell distribution width (RDW): normal or decreased
- Reticulocyte count: increased
- Hemoglobin electrophoresis: used for diagnosis
- Serum ferritin level: normal or increased depending on diet
- Skull and long bone x-rays: cortical thinning and widening of the marrow space

β-thalassemia minor:

- Hemoglobin: slightly decreased or normal
- Hematocrit: 28-40%
- Peripheral smear: microcytosis, hypochromia
- Serum ferritin level: normal or increased
- Hemoglobin electrophoresis: Hgb A_2 increased
- Total iron binding capacity (TIBC): normal
- RBC count: normal or increased
- Reticulocyte count: normal or slightly increased

α-thalassemia trait:

- Peripheral smear: microcytosis, hypochromia
- Hematocrit: 28-40%
- Hemoglobin electrophoresis: used for diagnosis
- Hemoglobin electrophoresis: Hb A_2 normal; Hb F increased

PREVENTION

- Genetic counseling before conception for persons who carry or may be at risk of carrying the gene
- Amniocentesis after 14 weeks gestation

NONPHARMACOLOGIC MANAGEMENT

- Monitor mild cases (alpha and beta thalassemia minor); usually no intervention needed, except, low iron diet
- Regular blood transfusions to maintain hemoglobin >10 g/dL (thalassemia major)
- Splenectomy if hypersplenism is increasing need for transfusions
- Drinking tea will chelate iron and so may be helpful for patients with high iron in diet
- Evaluation of children of adults with thalassemia
- Regular preventive dental care

PHARMACOLOGIC MANAGEMENT

- Deferoxamine (Desferal®): iron chelation therapy for iron overload
- Polyvalent pneumococcal vaccine

PREGNANCY/LACTATION CONSIDERATIONS

- Degree of anemia exacerbated during pregnancy

CONSULTATION/REFERRAL

- Refer for genetic counseling
- Hematologist referral

FOLLOW-UP

- Frequent lifelong monitoring

EXPECTED COURSE

- Thalassemia major: average lifespan 17 years
- Heart failure and infection are leading causes of death
- Thalassemia minor: normal life span

POSSIBLE COMPLICATIONS

β-thalassemia major:
- Chronic hemolysis
- Complications from splenectomy if needed
- Infections, skin ulcerations
- Jaundice
- Enlarged heart
- Cholelithiasis
- Impaired vertical growth
- Delayed onset of puberty
- Hepatomegaly
- Iron overload
- Splenomegaly

VITAMIN B_{12} DEFICIENCY ANEMIA
(Pernicious Anemia, Cobalamin Deficiency)

DESCRIPTION

Macrocytic anemia due to vitamin B_{12} deficiency

Macrocytosis: red blood cell is larger than average (<100 fl)

ETIOLOGY
- Atrophic gastric mucosa
- GI surgery
- Impaired absorption
- Drug induced
- Breastfed infants whose mothers have deficient diets or pernicious anemia

INCIDENCE

- Found mostly in adults >60 years
- Males = Females
- Most prevalent in Scandinavian and English speaking populations

RISK FACTORS

- Inadequate dietary intake (alcoholics, strict vegetarians)
- GI surgery
- Tapeworm infestation
- Malabsorption syndromes (Sprue, Zollinger-Ellison syndrome)
- Medications (e.g., colchicines, oral chelating agents, biguanides, proton pump inhibitors)
- Chronic disease

ASSESSMENT FINDINGS

- Onset gradual, months to years

A Vitamin B_{12} diagnosis starts with an index of suspicion by the health care provider.

Neurological abnormalities:
- Abnormal reflexes
- Ataxia
- Disorientation, memory loss
- Positive Babinski reflex, Romberg's sign
- Dementia
- Weakness/spasticity
- Extremity numbness
- Paresthesias
- Poor finger coordination
- Decreased position and vibratory sense
- Vertigo

Other findings:
- Atrophic glossitis
- Depression
- Dyspnea on exertion
- Hepatomegaly/splenomegaly
- Prematurely graying hair

- Skin becomes waxy
- GI symptoms: diarrhea, constipation, indigestion, anorexia

DIFFERENTIAL DIAGNOSIS

- Alcoholism
- Folic acid deficiency anemia
- Other macrocytic anemias
- Other neurological disorders
- Hepatic dysfunction
- Polypharmacy

DIAGNOSTIC STUDIES

- Mean corpuscular volume (MCV): >110 fl
- Serum vitamin B_{12} level: <100 pg/ml
- Schilling test: decreased vitamin B_{12} absorption
- Peripheral smear: anisocytosis, poikilocytosis

Anisocytosis: variation in red blood cell size
Poikilocytosis: variation in red blood cell shape

- Folate level: 60% of patients with Vitamin B_{12} deficiency have low folate levels (low folate levels impair B_{12} absorption)
- Gastric analysis: achlorhydria
- Howell-Jolly bodies
- Indirect bilirubin: increased
- LDH: increased
- WBC with differential: hypersegmented neutrophils, decreased WBCs
- Serum ferritin: increased or normal
- Platelets: decreased
- Hemoglobin: normal
- Total iron binding capacity (TIBC): normal

PREVENTION

- Index of suspicion, early detection

NONPHARMACOLOGIC MANAGEMENT

- Increased dietary intake of meats, peas and beans, and other protein rich foods
- Educate about lifelong nature of treatment
- Teach patients to give self-injections of vitamin B_{12}

PHARMACOLOGIC MANAGEMENT

- Vitamin B_{12} (cyanocobalamin) intramuscularly administered every day for one week, then weekly for one month, then monthly for life
- Oral Vitamin B_{12} supplementation (not as well absorbed as via intramuscular route)

PREGNANCY/LACTATION CONSIDERATIONS

- Deficiency may be seen secondary to increased demand

CONSULTATION/REFERRAL

- Consult hematologist if resistant to B_{12} therapy

FOLLOW-UP

- Re-evaluate 2 weeks after beginning therapy to determine response
- Monthly vitamin B_{12} injections
- Endoscopy every 5 years (3 fold increase in gastric carcinoma)

EXPECTED COURSE

- Anemia is reversible, but neurologic deficits may not be reversible with treatment if symptoms > 6 months and severe
- Reticulocyte count rapidly increases and peaks in 7-10 days after treatment initiated
- Hematocrit begins to rise within 1 week after beginning treatment

POSSIBLE COMPLICATIONS

- Hypokalemia
- Gastric polyps
- Gastric cancer

FOLIC ACID DEFICIENCY ANEMIA

DESCRIPTION

Macrocytic anemia due to folic acid deficiency

ETIOLOGY

- Inadequate folic acid intake, especially in the elderly, chronically ill, alcoholics, infants on goat's milk, kwashiorkor, marasmus
- Malabsorption syndromes (e.g., sprue, short-bowel syndrome, Celiac disease)
- Increased demand for folic acid (e.g., pregnancy, malignancy, severe psoriasis, rapid growth)
- Decreased folic acid utilization with some drugs (e.g., methotrexate, TMPS (Bactrim®), triamterene, phenytoin)

INCIDENCE

- Most common during ages 60-70 years
- Peak incidence in children is at 4-7 months of age

RISK FACTORS

- *See* Etiology
- Low birthweight infant

ASSESSMENT FINDINGS

- Insidious onset
- Similar clinical and hematologic features as vitamin B_{12} deficiency anemia, but neurological lesions do not occur
- Atrophic glossitis (tongue is red and shiny)
- GI symptoms: indigestion, constipation, diarrhea

Infants:
- Irritability
- Failure to thrive
- Chronic diarrhea

DIFFERENTIAL DIAGNOSIS

- Pernicious anemia

DIAGNOSTIC STUDIES

- Mean corpuscular volume (MCV): >100 fl
- Hematocrit: decreased
- Hemoglobin: normal
- Red cell distribution width (RDW): elevated
- Reticulocyte count: decreased
- Serum folic acid level: decreased, <3 ng/ml
- RBC folate level < 150mg/ml
- Homocysteine levels: elevated because folate needed to convert homocysteine to methionine
- Serum ferritin level: normal
- Total iron binding capacity (TIBC): normal
- Lactic acid dehydrogenase (LDH): elevated
- Vitamin B_{12} level: normal

PREVENTION

- Avoid medications which interfere with folic acid absorption
- Adequate dietary intake of folic acid

NONPHARMACOLOGIC MANAGEMENT

- Increased folic acid intake in diet
- Dietary counseling about foods that are high in folic acid:
  - ◊ green leafy vegetables
  - ◊ fruits
  - ◊ nuts
  - ◊ liver
  - ◊ yeast
  - ◊ mushrooms

PHARMACOLOGIC MANAGEMENT

- Folic acid supplementation orally or parenterally

PREGNANCY/LACTATION CONSIDERATIONS

- Increased demand for folic acid
- Adequate folic acid intake before and during pregnancy important for prevention of neural tube defects in fetus

- Recommended dosage prepregnancy is 0.4-1.0 mg/day

CONSULTATION/REFERRAL

- Usually not needed

FOLLOW-UP

- Re-evaluate in 2 weeks to determine response to therapy and then every month until stable

EXPECTED COURSE

- Rapid increase in reticulocyte count with peak in 7-10 days after therapy started
- Hematocrit should rise within 1 week of initiation of therapy

POSSIBLE COMPLICATIONS

- Failure to thrive

LEUKEMIA
(ALL, ANLL, CML, CLL)

DESCRIPTION

Hyper/hypo proliferation of blast cells in the bone marrow and other tissues with resultant bone marrow failure. The specific type of leukemia is categorized according to the course of the disease and the type of blast cell which predominates.

- Acute lymphocytic leukemia (ALL): principal type of leukemia in children
- Acute nonlymphoblastic leukemia (ANLL)
- Chronic myelocytic leukemia (CML)
- Chronic lymphocytic leukemia (CLL)

ETIOLOGY

- Exact cause unknown
- Some have familial tendency

INCIDENCE

- Account for 33% of pediatric malignancies
- ALL: 75% of all pediatric cases; peaks at 4 years of age
- ANLL: 20% of all cases
- Males > Females
- 70% occurs in adults (CLL and ANLL)

RISK FACTORS

- Family history
- Chromosomal abnormalities
- Exposure to teratogens, carcinogens
- Immunocompromised state
- Chemical and drug exposure, especially nitrogen mustard and benzene
- Cigarette smoking

ASSESSMENT FINDINGS

ALL:

- Symptoms appear acutely and progress rapidly
- Fever
- Bleeding tendencies: petechiae, delayed clotting after injury
- Lymphadenitis
- Pallor
- Fatigue
- Hepatosplenomegaly
- Lymphadenopathy
- Gingival swelling

ANLL:

- Pallor
- Fever
- Infection
- Bleeding
- Hepatomegaly
- Gingival hypertrophy

CML:

- Onset usually insidious
- Splenomegaly
- Weight loss
- Fatigue
- Low grade fever
- Anorexia
- Night sweats
- Visual disturbances

- Priapism

DIFFERENTIAL DIAGNOSIS

- Other diseases of the bone marrow
- Viral or drug induced bone marrow dysfunction

DIAGNOSTIC STUDIES:

- WBC: decreased
- Differential: increased lymphocytes and blast cells
- Platelets: decreased
- Hemoglobin: decreased
- Reticulocyte count: <0.5%
- Erythrocyte sedimentation rate: usually elevated
- LFTs: may be abnormal
- Coagulation profile: can be abnormal; especially in ANLL
- Bone marrow aspiration used for specific diagnosis
- Chest X ray: mediastinal mass

PREVENTION

- Avoidance of known risk factors

NONPHARMACOLOGIC MANAGEMENT

- Radiation/chemotherapy
- Keep well hydrated
- Platelet transfusion if count <20,000 mm^3
- RBC transfusion if patient has symptomatic anemia
- Patient/family education
  - ◊ Screen other family members
  - ◊ Avoid aspirin products
  - ◊ Close temperature monitoring if WBC count <1000
  - ◊ No intense activity or contact sports
  - ◊ Aggressive treatment of infections and potential infections
- Refer patient and family to Leukemia Society of America for educational and supportive resources

PHARMACOLOGIC MANAGEMENT

- Chemotherapy regimens specific for type of leukemia

PREGNANCY/LACTATION CONSIDERATIONS

- Chemotherapy may be used in the second and third trimesters, but plan is specific for type of leukemia

CONSULTATION/REFERRAL

- Refer to oncologist for treatment

FOLLOW-UP

- Close monitoring of WBCs, RBCs, and platelets, other indices as indicated
- Bone marrow studies every week or as appropriate for status
- Follow up bone scans, CT, MRIs as indicated

EXPECTED COURSE

ALL:

- Remission rate is greater than 90% with treatment
- Long-term survival is typical in children

ANLL:

- Remission rate is 60-80% with 20-40% long-term survival

CML:

- Acute form apparent by 24 months
- Poor long term prognosis

CLL:

- Usually asymptomatic early in course of the disease.
- Overall survival is about 9 years after diagnosis

POSSIBLE COMPLICATIONS

- Infection
- Blast crisis

LYMPHOMA

DESCRIPTION

Malignancy of lymphatic system. Two common types:

- Hodgkin: malignant disease of the lymphatic system characterized by presence of Reed-Sternberg cells
- Non-Hodgkin: diverse group of lymphomas

ETIOLOGY

- Unknown
- Evidence of links to viral infections

INCIDENCE

Hodgkin:
- 7900 cases annually
- Males > Females
- Two peak ages: during twenties and again during sixties
- Increased incidence in first-degree relatives and siblings of patients with Hodgkin

Non-Hodgkin:
- Twice as common as Hodgkin
- Peak incidence during sixties

RISK FACTORS

- Immunodeficiency (acquired or inherited)
- Autoimmune disease (lupus, others)
- HIV infection

ASSESSMENT FINDINGS

- Firm, nontender, enlarged lymph nodes in cervical, supraclavicular, axillary, or inguinal areas
- Freely mobile nodes (less common)
- Fever
- Cough
- Night sweats
- Weight loss >10%
- Pruritus
- Fatigue
- Hepatomegaly
- Splenomegaly
- Adenopathy usually asymmetric in Hodgkin
- Non-Hodgkin often has disseminated adenopathy

DIFFERENTIAL DIAGNOSIS

- Hodgkin vs. Non-Hodgkin disease
- Infectious lymphadenopathy (Cat scratch disease)
- Tumor metastasis from other site
- Autoimmune diseases
- Drug reaction

DIAGNOSTIC STUDIES

- Reed-Sternberg cells on biopsy (pathognomonic)
- CBC with differential: anemia
- Peripheral smear
- Chemistry profile
- Erythrocyte sedimentation rate (ESR): elevated
- Liver function tests: elevated
- Renal function tests
- Chest x-ray: mediastinal mass possible
- CT of chest if chest x-ray abnormal
- Bone scan
- Abdominal ultrasound and CT
- Lymph node biopsy
- Bone marrow biopsy

NONPHARMACOLOGIC MANAGEMENT

- Radiation therapy alone or in combination with chemotherapy
- Splenectomy may be done for staging of illness
- Autologous bone marrow transplantation
- Excellent oral hygiene

PHARMACOLOGIC MANAGEMENT

- Chemotherapy
- Interferon
- Polyvalent pneumococcal vaccine

- Influenza immunization

PREGNANCY/LACTATION CONSIDERATIONS

- Diagnosis during pregnancy does not have a negative impact on Hodgkin disease
- Hodgkin does not have a deleterious affect on fetus

CONSULTATION/REFERRAL

- Referral to oncologist/hematologist

FOLLOW-UP

- Monitor CBC and hydration status
- Periodic examination of involved nodes to monitor response to therapy
- Careful follow-up for early detection of relapse

EXPECTED COURSE

Hodgkin:

- Dependent on stage
- 75% overall survival
- Stage I (single node group): 90% five-year survival
- Stage II (two or more node groups on same side of diaphragm): 90% five-year survival
- Stage III (node groups on both sides of the diaphragm): 75% ten-year survival
- Stage IV (dissemination involving extralymphatic organs): 66% ten-year survival

Non-Hodgkin:

- Survival rates not as high as in Hodgkin

POSSIBLE COMPLICATIONS

- Infertility
- Secondary malignancy

IDIOPATHIC THROMBOCYTOPENIA PURPURA (ITP)

DESCRIPTION

Decrease in the number of platelets in the absence of an identifiable cause; all other causes of thrombocytopenia must be ruled out before a diagnosis of ITP can be made.

ETIOLOGY

- Underlying cause unknown
- Defect is due to IgG autoantibodies on platelet surfaces which precipitates autoimmune response

INCIDENCE

- 1/10,000 in U.S.

Acute ITP:

- Predominant age: 2-9 years old
- Increased incidence in fair-skinned children

Chronic ITP:

- Predominant age: > 45 years old
- Females > Males (2:1)

RISK FACTORS

- Acute infection
- Cardiopulmonary bypass
- Hypersplenism
- Pre-eclampsia

ASSESSMENT FINDINGS

- Onset is often acute
- History of viral illness 1-4 weeks prior to onset common in children
- Bleeding can occur with minor accident once platelet count reaches 40,000-60,000 mm^3
- Petechiae, purpura, and/or bruising
- Unusual bleeding in GI and GU tracts
- Epistaxis
- Nonpalpable spleen (if palpable, probably not idiopathic)
- Spontaneous bleeding can occur if platelet count <20,000 mm^3

DIFFERENTIAL DIAGNOSIS

- Thrombocytopenia secondary to another cause
- Medications: > 150 have been identified
- Hemophilia
- Von Willebrand's disease
- Meningococcemia
- Vitamin K deficiency
- Alcohol ingestion
- Lymphoma
- Systemic lupus erythematosus
- Disseminated intravascular coagulation (DIC)

DIAGNOSTIC STUDIES

- Platelet bound IgG antibody: positive in 80% of patients with ITP
- Platelet count: 5,000-75,000/mm^3
- WBC: normal
- Bleeding time: prolonged
- Hematocrit and hemoglobin: normal unless significant blood loss has occurred
- PT, PTT: normal
- Peripheral smear: megathrombocytes
- Bone marrow aspiration: megakaryocytes

PREVENTION

- Avoid unnecessary exposure to medications that inhibit platelet function (e.g., aspirin, heparin), suppress bone marrow

NONPHARMACOLOGIC MANAGEMENT

- Hospitalization for patients with active bleeding
- Consider platelet transfusions
- Splenectomy in patients that fail medical therapy and need prednisone daily to preserve platelets

Pneumococcal vaccine should be administered at least 2 weeks prior to splenectomy.

- Minimal activity to prevent injury or bruising
- No contact sports; especially if spleen is enlarged

PHARMACOLOGIC MANAGEMENT

- Prednisone for 4-6 weeks, then taper off, may need repeat course for chronic ITP

PREGNANCY/LACTATION CONSIDERATIONS

- Prednisone for 10-14 days before delivery
- Thrombocytopenia may be secondary to pre-eclampsia
- Increased fetal mortality

CONSULTATION/REFERRAL

- Surgical referral for splenectomy with medical failure
- Referral to hematologist; especially during pregnancy

FOLLOW-UP

- Frequent platelet counts (daily to weekly depending on severity)

EXPECTED COURSE

Acute ITP:

- 80-85% recover within 4-8 weeks of onset
- 15-20% develop chronic ITP

Chronic ITP:

- Rare spontaneous recovery

POSSIBLE COMPLICATIONS

- 1% mortality due to intracranial bleeding
- Severe blood loss

NEONATAL HYPERBILIRUBINEMIA
(Neonatal Jaundice)

DESCRIPTION

An accumulation of unconjugated bilirubin from destruction of fetal erythrocytes and decreased ability of the liver to excrete this. It is deposited in the skin and sclera and the characteristic yellow color appears.

ETIOLOGY

- Physiologic jaundice
- ABO incompatibility
- Rh incompatibility
- Sepsis
- Breastfeeding

INCIDENCE

- 60% of term infants and 80% of premature infants exhibit jaundice in the first week of life

RISK FACTORS

- Prematurity
- Rh-positive infant of Rh-negative mother
- ABO incompatibility between mother and fetus
- Family history of hemolytic disease

ASSESSMENT FINDINGS

- Yellow tone to sclera, mucous membranes, skin
- Jaundice appears on the head and face first and then progresses to the trunk and extremities
- It resolves in the opposite direction (extremities, trunk, face)

Diagnosis is aided by applying gentle pressure to the baby's skin. Blanching reveals the normal skin color and the contrast in skin color becomes more evident.

- Bright yellow stools
- Jaundice occurs usually on day 2-3 of life in physiological jaundice
- If jaundice occurs within the first 24 hours of life or after the third day, other causes must be investigated

DIFFERENTIAL DIAGNOSIS

- *See* Etiology

DIAGNOSTIC STUDIES

Findings suggesting nonphysiologic hyperbilirubinemia:
- Serum bilirubin rising at rate greater than 5 mg/dL in 24 hours
- Serum bilirubin >20 mg/dL in term infant or 10-14 mg/dL in preterm infant

Elevated bilirubin levels can be neurotoxic.

Other studies:
- Liver function tests
- Coombs' (direct and indirect) to evaluate for Rh and/or ABO isoimmunization
- CBC to assess for infection

PREVENTION

- Early frequent feedings

NONPHARMACOLOGIC MANAGEMENT

- Monitor status closely as long as serum bilirubin levels are < 20 mg/dL
- Good hydration
- Exposure to sunlight
- Phototherapy
- Exchange transfusion
- Treatment of underlying cause if nonphysiologic

EXPECTED COURSE

- Physiologic jaundice resolves spontaneously without sequelae

- 33% of all infants with untreated hemolytic disease and bilirubin levels >30 mg/dL will develop kernicterus

COMPLICATIONS

- Kernicterus
- Mental retardation
- Deafness
- Quadriplegia
- Complications from phototherapy or exchange transfusion

RH INCOMPATIBILITY

DESCRIPTION

- Anti-Rh antibody production in Rh-negative person after exposure to Rh antigen

ETIOLOGY

- Most commonly occurs when an Rh-negative woman carries an Rh-positive fetus

- Blood transfusion of Rh-positive blood to Rh-negative recipient

INCIDENCE

- 15% of Caucasian population is Rh negative
- < 5% of all populations is Rh negative

RISK FACTORS

- Rh-negative mother with Rh-positive fetus
- Any maternal fetal hemorrhage
- Ectopic pregnancy
- Placenta abruptio
- Placenta previa
- Spontaneous/induced abortion
- Blood transfusion

ASSESSMENT FINDINGS

- Jaundice in newborn
- Hemolytic transfusion reaction
- Congenital anemia
- Fetal hydrops

DIFFERENTIAL DIAGNOSIS

- ABO incompatibility
- Isoimmunization from another cause

DIAGNOSTIC STUDIES

- Indirect Coombs': positive in mother
- Direct Coombs': positive in infant

PREVENTION

- Rho(D) immune globulin (RhoGAM®) administered to Rh-negative women:
  - ◊ Routinely at 28 weeks gestation
  - ◊ Routinely within 72 hours after delivery of Rh-positive infant
  - ◊ Anytime maternal fetal hemorrhage occurs
  - ◊ After ectopic pregnancy
  - ◊ After spontaneous/induced abortion

RhoGAM® administration does not eliminate the possibility of incompatibility but decreases the likelihood to less than 1%.

NONPHARMACOLOGIC MANAGEMENT

- Phototherapy
- Exchange transfusion
- Early delivery of affected fetus
- Intrauterine transfusion

PHARMACOLOGIC MANAGEMENT

- Diuretics and digoxin for infant that has developed hydrops fetalis

FOLLOW-UP

- Antibody titer measured frequently during pregnancy in Rh-negative women
- Nonstress testing to determine status of fetus
- Biophysical profile to determine status of fetus

EXPECTED COURSE

- Survival rate of severely affected pregnancies with proper management: 80%-90%
- Fetuses affected by hydrops fetalis have poor prognosis
- Once a woman is isoimmunized, each subsequent pregnancy more severely affected

POSSIBLE COMPLICATIONS

- Hydrops fetalis
- Kernicterus
- Pregnancy loss
- Severe anemia of infant

References

Behrman, R.E., Kliegman, R.M., Arvin, A.M., & Nelson, W.E. (Eds.). (1995). *Nelson textbook of pediatrics* (15th ed.). Philadelphia: W.B. Saunders.

Bickley, L.S., & Szilagyi, P.G. (2003). *Bates' guide to physical examination and history taking* (8th ed.). Philadelphia: Lippincott Williams & Wilkins.

Branch, W.T. (2003). *Office practice of medicine* (4th ed.). Philadelphia: Saunders.

Burns, C.E., Brady, M.A., Blosser, C., Starr, N.B., & Dunn, A.M. (2004). *Pediatric primary care: A handbook for nurse practitioners* (3rd ed.). Philadelphia: W.B. Saunders.

Centers for Disease Control and Prevention. (1997). *Screening young children for lead poisoning: Guidance for state and local health officials.* Atlanta, GA: Centers for Disease Control and Prevention.

Centers for Disease Control and Prevention. (2003). *Surveillance for elevated blood lead levels among children. MMWR,* vol. 52, SS-10.

Dambro, M.R. (2005). *Griffith's 5 minute clinical consult.* Philadelphia: Lippincott Williams & Wilkins.

DeCherney, A.H., & Nathan, L. (2002). *Current obstetric and gynecologic diagnosis and treatment.* New York: McGraw Hall Education.

Goroll, A. H., & Mulley, A. G., Jr. (Eds.). (2000). *Primary care medicine: Office evaluation and management of the adult patient* (4th ed.). Philadelphia: Lippincott Williams Wilkins.

Graber, M.A., & Lanternier, M.L. (Eds.) (2001). *The family practice handbook.* (4th ed.). St. Louis: Mosby.

Griffith, C.J. (1996). Evaluation and management of anemia: A cost-effective approach. *Advance for Nurse Practitioners, 4*(5), 28-35.

Hay, W.W., Levin, M.J., Sondheiner, J.M., & Deterding, R.R. (2004). *Current Pediatric Diagnosis and Treatment* (17th ed.). New York: McGraw-Hill Medical.

Macey, W. H. (2000). A primary care approach to cutaneous T-cell lymphoma. *The Nurse Practitioner*, 25(4): 82-98.

Mangion, S. (2000). *Physical diagnosis secrets.* Philadelphia: Hanley and Belfus.

Manning-Dimmitt, L.L., Dimmitt, S.G., & Wilson, G.R. (2005). Diagnosis of gastrointestinal bleeding in adults. *American Family Physician, 71*, 1339-1345.

Mladenovic, J. (Ed.). (2003). *Primary care secrets.* (3rd Ed.). Philadelphia: Hanley and Belfus.

Rakel, R.E. (Ed.). (1998). *Essentials of family practice.* (2nd ed.). Philadelphia: WB Saunders.

Richer, S. (1997). A practical guide for differentiating between iron deficiency anemia and anemia of chronic disease in children and adults. *The Nurse Practitioner, 22*(4), 82-98.

Schwartz, M.W. (Ed.). (2002). *The 5 minute pediatric consult.* (2nd ed.) Philadelphia: Lippincott Williams & Wilkins.

Shine, J.W. (1997). Microcytic anemia. *American Family Physician, 55*, 2455-2462.

Sickle Cell Disease Guideline Panel. (1993). *Sickle cell disease: Screening, diagnosis, management, and counseling in newborns and infants.* Clinical Practice Guideline No. 6. AHCPR Pub. No. 93-0562. Rockville, MD: Agency for Health Care Policy and Research, Public Health Service, U.S. Department of Health and Human Services.

Staudinger, K., & Rother, V.S. (1998). Occupational lead poisoning. *American Family Physician, 57*(4), 719-726.

Tierney, L.M.,Jr., McPhee, S.J., Papadahis, M.A. (2004) *Current medical diagnosis and treatment* (44th ed.). New York: McGraw-Hill Professional Publishing.

Uphold, C.R., & Graham, M.V. (2003). *Clinical guidelines in family practice.* (4th ed.). Gainesville, FL: Barmarrae Books.

U.S. Preventive Services Task Force. (1996). *Guide to clinical preventive services.* (2nd ed.) Washington, D.C.: Office of Disease Prevention and Health Promotion, U.S. Government Printing Office.

Zollo, A.J., Jr (Ed.). (2004). *Medical Secrets.* (4th ed.), St. Louis, MO: Mosby-Year Book.

10

INFECTIOUS DISEASES

OF THE SKIN, HAIR, NAIL, AND MUCOUS MEMBRANE

Infectious Diseases

Of the Skin, Hair, Nail, and Mucous Membrane

ACNE VULGARIS
(Acne)

DESCRIPTION

Inflammatory disorder of the androgen-dependent sebaceous glands in which excessive amounts of sebum are produced which can lead to comedones, pustules, papules, and scarring.

ETIOLOGY

- Increase in androgen production, especially during puberty; but may have normal androgen production with hypersensitivity
- Increased rate of keratin production which blocks movement of sebum out of the cell
- Presence of bacteria (*Propionibacterium acnes*) which increase inflammatory response

INCIDENCE

- Adolescence (virtually 100% are affected)
- Females > Males in adolescence
- Males may be more severely affected
- Improves in summer

RISK FACTORS

- Family history: 50% have family history
- Adolescence (nearly 100% are affected at some point)
- Caucasians
- Oil-based cosmetics
- Touching face and skin with hands
- Skin contact with chin straps, shoulder pads, telephone receiver
- Hot, humid climates
- Worsens with stress, menses

ASSESSMENT FINDINGS

	Comedonal Acne	Inflammatory Acne	Nodulocystic
Age	Pre-teens and early adolescence	Adolescence and early 20s	Adolescence
Characteristics	Whiteheads (closed comedones)	Pustules Papules, minimal scarring Mild inflammation	Nodules, cysts Moderate to severe inflammation
Infection with P. acnes	Not usually	Usually	Usually

- ***Whiteheads*** (closed comedones) are noninflammatory papules which result from blockage at the follicle neck
- ***Blackheads*** (open comedones) are noninflammatory papules which result from blockage at the follicle mouth. Black color is from oxidized melanin.
- ***P. acnes*** instrumental in inflammation

DIFFERENTIAL DIAGNOSIS

- Acne rosacea
- Folliculitis
- Occupational exposure to grease, tar, or other agents

DIAGNOSTIC STUDIES

- Usually none are indicated

PREVENTION

- Avoid occupational irritants
- Good hand-face hygiene
- Frequent cleansing of the skin and area (too frequent cleansing may lead to irritation)
- Rapid treatment if inflammatory and cystic to prevent scarring

NONPHARMACOLOGIC MANAGEMENT

- Avoid rubbing the skin with hands; avoid occluding the skin with materials like cosmetics, face creams, oily topical preparations (e.g., suntan lotion)
- Cleanse affected area twice daily with mild soap to decrease oil accumulation
- Avoid picking or squeezing lesions
- Reassure patient that acne may take months to improve, but usually will show improvement in 4 weeks
- Sun exposure may help
- Address psychosocial concerns of patient
- Discuss stress management if stress precipitates outbreaks
- Counsel regarding good nutrition (there is no evidence that fatty foods, chocolate, etc. cause acne)

PHARMACOLOGIC MANAGEMENT

Dry or sensitive skin: cream
Oily skin: gel or solution
Hairy area (scalp, eyebrows): lotion

- Systemic antibiotics: oral tetracycline or erythromycin are most commonly used (exhibit anti-inflammatory properties)
- Inflammatory acne (nodulocystic acne)
  - ◊ Treat with isotretinoin (Accutane®) if unresponsive to other measures. Must monitor monthly lipids, liver function tests, and pregnancy status
- Oral contraceptives may be used

AGENT	ACTION	COMMENTS
Keratinolytic Agent ***Tretinoin*** *Example:* Retin-A®	Accelerate turnover of keratin plugs and decreases comedone formation	Do not apply around eyes, nose, and mucous membranes. Increases photosensitivity. Careful use in patients who take other drugs which increase photosensitivity (tetracyclines, thiazides, sulfonamides, fluoroquinolones).
Benzoyl peroxide *Examples:* Benzac®, Brevoxyl®, PanOxyl®	Decrease number of anaerobic bacteria by oxidizing bacterial proteins in the sebaceous follicles	May cause excessive dryness, peeling, and skin irritation. May bleach colors from fabrics. Avoid excessive sun exposure.
Topical Antibiotics ***Clindamycin topical*** *Example:* Clindagel®	Inhibit protein synthesis by binding to the 5OS ribosomal subunits of bacteria	May cause skin to be dry, red, and scaly. Little or no systemic absorption.
Sulfacetamide topical *Examples:* Plexion®, Rosula®, Sulfacet-R®	Inhibit bacterial growth by antagonizing PABA (para-aminobenzoic acid) essential for bacterial growth	Do not use in patients with a sulfa allergy. Avoid contact with eyes, lips, mucous membranes.
Erythromycin topical *Examples:* A/T/R®, Erygel®	Inhibit bacterial protein synthesis by binding to the 5OS ribosomal subunit	May cause skin to be red, dry, or itch. Avoid contact with eyes, lips, mucous membranes.

PREGNANCY/LACTATION CONSIDERATIONS

- Do not use tetracycline in breastfeeding women or pregnant patients
- Isotretinoin (Accutane®)

Isotretinoin (Accutane®) is absolutely contraindicated in pregnancy: associated with severe fetal anomalies. Contraceptive therapy should be used one month before, during, and after treatment with isotretinoin.

- Erythromycin may be safely used during pregnancy; topical preferred over systemic
- Pregnancy may cause remission or exacerbation of acne
- Some oral antibiotics may reduce effectiveness of oral contraceptives

CONSULTATION/REFERRAL

- Severe acne
- Unresponsive acne

FOLLOW-UP

- Monthly visits until adequate response achieved

EXPECTED COURSE

- 4-6 weeks before improvement can be seen
- Treatment may last for months or years
- Gradual improvement as adolescence progresses

POSSIBLE COMPLICATIONS

- Scarring
- Damage to self-image and self-esteem

BACTERIAL INFECTIONS OF THE SKIN (Folliculitis, Furunculosis, Carbunculosis)

DESCRIPTION

Folliculitis	Superficial infection/irritation of the hair follicles. Lesions consist of a pustular or inflammatory nodule which surrounds the hair follicle.
Furunculosis (boils)	Deep infection of the hair follicle. The nodule becomes a pustule which contains necrotic tissue and purulent exudate. Neck, face, buttocks, waistline and breasts are common areas.
Carbunculosis (a cluster of furuncles)	Deep suppurative lesion with extension into the subcutaneous area. The nape of the neck and posterior thigh are common areas.

ETIOLOGY

- Folliculitis, Furunculosis, Carbunculosis: *Staphylococcus aureus* is the most common causative organism; consider MRSA (methicillin resistant *Staph aureus*) very common outpatient pathogen
- Hot tub folliculitis: *Pseudomonas aeruginosa*

INCIDENCE

Folliculitis	Very common in all age groups Tends to recur frequently
Furunculosis (boils)	Common in teenagers & adults Tend to be recurrent
Carbunculosis (a cluster of furuncles)	Males > females Common in at-risk populations (e.g., patients with chronic diseases, the elderly, the immunocompromised)

RISK FACTORS

- *Folliculitis*: poor hygiene, shaving, tight jeans
- *Furunculosis*: adolescence, prior furunculosis, crowded quarters, poor hygiene, diabetes
- *Carbunculosis*: chronic disease, diabetes, alcoholism, advancing age

ASSESSMENT FINDINGS

Folliculitis	Superficial pustule, hair easily removed, mild erythema, inflammation
Furunculosis (boils)	Pustular lesion with central necrosis and a core of purulent exudate, pain, inflammation, and erythema; sometimes spontaneous drainage, but may need incision and drainage
Carbunculosis (a cluster of furunculosis)	Cluster of furunculosis, slow development, fever, local sloughing of tissues, drainage from multiple openings, pain; usually requires incision and drainage

DIFFERENTIAL DIAGNOSIS

- ***Folliculitis***: pseudofolliculitis, furunculosis
- ***Furunculosis***: folliculitis, carbunculosis, hidradenitis suppurativa
- ***Carbunculosis***: folliculitis, hidradenitis suppurativa

DIAGNOSTIC STUDIES

- ***Folliculitis***: usually none
- ***Furunculosis***: usually none; may culture for frequent recurrences
- ***Carbunculosis***: culture

PREVENTION

- Good hygiene
- For recurrent, severe infections
  - ◊ Culture nares, skin, axilla
  - ◊ Use povidone-iodine (Betadine®) or chlorhexidine (Hibiclens®) for full body showers for 1-3 weeks (may cause severe drying of skin)
  - ◊ WARNING: Hibiclens® can cause eye damage!
  - ◊ Change towels and sheets daily
  - ◊ Frequent hand washing

NONPHARMACOLOGIC MANAGEMENT

- ***Folliculitis***
  - ◊ Warm, moist compresses intermittently
  - ◊ Allow spontaneous drainage (excision may cause spread)
  - ◊ Frequent hand washing
- ***Furunculosis***
  - ◊ Warm moist compresses intermittently for pain and to promote spontaneous drainage
  - ◊ Good hygiene and preventive measures listed above
  - ◊ Possible incision and drainage
  - ◊ Consider culture and sensitivity
- ***Carbunculosis***
  - ◊ Good hygiene and preventive measures listed above
  - ◊ Warm moist compresses intermittently
  - ◊ Possible incision and drainage
  - ◊ Packing will promote drainage if wound is deep
  - ◊ Strongly consider culture and sensitivity; especially if immunocompromised or diabetic

PHARMACOLOGIC MANAGEMENT

- ***Folliculitis***
  - ◊ Treatment with an oral antibiotic usually not indicated
  - ◊ May use 5% benzoyl peroxide or a topical antibiotic (mupirocin)
- ***Furunculosis***
  - ◊ Systemic antibiotics do not shorten the duration, but consider for lesions in the facial area; empirically treated with a first-generation cephalosporin; consider TMPS or quinolone for MRSA
- ***Carbunculosis***
  - ◊ Systemic antibiotics (consider first generation cephalosporin: or TMPS or quinolone for MRSA
  - ◊ Warm moist compresses intermittently

AGENT	ACTION	COMMENTS
Cephalosporins (first generation) *Examples:* cephalexin (Keflex®) cefadroxil (Duricef®)	Inhibit cell wall synthesis by bacteria More effective against rapidly reproducing organisms with cell walls	Approximately 2-10% cross-sensitivity between the penicillins (PCN). Inquire about the type of penicillin allergy and do not prescribe cephalosporins if PCN allergy was anaphylactic (Type I).
Sulfa Agent *Examples:* Trimethoprim (TMP)-sulfamethoxazole (SMZ) (Bactrim®, Septra®)	Block synthesis of folic acid by bacteria and thus inhibit bacterial replication	Do not give to pregnant women. Do not use to treat Strep infections. Hypersensitivity reactions like Stevens-Johnson epidermal necrolysis and blood dyscrasias have been associated with sulfa use. Photosensitivity may occur with these drugs.

CONSULTATION/REFERRAL

- Consider referral for furunculosis on face, scalp, and neck
- Consider referral for immunocompromised individuals, diabetics, others with chronic diseases

FOLLOW-UP

- Depends on severity and comorbid conditions

EXPECTED COURSE

- Complete resolution expected
- Recurrences are common
- For recurrences, consider nasal/skin carriage of organism

POSSIBLE COMPLICATIONS

- Cellulitis
- Sepsis
- Scarring

CELLULITIS

DESCRIPTION

Acute, spreading infection of the skin and its subcutaneous structures

ETIOLOGY

- Group A *Streptococcus*
- *Staphylococcus aureus*
- *Haemophilus influenza* (more common in children and often associated with an upper respiratory infection)
- Other organisms depending on cause

INCIDENCE

- Unknown
- Facial (periorbital) cellulitis common in children, elderly

RISK FACTORS

- Prior trauma
- Untreated, undertreated furunculosis
- Burns
- Diabetes mellitus
- Upper respiratory infection in children
- Immunocompromised state

ASSESSMENT FINDINGS

- Most common sites are lower legs and face (face is common site in children)
- Erythema
- Warmth
- Edema
- Pain
- Fever
- Lymphadenopathy

DIFFERENTIAL DIAGNOSIS

- Gout
- Erysipelas (superficial cellulitis)
- Contact dermatitis
- Ruptured Baker's cyst
- Thrombophlebitis

DIAGNOSTIC STUDIES

- Culture and sensitivity
- CBC: mild leukocytosis with a shift to the left
- Blood culture if sepsis suspected
- ESR: elevated

PREVENTION

- Good skin hygiene, especially when there is a break in the skin
- Avoid swimming when skin abrasion present
- Early treatment of upper respiratory infections

NONPHARMACOLOGIC MANAGEMENT

- Elevation of extremity to help prevent edema
- Moist heat for pain relief

PHARMACOLOGIC MANAGEMENT

- Antibiotic specific for organism if culture obtained
- Consider penicillin initially. If allergic, consider first generation cephalosporin or macrolide.

AGENT	ACTION	COMMENTS
Penicillin agents *Examples:* Penicillin-G (Bicillin® L-A) Oxacillin (various) Amoxicillin/clavulanate (Augmentin®)	Inhibit cell wall synthesis of bacteria and are most effective against rapidly reproducing organisms with cell walls	Oxacillin is better choice if suspected organism is Staph. PCN is drug of choice to eradicate Strep. Hypersensitivity reactions to PCN are common. (1-10% occurrence). Monitor for urticaria, bronchospasm. Amoxicillin-clavulanate (Augmentin®) for bites and upper respiratory infection in children because of likelihood of *H. influenzae*

CONSULTATION/REFERRAL

- Consider referral for infections of the face, scalp, or neck; or if sepsis is suspected
- Consider referral for patients with chronic illnesses or who are immunocompromised

FOLLOW-UP

- 48 hours after initial treatment and then as patient condition indicates

EXPECTED COURSE

- Complete resolution expected with appropriate treatment

POSSIBLE COMPLICATIONS

- Septicemia/bacteremia
- Meningitis (from facial cellulitis in children) and cavernous sinus thrombosis
- Superinfection with gram negative organisms

HIDRADENITIS SUPPURATIVA

DESCRIPTION

Inflammation of apocrine glands of the skin which produce tender, cyst-like abscesses. Common sites are the axilla, groin, trunk, and the scalp. They tend to recur.

ETIOLOGY

- Blockage of the apocrine glands leading to rupture of the ducts

INCIDENCE

- Common from late puberty to age 40 years
- Rare in children

RISK FACTORS

- Obesity
- Diabetes mellitus
- African-American females
- Female

ASSESSMENT FINDINGS

- Most frequent place of occurrence: axilla, groin, nipples, and anus
- Pain
- Warmth
- Erythema
- Discharge
- Papules, nodules (1-3 cm)
- Fluctuance (a wave-like impulse felt on palpation) in larger lesions

DIFFERENTIAL DIAGNOSIS

- Furunculosis

DIAGNOSTIC STUDIES

- Culture and sensitivity of lesion exudate

PREVENTION

- Avoid constrictive clothing; especially tight jeans
- Weight loss if indicated
- Good hygiene

NONPHARMACOLOGIC MANAGEMENT

- Aspirate; culture and sensitivity
- Good hygiene
- Avoid antiperspirants (if lesion is in axilla) or other irritants
- Rest
- Moist heat
- Surgical excision for large persistent lesions

PHARMACOLOGIC MANAGEMENT

- Systemic antibiotics not curative; relapse almost always results, base treatment on culture results
- Topical clindamycin
- Oral retinoids: isotretinoin (Accutane®) if recurrent and severe

PREGNANCY/LACTATION CONSIDERATIONS

Isotretinoin (Accutane®) is ABSOLUTELY CONTRAINDICATED in pregnancy: associated with severe fetal anomalies. Contraceptive therapy should be used one month before, during, and after treatment with isotretinoin.

- Do not use tetracycline in pregnant or lactating women

CONSULTATION/REFERRAL

- Consider referral for large lesions and slow healing lesions

FOLLOW-UP

- Depends on severity and patient condition

EXPECTED COURSE

- Rare spontaneous resolution
- Lesions may take a month or more to heal

POSSIBLE COMPLICATIONS

- Scarring
- Recurrences may take years to heal

IMPETIGO

DESCRIPTION

Superficial infection of the skin which begins as small superficial vesicles which rupture and form honey-colored crusts

Superficial infections are usually treated with topical agents unless they span a large surface area. Then, oral agents are usually, more economical.

ETIOLOGY

- *Staphylococcus aureus* (predominant organism)
- Group A β-hemolytic *Streptococcus* (presents in 10-20% of cases)

INCIDENCE

- Common
- Most prevalent in ages 2-5 years
- Summer and fall

RISK FACTORS

- Residing in warm, humid climates
- Insect bites, minor cuts
- Infected family member
- Direct contact with lesions
- Poor hygiene

ASSESSMENT FINDINGS

- 1-2 mm vesicles which rupture
- Honey-colored crusts
- Weeping shallow red ulcer
- Common on mouth, face, nose, or site of insect bites or trauma

DIFFERENTIAL DIAGNOSIS

- Chickenpox
- Folliculitis
- Herpes simplex
- Insect bites
- Dermatitis

DIAGNOSTIC STUDIES

- Usually none required

PREVENTION

- Good hygiene
- Good hand washing, especially by household members

NONPHARMACOLOGIC MANAGEMENT

- Washing of lesions 2-3 times per day
- Good hygiene
- Good hand washing, especially by household members

PHARMACOLOGIC MANAGEMENT

- Antibacterial soap to cleanse lesions
- Topical is preferred: mupirocin ointment (Bactroban®)
- First or second-generation cephalosporin for large area of infection; may consider macrolide if unable to use cephalosporin
- Some resistance to erythromycin encountered in U.S., dicloxacillin (Dynapen®) may be substituted

AGENT	ACTION	COMMENTS
Cephalosporins (first generation) *Examples:* cephalexin (Keflex®) cefadroxil (Duricef®)	Inhibit cell wall synthesis by bacteria	First generation agents are effective against Gram positive organisms like Staph & Strep.
Cephalosporin (second generation) *Examples:* cefprozil (Cefzil®) cefuroxime (Ceftin®)	Inhibit cell wall synthesis by bacteria	Second generation agents are effective against Gram positive and some Gram negative organisms. First and second generation agents will be effective, but > 90% eradication with second-generation agents.

CONSULTATION/REFERRAL

- None usually needed
- Refer for slow to resolve infections

FOLLOW-UP

- 10-14 days from start of treatment
- If no improvement, culture and sensitivity

EXPECTED COURSE

- Complete resolution 7-10 days with treatment

POSSIBLE COMPLICATIONS

- Ecthyma: entire epidermis is infected, crusts are dark-colored
- Poststreptococcal acute glomerulonephritis
- Cellulitis

WARTS

DESCRIPTION

Painless, benign skin tumors

ETIOLOGY

- Human papillomavirus (HPV)
- Different genotypes cause different warts
  - ◊ Common wart: verruca vulgaris
  - ◊ Plantar wart: verruca plantaris

INCIDENCE

- Common, approximately 7-10% of population in U.S.
- Occurs in children and young adults predominantly
- Females > Males

RISK FACTORS

- Skin trauma
- Contact with wart exudate after treatment
- Immunocompromised state

ASSESSMENT FINDINGS

- Common wart: rough surface, elevated, flesh-colored papules
- Plantar wart: rough, flat surface, flesh-colored, 2-3 cm in diameter usually located on sole of foot

DIFFERENTIAL DIAGNOSIS

- Molluscum contagiosum
- Seborrheic keratoses
- Corns
- Basal cell carcinoma
- Condyloma lata

DIAGNOSTIC STUDIES

- Usually none needed

PREVENTION

- Avoid contact with wart exudate from self (auto-inoculation) and others by covering wart
- Avoid skin trauma

NONPHARMACOLOGIC MANAGEMENT

- Paring and debridement of wart prior to any treatment
- Soaking of wart in warm water to soften and moisten it
- Occlude the wart with waterproof tape for one week, leave open to air for 8-12 hours, then re occlude for one week. This creates an environment that is not conducive to growth. Best used for periungual warts.
- Cryotherapy
- Excision

PHARMACOLOGIC MANAGEMENT

- Lactic-salicylic acid (DuoFilm®) daily for 3 months
- Salicylic acid in propylene glycol (Keralyt®): rub into wart daily
- Salicylic acid (Trans-Ver-Sal®) transdermal delivery system
- Benzoyl peroxide BID for 4-6 weeks
- Cimetidine for 3 months
- Podophyllin
- Trichloroacetic acid
- Imiquimod (Aldara®)

CONSULTATION/REFERRAL

- Dermatologist or surgeon for removal if large or if possibility of scarring is likely
- Refer all warts unresponsive to treatment

FOLLOW-UP

- Usually none needed

EXPECTED COURSE

- Resolution with or without treatment

POSSIBLE COMPLICATIONS

- Scarring
- Auto-inoculation
- Nail deformity

HERPES ZOSTER
(SHINGLES)

DESCRIPTION

A reactivation of the varicella-zoster virus (chickenpox virus) that has lain dormant in nerve cells. This involves the skin of a single dermatome or less commonly, several dermatomes.

ETIOLOGY

- Varicella-zoster virus

INCIDENCE

- 215/100,000 annually
- Higher incidence in the elderly, neonates, and immunocompromised patients

- Rarely occurs in children unless immunocompromised

RISK FACTORS

- Advancing age
- Majority of patients have no risk factors
- Immunocompromised status
- Emotional stress
- Spinal surgery or spinal radiation

ASSESSMENT FINDINGS

- *Prodrome*
  - ◊ Itching
  - ◊ Burning
  - ◊ Photophobia
  - ◊ Fever, headache, malaise
- *Acute Phase*
  - ◊ Dermatomal rash erupts over 3-4 days: expect unilateral
  - ◊ Fever, malaise, headache

- ◊ Maculopapular rash which progresses to grouped vesicles on an erythematous base, and then pustules in 3-4 days. Successive crops of vesicles may appear for a week.
- ◊ Pain, possibly severe
- *Convalescent Phase*
  - ◊ Within 2-3 weeks, rash resolves
  - ◊ Pain
  - ◊ May be prolonged in elderly and immunocompromised patients
  - ◊ Postherpetic neuralgia (pain longer than 1 month after rash has resolved) common in the elderly, may last for months

DIFFERENTIAL DIAGNOSIS

- Other viral infections: coxsackievirus, herpes simplex virus, varicella
- Contact dermatitis
- Herniated disc
- Poison ivy
- Early HIV

DIAGNOSTIC STUDIES

- Usually none needed
- Consider HIV testing if patient is young or has multiple eruptions across several dermatomes
- Direct immunofluorescence of viral exudate

PREVENTION

- None at this time
- Elderly, neonates, and immunocompromised should avoid persons with known shingles until lesions have crusted over

NONPHARMACOLOGIC MANAGEMENT

- Wet compresses of Domeboro solution several times per day
- Avoid contact with known patients if member of high-risk group (they can develop chickenpox)

PHARMACOLOGIC MANAGEMENT

- NSAIDs or narcotic analgesics for pain
- Antiviral agents if patient presents within 72 hours of symptoms and is a member of a high-risk group
- Silver sulfadiazine (Silvadene®) or mupirocin (Bactroban®) for secondary infections
- Capsaicin cream (Zostrix®) for postherpetic neuralgia
- Avoid corticosteroids (no decrease in severity, duration, or symptoms) and may increase dissemination
- Amitriptyline, gabapentin may reduce incidence and pain associated with postherpetic neuralgia

AGENT	ACTION	COMMENTS
Antiviral *Examples:* acyclovir (Zovirax®) famciclovir (Famvir®) valacyclovir (Valtrex®)	Inhibit viral DNA synthesis and thus viral DNA replication	Cautious use in patients with renal or hepatic dysfunction. Generally well tolerated. All are Category B drugs.

PREGNANCY/LACTATION CONSIDERATIONS

- Acyclovir, famciclovir, and valacyclovir are all pregnancy category B drugs

CONSULTATION/REFERRAL

- Consult specialist for dermatomes involving the eye, face
- Consider referral for elderly, neonatal, or immunocompromised patients

FOLLOW-UP

- Usually recheck in 3-5 days after diagnosis, then in 1-2 weeks

EXPECTED COURSE

- Resolution of acute phase usually 14-21 days
- Postherpetic neuralgia may last for months

POSSIBLE COMPLICATIONS

- Postherpetic neuralgia
- Superinfection of skin lesions

- Cranial nerve syndromes, especially if the facial or ophthalmic nerves are involved
- Guillain-Barré syndrome
- Corneal ulceration

PARONYCHIA

DESCRIPTION

Skin surrounding finger (nail folds) or toenails becomes infected. May be acute or chronic.

ETIOLOGY

- *Staphylococcus aureus* (most common pathogen)
- *Streptococcus* sp.
- *Pseudomonas* sp.
- *Candida albicans* (chronic paronychia)

INCIDENCE

- Common all ages
- Increased incidence in diabetics
- Female > Male 3:1

RISK FACTORS

- Diabetes
- Trauma to skin around nail or ingrown nails
- Nail biting
- Frequent and continuous wet hands: certain occupations (e.g., hairdressers, dishwashers) are at high risk

ASSESSMENT FINDINGS

- Nail fold separates from nail plate
- Pain around skin of nail plate
- Erythema, tenderness around nail plate
- Changes in nail plate or nail

DIFFERENTIAL DIAGNOSIS

- Psoriasis
- Herpetic whitlow

DIAGNOSTIC STUDIES

- Usually none
- KOH for suspected fungal infection
- Gram stain

PREVENTION

- Avoid long term contact with moisture to hands
- Wear gloves to wash dishes
- Adequate glycemic control in diabetics

NONPHARMACOLOGIC MANAGEMENT

- Keep fingers dry
- Warm compresses or soaks for acute infection
- Incision and drainage if abscess present
- Possible nail removal if severe

PHARMACOLOGIC MANAGEMENT

- Oral antibiotic: dicloxacillin (Dynapen®), erythromycin, cephalexin (Keflex®)
- Topical antifungal for fungal infection
- Oral antifungal for severe fungal infection

CONSULTATION/REFERRAL

- Dermatologist for infection/inflammation which does not resolve after routine treatment

FOLLOW-UP

- Recheck as needed by patient condition

EXPECTED COURSE

- Nails grow slowly, complete resolution when nail plate is effected may take weeks to months

POSSIBLE COMPLICATIONS

- Nail loss
- Thickening and hardening of nail
- Subungual abscess

SCABIES

DESCRIPTION

Infection of human skin by mites

ETIOLOGY

- Infection with *Sarcoptes scabiei*, a human skin mite

INCIDENCE

- Common
- Usually infects children and young adults

RISK FACTORS

- Crowded living conditions
- Skin-to-skin contact with infected patients or infected bedding, cloth furniture, etc.
- Immunocompromised patients

ASSESSMENT FINDINGS

- Itching (more noticeable at nighttime)
- Small itching blisters in a thin line
- Mite burrows between finger webbing, feet, wrists, axilla, scrotum, penis, waist, and or buttocks
- Scaling
- Erythema
- Vesicles, papules
- Vesicles and papules more common on soles and palms in infants
- Mite may be recovered from the burrow

PREVENTION

- Treat all intimate contacts, household contacts, roommates, etc.
- Maintain good personal hygiene
- Launder clothes often
- Wash hands

DIFFERENTIAL DIAGNOSIS

- Atopic dermatitis
- Contact dermatitis
- Insect bites
- Psychogenic causes

DIAGNOSTIC STUDIES

- Burrow ink test (apply a drop of black ink to the rash, then wash off with alcohol, the burrow will remain stained)
- Recovery of mite from the burrow using a 25 gauge needle or #15 surgical blade, visualize microscopically

NONPHARMACOLOGIC MANAGEMENT

- Wash all clothing, bedding, towels, etc.
- Wash toys used prior to treatment and during treatment
- Carpets, floors do NOT need special treatment under usual circumstances

PHARMACOLOGIC MANAGEMENT

- Alternative treatment: lindane (Kwell®) 1% applied to skin (not head) and washed off in 10-12 hours (avoid using in infants)
- Oral antihistamines for itching

AGENT	ACTION	COMMENTS
Topical Scabicides *Example:* permethrin (Elimite®, Rid® spray, Nix®)	Inhibit nerve cell function in the mites/lice producing paralysis and death of the mite/louse	Apply cream or lotion from head to toe excluding mucous membranes. Leave on at least 6 hours before showering off (10 minutes if applied to scalp). Must treat all household members and sexual contacts at the same time. Clothing, bedding, cloth furniture must all be treated. Spray may be used on furniture, mattress, etc.

PREGNANCY/LACTATION CONSIDERATIONS

- Lindane should be used cautiously (if at all) in pregnancy due to the potential neurotoxic effects and potential for convulsions
- Lindane should NOT be used more than twice during pregnancy

CONSULTATION/REFERRAL

- Consider referral to dermatologist for cases resistant to treatment

FOLLOW-UP

- Recheck patient if itching is persistent

EXPECTED COURSE

- Complete resolution after appropriate treatment
- Geriatric patients may itch more severely than other patients
- Itching may prevail beyond infectious period. This is due to antigenic reaction to dead mites and debris which is present under the skin. This does not indicate persistent infection.

POSSIBLE COMPLICATIONS

- Bacterial secondary infections

PEDICULOSIS
(LICE)

DESCRIPTION

An infestation of the body, head, or pubic area by lice

ETIOLOGY

- Lice are ectoparasites which feed on human blood. Nits are the eggs laid by the females which may survive up to 3 weeks when removed from the human host.

Head lice: *Pediculus humanus capitis*
Body lice: *Pediculus humanus corporis*
Pubic lice: *Phthirus pubis*

INCIDENCE

- Head and body lice are more common in children
- Pubic lice are more common in adults
- Females > Males

RISK FACTORS

***Head lice*:**
Crowded conditions, sharing of hats, combs, etc.; poor hygiene is NOT a risk factor
***Body lice*:**
Poor hygiene, infrequent laundering of clothes (lice live and multiply in the seams of clothing), crowded conditions, contact with infected bed linen, towels, clothing etc.
***Pubic lice*:**
Sexual contact with an infected person

ASSESSMENT FINDINGS

- ***Head lice***
  - ◊ Itching, prickly sensation on the scalp
  - ◊ "Dandruff that moves"
  - ◊ Nits are tiny, white spheres (<1 mm long) which are attached to the hair shaft and are immovable. They are found in greater numbers than adult lice.
  - ◊ Back of head, neck, and behind ears are common places of attachment because these are warmer areas of the hair

- ***Body lice***
  - ◊ Pruritus
  - ◊ Papules 2-4 mm in diameter
  - ◊ Skin of the axilla, trunk, and groin are common sites of attachment
- ***Pubic lice***
  - ◊ Pruritus ani
  - ◊ Nits found at the base of pubic hair shafts
  - ◊ Inflammation in groin area, adenopathy
  - ◊ Macular rash in area of infestation
  - ◊ Commonly found in pubic hair but may be spread to other hairy parts of the body

DIFFERENTIAL DIAGNOSIS

- Lice vs. mite infestation
- Dandruff

DIAGNOSTIC STUDIES

- Wood's lamp
  - ◊ Live nits fluoresce white
  - ◊ Empty nits fluoresce gray

PREVENTION

- Launder clothes in hot water
- Nit removal: soak hair in equal parts water & white vinegar for at least 15 minutes
- Good hygiene
- Careful monitoring/treatment by parents and school personnel after lice discovered
- Washing/not sharing combs, hats, bed linens, towels, etc.

NONPHARMACOLOGIC MANAGEMENT

- Patient education about means of transmission and mechanism to break life cycle
- *See* Prevention

PHARMACOLOGIC MANAGEMENT

- ***Head lice***
  - ◊ Synergized pyrethrins: piperonyl butoxide (Rid®) (wash off in 10 minutes)
  - ◊ 1% permethrin (Nix®): most effective treatment
  - ◊ Frequently need repeat treatments
  - ◊ Alternative treatment: lindane (Kwell®): avoid use in pregnant women and infants
- ***Body lice***
  - ◊ Lindane (Kwell®): avoid use in pregnant women and infants
- ***Pubic lice***
  - ◊ Synergized pyrethrins: piperonyl butoxide (Rid®)
  - ◊ 1% permethrin (Nix®): most effective treatment
  - ◊ Alternative treatment: lindane (Kwell®), avoid use in pregnant women and infants
- Eyelash infestation

DO NOT USE ANY MEDICATION LISTED ABOVE!

  - ◊ Manual removal of nits necessary
  - ◊ May use petroleum jelly 3-4 times per day for a week

PREGNANCY/LACTATION CONSIDERATIONS

- Lindane (Kwell®): avoid use in pregnant women due to potential neurotoxic effects and seizure potential

CONSULTATION/REFERRAL

- School personnel
- Parents
- Consult dermatologist for lice unresponsive to treatment

FOLLOW-UP

- Recheck head lice 2-3 days after treatment for presence of nits. If not clear, retreat until clear.

EXPECTED COURSE

- Complete resolution if appropriate treatment and other measures taken

POSSIBLE COMPLICATIONS

- Spread of pubic lice to other area of the body
- Check for STDs if pubic lice present
- Bacterial secondary infections from scratching

TINEA INFECTIONS
(RINGWORM)

DESCRIPTION

Fungal infections affecting various parts of the body.

ETIOLOGY

- *Trichophyton* sp.: most common
- *Microsporum* sp.
- *Epidermophyton* sp.: causative agent for some tinea cruris and tinea pedis infections
- *Pityrosporum* sp.: causative agent for tinea versicolor

INCIDENCE

- Common
- More prevalent in summer months, warm climates

RISK FACTORS

- ***Tinea capitis***
  - ◊ Daycare age group
  - ◊ Contact with infected items (e.g., combs, brushes, hats)
  - ◊ Poor hygiene
- ***Tinea corporis***
  - ◊ Close contact with animals
  - ◊ Warm climates
  - ◊ Obesity
  - ◊ Prolonged use of topical steroids
  - ◊ Immunocompromised state
- ***Tinea cruris***
  - ◊ Wearing wet clothing
  - ◊ Excessive sweating
  - ◊ Obesity
  - ◊ Prolonged use of topical steroids
  - ◊ Immunocompromised state
- ***Tinea pedis***
  - ◊ Occlusive footwear
  - ◊ Damp footwear
  - ◊ Prolonged use of topical steroids
  - ◊ Immunocompromised state
- ***Tinea versicolor***
  - ◊ Hot, humid climates
  - ◊ Wearing wet clothing
  - ◊ Prolonged use of topical steroids
  - ◊ Immunocompromised state

ASSESSMENT FINDINGS

- ***Tinea capitis***
  - ◊ Round patchy scales on scalp
  - ◊ Occasionally alopecia will develop
  - ◊ Most commonly found in pediatric patients
- ***Tinea corporis***
  - ◊ Rash
  - ◊ Pruritus
  - ◊ Well-circumscribed, red, plaque usually found on the trunk
  - ◊ May occur in groups of 3 or more
- ***Tinea cruris***
  - ◊ Pruritus
  - ◊ Well marginated half-moon plaques in the groin and/or upper thighs
  - ◊ May take on eczematous appearance from chronic scratching
  - ◊ Does not affect the scrotum or penis
  - ◊ May appear as vesicles
  - ◊ Rare in pediatric patients before puberty
- ***Tinea pedis***
  - ◊ Itching in interdigital spaces
  - ◊ Maceration in affected areas
  - ◊ Scaling
  - ◊ Can affect the sole and arch
  - ◊ Elderly more susceptible
- ***Tinea versicolor***
  - ◊ Well-marginated lesions of varying colors (white, red, brown); hence the name "versicolor"
  - ◊ Rare itching
  - ◊ Common in axilla, shoulders, chest, back (sebum rich areas)

DIFFERENTIAL DIAGNOSIS

- ***Tinea capitis***: alopecia areata, psoriasis, seborrhea, trichotillomania
- ***Tinea corporis***: pityriasis rosea, psoriasis, atopic dermatitis

- *Tinea cruris*: candidiasis, intertrigo, psoriasis
- *Tinea pedis*: intertrigo, dyshidrosis, psoriasis
- *Tinea versicolor*: pityriasis alba, vitiligo

DIAGNOSTIC STUDIES

- KOH scraping
- Wood's lamp exam (some tinea will not fluoresce, most forms of tinea capitis will not fluoresce)

PREVENTION

- Good personal hygiene
- Identification and treatment of infected humans and pets (tinea capitis and corporis)
- Remove wet clothes as soon as possible
- Dry between toes after showering and bathing
- Avoid direct contact with surfaces in public bathing facilities

NONPHARMACOLOGIC MANAGEMENT

- *Tinea capitis*
  - ◊ Good hygiene
  - ◊ Consider liver function test monitoring for treatment with griseofulvin or another oral antifungal
  - ◊ Teach patients to wear sunscreen and minimize sun exposure because of increased photosensitivity when taking griseofulvin
  - ◊ Treat family members and infected pets
  - ◊ Shaving of head is not necessary for treatment
- *Tinea corporis*
  - ◊ Good hygiene
  - ◊ Avoid contact with lesions
- *Tinea cruris*
  - ◊ Keep area as dry as possible
  - ◊ Do not scratch
- *Tinea pedis*
  - ◊ Dry between toes
  - ◊ Trim dead skin
- *Tinea versicolor*
  - ◊ Keep area as dry as possible

PHARMACOLOGIC MANAGEMENT

- *Tinea capitis*
  - ◊ Oral griseofulvin (Fulvicin®) for 4-6 weeks
  - ◊ Topical antifungals are of no benefit but may decrease time of infectivity
- *Tinea corporis*
  - ◊ Topical antifungal cream: clotrimazole miconazole, others for 2 weeks then re-evaluate
  - ◊ Use for one week after resolution Occurs
- *Tinea cruris*
  - ◊ Topical antifungal creams: tolnaftate, miconazole
  - ◊ Use for at least 10 days even if resolution occurs
- *Tinea pedis*
  - ◊ Topical antifungal cream (clotrimazole, tolnaftate, miconazole, others)
- *Tinea versicolor*
  - ◊ Selenium sulfide shampoo
  - ◊ Topical antifungal creams: clotrimazole, ketoconazole, others for several weeks

AGENT	ACTION	COMMENTS
Topical antifungal agents *Examples:* clotrimazole (Lotrimin®) miconazole (Monistat®) ketoconazole (Nizoral®)	Variety of mechanisms of action, but alter cell wall permeability resulting in disruption of cell wall membranes	Monitor for pruritus and stinging in effected areas. Generally need 10-21 days of treatment on skin to eradicate infection. To facilitate resolution keep effected area dry, open to air, clean. Monitor glucose in diabetics.

PREGNANCY/LACTATION CONSIDERATIONS

- Oral antifungals are contraindicated in pregnancy

CONSULTATION/REFERRAL

- Dermatologist for cases which are not responsive to treatment

FOLLOW-UP

- If on oral anti-fungal medication, consider liver function tests; recheck after 2 weeks and then in 6 weeks
- Recheck as needed for conditions requiring topical therapy

EXPECTED COURSE

- ***Tinea capitis***
  - ◊ Will resolve completely in about 4 weeks with appropriate treatment
- ***Tinea corporis***
  - ◊ Complete resolution in 1-2 weeks following treatment
- ***Tinea cruris***
  - ◊ Complete resolution in 1-2 weeks with appropriate treatment
- ***Tinea pedis***
  - ◊ Symptoms become controlled, but cure never occurs
  - ◊ Frequent recurrences
- ***Tinea versicolor***
  - ◊ Frequent recurrences, especially during springtime

POSSIBLE COMPLICATIONS

- ***Tinea capitis***
  - ◊ Possible permanent alopecia and/or scarring
- ***Tinea corporis***
  - ◊ Bacterial secondary infection from scratching
- ***Tinea cruris***
  - ◊ Bacterial secondary infection
- ***Tinea pedis***
  - ◊ Frequent recurrences
- ***Tinea versicolor***
  - ◊ None

CAT SCRATCH FEVER

DESCRIPTION

Subacute lymphadenitis following contact with a cat (99% of the time), usually a scratch

ETIOLOGY

- *Bartonella henselae*
- No person-to-person transmission

INCIDENCE

- 24,000 cases annually in the U.S.
- Most common in people < 21 years

RISK FACTORS

- Contact with a cat, (a scratch is the most usual means of inoculation) most often a kitten. Animals are usually described as "well".

ASSESSMENT FINDINGS

- Mild symptoms of malaise, anorexia, aches, headache, and occasionally fever
- Erythematous, crusty papule (2-6 mm in diameter) 3-10 days after inoculation
- Unilateral lymphadenopathy evident within 1-2 weeks of scratch
- Nodes are tender and firm for several weeks

DIFFERENTIAL DIAGNOSIS

- Hodgkin's and non-Hodgkin's lymphoma
- Kawasaki disease

DIAGNOSTIC STUDIES

- Culture of primary papule
- Direct fluorescence antibody testing for detection of antibodies to *B. henselae*

- Cat scratch antigen skin test when diagnosis is uncertain

PREVENTION

- Cleanse cat scratches as soon as possible after they occur
- Supervise children around animals

NONPHARMACOLOGIC MANAGEMENT

- Treatment is symptomatic usually
- Local heat to painful nodes
- Limit vigorous activity

PHARMACOLOGIC MANAGEMENT

- Analgesics
- Antibiotic treatment in immunocompromised: azithromycin; but antibiotic treatment controversial: will resolve in 2-6 months without treatment

PREGNANCY/LACTATION CONSIDERATIONS

- Pregnant women should maintain cautious contact with cats, especially litter boxes

CONSULTATION/REFERRAL

- Consult physician for immunocompromised patients or patients with lymphadenopathy of uncertain origin

FOLLOW-UP

- Usually none needed
- Individualize follow up for severe cases or in immunocompromised patients

EXPECTED COURSE

- Usually benign without any complications within 2 weeks of onset of symptoms

POSSIBLE COMPLICATIONS

- Chronic lymphadenopathy
- Encephalitis/encephalopathy
- Erythema nodosum

LYME DISEASE

DESCRIPTION

Multisystem infection transmitted by a tick. Disease ranges in severity from mild to severe.

ETIOLOGY

- *Borrelia burgdorferi* is the spirochete transmitted by the Ixodid tick

INCIDENCE

- 4.4/100,000 population
- States with highest prevalence: Connecticut, New York, New Jersey, Pennsylvania, Rhode Island, Wisconsin, Maryland, Minnesota but is found in almost every state in the U.S.

RISK FACTORS

- Exposure to the bite of infected ticks during May to September
- Exposure to outdoors, hunting, hiking, camping, or living in wooded areas

ASSESSMENT FINDINGS

Stage 1	Asymptomatic Erythema migrans (60-80%) Headache Fever Myalgias and arthralgias
Stage 2 Involves multiple organs or systems	Erythema migrans Aseptic meningitis, iritis Heart block, pericarditis Orchitis Hepatitis Arthritis of the large joints
Stage 3	Aches and pains of the joints and soft tissues Neurological impairment (memory loss, dementia, confusion, difficulty concentrating, peripheral neuropathies) Iritis, optic neuritis

DIFFERENTIAL DIAGNOSIS

- Arthritis
- Multiple sclerosis
- Parkinson's disease
- Ophthalmic disorders
- JRA
- Viral disorders
- Systemic lupus erythematosus

DIAGNOSTIC STUDIES

- ELISA for *Borrelia burgdorferi* antibodies
- Lumbar puncture for neuro symptoms
- ELISA of CSF for *Borrelia burgdorferi* antibodies

PREVENTION

- Teach patients to protect themselves from ticks while in potentially tick- infested areas (e.g., wearing of clothing that protects ankles)
- Use of insect repellents
- Self-examination after exposure in tick infested areas
- Prompt removal of ticks with tweezers

NONPHARMACOLOGIC MANAGEMENT

- Self-examination for ticks; examination of backs of ears and neck
- Remove ticks by using tweezers and grasping the tick as near to the skin as possible. Do not twist! Do not use a lighted match on the tick.
- Examine area for remaining tick parts. Attempt to remove. Occasionally there can be a local reaction to remaining parts.
- Teach patient that to contract Lyme disease, tick must be infected and remain in place for at least 24 hours.

PHARMACOLOGIC MANAGEMENT

Stage 1	doxycycline (Vibramycin®) 14-21 days *OR* amoxicillin for 14-21 days
Stage 2 (no CSF involvement)	doxycycline *OR* amoxicillin for 28 days short course (one week) of steroids
Stage 2 (CSF involvement)	ceftriaxone (Rocephin®) *OR* cefotaxime (Claforan®) *OR* penicillin G for 21-28 days
Stage 3	doxycycline *OR* amoxicillin for 28 days If oral treatment fails, intravenous ceftriaxone (Rocephin®) *OR* cefotaxime (Claforan®) *OR* penicillin G for 14-21 days

- Do not use doxycycline in children <9 years

PREGNANCY/LACTATION CONSIDERATIONS

- Do not use doxycycline during pregnancy or during breastfeeding.
- *Borrelia burgdorferi* can cross the placenta, therefore, treat with intravenous antibiotics.
- Oral contraceptives may be less effective if tetracycline is taken.

CONSULTATION/REFERRAL

- Refer patients with cardiac or neurological involvement
- Consult obstetrician for pregnant patients

FOLLOW-UP

- Depends on stage and severity
- Follow up for Stage 2 and 3 patients may be months to years

EXPECTED COURSE

- Stage 1 infection responds well to antibiotics
- Stages 2 and 3 have a variable response and depend on the severity

POSSIBLE COMPLICATIONS

- Persistent neurological symptoms
- Persistent arthralgias and myalgias
- Heart block

ORAL CANDIDIASIS

Thrush

DESCRIPTION

Fungal infection of the mucus membranes of the mouth which may involve the throat, esophagus, trachea, and angles of the mouth

ETIOLOGY

- Usually *Candida albicans*: normal flora of the mouth that flourishes under warm, moist, and glucose-rich environment

INCIDENCE

- Most common in newborns, infants, and elderly, and immunocompromised patients

RISK FACTORS

- Age extremes (very young and very old)
- Recent antibiotic use
- Immunocompromised status
- Presence of chronic disease(s)

ASSESSMENT FINDINGS

- White oral plaques on an erythematous base
- May have concurrent diaper candidiasis

DIFFERENTIAL DIAGNOSIS

- Geographic tongue
- Leukoplakia
- Stomatitis
- Other yeasts

DIAGNOSTIC STUDIES

- Usually none indicated
- 10% KOH wet prep: demonstrates pseudohyphae and spores
- Culture
- Consider tests to rule out HIV and/or diabetes in patients with recurrent candidiasis

PREVENTION

- Discourage thumb sucking to prevent spread to nails
- Oral hygiene

NONPHARMACOLOGIC MANAGEMENT

- *See* Prevention

PHARMACOLOGIC MANAGEMENT

- Nystatin oral suspension in each cheek after feedings four times a day
- For adults: clotrimazole buccal troches for 2 weeks; fluconazole

PREGNANCY/LACTATION CONSIDERATIONS

- Exercise good hygiene of lactating mother's nipples if baby has thrush
- Do not prophylactically treat mother (controversial)

CONSULTATION/REFERRAL

- Consult physician for disease which persists
- Consult physician for HIV-positive or other immunocompromised patients

FOLLOW-UP

- Usually none needed if resolution occurs by 2 weeks
- Return if thrush worsens while on medication or if unresolved after 2 weeks

EXPECTED COURSE

- Usually resolves with appropriate treatment
- Frequently recurs

POSSIBLE COMPLICATIONS

- Systemic infection (rare)

References

Achar, S. (1996). Principles of skin biopsies for the family physician. *American Family Physician, 54*(8), 2411-2422.

American Academy of Pediatrics. (2003). *Red book: Report of the committee on infectious disease* (26th ed.). Elk Grove Village, IN: American Academy of Pediatrics.

Anderson, M.L. (2005). Atopic dermatitis: More than a simple skin disorder. *Journal of the American Academy of Nurse Practitioners, 17*, 249-255.

Bickley, L.S., & Szilagyi, P.G. (2003). *Bates' guide to physical examination and history taking* (8th ed.). Philadelphia: Lippincott Williams & Wilkins.

Branch, W.T. (2003). *Office practice of medicine* (4th ed.). Philadelphia: Saunders.

Bratton, R.L., & Corey, G.R. (2005). Tick-borne disease. *American Academy of Family Physicians, 71,* 2323-2330.

Burns, C.E., Brady, M.A., Blosser, C., Starr, N.B., & Dunn, A.M. (2004). *Pediatric primary care: A handbook for nurse practitioners* (3rd ed.). Philadelphia: W.B. Saunders.

Dambro, M.R. (2005). *Griffith's 5 minute clinical consult.* Philadelphia: Lippincott Williams & Wilkins.

Depietropaolo, D.L., Powers, J.H., Gill, J.M., & Foy, A.J. (2005). Diagnosis of lyme disease. *American Academy of Family Physicians, 72,* 297-304.

Diehl, K.B. (1996). Topical antifungal agents: An update. *American Family Physician, 54,* 1687-1692.

Elston, D.M. (2005). Bites and stings: Be prepared to respond quickly. *Clinical Advisor, 8(7)* 20-32.

Epstein, E. (2001). *Common Skin Disorders.* (5th ed.). Philadelphia: WB Saunders.

Gilber, D.N., Moellering, R.C., Eliopoulos, G.M., & Sande, M.A. (Eds.). (2004). *Sanford Guide to Antimicrobial Therapy* (34th ed.). Hyde Park, VT: Antimicrobial Therapy.

Graber, M.A., & Lanternier, M.L. (Eds.) (2001). *The family practice handbook.* (4th ed.). St. Louis: Mosby.

Johnson, C.E., Stancin, T., Fattlar, D., Rowe, L.P., & Kumar, M.L. (1997). A long-term prospective study of varicella vaccine in healthy children. *Pediatrics, 100*, 761-766.

Kasper, D.L., Braunwald, E., Fauci, A.S., Hauser, S.L., Longo, D.L., Jameson, J.L., et al. (2004). *Harrison's principles of internal medicine* (16th ed.). New York: McGraw-Hill.

Kliegman, R.M., Greenbaum, L.A., & Lye, P.S. (2004). *Practical strategies in pediatric diagnosis and therapy* (2nd ed.). Philadelphia: W.B. Saunders.

Lobato, M.N., Vugia, D.J., & Friede, I.J. (1997). Tinea capitis in California children: A population-based study of a growing epidemic. *Pediatrics, 99*, 551-554.

Mangion, S. (2000). *Physical diagnosis secrets.* Philadelphia: Hanley and Belfus.

Mladenovic, J. (Ed.). (2003). *Primary care secrets.* (3rd Ed.). Philadelphia: Hanley and Belfus.

Nicol, N.H. (2000). Managing atopic dermatitis in children and adults. *The Nurse Practitioner, 25*(4), 58-76.

Noronha., P.A., & Zubkov, B. (1997). Nails and nail disorders in children and adults. *American Family Physician, 55*, 2129-2140.

Olson, A.L., Dietrich, A.J., Sox, C.H., Stevens, M.M., Winchell, C.W., & Ahles, T.A. (1997). Solar protection of children at the beach. *Pediatrics Electronic Pages.* [On-line serial]. Available: www.pediatrics.come1.

Rakel, R.E. (1998). *Essentials of family practice.* (2nd ed.). Philadelphia: WB Saunders.

Reifsnider, E. (1997). Adult infectious skin conditions. *The Nurse Practitioner, 22*(11), 17-33.

Scheinfeld, N.S. (2005). Psoriasis: The "Nuts and bolts" of management. *Consultant, 45,* 798-807.

Schwartz, M.W. (Ed.). (2002). *The 5 minute pediatric consult.* (2nd ed.) Philadelphia: Lippincott Williams & Wilkins.

Singleton, J.K. (1997). Pediatric dermatoses: Three common skin disruptions in infancy. *The Nurse Practitioner, 22*(6), 32-50.

Stein, D.H. (1998). Tineas-superficial dermatophyte infections. *Pediatric Review, 19,* 368-372.

Supple, K. (2005). An overview of burn injury. *Advance for Nurse Practitioners, 13*(7), 24-29

Temple, M.E. (1999). Pharmacotherapy of tinea capitis. *Journal of the American Board of Family Practice, 12*(3), 236-242.

Treadwell, P.A. (1997). Dermatoses in newborns. *American Family Physician, 56,* 443-454.

Uphold, C.R., & Graham, M.V. (2003). *Clinical guidelines in family practice.* (4th ed.). Gainesville, FL: Barmarrae Books.

U.S. Preventive Services Task Force. (1996). *Guide to clinical preventive services.* (2nd ed.) Washington, D.C.: Office of Disease Prevention and Health Promotion, U.S. Government Printing Office.

Verdon, M.E., & Sigal, L.H. (1997). Recognition and management of Lyme disease. *American Family Physician, 56,* 427-438.

Zollo, A.J., Jr (Ed.). (2004). *Medical Secrets.* (4th ed.), St. Louis, MO: Mosby-Year Book.

Zoltan, T.B., Taylor, K.S., & Achar, S.A. (2005). Health issues for surfers. *American Academy of Family Physicians, 71,* 2313-2317.

11

LACTATION

Lactation

BENEFITS OF BREASTFEEDING

MATERNAL

- Economical
- Accelerates uterine involution and decreases postpartal bleeding
- Exerts protective effect against endometrial and breast cancer
- No preparation of milk or bottles needed

INFANT

- Decreases rate of respiratory, gastrointestinal, and middle ear infections
- Easy to digest
- Enhances bonding and encourages a close relationship between mother and infant
- May decrease development of allergies
- Decreases constipation

DISADVANTAGES OF BREASTFEEDING

- Mother may perceive it as an inconvenience
- Time commitment may be perceived as a disadvantage
- Only mother can feed baby

CONTRAINDICATIONS TO BREASTFEEDING

- HIV positive mother
- Active tuberculosis
- Newly diagnosed breast cancer
- Drug abuse by mother
- Infant galactosemia
- Herpes lesion on mother's breasts
- Mother receiving medications that are contraindicated for infant

PHYSIOLOGY OF LACTATION

- Decline of estrogen and progesterone after delivery of placenta initiates increased milk production
- Oxytocin and prolactin are two of the major hormones responsible for lactation
- Oxytocin is responsible for let-down reflex which is necessary for successful breastfeeding
- Prolactin is released as nipple stimulation occurs during sucking
- Day 0-2: colostrum is secreted: a thick, sticky, yellow fluid rich in immunoglobulins, vitamin E, and leukocytes. It is higher in protein, fat-soluble vitamins, and minerals than mature milk
- Day 2-4: transitional milk is thinner, more plentiful milk with increased lactose, fat, calories, and water-soluble vitamin content
- Day 4: mature milk: consists of fore milk (first milk expressed from breast at each nursing) and hind milk (milk higher in fat and calories); expressed after the let-down reflex occurs and is essential for adequate infant nutrition

BREASTFEEDING TECHNIQUE

- Infant should be placed facing the mother (belly-to-belly)
- Teach breastfeeding woman different positions for breastfeeding:
  - ◊ Cradle position
  - ◊ Football hold
  - ◊ Side-lying position
- Position should be rotated frequently, especially first few weeks of breastfeeding
- Generally, newborns should breastfeed 8-12 times in 24 hours
- Nursing time: varies widely with each infant; limiting nursing time may increase engorgement. Breast will be emptied usually after 10-20 minutes of nursing.
- Removing infant from breast: break suction with finger before removing infant to prevent sore nipples
- Burp infant when changing breasts and after feeding
- Avoid use of pacifiers and bottles which may cause nipple confusion in infant
- Supplemental feedings including water are not usually needed for adequate nutrition

MATERNAL NUTRITION

- Increased fluids are required
- Avoid caffeine (may stimulate infant)
- Increased calorie intake by 500 kcal over prepregnancy requirements
- Continue prenatal vitamins
- Iron supplementation may be needed if diet inadequate
- Calcium supplement if not taking in adequate amounts in diet

VITAMIN SUPPLEMENTATION OF THE BREASTFED INFANT

- Iron supplementation after 6 months of age
- Fluoride started after 6 months of age if living in an area where water is not fluoridated
- Supplementation with vitamin D if mother is deficient

DETERMINATION OF ADEQUATE INTAKE

- Appropriate weight gain of infant (about one ounce per day for first 6 months)
- Breasts feel hard before nursing and soft afterwards
- Infant has 6-8 wet diapers in a 24 hour period
- Infant satisfied
- Infant has at least two soft stools per day
- Audible swallowing while nursing

BREAST CARE

- Wear comfortable, well-fitting bra
- Wash breasts with warm water
- Avoid use of soap due to its drying effect
- Lanolin may be used for soothing and healing

STORAGE OF BREAST MILK

- Store in sterilized polypropylene plastic containers
- Write date on container
- Refrigerate or freeze milk immediately after expressing
- Freeze milk that will not be used within 2 days
- Use milk within 3 months if stored in a self-defrosting freezer
- Use milk stored in a traditional freezer within 12 months
- Use oldest milk first
- Thaw under warm running water. Do not heat milk on stove or in microwave
- Do not refreeze breast milk

WEANING

- Breastfeeding alone is adequate until infant is 6 months of age. At this time solid foods may be introduced slowly.
- To wean infant, substitute a bottle or cup feeding for a breastfeeding every few days until infant is completely off breast

DRUGS/MEDICATIONS

- Many drugs are excreted in breast milk and have the potential to affect infant
- Health care provider should be consulted before taking any medications
- When a medication must be taken by the lactating woman, take it immediately after breastfeeding so that the infant receives the least amount possible

ALCOHOL

- Discouraged during lactation
- May impair let-down reflex

SMOKING

- Smoking decreases breast milk volume
- Nicotine is excreted in breast milk to infant
- Smoking cessation is recommended

COMMON PROBLEMS OF LACTATION

PLUGGED MILK DUCT

CAUSE

- Infrequent nursing
- Engorgement

ASSESSMENT FINDINGS

- Sore lump in one or both breasts
- No fever

MANAGEMENT

- Moist hot packs to breast lump before and during nursing
- More frequent nursing, especially on affected side
- Do not stop breastfeeding
- Pump or express milk after feeding if infant not emptying breasts
- Breast massage
- Breastfeeding in various nursing positions

SORE NIPPLES

CAUSE

- Improper positioning of infant
- Removing infant from breast without first breaking suction with finger
- Nipples remaining wet after feeding
- Inappropriate use of breast creams and soaps
- Thrush
- Infant nursing on tip of nipple

ASSESSMENT FINDINGS

- Complaint of pain when infant nurses
- Nipples tender, raw, swollen, or traumatized

MANAGEMENT

- Expose breasts to air or sunlight for short period several times a day. Avoid washing breasts with soap and water.
- Avoid use of breast creams
- Breastfeed frequently to avoid vigorous nursing by infant
- Make sure nipple is in the posterior portion of infant's mouth
- Limit nursing time on sore nipple
- Nurse on the least sore side first
- Change bra pads frequently to keep nipples dry
- Wear vented breast shells to protect and dry nipples between feedings
- Avoid use of rubber nipple shield
- Mild analgesics may be required
- Educate regarding positioning and breaking suction with finger when taking infant off breast
- For patients with cracking, blistering, bleeding, or severe pain of nipples, a consultation or referral to a lactation consultant is recommended

FLAT OR INVERTED NIPPLES

CAUSE

- Adhesions of the nipple causing retraction or inversion

ASSESSMENT FINDINGS

- Inverted nipples retract inward when stimulated

MANAGEMENT

- Should be assessed during pregnancy
- Specially designed, vented breast shells with a hole in the center can be worn during the last month of pregnancy. These shells provide slight, constant pressure to draw the nipple out.
- Manually pull the nipple out before feeding
- Use a breast pump for a short while before feeding
- Application of ice before nursing to draw out nipple
- Referral to lactation consultant usually necessary

ENGORGEMENT

CAUSE

- Milk stasis in the breast from inadequate emptying

ASSESSMENT FINDINGS

- Pain in breasts
- Hard, warm, lumpy breasts
- Feeling of fullness in breasts
- Flattened nipples
- Usually occurs in first few weeks of nursing

MANAGEMENT

- Increase frequency of nursing
- Avoid long periods without nursing
- Manual expression of milk
- Hot shower allowing water to flow over breasts
- Apply warm compresses to breasts before nursing
- Apply ice to breasts for relief after nursing
- Hand expression of some milk before feeding to soften breast and facilitate infant attaching to breasts
- Breast massage

MASTITIS

CAUSE

- Plugged milk ducts leading to infection
- Usually caused by staphylococcal or streptococcal organisms
- Predisposing factors
  - ◊ Fatigue, stress
  - ◊ Cracked nipples
  - ◊ Improper-fitting bra
  - ◊ Inadequate emptying of breast
  - ◊ Abrupt weaning

ASSESSMENT FINDINGS

- Breast tenderness and pain
- Lump in one or both breasts
- Fever, chills
- Erythema overlying sore area
- Flu-like symptoms
- Fatigue

MANAGEMENT

- Moist hot packs or warm shower before and during nursing
- More frequent nursing on affected side
- Do not stop breastfeeding
- Antibiotics to cover *Staphylococcus aureus*, the most common causative organism
- Rule out other sources of fever
- Acetaminophen for fever
- Analgesics for pain
- Increased rest
- Increased fluids
- If abscess occurs, surgical drainage is required
- Do not wean abruptly

LEAKING

CAUSE

- Let-down reflex stimulated by crying infant or even the sight of an infant
- Overly full breasts

MANAGEMENT

- Tight-fitting bra
- Wearing breast pads without plastic liners; should be changed frequently
- Pressure against nipple with heel of hand when feel let-down sensation
- Increased feeding

- Manual expression of milk if breast overly full

INADEQUATE LET-DOWN REFLEX

CAUSE

- Multifactorial
- Inadequate relaxation
- Fatigued or tense mother
- Infant not nursing long enough

ASSESSMENT FINDINGS

- Breasts not completely emptying

MANAGEMENT

- Allow infant ample time to nurse
- Massage breasts before nursing
- Use relaxation and breathing techniques
- Adequate rest and nutrition
- Oxytocin nasal spray during feeding
- Referral to lactation consultant often necessary

CANDIDAL INFECTION OF NIPPLES

CAUSE

- Infection with *Candida albicans*
- May be contracted by infant during delivery and transmitted to mother's breast

ASSESSMENT FINDINGS

- White patches on nipple and areola and/or infant's mouth
- Patches do not rub off
- Pain and burning of breasts

MANAGEMENT

- Treat infant with oral nystatin (Mycostatin®) and mother with topical agent to breast
- Keep nipples clean and dry
- Wash nystatin off breast before breastfeeding

JAUNDICE

CAUSE

- Thought to be due to enzyme found in breast milk which leads to increased reabsorption of unconjugated bilirubin in the intestine causing hyperbilirubinemia and jaundice

ASSESSMENT FINDINGS

- Yellow skin tone
- Yellow sclera
- Usually occurs after third day of life
- Infant healthy and thriving

MANAGEMENT

- Serum bilirubin measurement
- Rule out pathological causes of jaundice
- Continue breastfeeding
- Usually resolves without harm to infant

References

American Academy of Pediatrics. (2003). *Red book: Report of the committee on infectious disease* (26th ed.). Elk Grove Village, IN: American Academy of Pediatrics.

Bickley, L.S., & Szilagyi, P.G. (2003). *Bates' guide to physical examination and history taking* (8th ed.). Philadelphia: Lippincott Williams & Wilkins.

Branch, W.T. (2003). *Office practice of medicine* (4th ed.). Philadelphia: Saunders.

Burns, C.E., Brady, M.A., Blosser, C., Starr, N.B., & Dunn, A.M. (2004). *Pediatric primary care: A handbook for nurse practitioners* (3rd ed.). Philadelphia: W.B. Saunders.

Cunningham, F.G.,Gant, N.F., Leveno, K.J., Gilstrap, L.C., Hauth, J.C., & Wenstrom, K.D. (2005). *Williams obstetrics* (22th ed.). New York: McGraw-Hill

Dambro, M.R. (2005). *Griffith's 5 minute clinical consult.* Philadelphia: Lippincott Williams & Wilkins.

Lawrence, R.A., & Lawrence, R.M. (1998). *Breastfeeding: A guide for the medical profession* (5th ed.). St. Louis, MO: Mosby.

Olds, S.B., London, M.L., & Ladewig, P.W. (1999). *Maternal-newborn nursing: A family-centered approach* (5th ed.). Upper Saddle River, NJ: Prentice Hall.

Uphold, C.R., & Graham, M.V. (2003). *Clinical guidelines in family practice* (4th ed.). Gainesville, FL: Barmarrae Books.

12

MEN'S HEALTH

Men's Health

BENIGN PROSTATIC HYPERPLASIA (BPH)

DESCRIPTION

Noncancerous enlargement of the prostate gland

ETIOLOGY

- Exact cause unknown
- The presence of androgens is necessary for the development of BPH

INCIDENCE

- Uncommon < 40 years of age
- >50% of men aged 60 years and 80% of men by age 70 years have some degree of BPH
- High prevalence that progresses with age

RISK FACTORS

- Presence of androgens
- Increasing age

ASSESSMENT FINDINGS

- Weak urinary stream
- Hesitancy and post-void dribbling
- Incomplete emptying of bladder
- Frequency and urgency
- Nocturia
- Incontinence
- Urinary retention
- Hematuria: gross or microscopic
- Firm, smooth, symmetrically enlarged prostate

DIFFERENTIAL DIAGNOSIS

- Prostatitis
- Prostate cancer
- Urethral stricture
- Neurogenic bladder
- Effect of medications (e.g., sympathomimetics)
- Urinary tract infection
- Bladder cancer

DIAGNOSTIC STUDIES

- Use of American Urological Association Symptom Index (a self-administered tool consisting of seven questions about symptoms of prostatism including incomplete emptying, frequency, intermittency, urgency, a weak stream, hesitancy, and nocturia) for initial evaluation. The index is scored from 0-35 depending on symptoms:
  - ◊ Mild symptoms: score of 0-7
  - ◊ Moderate symptoms: score of 8-19
  - ◊ Severe symptoms: score of 20-35
- Urinalysis: pyuria if residual urine present
- Creatinine for assessment of renal function
- Postvoid residual urine measurement (> 100 ml)
- Prostate specific antigen (PSA): may be elevated, but <10 ng/ml
- Ultrasound of prostate
- Needle biopsy
- IVP, CT or MRI of the prostate

NONPHARMACOLOGIC MANAGEMENT

- Lifestyle modifications may provide relief for patients with mild symptoms (AUA score 0-7)
  - ◊ Limit fluids before bedtime
  - ◊ Frequent voiding
  - ◊ Avoid sympathomimetic or anticholinergic medications (e.g., decongestants) due to increased risk of urinary retention
  - ◊ Avoid caffeine, alcohol, and other beverages that produce diuresis
- Surgical options for patients with moderate to severe symptoms:
  - ◊ Transurethral resection of the prostate (TURP)
  - ◊ Transurethral incision of the prostate (TUIP): may be better option for younger men
  - ◊ Open prostatectomy may be needed for very large prostates

- Indications for surgery: severe symptoms, refractory urinary retention, recurrent urinary tract infections, recurrent hematuria, bladder stones, renal insufficiency due to BPH
- Balloon dilation of the prostate in selected patients with smaller prostates

PHARMACOLOGIC MANAGEMENT

- Pharmacologic therapy is indicated in mild to moderate disease (AUA score >8)

AGENT	ACTION	COMMENTS
Alpha adrenergic antagonists *Example:* terazosin (Hytrin®) doxazosin (Cardura®) tamsulosin (Flomax®)	Blockade of the alpha adrenergic receptors causes relaxation of smooth muscle in the prostate and neck of the bladder	May cause orthostatic hypotension. Cautious use in patients with cardiac or cerebrovascular diseases. Contraindicated in patients taking Levitra®,Viagra®, and Cialis®.
Antiandrogenic agents *Examples:* finasteride (Proscar®) dutasteride (Avodart®)	Inhibit conversion of testosterone to the androgen, DHT. Enlargement of the prostate gland is caused by DHT.	Hormones may cause impotence. At least 6-12 months are needed to adequately assess benefit of therapy. Pregnant patients should never handle crushed or broken tablets. PSA will decrease while taking this drug.

CONSULTATION/REFERRAL

- Refer for urological evaluation if refractory to treatment, evidence of renal complications, or if surgery indicated

FOLLOW-UP

- Digital rectal exam annually
- PSA annually

EXPECTED COURSE

- Symptoms improve or stabilize in 70-80% of patients
- 20-30% require treatment due to worsening of symptoms

POSSIBLE COMPLICATIONS

- Acute urinary retention
- Urinary incontinence
- Urinary tract infection
- Prostatitis
- Hydronephrosis
- Impotence from pharmacologic or surgical treatment

ACUTE BACTERIAL PROSTATITIS

DESCRIPTION

Acute inflammatory condition of the prostate

ETIOLOGY

- Translocation of bacteria up the urethra
- Urinary reflux into prostate ducts
- Common organisms: *Chlamydia trachomatis, Trichomonas vaginalis, N. gonorrhoea, E. coli, Pseudomonas, Klebsiella, Proteus*

INCIDENCE

- Most common in ages 30-50 years

RISK FACTORS

- Sexual activity
- Multiple sexual partners
- Urinary tract infection

ASSESSMENT FINDINGS

- Abrupt onset
- Fever, chills, malaise
- Enlarged, boggy, and tender prostate
- Low back pain
- Perineal pain
- Decreased urinary stream
- Frequency, urgency, dysuria
- Nocturia
- Pain upon defecation and ejaculation

DIFFERENTIAL DIAGNOSIS

- Benign prostatic hyperplasia
- Chronic prostatitis
- Urinary tract infection
- Sexually transmitted disease
- Malignancy
- Acute urinary retention

DIAGNOSTIC STUDIES

- Fractional urine examination: third specimen (after prostate massage) has 10-15 WBCs/high-powered field
- Urinalysis: WBCs, bacteria, hematuria
- Urine culture
- Gram stain, culture and sensitivity of expressed prostatic secretions
- PSA will be increased during acute infection, therefore, do not consider screening for prostate cancer until 4 weeks post treatment

> **Never perform vigorous prostate massage because this can potentially cause bacteremia.**

PREVENTION

- Safer sex practices

NONPHARMACOLOGIC MANAGEMENT

- Good hydration
- Sitz bath for pain relief
- Avoid vigorous prostate massage
- Hospitalization may be required if infection severe

PHARMACOLOGIC MANAGEMENT

- Antibiotic treatment for 4 weeks using culture and sensitivity as guide in antibiotic selection
- Consider:
  - ◊ trimethoprim-sulfamethoxazole (Bactrim®)
  - ◊ ciprofloxacin (Cipro®) *OR*
  - ◊ doxycycline (Vibramycin®)
- Analgesics
- Antipyretics
- Stool softeners

CONSULTATION/REFERRAL

- Refer patient with possible abscess or systemic illness to urologist

FOLLOW-UP

- Urinalysis and culture 4-6 weeks after initiating therapy

EXPECTED COURSE

- Variable cure rate

POSSIBLE COMPLICATIONS

- Bacteremia
- Urinary tract infection, epididymitis
- Urinary retention
- Renal parenchymal disease

CHRONIC PROSTATITIS

DESCRIPTION

Chronic inflammatory condition of the prostate

ETIOLOGY

- *See* Bacterial Prostatitis

INCIDENCE

- Most common over 50 years of age

RISK FACTORS

- Age over 50 years
- Urinary tract infection

ASSESSMENT FINDINGS

- Asymptomatic, but not usually
- Frequency, urgency, dysuria
- Dribbling, hesitancy
- Decreased force of urinary stream
- Pain
  - ◊ With defecation or ejaculation
  - ◊ Perineum
  - ◊ Lower abdomen
  - ◊ Low back
  - ◊ Scrotum
  - ◊ Penis
- Hematuria: gross or microscopic
- Mildly tender prostate gland with enlargement

DIFFERENTIAL DIAGNOSIS

- Acute bacterial prostatitis
- Acute urinary retention
- Benign prostatic hyperplasia
- Prostate cancer
- Urinary tract infection

DIAGNOSTIC STUDIES

- Fractional urine examination: third specimen has 10-15 WBCs/high-powered field
- Urinalysis: WBCs, blood, bacteria
- Urine culture and sensitivity
- Culture of prostatic secretions
- CT and/or ultrasound if indicated to rule out malignancy
- PSA: frequently elevated
- BUN and creatinine
- Cystoscopy (refer to urologist)

NONPHARMACOLOGIC MANAGEMENT

- Sitz bath to relieve pain
- Good hydration
- Avoid coffee, tea, alcohol, and other beverages which can cause diuresis
- Avoid anticholinergics and sympathomimetics which can cause urinary retention
- Surgical resection of prostate for intractable chronic disease in older men

PHARMACOLOGIC MANAGEMENT

- Fluoroquinolone daily (e.g., norfloxacin, ciprofloxacin, levofloxacin) for 6-24 weeks
- Suppression therapy may be needed if a cure is not attainable: trimethoprim-sulfamethoxazole (Bactrim DS®) one tablet daily

CONSULTATION/REFERRAL

- Consultation with urologist if unresponsive to antibiotic therapy or cystoscopy needed

FOLLOW-UP

- Urinalysis and urine culture every 30 days until resolved (may be chronic)

EXPECTED COURSE

- May take several months to cure

POSSIBLE COMPLICATIONS

- Bacteremia
- Urinary tract infection, epididymitis
- Urinary retention
- Renal parenchymal disease

PROSTATE CANCER

DESCRIPTION

- Malignancy of prostate gland

ETIOLOGY

- Unknown

INCIDENCE

- Leading cause of cancer in men
- Incidence increases with age, most common after age 60 years

RISK FACTORS

- Family history, especially first degree relative
- Increasing age
- African-American

ASSESSMENT FINDINGS

- Asymptomatic
- Prostate feels hard upon digital examination
- Prostatic nodules may be palpated
- Acute urinary retention possible
- Hematuria possible
- Urinary tract infection
- Anemia
- Lymphedema
- Lymphadenopathy

DIFFERENTIAL DIAGNOSIS

- Prostatitis
- Benign prostatic hyperplasia
- Benign prostatic nodules
- Prostate stones

DIAGNOSTIC STUDIES

- Prostatic ultrasound
- Prostate specific antigen (PSA): can be normal but if elevated, usually > 10 ng/ml
- Alkaline phosphatase: elevated with metastasis
- CT
- MRI not helpful
- Biopsy

PREVENTION

- Annual digital rectal examination beginning at age 40 years
- Annual PSA and digital rectal examination beginning at age 50 years
- Consider screening at age 45 years for those at high risk (first degree relative with prostate cancer, African-American heritage)

NONPHARMACOLOGIC MANAGEMENT

- Surgical intervention: TURP or radical prostatectomy and orchiectomy
- Radiation therapy

PHARMACOLOGIC MANAGEMENT

- Leuprolide (Lupron®) or Flutamide (Eulexin®) for androgen ablation
- Estrogen therapy
- Chemotherapy

CONSULTATION/REFERRAL

- Refer to urologist

FOLLOW-UP

- Clinical examination every 3 months for one year; then every 6 months for one year; then annually
- PSA every 3 months for one year; then every 6 months for one year, then annually

EXPECTED COURSE

- Depends on stage at time of diagnosis
- Usually grows slowly
- Cancer confined to prostate: 5-year survival rate is 98%
- Cancer which has spread outside of the prostate: 5-year survival rate is 29%

POSSIBLE COMPLICATIONS

- Urinary retention

- Metastasis
- Pathologic fracture
- Impotence secondary to radical prostatectomy
- Postoperative incontinence

CRYPTORCHIDISM
(Undescended Testicle)

DESCRIPTION

Incomplete descent of one or both testicles into the scrotum

ETIOLOGY

- Not completely understood
- May involve hormonal, mechanical, and/or neural factors

INCIDENCE

- 3% of full term male infants
- 33% of premature male infants

RISK FACTORS

- Family history of cryptorchidism
- Premature birth (testicles usually descend in 7th or 8th month gestationally)
- Hypospadias

ASSESSMENT FINDINGS

- Absence of one or both testes upon palpation of scrotum (assess with child or infant in sitting, squatting, and standing positions)
- One or both testicles in a site other than scrotum

DIFFERENTIAL DIAGNOSIS

- Retractile testis (normal testis that ascends into inguinal canal as a result of cremasteric reflex)
- Atrophic testis
- Anorchia: complete absence of testis

DIAGNOSTIC STUDIES

- Ultrasound to identify location of testicle(s)

NONPHARMACOLOGIC MANAGEMENT

- Orchiopexy usually performed by age one year
- Teach self-testicular examination when older
- Educate regarding increased risk of testicular cancer and infertility

PHARMACOLOGIC MANAGEMENT

- Human chorionic gonadotropin (hCG) sometimes recommended for older children (may induce precocious puberty)

CONSULTATION/REFERRAL

- Refer for urological evaluation if testicle(s) not descended by 6 months of age

FOLLOW-UP

- Follow closely before surgical correction to determine if dissension has occurred
- Follow closely after surgical correction to evaluate testicular growth

EXPECTED COURSE

- Spontaneous descent, if it occurs, will usually do so in first 6 months of life (and usually by 3 months of age)
- Usually corrected with surgical therapy
- Lifelong consequence of increased testicular cancer risk (20-46 times higher) even after correction

POSSIBLE COMPLICATIONS

- Testicular cancer
- Decreased fertility rate even with treatment
- Hernia development
- Testicular torsion

EPIDIDYMITIS

DESCRIPTION

Inflammation of the epididymis usually occurring from ascension of pathogens from urethra or prostate

ETIOLOGY

Prepubertal boys:
- Bacterial urinary tract infection
- Underlying congenital defect

Younger than 35 years:
- Usually *Chlamydia trachomatis* or *Neisseria gonorrhoeae* in men <35 years

Older than 35 years:
- Bacterial urinary tract infection
- Prostatitis, urinary instrumentation, or structural lesion

INCIDENCE

- Common, especially in younger, sexually active men or older men with urinary tract infection

RISK FACTORS

- Recent trauma to scrotum
- Multiple sexual partners
- Urinary tract infection
- Indwelling urinary catheter
- Urethral instrumentation or surgery

ASSESSMENT FINDINGS

- Gradual development of scrotal pain
- Urethral discharge
- Dysuria, frequency
- Hematuria
- Epididymis very tender, enlarged, and indurated (epididymis is located posterior to testicle)
- Discomfort decreases with elevation of testes
- Scrotal edema and erythema
- Fever, chills
- Cremasteric reflex present
- Presentation in children not as dramatic as in older males

DIFFERENTIAL DIAGNOSIS

- Testicular torsion
- Orchitis
- Testicular tumor
- Testicular trauma
- Epididymal cyst or tumor
- Spermatocele
- Hydrocele
- Varicocele
- Insect bites to scrotum
- Tuberculous or fungal infection

DIAGNOSTIC STUDIES

- Doppler ultrasound of scrotum
- Urinalysis: pyuria, hematuria
- Urine and urethral Gram stain and culture with sensitivity
- Urethral discharge for chlamydia and gonorrhea testing
- HIV screen
- Syphilis serology

PREVENTION

- Antibiotic prophylaxis before urethral instrumentation or surgery

NONPHARMACOLOGIC MANAGEMENT

- Elevation of scrotum with athletic supporter
- Cool compresses to scrotum or ice packs
- Treat sexual partner if causative agent *N. gonorrhoeae* or *C. trachomatis*

PHARMACOLOGIC MANAGEMENT

- NSAIDs for pain/discomfort

Prepubertal boys:
- Trimethoprim-sulfamethoxazole (Bactrim®)

Postpuberty to age 35 years:

- Doxycycline (Vibramycin®) *AND* ceftriaxone (Rocephin®) intramuscular
- Treat sexual partners

Older men:

- Trimethoprim-sulfamethoxazole (Bactrim®) *OR* ciprofloxacin (Cipro®) *OR* ofloxacin (Floxin®) *OR* norfloxacin (Noroxin®)

CONSULTATION/REFERRAL

- Immediate referral if testicular torsion cannot be ruled out
- Consult urologist in prepubertal patients, for recurrence, and if unresponsive to therapy

FOLLOW-UP

- Urine cultures posttreatment in prepubertal boys and older men
- Evaluation of prepubertal boys for genitourinary anomaly

EXPECTED COURSE

- Expect improvement within 72 hours if on appropriate antibiotic
- Infection and pain resolve over 2-4 weeks with appropriate treatment

POSSIBLE COMPLICATIONS

- Recurrent epididymitis
- Infertility
- Abscess

TESTICULAR TORSION

DESCRIPTION

An acute ischemic event that occurs when the testis and spermatic cord twist

ETIOLOGY

- Usually occurs suddenly with no known cause
- History of trauma may be reported; especially a kick to the groin or falling on a hard object
- May be associated with exercise, very cold temperatures, or sexual stimulation

INCIDENCE

- 1/160 males
- 2/3 of cases occur in adolescents
- Accounts for 40% of cases of acute scrotal pain and swelling

RISK FACTORS

- May be more common in winter
- Paraplegia
- Commonly occurs at puberty
- Bell-clapper deformity

ASSESSMENT FINDINGS

- Sudden, severe, unilateral scrotal pain
- Scrotal edema and erythema
- Firm tender mass which may appear retracted upward
- No relief of pain with testicular elevation
- Lower abdominal pain
- Nausea and vomiting
- Testis is very tender
- Cremasteric reflex absent

DIFFERENTIAL DIAGNOSIS

- Epididymitis
- Orchitis
- Hydrocele, varicocele, spermatocele
- Testicular tumor
- Incarcerated inguinal hernia
- Trauma

DIAGNOSTIC STUDIES

- Doppler ultrasound of scrotum
- Urinalysis: normal in 90% of cases

NONPHARMACOLOGIC MANAGEMENT

- Manual relief of torsion

- Surgical exploration and detorsion or orchiectomy if nonviable testis
- Bilateral orchiopexy

PHARMACOLOGIC MANAGEMENT

- Analgesics

CONSULTATION/REFERRAL

- Immediate urological referral for correction

FOLLOW-UP

- By urologist at 1-2 weeks post correction
- Annual visits to evaluate for testicular atrophy until adolescence

EXPECTED COURSE

- Duration of torsion determines if testicle remains viable:
  - ◊ 80-100% salvage if blood flow re-established within 6 hours
  - ◊ <20% if greater than 24 hours
  - ◊ Decreased spermatogenesis vast majority of time
  - ◊ 66% of salvaged testicles may atrophy in first 2-3 years post-torsion

POSSIBLE COMPLICATIONS

- Infertility, decreased sperm counts
- Testicular atrophy

HYDROCELE

DESCRIPTION

Collection of peritoneal fluid within scrotum

ETIOLOGY

Infants:
- Usually *communicating*: represents an incomplete closure of processus vaginalis which results in temporary trapping of peritoneal fluid

Adults:
- Usually *non-communicating*: represents closure of the processus vaginalis which traps peritoneal fluid
- Neoplasms
- Infection
- Trauma

INCIDENCE

- 1% of adult males
- Not uncommon in infancy especially in premature infants

RISK FACTORS

- Unknown in many cases
- Exstrophy of bladder
- Peritoneal dialysis

ASSESSMENT FINDINGS

- Painless, swelling in the scrotum
- Fluctuation in size of scrotum in communicating hydrocele
- Scrotum feels heavy and enlarged
- Transillumination of scrotum

DIFFERENTIAL DIAGNOSIS

- Communicating vs. non-communicating hydrocele
- Scrotal trauma; such as falling on a hard object
- Spermatocele
- Varicocele
- Inguinal hernia
- Orchitis, epididymitis
- Scrotal tumor

DIAGNOSTIC STUDIES

- Scrotal ultrasound to differentiate hernia from hydrocele

NONPHARMACOLOGIC MANAGEMENT

Communicating hydrocele:
- Observation and reassurance until one to two years of age

- Surgical correction if not closed by one to two years of age

Non-communicating hydrocele:

- Surgical drainage of fluid and ligation of processus vaginalis
- Therapy not always required in adults unless causing discomfort or other complication

CONSULTATION/REFERRAL

- Refer for surgical evaluation if hydrocele has not absorbed by one year of age or for new hydroceles in adults

FOLLOW-UP

- Follow at 3 month intervals in infants until resolved or referral made

EXPECTED COURSE

- Communicating hydrocele usually absorbs within first year of life
- Non-communicating hydroceles rarely resolve spontaneously

POSSIBLE COMPLICATIONS

- Inguinal hernia

SPERMATOCELE

DESCRIPTION

A well circumscribed mass located in the scrotum along the spermatic cord which contains sperm (often found in the head of the epididymis)

ETIOLOGY

- Unknown
- May be due to blockage of the epididymal ducts

ASSESSMENT FINDINGS

- Freely movable, painless, cystic mass
- Maybe tender when palpated
- Located posterior and superior to testicle
- Easily transilluminates
- Circumscribed mass in scrotum

DIFFERENTIAL DIAGNOSIS

- Varicocele
- Hydrocele
- Testicular tumor
- Epididymitis
- Orchitis

DIAGNOSTIC STUDIES

- Scrotal ultrasound
- Aspiration reveals nonviable sperm

MANAGEMENT

- No therapy necessary unless mass becomes bothersome

CONSULTATION/REFERRAL

- Refer to urologist if causing discomfort to patient

EXPECTED COURSE

- Benign

VARICOCELE

DESCRIPTION

Collection of abnormally large dilated veins (usually the internal spermatic vein) in the scrotum, usually situated above the testis

ETIOLOGY

- Poorly functioning anti-reflux valves of the spermatic veins

INCIDENCE

- Usually found in older adolescents, but may occur at any age
- 80-90% occur on left
- Present in 20% of male population

RISK FACTORS

- Abdominal pathology
- Renal tumor
- Venous obstruction

ASSESSMENT FINDINGS

- Asymptomatic usually
- Presenting complaint is often infertility
- Scrotum resembles "bag of worms"
- Bluish discoloration of scrotum
- Varicocele increases in size when patient standing and with Valsalva maneuver
- Testis nontender
- Feeling of heaviness in scrotum

Sudden appearance of a left-sided varicocele in an adult male should prompt evaluation for possible renal tumor.

DIFFERENTIAL DIAGNOSIS

- Hydrocele
- Spermatocele
- Testicular tumor
- Epididymal cyst

DIAGNOSTIC STUDIES

- Doppler ultrasound
- Sperm count: decreased
- Intravenous pyelography to rule out renal tumor or venous obstruction

MANAGEMENT

- If mild, left-sided varicocele present in an adult without infertility, observation is indicated
- Scrotal support
- Surgical correction if infertility present

CONSULTATION/REFERRAL

- Consult urologist in the following situations
  - ◊ Right-sided varicoceles
  - ◊ New onset in adults
  - ◊ Large varicocele
  - ◊ Does not disappear when supine
  - ◊ Pain
  - ◊ Testicular atrophy
  - ◊ Rapidly increasing in size
  - ◊ Infertility
  - ◊ Prepubertal boys
  - ◊ Older males (increased risk of renal tumors)

EXPECTED COURSE

- Surgical intervention will alleviate symptoms, but infertility is rarely reversed

POSSIBLE COMPLICATIONS

- Causes 40% of male infertility
- Testicular atrophy especially post surgery
- Prepubertal boys: failure to develop secondary sex characteristics

TESTICULAR CANCER

DESCRIPTION

Malignant tumor of the testicle. Two types:

- Seminomas account for 40-50% of cases
- Non seminomas: embryonal cell carcinoma, teratoma, choriocarcinoma

CLINICAL STAGING (Skinner/Walter Reed)

- A: tumor limited to testis and cord
- B: tumor of testis and retroperitoneal nodes
- B1: < 6 nodes all < 2 cm
- B2: > 6 nodes all > 2 cm

- B3: positive retroperitoneal nodes > 5 cm
- C: metastases above diaphragm or involving solid abdominal organs

ETIOLOGY

- Unknown

INCIDENCE

- Most common malignancy in males aged 15-35 years
- Peak incidence between ages 20-40 years
- Accounts for 1-2% of all cancers in males

RISK FACTORS

- History of cryptorchidism (even if repaired)
- Testicular atrophy
- Caucasian race; rare in African-Americans
- HIV positive status

ASSESSMENT FINDINGS

- Solid, firm, nontender testicular mass
- Sensation of fullness or heaviness in scrotum
- Previous small testicle enlarging to size of normal testicle
- Hydrocele
- Gynecomastia
- Mass does not transilluminate

DIFFERENTIAL DIAGNOSIS

- Hernia
- Hydrocele, spermatocele, varicocele
- Epididymitis
- Benign testicular mass
- Testicular torsion

DIAGNOSTIC STUDIES

- α-fetoprotein: elevated
- β-human chorionic gonadotropin (β-hCG): elevated
- Scrotal ultrasound
- Abdominal and chest CT scan
- Biopsy

PREVENTION

- Monthly self-testicular examination beginning in adolescence

MANAGEMENT

- Dependent on staging
- Radiation therapy
- Chemotherapy
- Surgical intervention: radical orchiectomy

CONSULTATION/REFERRAL

- Refer to urologist for evaluation and treatment

FOLLOW-UP

- Close monitoring of hCG and α-fetoprotein for indication of response to therapy and recurrence
- Periodic chest and abdominal CT for detection of metastasis

EXPECTED COURSE

- Usually complete cure in patients with limited disease
- 70-80% cure in patients with advanced disease
- 5-year survival rate: about 95%

POSSIBLE COMPLICATIONS

- Metastasis
- Complications associated with radiation, chemotherapy, and surgery

INGUINAL HERNIA

DESCRIPTION

- Two types:
  - ◊ Indirect: hernial sac protrudes through the internal inguinal ring into the inguinal canal often descending into the scrotum
  - ◊ Direct: hernial sac protrudes directly through the abdominal wall in the region of Hesselbach's triangle

TERMS

- Incarcerated: one in which the hernia's contents cannot be replaced into the abdomen
- Strangulated: incarcerated hernia in which the blood supply to the entrapped bowel has been diminished; a surgical emergency
- Reducible: the hernia is easily replaced into the abdomen using gentle pressure or may occur spontaneously

ETIOLOGY

- Congenital defect
- Injury

INCIDENCE

- 80% of all hernias are inguinal

Indirect:
- 3.5-5.5% of full term infants; increased incidence in premature infants
- 50% of all hernias in adults are indirect
- Males > Females

Direct:
- More common in middle and later years of life
- Rare in pediatric population

RISK FACTORS

- Male
- Weak abdominal musculature
- Premature
- Twin gestation

ASSESSMENT FINDINGS

- Feeling of heaviness in groin
- Painful or painless swelling or lump in groin or into scrotum which increases when standing or straining
- In women, bulge may be seen in the labia majora
- Strangulated hernia:
  - ◊ Colicky abdominal pain
  - ◊ Nausea and vomiting
  - ◊ Abdominal distention

DIFFERENTIAL DIAGNOSIS

- Hydrocele/varicocele/spermatocele
- Epididymitis
- Testicular tumor
- Undescended testicle
- Lymphadenopathy

DIAGNOSTIC STUDIES

- Ultrasound

NONPHARMACOLOGIC MANAGEMENT

- Educate about signs and symptoms of strangulation
- Do not attempt to reduce a strangulated hernia
- Hernia will not resolve spontaneously, surgical correction (herniorrhaphy) is required

CONSULTATION/REFERRAL

- Refer to surgeon for evaluation
- Refer immediately if strangulated

EXPECTED COURSE

- Complete recovery without sequelae if treated promptly and appropriately

POSSIBLE COMPLICATIONS

- Strangulation of hernia

HYPOSPADIAS

DESCRIPTION

Congenital abnormality in which the urethral opening is on the underside of the penis (ventral surface)

ETIOLOGY

- Multifactorial

INCIDENCE

- Occurs in 1/300 male infants

RISK FACTORS

- Family history
- Increased incidence in whites
- Exogenous progesterone intake by mother during pregnancy
- Increased risk of undescended testicles, inguinal hernia, and hydrocele

ASSESSMENT FINDINGS

- Urethra located on ventral surface of penis
- Urinary stream aims downward
- Foreskin may not be present
- Chordee (bowing of the penis due to fibrous band of tissue pulling on penis)

DIFFERENTIAL DIAGNOSIS

- Ambiguous genitalia

DIAGNOSTIC STUDIES

- None usually needed

MANAGEMENT

- Circumcision must NOT be done, foreskin may be needed for surgical repair
- Surgical repair usually at age 6-18 months

CONSULTATION/REFERRAL

- Refer to urologist for surgical repair

EXPECTED COURSE

- Usually excellent prognosis

POSSIBLE COMPLICATIONS

- Erectile dysfunction if chordee present

PHIMOSIS

DESCRIPTION

Foreskin which is too tight, preventing retraction over the glans penis

ETIOLOGY

- Physiologic: present at birth and resolves spontaneously by 3 years of age
- Congenital: unresolved physiologic phimosis
- Acquired: recurrent infection or irritation

INCIDENCE

- 1% of adolescent males

RISK FACTORS

- Poor hygiene
- Diabetes mellitus
- Presence of an STD

ASSESSMENT FINDINGS

- Unretractable foreskin
- Pain with erection
- Balanitis may be present

DIFFERENTIAL DIAGNOSIS

- Allergic reaction

DIAGNOSTIC STUDIES

- None usually needed

PREVENTION

- Good hygiene
- Parental education about care of uncircumcised infant
- Circumcision at birth (controversial)

NONPHARMACOLOGIC MANAGEMENT

- Normal cleansing and gentle stretching of foreskin
- Often nocturnal erections will stretch ring and problem resolves without other intervention
- Circumcision if there is urinary obstruction

CONSULTATION/REFERRAL

- Refer for surgical evaluation for circumcision

EXPECTED COURSE

- Complete resolution if treated appropriately

POSSIBLE COMPLICATIONS

- Urinary tract infection
- Stricture
- Inflammation of the prepuce
- Balanitis

ERECTILE DYSFUNCTION

DESCRIPTION

Inability to achieve or maintain an erection satisfactorily to effect penetration and ejaculation. Transient or occasional impotence is common and not necessarily evidence of pathology. A pattern of repeated (>25%) episodes over more than a month should be investigated, however.

ETIOLOGY

- 50% organic in nature
    - ◊ Spinal cord injury
    - ◊ Surgical procedures
    - ◊ Diabetes mellitus: reported in up to 50% of men with diabetes
    - ◊ Heavy metal toxicity
    - ◊ Medications (e.g., phenothiazines, tricyclic antidepressants, selective serotonin-reuptake inhibitors, exogenous estrogen, many antihypertensives)
    - ◊ Drug abuse (e.g., heroin, morphine, methadone, barbiturates)
    - ◊ Chronic alcoholism
    - ◊ Heavy smoking
    - ◊ Hypo/hyperthyroidism
    - ◊ Addison's disease
    - ◊ Cushing's syndrome
    - ◊ Acromegaly
    - ◊ Hyperprolactinemia
    - ◊ Prostatic cancer
    - ◊ Arterial insufficiency
- Psychogenic

INCIDENCE

- Affects up to 10% of men at any given point in time, but much higher incidence in treatment of hypertension

RISK FACTORS

- *See* Etiology

ASSESSMENT FINDINGS

- Dependent on underlying etiology
- Inability to achieve or maintain an erection
- Absence of nocturnal erection may indicate organic cause

DIAGNOSTIC STUDIES

- Determined by suspected underlying etiology
- CBC and complete metabolic panel
- Hormone levels: free testosterone, prolactin level
- Fasting blood sugar
- Thyroid stimulating hormone
- Testing of nocturnal erection at home with use of a "snap gauge" or a formal tumescence study in a sleep laboratory (tends to be intact with psychogenic causes)
- Doppler estimation of penile blood flow if vascular cause suspected

PREVENTION

- Good glucose control in diabetes mellitus
- Avoid (if possible) medications which may cause impotence (marijuana)

NONPHARMACOLOGIC MANAGEMENT

- Psychologic support
- Education regarding causes
- Change in medications which may cause impotence
- Penile implants for patients with refractory impotence
- Vacuum suction device
- Vascular surgery for those with vascular insufficiency

PHARMACOLOGIC MANAGEMENT

- Sildenafil (Viagra®), vardenafil (Levitra®), tadalafil (Cialis®),
- Intracavernosal injection therapy with papaverine and phentolamine for those with vascular disease, diabetes, neurological dysfunction
- Testosterone therapy for patients with hypogonadism

CONSULTATION/REFERRAL

- Referral to urologist, vascular surgeon, neurologist depending on underlying pathology

FOLLOW-UP

- Frequent follow-up is indicated

EXPECTED COURSE

- Dependent on underlying cause

POSSIBLE COMPLICATIONS

- Complications from treatments (e.g., priapism)
- Low self-esteem
- Disruption in sexual relationships

References

Bhatnagar, V., & Kaplan, M. (2005). Treatment options for prostate cancer: Evaluating the evidence. *American Family Physician, 71,* 1915-1922.

Bickley, L.S., & Szilagyi, P.G. (2003). *Bates' guide to physical examination and history taking* (8th ed.). Philadelphia: Lippincott Williams & Wilkins.

Branch, W.T. (2003). *Office practice of medicine* (4th ed.). Philadelphia: Saunders.

Burns, C.E., Brady, M.A., Blosser, C., Starr, N.B., & Dunn, A.M. (2004). *Pediatric primary care: A handbook for nurse practitioners* (3rd ed.). Philadelphia: W.B. Saunders.

Centers for Disease Control and Prevention. (1998). Sexually transmitted diseases treatment guidelines. *MMWR, 47,* (RR-1).

Campbell, M.F., Walsh, P.C., & Retnick, A.B.(Eds.). (2002). *Campbell's urology.* (8th ed.). Philadelphia: WB Saunders.

Dambro, M.R. (2005). *Griffith's 5 minute clinical consult.* Philadelphia: Lippincott Williams & Wilkins.

Dufour, J. L. (2001). Assessing and treating epididymitis. *The Nurse Practitioner, 26*(3), 23-24.

Gilber, D.N., Moellering, R.C., Eliopoulos, G.M., & Sande, M.A. (Eds.). (2004). *Sanford Guide to Antimicrobial Therapy* (34th ed.). Hyde Park, VT: Antimicrobial Therapy.

Golden, W.E. (2003). BPH diagnosis and management. *Internal Medicine News, 36*(19), 27.

Goroll, A. H., & Mulley, A. G., Jr. (Eds.). (2000). *Primary care medicine: Office evaluation and management of the adult patient* (4th ed.). Philadelphia: Lippincott Williams Wilkins.

Graber, M.A., & Lanternier, M.L. (Eds.) (2001). *The family practice handbook.* (4th ed.). St. Louis: Mosby.

Junnila, J., & Lassen, P. (1998). Testicular masses. *American Family Physician, 57,* 685-692.

Mangion, S. (2000). *Physical diagnosis secrets.* Philadelphia: Hanley and Belfus.

McConnell, J.D., Barry, M.J., Bruskewitz, R.C., et.al. (1994). *Benign prostatic hyperplasia: Diagnosis and treatment.* Clinical Practice Guideline, No. 8. AHCPR Publication No. 94-0582. Rockville, MD: Agency for Health Care Policy and Research, Public Health Service, U.S. Department of Health and Human Services.

McVary, K.T. (2005). Managing sexual dysfunction in the andropause. *Clinical Advisor, 8*(7) (Suppl.), 3-11.

Mladenovic, J. (Ed.). (2003). *Primary care secrets.* (3rd Ed.). Philadelphia: Hanley and Belfus.

Proceedings of 94th annual American Urological Association Meeting, Dallas, 1999.

Rakel, R.E. (Ed.). (1998). *Essentials of family practice.* (2nd ed.). Philadelphia: WB Saunders.

Randrup, E.R., & Baum, N. (1997). Pharmacologic management of benign prostatic hyperplasia. *Hospital Medicine, 33*(11), 43-53.

Uphold, C.R., & Graham, M.V. (2003). *Clinical guidelines in family practice.* (4th ed.). Gainesville, FL: Barmarrae Books.

U.S. Preventive Services Task Force. (1996). *Guide to clinical preventive services.* (2nd ed.) Washington, D.C.: Office of Disease Prevention and Health Promotion, U.S. Government Printing Office.

Men's Health

Zollo, A.J., Jr (Ed.). (2004). *Medical Secrets*. (4th ed.), St. Louis, MO: Mosby-Year Book.

13

NEUROLOGICAL DISORDERS

Neurological Disorders

* *Denotes pediatric diagnosis*

HEADACHES
(Cephalgia)

DESCRIPTION

Pain in the head caused by multiple etiologies

ETIOLOGY

Due to stimulation, traction, tension, pressure on any pain sensitive structures of the head

- Abnormal metabolism of serotonin, norepinephrine, dopamine
- Hypertension
- Sinus infections
- Tooth abscesses
- Lesions of the oral cavity
- Ear infections
- Eye strain or other eye lesions
- Dilation of cerebral blood vessels by drugs
- Space-occupying tumors
- Increased intracranial pressure from hematomas
- Hemorrhage within the cranium
- Temporal arteritis
- Uremia
- Meningitis
- TB
- Syphilis
- Carbon monoxide poisoning
- Anxiety, hysteria, etc.

INCIDENCE

- Very common
- Cluster headaches: 0.5-1.0% of adults, rarely occur in children, very rare during pregnancy
- Tension headaches: 60% have onset after age 20 years, rarely have onset after age 50 years, 15% of pediatric patients will have onset before age 10 years, no documented relationship between tension headaches and pregnancy
- Migraine headaches: 17.6% of females, 5.6% of males in U.S.
- Pediatric migraines: 3-5% of all children in U.S. increase to 10-20% during the second decade

Headaches of new onset in the elderly tend to have a secondary cause: tumor, bleed, etc.

RISK FACTORS

- Cluster headaches
- Male gender (6:1)
- Age >30 years
- Alcohol intake
- Use of nitroglycerine
- Tension headaches
- Excessive intake of caffeine, nicotine
- Stressful situations
- Migraine headaches
- Family history (>80% have positive family history)
- Female gender
- First headache in early childhood but grossly under reported
- Excessive sleep
- Ingestion of certain foods
    * Tryptophan or tyramine rich foods: ripe cheeses, red wine, and chocolate
- Alcohol
- Estrogen replacement
- Missing meals

A cluster headache is sometimes referred to as a suicide headache because there is a high rate of suicide or self-harm in these individuals during the headache cycle.

ASSESSMENT FINDINGS

- *Cluster headache*
    - ◊ Pain peaks within 15 minutes, usually lasts <3 hours
    - ◊ Sudden, severe and unilateral
    - ◊ Eye, temple, face, or neck involvement
    - ◊ Lacrimation and/or rhinorrhea

- ◊ Ptosis
- ◊ Injected conjunctiva
- ◊ Nasal stuffiness
- ◊ Attacks may occur at the same time for several days
- ◊ Attack may occur within 90 minutes of falling asleep

- *Tension Headaches*
  - ◊ Bilateral in 90% of cases
  - ◊ Dull, vice-like, pressure around head
  - ◊ May be frontal-occipital
  - ◊ May be intermittent; may be present all day ranging in intensity from mild to severe
  - ◊ Palpable muscle tightness, soreness, or stiffness in neck, upper shoulders, or scalp
- *Migraine*: 5 phases may occur
  - ◊ Prodrome
    - * Mood swings
    - * Fatigue
    - * Food craving
    - * Yawning
  - ◊ Aura
    - * Visual disturbances: visual field cuts, flashing lights, zigzag patterns, floaters
    - * Headache begins within one hour and is usually generalized
  - ◊ Headache (lasts 4-72 hours)
    - * Unilateral, bilateral, or generalized
    - * Throbbing (or not)
    - * Anorexia, nausea, vomiting
    - * Photophobia, phonophobia, lightheadedness
    - * Vertigo
  - ◊ Termination of headache
    - * Usually occurs with sleep or medication
  - ◊ Postdrome
    - * Lingering symptoms: fatigue, malaise, inability to problem solve

Not all patients with migraine will experience all 5 phases.

ASSESSMENT FINDINGS CHARACTERISTIC OF SECONDARY HEADACHES

- "Worst headache of my life": subarachnoid hemorrhage
- Headache worse in the morning, deep pain, aggravated by coughing, sneezing: brain tumor
- Morning headaches worse in the occipital region: hypertension
- Headaches worse with bending over, nasal congestion, facial tenderness: sinusitis
- Severe headache, tachycardia, diaphoresis: pheochromocytoma
- Orbital headache: acute angle glaucoma

DIFFERENTIAL DIAGNOSIS

- Headache disorders
- Secondary headaches
- Giant cell arteritis
- Drug-seeking patients
- Psychiatric disease

DIAGNOSTIC STUDIES

- Depends on patient's symptoms and presumed etiology
- CT and/or MRI (reserve for patients with neurological deficits, sudden onset of severe headache, or change in frequency and occurrence of headaches)
- Consider sinus series
- CBC, complete metabolic panel, TSH
- Cervical x-rays
- EEG
- Lumbar puncture
- Sedimentation rate

PREVENTION/AVOIDANCE

Cluster headache	Avoid triggering substance (e.g., alcohol) Temper strong emotions Maintain usual sleep/wake hours Pharmacologic interventions for prophylaxis (*see* Pharmacologic Management) Avoidance of vasodilators (NTG, alcohol)
Tension headache	Relaxation therapy Stress management
Migraine headache	Avoid precipitating factors Avoid foods which may precipitate headaches: * Nitrite-containing foods (e.g., hot dogs) * Monosodium glutamate-containing foods (e.g., Chinese food) * Tyramine-containing foods (e.g., chocolate, cheese, red wine, caffeine containing beverages) Pharmacologic prophylaxis (*see* Pharmacologic Management)

NONPHARMACOLOGIC MANAGEMENT

- *See* Prevention/Avoidance
- Application of ice, cool compresses to head, face, scalp, or neck
- Darkened room
- Quiet atmosphere
- β-blockers or calcium channel blockers daily for prophylaxis

PHARMACOLOGIC MANAGEMENT

Cluster headache	◊ 100% oxygen 7-10 liters for 10-15 minutes at onset ◊ Sumatriptan (Imitrex®) for abortive therapy ◊ Prophylactic management: verapamil (Calan®), lithium (Lithobid®), ergotamine (Cafergot®), indomethacin (Indocin®), nifedipine (Procardia®), nimodipine (Nimotop®), others ◊ Prednisone used while waiting for other therapy (oral medications) to become effective ◊ Intranasal lidocaine 4% topical on same side as symptoms
Tension headache	◊ NSAIDs: naproxen sodium, ibuprofen, ketoprofen, aspirin ◊ Prophylaxis for chronic headache: amitriptyline (Elavil®), imipramine (Tofranil®), non-specific beta blockers
Migraine headache	◊ Triptans ◊ Ergotamines: dihydroergotamine (DHE®) ◊ Combination medications: ergotamine-caffeine (Cafergot®), isometheptene-dichloralphenazone-acetaminophen (Midrin®), butalbital-acetaminophen (Fioricet®) ◊ NSAIDs: aspirin, ibuprofen, naproxen, ketoprofen ◊ TCA: off label use for prophylaxis

AGENT	ACTION	COMMENTS
Abortive agents ***Serotonin 5HT$_1$ receptor agonists ("Triptans")*** *Example:* sumatriptan (Imitrex®) almotriptan (Axert®) frovatriptan (Frova®) naratriptan (Amerge®)	Triptans cause constriction of the cerebral vessels	May cause coronary artery vasoconstriction, arrhythmias, stroke or MI. Expect elevation in patient's blood pressure after triptan consumption. Potential drug interactions with MAOI, cimetidine, SSRIs, propanolol.
Analgesic Agents ***NSAID*** *Examples:* ibuprofen naproxen ketoprofen	Inhibit cyclooxygenase (COX) activity and inhibit prostaglandin synthesis	COX_1 and COX_2 are isoenzymes. Inhibition of COX_1 responsible for major GI toxic effect. COX_2 produced during pain and inflammatory states.
Prophylactic Agents (some are off label use) ***Nonselective beta blockers*** *Examples:* propanol (Inderal®) timolol (Blocadren®)	Mechanism of action is poorly understood	Nonselective beta blockers are better prophylactic agents than the cardioselective agents.
Calcium channel blockers *Examples:* verapamil (Calan®)	Mechanism of action is poorly understood	Watch for drug interactions with grapefruit juice.
TCA *Examples:* amitriptyline nortriptyline	Inhibit the re-uptake of serotonin and/or norepinephrine	Used off-label once daily at bedtime for migraine prophylaxis. Watch for drug interactions: MAOI, SSRI, cimetidine, quinolones

SPECIAL CONSIDERATIONS

- Avoid triptans in patients with coronary artery disease, poorly controlled hypertension
- Triptans most effective if given during early headache phase
- Avoid concomitant use of triptans and ergotamine within a 24-hour period
- Reserve narcotics for infrequent use due to addiction potential

PREGNANCY/LACTATION CONSIDERATIONS

- Triptan pregnancy category C drug
- Avoid use of ergotamine
- Number and intensity of migraine headaches may decrease during 2nd and 3rd trimester

CONSULTATION/REFERRAL

- Refer to neurologist for severe headaches or those that are unresponsive to drug therapy

FOLLOW-UP

- Return to clinic or emergency department if headache unresolved after treatment, becomes more severe, or varies from the usual pattern

EXPECTED COURSE

- Cluster headache: recurrent attacks are usual until cycle can be interrupted
- Tension headache: most follow a chronic course if stressors are not eliminated
- Migraine headache: most resolve within 72 hours; decrease in frequency and duration as patient ages

POSSIBLE COMPLICATIONS

- Cluster headache: suicide or self-injury during an attack, risk of addiction to narcotic analgesics
- Tension headache: GI bleed from continued use of NSAIDs
- Migraine headache: risk of addiction to narcotic analgesics, iatrogenic complications from treatment (e.g., angina from triptans)

TRIGEMINAL NEURALGIA
Tic Douloureux

DESCRIPTION

A disorder of the 5th cranial nerve (trigeminal nerve) which produces severe pain in the lip, gum, cheek, and/or face.

ETIOLOGY

- Compression of the 5th cranial nerve from unknown causes, tumors, or vascular malformations

INCIDENCE

- 16/100,000 in U.S.
- Females > Males (2:1)
- Peak age is 60 years

RISK FACTORS

- None known

ASSESSMENT FINDINGS

- Severe pain in the lip, face, mouth, gum, cheek
- Wincing
- Pain may be in "bursts" with pain free period after burst
- Pain may be elicited by touch, changes in temperature, or a light breeze on the cheek
- Lacrimation, flushing, salivation

Pain can be reported as "unbearable" and often thought to be of dental origin initially.

DIFFERENTIAL DIAGNOSIS

- Other form of neuralgia
- Migraine

DIAGNOSTIC STUDIES

- MRI or CT scan to rule out neoplasm

PREVENTION/AVOIDANCE

- Withdraw medications used for management slowly (4-6 weeks)
- Restart at highest level if pain resumes
- Avoidance of breeze, heat, cold on facial areas

NONPHARMACOLOGIC MANAGEMENT

- Avoidance of breeze, heat, cold on facial areas
- Surgical decompression or nerve ablation
- Peripheral nerve block of the 5th cranial nerve

PHARMACOLOGIC MANAGEMENT

- Carbamazepine (Tegretol®) *OR* phenytoin (Dilantin®) *OR* clonazepam (Klonopin®) *OR* valproic acid (Depakene®)
- Neurontin®
- Clonidine
- Injectable numbing agents or nerve block

CONSULTATION/REFERRAL

- Neurologist

FOLLOW-UP

- Check carbamazepine and phenytoin levels
- Check liver and hematopoietic (LFT and CBC) functions if carbamazepine prescribed

EXPECTED COURSE

- Prognosis good
- Exacerbations in spring and fall

POSSIBLE COMPLICATIONS

- Sedation from medications
- Vertigo from carbamazepine

SYNCOPE
(Faint)

DESCRIPTION

A sudden, brief loss of consciousness with a spontaneous recovery

ETIOLOGY

Vasovagal	Due to decreased cardiac output from peripheral vasodilation and bradycardia
Orthostatic hypotension	Due to medications, hypovolemia, autonomic dysfunction
Situational syncope	Due to coughing, micturition, or defecation
Cardiac	Due to sudden decrease in cardiac output ◊ Aortic stenosis ◊ Arrhythmias (heart blocks, ventricular tachycardia)
Carotid sinus syncope	Due to manual pressure/stimulation of the carotid arteries
Cerebrovascular disease	Due to decreased perfusion of the vertebrobasilar system
Other causes	Depression, alcohol ingestion, drug abuse, psychogenic, subclavian steal syndrome, cardiomyopathy

INCIDENCE

- 6% in persons over age 75 years
- More common in the elderly
- Unidentifiable cause in 48% of patients

RISK FACTORS

- Underlying cardiac disease
- Patients on antihypertensive agents, antiarrhythmics, antidepressants, diuretics, phenothiazines, vasodilators
- Malfunctioning pacemaker

ASSESSMENT FINDINGS

- General findings
  - ◊ Feelings of lightheadedness, weakness, nausea, vomiting, diaphoresis
  - ◊ Loss of consciousness
  - ◊ Loss of postural tone
  - ◊ Spontaneous recovery
- Vasovagal
  - ◊ Fear, anxiety, or sudden emotion may precipitate syncopal episode
  - ◊ Sudden onset of weakness, sweating, nausea
- Orthostatic hypotension
  - ◊ Occurs when patient stands
- Situational syncope
  - ◊ May be precipitated by swallowing, coughing, micturition, defecation
- Cardiac arrhythmias
  - ◊ Usually abrupt onset without warning
  - ◊ Related to physical activity
  - ◊ May be precipitated by electrolyte imbalance (especially potassium, calcium, or magnesium), malfunction

of prosthetic heart valve or pacemaker, hypoxia, coronary artery disease

- Carotid sinus syncope
    - ◊ Bradycardia often precipitates syncope
    - ◊ Turning of neck may precipitate syncope
- Cerebrovascular disease
    - ◊ May experience auditory, visual, or vestibular symptoms prior to syncope
    - ◊ May have history of previous transient ischemic attack

DIFFERENTIAL DIAGNOSIS

- Vertigo
- Seizure activity
- Cerebellar disease
- Space-occupying lesion in the cranial cavity
- Psychological stress
- Cardiac vs. noncardiac syncope

DIAGNOSTIC STUDIES/PHYSICAL EXAMINATION

- Complete metabolic panel: Sodium, calcium, glucose needed
- 24-hour ECG monitoring (helpful 4-15% of the time)
- Blood pressure measurements in both arms: difference of 20 mm Hg or more is considered abnormal
- Blood pressure measurements lying and standing: normal findings are systolic pressure decrease of less than 10 mm Hg, increase in diastolic 2-5 mm Hg, and increase in heart rate 5-20 beats. If heart rate does not increase, consider cardiac origin.
- Flexion/extension of neck 10 times to simulate vertebrobasilar insufficiency
- Flexion/extension of arms to simulate symptoms of subclavian steal syndrome
- Complete neurological examination; if abnormal, consider CT, MRI, EEG
- Complete cardiac examination
- Carotid auscultation/studies for suspected carotid artery disease: bruit indicates probable blockage
- Echocardiogram if valvular or cardiomyopathy is suspected
- Tilt testing

After thorough examination, only 50-60% of patients will have an identifiable cause.

PREVENTION

- Rise slowly from lying or sitting to standing

NONPHARMACOLOGIC MANAGEMENT

- Elevate patient's legs if due to vasovagal or hypotension
- Elastic support stockings to prevent orthostatic hypotension
- Changing positions slowly, especially to an upright position
- Teach patient about measures to take to ensure safety (e.g., do not climb on stools, don't operate dangerous machinery, avoid bathing in tub of very hot water, etc.), especially if a particular activity may precipitate syncopal episode
- Other actions dependent on underlying cause of syncope
- Increased sodium intake to help expand volume

PHARMACOLOGIC MANAGEMENT

- Depends on underlying cause
- β-blockers may prevent recurrent vasovagal symptoms
- Antiarrhythmic drugs for documented arrhythmias

PREGNANCY/LACTATION CONSIDERATIONS

- Vasovagal syncope may present in pregnant women from compression of the vena cava and aorta
- Positioning the pregnant woman on her left side should relieve the compression and the symptoms

CONSULTATION/REFERRAL

- Refer to cardiologist, neurologist, depending on etiology

FOLLOW-UP

- Depends on etiology

EXPECTED COURSE

- Depends on etiology

POSSIBLE COMPLICATIONS

- Head injury from falls during episode
- Sudden death (more common if cardiac etiology)

TRANSIENT ISCHEMIC ATTACK (TIA)

DESCRIPTION

A sudden onset of neurological deficits which is caused by cerebral ischemia and lasts < 24 hours

ETIOLOGY

- Atherosclerotic disease within the brain and/or carotid arteries
- Microemboli from atrial fibrillation, cardiac valve disorders
- Hypercoagulable states
- Spontaneous
- Cerebral artery vasospasm
- Use of oral contraceptive

INCIDENCE

- 30/100,000 in U.S.
- Male > Female 3:1

RISK FACTORS

- Hypertension
- Advanced age
- Prior TIA
- Smoking
- Diabetes
- Hyperlipidemia
- Cardiac disease
- Atrial fibrillation
- Family history of TIA or stroke
- Oral contraceptive use

ASSESSMENT FINDINGS

- Aphasia
- Visual field defects
- Confusion
- Amnesia
- Diplopia
- Dysphagia
- Dysarthria
- Unilateral weakness
- Neurological deficits usually last <24 hours

Any sudden onset of neurological symptoms should prompt an evaluation for stroke.

DIFFERENTIAL DIAGNOSIS

- Stroke
- Seizure
- Hypoglycemia

DIAGNOSTIC STUDIES

- CT, MRI of head: rule out hemorrhage, CVA
- Carotid studies (ultrasound and/or angiography): >70% blockage may cause symptoms
- Cerebral angiography: may demonstrate atherosclerosis
- ECG, 24-hour Holter monitor, echocardiogram if underlying cardiac problem suspected
- EEG if seizure suspected

PREVENTION

- Control blood pressure, lipids, diabetes
- Antiplatelet therapy
- ACE inhibitors
- Statins
- Aspirin or ticlopidine (Ticlid®)

NONPHARMACOLOGIC MANAGEMENT

- Control risk factors: hypertension, hyperlipidemia, diabetes
- Patient education regarding importance of stopping smoking, taking medications as prescribed (e.g., antihypertensives, lipid lowering agents, anticoagulants)
- Endarterectomy

PHARMACOLOGIC MANAGEMENT

- Aspirin or Ticlopidine (Ticlid®)
- Clopidogrel (Plavix®)

PREGNANCY/LACTATION CONSIDERATIONS

- Pregnancy may produce a state of hypercoagulation

CONSULTATION/REFERRAL

- Cardiologist if underlying cardiac disorders
- Neurologist

FOLLOW-UP

- Depends on etiology

EXPECTED COURSE

- Increased risk of stroke with presence of additional risk factors (e.g., hypertension, hypercholesterolemia, smoking)

POSSIBLE COMPLICATIONS

- Stroke
- Injury from fall

SEIZURE DISORDERS
(Convulsions, Epilepsy)

DESCRIPTION

A transient alteration in behavior with or without loss of consciousness, sensory perception, motor function, and/or autonomic function. Seizures are due to excessive rate of neuronal discharges. Seizures which are recurrent are termed *epilepsy*.

TYPES OF SEIZURES

Seizures are classified by the location of their onset
Partial (begins with motor symptoms characterized by recurrent contractions of muscles in one part of the body ◊ Jacksonian-type seizures begin in one part of the body and progress to contiguous body parts over seconds or minutes ◊ Simple partial (consciousness not impaired)
Generalized (without local onset and bilaterally symmetrical) ◊ Absence: brief arrest of activity and loss of consciousness ◊ Myoclonic: muscle movements are repetitive ◊ Clonic: seizure associated with intermittent contraction and relaxation of muscles ◊ Tonic: sustained muscle contraction during seizure ◊ Atonic: seizure associated with an absence of muscle tone ◊ Tonic-clonic ◊ Other types

ETIOLOGY

- Idiopathic
- Alcohol intoxication or withdrawal
- Brain tumor
- Hypoxia
- Brain attack (formerly called stroke)
- Breath holding spells
- Exposure to toxic agents
- Eclampsia
- Fever (*see* Febrile Seizures)
- Head injury
- Hyperthermia
- Hyperventilation
- Meningitis
- Migraine

INCIDENCE

- Highest incidence is in children
- 4-6% of children will have a seizure before age 16 years
- 1.5 million people in U.S. have epilepsy
- 1.2/1000 in U.S. for all types of seizures
- 10% of general population has isolated seizures

Patients most likely to have seizures are pediatric and geriatric patients.

RISK FACTORS

- Previous history of seizure
- Family history
- Brain tumor
- History of neurological insult (e.g., brain attack, intracranial hemorrhage, head trauma, meningitis)
- Withdrawal from anticonvulsant medications

ASSESSMENT FINDINGS

- Seizure with or without loss of consciousness, with or without loss of posture

DIAGNOSTIC CLUES

- Fever: infectious etiology
- Headache: infectious etiology, hemorrhage, tumor
- Meningismus (irritation of the brain and spinal cord without meningitis): CNS infection
- Papilledema: increased intracranial pressure from tumor, bleed
- Focal neurologic finding: tumor or localized injury to specific site in brain

DIFFERENTIAL DIAGNOSIS

Newborn to 2 years of age	Metabolic (hypoglycemia, hypocalcemia, hypo-magnesemia, phenylketonuria) Infection Birth injury Febrile seizure
2 to 10 years of age	**Febrile seizure** **Tumor** **CNS infection** **Trauma** **Idiopathic**
10 to 18 years of age	Tumor Trauma Arteriovenous malformation Drug or alcohol related Idiopathic
18 to 25 years of age	Tumor Trauma Infection, meningitis Drug or alcohol intoxication or withdrawal Idiopathic
25 to 60 years of age	Tumor Trauma Drug or alcohol related
Over 60 years of age	Tumor Metabolic (hypoglycemia, hypocalcemia, hypomagnesemia, uremia)

DIAGNOSTIC STUDIES

- Complete metabolic panel to assess for glucose, electrolytes, BUN, ammonia
- Toxicology screens: presence of drugs or alcohol
- Complete blood count: elevated WBC if infection present
- Anticonvulsant levels if patient is on anticonvulsant
- MRI or CT of brain: MRI preferred because it provides more detailed information, but CT is faster, may be more easily accessible, and easier to obtain if patient is medically unstable
- EEG usually indicated for all children with a first nonfebrile seizure
- Lumbar puncture indicated for most children under 2 years of age or if CNS infection is suspected in any age

PREVENTION

- Usually none
- Fever management
- Maintain medication regimen if on anticonvulsants

NONPHARMACOLOGIC MANAGEMENT

- Monitor anticonvulsant levels if appropriate
- Patient education particular to type of anticonvulsant that patient is taking
- Provide safe environment during seizure
- Discussion regarding driving, swimming, other activities

PHARMACOLOGIC MANAGEMENT

- Phenytoin (Dilantin®)
- Carbamazepine (Tegretol®)
- Phenobarbital
- Valproic acid (Depakene®)
- Ethosuximide (Zarontin®)

PREGNANCY/LACTATION CONSIDERATIONS

- Monitor levels closely if on anticonvulsants
- Increased risk of congenital malformations in babies born to mothers on anticonvulsant therapy
- Breastfeeding is NOT a contraindication if mother is taking anticonvulsant (may necessitate checking levels in baby). Observe for sedation in baby.

CONSULTATION/REFERRAL

- Consult neurologist for all patients with first-time seizure

FOLLOW-UP

- Depends on etiology and severity
- Monitor anticonvulsant levels periodically

EXPECTED COURSE

- Depends on etiology

POSSIBLE COMPLICATIONS

- Drug toxicity from anticonvulsants
- Hypoxia from repetitive seizures with resultant neurological manifestations

FEBRILE SEIZURES

DESCRIPTION

Seizures which occur during a febrile episode. The seizure is not associated with any underlying disorder. They usually occur within the first 24 hours of an illness and do not necessarily occur when the fever is highest.

ETIOLOGY

- Fever lowers the seizure threshold
- Elevated temperature (usually >102.2°F, 39°C)

Rapidity with which body temperature rises or falls seems to be a greater predictor of seizure than the actual temperature.

INCIDENCE

- Highest incidence occurs between one and two years of age
- 85% occur before the age of 4 years
- 2-5% incidence overall
- Males slightly greater than females

RISK FACTORS

- Very rapid rise in temperature within 24 hours of a febrile illness (most common illnesses are viral upper respiratory and otitis media)
- Febrile seizure in a sibling (risk increased by 2-3 times)
- Recent MMR immunization (within 7-10 days) or DPT (previous 48 hours)

ASSESSMENT FINDINGS

- Fever of ≥102.2°F (39°C)
- First 24 hours of a febrile illness
- Seizure may be first sign of illness in child

DIFFERENTIAL DIAGNOSIS

- Syncopal episode
- Night terrors
- Breath-holding spells
- Febrile associated shivering or delirium
- Afebrile seizure which coincidentally occurs during a febrile event
- Sudden discontinuance of anticonvulsants
- Underlying CNS infection

DIAGNOSTIC STUDIES

- Lumbar puncture if child is younger than 12 months old
- Laboratory testing not done routinely for simple, febrile seizure
- Consider CBC, electrolytes, chemistries, urinalysis
- CBC, electrolytes, chemistries, EEG, MRI, CT if child appears toxic, has neurological deficits, multiple seizures, prolonged recovery, etc.

PREVENTION

- Antipyretics for fever >100.6°F (38.1°C)
- Tepid sponge bath for high fever

NONPHARMACOLOGIC MANAGEMENT

- Supportive care after seizure has occurred
- Patient/family education regarding
  - ◊ Emergency measures if seizures occur in the future
  - ◊ Fever management at home
  - ◊ Educate parents that febrile seizures do not cause developmental delays, learning problems or behavior problems

PHARMACOLOGIC MANAGEMENT

- Treatment for initial simple febrile seizure is not indicated. Cost-benefit ratio does not justify treatment.
- Only 33% of children with initial seizure have a recurrence
- Treat high fever with acetaminophen or other antipyretic
- Children's ibuprofen may be administered to children >6 months of age

Alternating ibuprofen and acetaminophen every 2 hours for fever management leads to medication errors and is not recommended by American Academy of Pediatrics.

CONSULTATION/REFERRAL

- Consult neurologist for suspected underlying cause (e.g., CNS infection, afebrile seizure)

FOLLOW-UP

- Depends on etiology of febrile illness and whether seizure was a simple febrile seizure
- If assessment indicates questionable underlying cause of seizure, follow-up by neurologist needed

EXPECTED COURSE

- 33% will develop recurrent seizures
- 95% of those that will have a recurrence do so within one year of initial episode

POSSIBLE COMPLICATIONS

- Slight increase in risk of development of epilepsy later in life

MENINGITIS

DESCRIPTION

Inflammation of the brain and spinal cord caused by infection with bacteria, viruses, and fungi. Occasionally parasites are responsible for meningitis.

ETIOLOGY

- *Bacterial meningitis*
  - ◊ Group B or D *Streptococcus*
  - ◊ *Streptococcus pneumoniae* (most common in adults)

- ◊ *Neisseria meningitidis*
- ◊ Other organisms
- *Viral meningitis*
  - ◊ Enterovirus is the most common cause, includes Coxsackie A and B, polioviruses, echoviruses
- *Fungal meningitis*
  - ◊ *Candida* species
  - ◊ *Aspergillus*
  - ◊ *Cryptococcus neoformans*

INCIDENCE

- *Bacterial*
  - ◊ Predominant age: extremes of age (very young, very old)
  - ◊ 80% occur in children under age 24 months
  - ◊ Males = Females
  - ◊ 3-10/100,000 in U.S.
- *Viral*
  - ◊ Most common in young adults
  - ◊ Effects all ages
  - ◊ About 10,000 cases annually in U.S.
  - ◊ Common in summer and early fall
- *Fungal*
  - ◊ Cryptococcal meningitis is most common in immunocompromised adults, especially those with AIDS
  - ◊ *Candida* species most common in premature infants and other immunocompromised adults

RISK FACTORS

- *Bacterial*
  - ◊ Immunocompromised hosts
  - ◊ Alcoholics
  - ◊ Neurosurgical patients
- *Viral*
  - ◊ Immunocompromised hosts
- *Fungal*
  - ◊ Immunocompromised hosts
  - ◊ Exposure to pigeon or bird droppings

ASSESSMENT FINDINGS

- *Bacterial*
  - ◊ Recent URI
  - ◊ Neck pain/stiff neck
  - ◊ Headache, fever
  - ◊ Nausea and vomiting, especially in children
  - ◊ Decreased level of consciousness, seizures
  - ◊ Meningococcemia rash
  - ◊ Nuchal rigidity
  - ◊ Positive Kernig and Brudzinski signs
    - * Kernig sign: complete extension of leg causes neck pain and flexion
    - * Brudzinski sign: flexion of legs if neck is passively flexed
  - ◊ In infants
    - * Irritable
    - * Sleeping more than usual
    - * Cries when moved
    - * Cries inconsolably
- *Viral*
  - ◊ Headache
  - ◊ Fever
  - ◊ Stiff neck
  - ◊ Photophobia
  - ◊ Rash
  - ◊ Seizures
  - ◊ Illness lasts 2-6 days
- *Fungal*
  - ◊ Worsening headaches over a period of days
  - ◊ Vomiting for days or weeks

A positive Kernig and Brudzinski signs are highly suggestive of meningitis.

DIFFERENTIAL DIAGNOSIS

- Bacterial vs. viral vs. fungal vs. tuberculous meningitis
- Meningitis caused by other infectious agents (e.g., syphilis, ameba)
- Seizure disorder
- Encephalopathy
- Brain abscess

Viral meningitis is rarely seen in the elderly. Strongly consider other differential diagnoses in the elderly.

DIAGNOSTIC STUDIES

- Lumbar puncture: cerebrospinal fluid (CSF) may be turbid, presence of WBCs, elevated protein levels

- CSF: decreased glucose if bacterial
- CSF Gram stain and cultures: presence of infectious agent
- CBC: elevated WBC
- Blood cultures: positive in 80% of bacterial meningitis patients
- Consider CT/MRI

PREVENTION

- Strict aseptic technique during neurosurgical dressing changes
- Treat URI infections promptly
- Administer meningococcal immunization as part of routine immunizations

NONPHARMACOLOGIC MANAGEMENT

- Vigorous supportive care
- Measures to prevent dehydration
- Good handwashing
- Anticipatory guidance for family

PHARMACOLOGIC MANAGEMENT

- Antibiotic specific for culture if available
- Empiric treatment with ampicillin *PLUS* third-generation cephalosporin; may need to add aminoglycoside
- Dexamethasone: may decrease morbidity and mortality
- Antipyretics
- Analgesics for headache
- Antiemetics
- Antiviral agents not recommended
- Depending on etiology: prophylaxis for contacts

CONSULTATION/REFERRAL

- Refer to emergency department/neurologist immediately

FOLLOW-UP

- Depends on severity

EXPECTED COURSE

- **Bacterial**
  - ◊ Overall fatality is 14%
  - ◊ Afebrile by 7-10 days
  - ◊ Headache and other symptoms may persist intermittently for 2 weeks
- **Viral**
  - ◊ Recovery in 2-7 days
  - ◊ Headache and other symptoms may persist intermittently for 2 weeks
- **Fungal**
  - ◊ poor prognosis usually related to overall health of patient

POSSIBLE COMPLICATIONS

- Seizures (common in bacterial meningitis, rare in viral)
- Unresolved neurologic deficits
- Sensorineural hearing loss
- Irritability
- Hydrocephaly

MULTIPLE SCLEROSIS (MS)

DESCRIPTION

A disease of the central nervous system (CNS) which is slow and progressive. It is characterized by demyelination of nerve cells in the brain and spinal cord which produces a variety of neurologic deficits.

ETIOLOGY

- Cause is unknown
  - ◊ Viral origin: supported by clusters in families, geographical clusters of cases
  - ◊ Immunologic: supported by presence of immunocytes in plaques
  - ◊ Environmental: supported by higher incidence in colder climates

INCIDENCE

- Age at onset 16-40 years
- Female > Male

- Approximately 25,000 new cases each year

RISK FACTORS

- Family history
- Northern European descent

ASSESSMENT FINDINGS

- Any of the following findings may present at various times during the illness
- Onset is insidious. Complaints may be present for months or years before diagnosis made.
- CNS complaints are intermittent with remissions and exacerbations. May be minor complaints or may be incapacitating.
- Paresthesias in extremities, weakness or clumsiness of a hand or leg
- Stiffness or unusual fatigability of a limb
- Transient blindness or pain in an eye
- Nystagmus common
- Speech may be slow with hesitancy at beginning of word (scanning speech)
- Mild emotional disturbances (e.g., apathy, lack of judgment, emotional lability) may be due to scattered CNS involvement
- Difficulty with bladder control (e.g., urgency, hesitancy, incontinence) may be present
- Deep tendon reflexes increased; superficial reflexes diminished
- Charcot's triad (i.e., scanning speech, nystagmus, tremor) common in later stages of disease

DIFFERENTIAL DIAGNOSIS

- Spinal cord or brain stem tumors
- Amyotrophic lateral sclerosis (ALS)
- CNS infections
- Compressed/ruptured intervertebral disk
- Multiple cerebral infarcts

DIAGNOSTIC STUDIES

- No specific test confirms diagnosis
- Diagnosis is from clinical and laboratory exam
- CSF: demonstrates total elevated IgG; protein and lymphocytes may be elevated
- Evoked potentials: recorded electrical responses to stimulation of a sensory system are abnormal in 75-97% of cases. May be an early finding.
- MRI (preferred) or CT: most sensitive technique; may show plaques or demyelination
- Syphilis serology: used to exclude this diagnosis

NONPHARMACOLOGIC MANAGEMENT

- Avoid factors which precipitate attack (e.g., hot weather, fatigue)
- Attempt to maintain as much patient independence as long as possible
- Extensive patient and family education regarding nature of disease
- Emotional support from family, health care provider
- Monitor for depression
- Occupational, physical therapy to help maintain range of motion, muscle flexibility, etc.
- Massage and passive movement of spastic limbs
- Teach self-catheterization if urinary retention is a problem
- High fiber diet to prevent constipation
- Possible custodial care for severe physical or cognitive impairments

PHARMACOLOGIC MANAGEMENT

- Immuno modulators (Avonex®, Betaseron®, Copaxone®)
  - ◊ Slow progression
  - ◊ Reduce relapses
- Intravenous prednisone may benefit during acute exacerbations
- Central muscle relaxants for spasticity (may exacerbate weakness, use cautiously)
- Constipation: stool softeners, bulk agents, laxatives
- Stimulate urination: propantheline (Pro-Banthine®), imipramine (Tofranil®), or oxybutynin chloride (Ditropan®)
- Neuropathic pain: NSAIDs, Neurontin®, Tegretol®
- Antidepressants as needed

- Chronic fatigue: amantadine (Symmetrel®) may be tried

PREGNANCY/LACTATION CONSIDERATIONS

- May be a triggering factor

CONSULTATION/REFERRAL

- Consult neurologist for suspected initial diagnosis and long-term management plan
- Physical, occupational therapy

FOLLOW-UP

- Depends on severity and frequency of exacerbations

EXPECTED COURSE

- Highly variable and unpredictable
- May have frequent exacerbations and remissions
- About 70% of patients lead very active lives but should avoid extreme fatigue
- Average illness lasts greater than 25 years

POSSIBLE COMPLICATIONS

- Urinary tract infections
- Depression
- Sexual impotence
- Decubitus ulcers if bedridden
- Severe depression
- Coma
- Optic nerve atrophy
- Paraplegia

PARKINSON DISEASE

DESCRIPTION

Idiopathic, neurodegenerative movement disorder characterized by 4 prominent features:

- Bradykinesia
- Muscular rigidity
- Resting tremor
- Postural instability

Diagnosis of PD supported by therapeutic response to levodopa.

ETIOLOGY

- There is a gradual loss of neurons in the substantia nigra which results in a decrease in production of the neurotransmitter dopamine

INCIDENCE

- 50,000 cases annually in U.S.
- Males > Females (1.4:1)
- Mean age of onset is 60 years
- Onset in childhood or adolescence is rare

RISK FACTORS

- Family history
- Unknown
- Ingestion of toxins, drugs, may produce a secondary Parkinson disease

ASSESSMENT FINDINGS

- "*Pill-rolling*" tremor is presenting sign of 50-80% of patients (30% do not present with tremor)
- Tremor is maximal at rest, minimal with activity, and absent during sleep
- *Bradykinesia* (movement initiation is difficult for patient): often the most disabling symptom and must be present for diagnosis
- *Cogwheel rigidity* with tremor
- Stooped posture
- Gait disturbances evidenced by shuffling with short steps and lack of arm swinging
- Steps may become quickened to keep from falling (festination)
- Loss of postural reflexes results in tendency to fall forward or backward

- Face becomes mask-like and there is decreased blinking in later stages
- Seborrhea
- Constipation, incontinence, sexual dysfunction
- Drooling from inability to swallow in later stages
- Dysphonia
- Depression

A patient who presents with tremor at rest, rigidity, and bradykinesia should be suspected as having Parkinson disease.

DIFFERENTIAL DIAGNOSIS

- Benign essential tremor
- Other movement disorders
- Parkinson disease from secondary causes (e.g., side effects from neuroleptic medications)

Benign essential tremor is relieved by alcohol ingestion and usually associated with a positive family history.

DIAGNOSTIC STUDIES

- CT or MRI can eliminate other causes of symptoms (e.g., brain tumor)

PREVENTION

- *See* Risk Factors

NONPHARMACOLOGIC MANAGEMENT

- Patient and family education
- Anticipatory guidance regarding progression of disease
- Encourage compliance with medication
- Physical, occupational, and speech therapy
- Adjustments in home environment to accommodate physical limitations (e.g., elevated toilet seat, elimination of floor objects which would increase likelihood of falls, elevated chair, elimination of stairs when possible, wheel chair ramp for later stages of disease)

PHARMACOLOGIC MANAGEMENT

AGENT	ACTION	COMMENTS
Dopamine Agonists *Example:* pramipexole (Mirapex®) ropinirole (Requip®) pergolide (Permax®) amantadine (Symmetrel®)	Stimulate the dopamine receptors and prevent catabolism of dopamine	Possibly neuroprotective by decreasing speed of progression of PD. May be used in combination with levodopa or as monotherapy initially. Monitor for hypotension and dyskinesias.
Dopaminergic Agents *Example:* carbidopa/levodopa (Sinemet SR®)	Supplement available dopamine and prevent its catabolism (carbidopa inhibits decarboxylation of levodopa)	Lowers levodopa dosage requirements. Used for patients with manifested disability. Monitor for dyskinesias, hallucinations, and hypotension. Increase every 4-7 days according to patient tolerance and symptoms.
MAO Inhibitors *Example:* Selegiline (Eldepryl®)	Inhibit the breakdown of dopamine in the brain and prolongs the action of levodopa	Helpful in diminishing the end of dose symptoms when levodopa begins to wear off. Many food-drug interactions.

Anticholinergics *Example:* trihexyphenidyl (Artane®) benztropine (Cogentin®)	Prolong the action of dopamine; reduce incidence and severity of dyskinesias, rigidity, and tremor	Contraindicated in glaucoma Older adults will be more sensitive to these drugs because of the anticholinergic effects. Cautious use in BPH. Monitor for tardive dyskinesias. Dry mouth very common.

A sudden worsening in the patient's status may indicate depression or non-compliance with medication.

CONSULTATION/REFERRAL

- Consult neurologist for Parkinson disease
- Allied health professionals: physical, occupational, and speech therapy
- Support groups

FOLLOW-UP

- Lifelong follow-up and medication adjustment will be needed

EXPECTED COURSE

- Chronic and progressive neurological disorder

POSSIBLE COMPLICATIONS

- Multiple falls
- Aspiration pneumonia
- Dementia
- Depression
- Accidents from falls

ALZHEIMER DISEASE

DESCRIPTION

The permanent or progressive decline in the intellectual functioning of a person that substantially interferes with his social and/or economic welfare. The decline in functioning is due to damage to the hippocampus, amygdala, or other areas of the brain.

INCIDENCE

- 50% of Alzheimer's patients have a family history of Alzheimer disease
- 40% of all patients over 85 years are affected
- Usually occurs after age 60

RISK FACTORS

- Aging
- Smoking (2-4x increase)
- Genetic markers on Chromosomes 1, 12, 14, 19, 21
- Family history

ASSESSMENT FINDINGS

- Recent memory loss (early finding)
- Impaired judgment, abstract thinking, memory, reasoning, orientation, attention
- Difficulty with speech and other forms of communications
- Inability to interpret sounds, speech, and use of objects
- Arousal disturbances: insomnia, daytime sleepiness
- Hyperactivity, wandering, restlessness
- Mood disturbances and emotional outbursts
- Urinary and/or fecal incontinence
- Paranoia, hallucinations, delusions (late findings)

DIFFERENTIAL DIAGNOSIS

- Normal aging process
- Hypothyroidism
- Depression
- Brain tumor

- Alcoholism
- Metabolic abnormalities
- Schizophrenia
- Delirium
- Other neurological conditions
- Side effects from medications

DIAGNOSTIC STUDIES

- To rule out reversible causes:
  - ◊ CBC
  - ◊ Electrolytes
  - ◊ Complete metabolic panel to include BUN, creatinine
  - ◊ Urinalysis
  - ◊ Liver function tests
  - ◊ Thyroid function tests
  - ◊ Vitamin B_{12} and folate levels
  - ◊ Syphilis serology
  - ◊ Consider CT or MRI
  - ◊ Others by history
- Mini Mental State Exam

PREVENTION

- None at this time

NONPHARMACOLOGIC MANAGEMENT

- Maintain routine and familiar environment to patient
- Attempt to maintain nutritional status by offering and encouraging regular meals of high nutritive value
- Display family pictures, calendars, clocks in prominent places
- Provide as much "accident-proofing" in the living environment as possible
- Emotional support and encouragement to family members
- Respite care for the caregivers
- Discuss advanced directives with family
- Offer information on support group for family

PHARMACOLOGIC MANAGEMENT

- No specific drug halts progression of disease
- Memory enhancement: Namenda®, Aricept®, Reminyl®, Exelon®
- Medications are used to treat symptoms
- Sun-downing, aggressive behavior: treat with antipsychotics such as haloperidol (Haldol®) or Risperdal®
- Sleep disturbance: temazepam (Restoril®), zolpidem (Ambien®)
- Depression: nortriptyline (Pamelor®), SSRIs
- Vitamin E

Depression develops in 33% of patients who are diagnosed with AD; therefore, remain alert for symptoms. Start treatment at low doses.

CONSULTATION/REFERRAL

- Consult neurologist for new-onset dementia
- Consult social services as needed for family
- Other consults as needed

FOLLOW-UP

- Depends on severity
- Periodic follow-up needed to assess rate of decline, predict prognosis, and assess caregiver coping

EXPECTED COURSE

- Alzheimer disease: variable rates of progression
- Average survival after diagnosis is 7-9 years

POSSIBLE COMPLICATIONS

- Accidents
- Malnutrition
- Caregiver exhaustion

ATTENTION DEFICIT DISORDER
ATTENTION DEFICIT HYPERACTIVITY DISORDER
(ADD, ADHD)

DESCRIPTION

Developmental disorder characterized by shortened attention span, impulsivity, and distractibility. Hyperactivity may or may not be present. When it is present, it is termed attention deficit hyperactivity disorder (ADHD).

ETIOLOGY

- Unknown
- Many factors seem to contribute: behavioral, biochemical, physiologic, and sensory and motor influences

INCIDENCE

- Estimated to affect 5-10% of school aged children
- Males > Females (5:1)
- Onset < 7 year of age
- Exists in to adolescence and adulthood

RISK FACTORS

- Family history
- Possible association with poor prenatal health (e.g., alcohol or drug abuse, smoking, preeclampsia)

ASSESSMENT FINDINGS

- DSM-IV R Criteria: symptoms must be present by age 7, last > 6 months, and be evident in 2 different settings (home, school)

ADHD **(hyperactivity with inattention)** *6 or more of the following must be present for diagnosis:*
◊ Fidgets, squirms, restless
◊ Difficulty remaining in seat
◊ Excessive activity
◊ Quiet play is difficult for child
◊ Acts as if "motorized"
◊ Excessive talking
◊ Impatient when forced to wait for turn
◊ Blurts out answers to questions before time
◊ Interrupts conversation

Note: Adapted from DSM-IV, 1994.

ADD **(Inattention)** *6 or more must be present for diagnosis:*
◊ Realizes careless mistakes when pointed out
◊ Exhibits difficulty maintaining attention
◊ Difficulty listening
◊ Does not finish tasks
◊ Organization skills are poor
◊ Tasks requiring sustained attention are difficult
◊ Forgetful
◊ Loses items (shoes, socks, school assignment)
◊ Easily distracted

Note: Adapted from DSM-IV, 1994.

DIFFERENTIAL DIAGNOSIS

- Learning disability
- Hearing/vision disorder
- Dysfunctional family situation
- Conduct disorder
- Poor parenting
- Inappropriate discipline
- Medication reaction (ex. decongestants)
- Absence seizures

DIAGNOSTIC STUDIES

- Diagnosis by DSM-IV criteria
- Other studies may be done to rule out other diagnoses, but no test is diagnostic

NONPHARMACOLOGIC MANAGEMENT

- Parent/teacher/patient education
- No dietary eliminations or additions are known to help. Some benefit may be gained for individual patients with elimination of sugar, dyes, and some additives.
- Educate parents about disorder
- Reinforce good behavior
- Singular task requests are more likely to be completed than multiple task requests
- Make eye contact when assigning tasks
- Time out
- Stop dangerous and threatening behavior before it reaches unmanageable levels
- Educate parents about risks and benefits of drug therapy
- Immediate consequences for broken rules
- Close monitoring of school activities and consistent reinforcement
- Education and support groups for parents and teachers

PHARMACOLOGIC MANAGEMENT

AGENT	ACTION	COMMENTS
Non-stimulant *Example:* atomoxetine (Strattera®)	Selective norepinephrine re-uptake inhibitor, but precise mechanism is unknown	Monitor liver enzymes. Can be used in children, adolescents, and adults. Do not use concurrently with MAOI. Careful use with SSRI. Monitor height and weight in children. May produce hypertension, heart rate. May impair sexual function. Has no street value.
Stimulants *Examples:* dexmethylphenidate (Focalin®) methylphenidate (Ritalin®, Concerta®, Metadate®) pemoline (Cylert®)	CNS stimulant but precise mechanism is unknown. Action is similar to amphetamines.	Monitor CBC, liver enzymes. Lowers threshold for seizures. May increase blood pressure or may worsen existing dryness. Long-term use may be associated with growth suppression. Remain alert for abuse. Supervised use because of potential for abuse and "street value".

Titrate to improved grades and behavior

PREGNANCY/LACTATION CONSIDERATIONS

- Avoid stimulant medications during pregnancy

CONSULTATION/REFERRAL

- Refer to personnel who can perform a psychometric evaluation for diagnosis
- Refer to neurologist if poor response to medication

FOLLOW-UP

- Close phone contact during initial and subsequent titration periods
- Monthly, quarterly, or every 6 months depending on severity and response
- Provide parents and teachers with regular support and encouragement
- Consult teachers regarding effectiveness of therapy
- Monitor growth and blood pressure, CBC periodically

EXPECTED COURSE

- More easily controlled as patient ages
- May last into and through adulthood

POSSIBLE COMPLICATIONS

- Children are at increased risk for abuse, social isolation, and depression
- Poor self-esteem and diminished self-confidence
- Failure in school

BELL'S PALSY
(Idiopathic Facial Paralysis)

DESCRIPTION

Facial nerve (Cranial Nerve VII) weakness or paralysis usually unilateral and idiopathic

ETIOLOGY

- Idiopathic
- Viral
- Exposure to cold
- Facial trauma causing inflammation of the facial canal

INCIDENCE

- 16 per 100,000 people in U.S.
- Age >30 years
- Males = Females

RISK FACTORS

- Lyme Disease
- 3rd trimester of pregnancy
- Family history
- Diabetes mellitus
- Herpes zoster

ASSESSMENT FINDINGS

- Numbness on effected side
- Sagging of eyebrow
- Mouth drawn to effected side
- Partial or total paralysis of facial muscles
- Hypersensitivity to sound
- Excessive tearing
- Inadequate tearing
- Ipsilateral loss of taste
- Ipsilateral ear pain, cheek pain
- Loss of nasolabial fold

DIFFERENTIAL DIAGNOSIS

- Stroke
- Lyme Disease
- Tumor
- Trauma
- Otitis media

DIAGNOSTIC STUDIES

- Usually diagnosed on clinical symptoms unless diagnosis is questionable
- Lyme titer if history of tick bite
- CT to rule out stroke or neoplasm
- Electromyographic (EMG) testing

PREVENTION

- None
- *See* Risk Factors

NONPHARMACOLOGIC MANAGEMENT

- Patient education regarding condition, expected outcomes, management
- Eyedrops to maintain lubrication (if inadequate tearing)
- Close and patch affected eye (especially at night)
- Warm, moist heat to affected side of face

PHARMACOLOGIC MANAGEMENT

- Tapered dosage of corticosteroids (must be initiated within 4 days of onset or corticosteroids are of little benefit)

- 80 mg prednisone daily for 3 days, then 60 mg daily for 3 days, then 40 mg daily for 3 days, then 20 mg daily for 3 days
- Possible benefit of oral anti-viral agent in conjunction with steroid

PREGNANCY/LACTATION CONSIDERATIONS

- Cautious use of steroids in pregnancy

CONSULTATION/REFERRAL

- Obstetrician for pregnant clients
- Refer to neurologist for serious comorbid conditions
- Ophthalmologist for actual or suspected corneal abrasions

FOLLOW-UP

- Re-evaluate in 3-5 days, then 2-4 weeks until resolved

EXPECTED COURSE

- Usually complete or partial recovery

POSSIBLE COMPLICATIONS

- Emergence of a subclinical infection from high dose steroid
- Corneal abrasion or ulceration if unable to blink eye

CARPAL TUNNEL SYNDROME (CTS)

DESCRIPTION

Entrapment neuropathy of the median nerve at the wrist due to inflammation of wrist tendons, transverse carpal ligament, and/or surrounding soft tissue.

> **This is also called "wake and shake syndrome".**

ETIOLOGY

- The median nerve is entrapped or compressed as it passes through a tunnel composed of the carpal bones and the transverse carpal ligament
- Any condition that results in edema may precipitate carpal tunnel syndrome (CTS)

INCIDENCE

- Common
- Females > Males (3-10:1)
- Predominant age is 40 to 60 years

RISK FACTORS

- Repetitive flexion, pronation, and supination of the wrist
- Tenosynovitis of the flexor tendons of the fingers
- Local trauma
- Prolonged improper positioning
- Weight gain
- Pregnancy or premenstrual edema
- Arthritis
- Hypothyroidism

ASSESSMENT FINDINGS

- Median paresthesias affecting the thumb, index finger, middle finger, and radial side of the ring finger
- Nocturnal paresthesias
- Positive Phalen's test
  - ◊ Hold flexed fingers against each other with wrists flexed at a 90° angle for 60 seconds
  - ◊ Considered positive if paresthesia occurs
  - ◊ Not highly sensitive
- Positive Tinel's test
  - ◊ Percuss over the median nerve on the volar aspect of the wrist
  - ◊ Considered positive if paresthesia occurs
  - ◊ Not highly sensitive

- Dull, aching sensation in hand, wrist, forearm, or upper arm
- Weakness and sensory loss, dropping objects from affected hand
- Affected hand may be cool to touch, pale in color, with dry skin
- Atrophy of thenar muscle

A blood pressure cuff blown up on the affected arm may precipitate symptoms.

DIFFERENTIAL DIAGNOSIS

- De Quervain's disease
- Cervical radiculopathy
- Lesion of the brachial plexus
- Peripheral neuropathy
- Thoracic outlet syndrome
- Multiple sclerosis
- CVA

DIAGNOSTIC STUDIES

- Nerve conduction studies of the median nerve: delayed latency across the wrist confirms diagnosis
- Consider EMG especially if nerve conduction studies are negative

PREVENTION

- Frequent rest periods when repetitive wrist motions are performed
- Proper hand/wrist positioning

NONPHARMACOLOGIC MANAGEMENT

- Correct underlying disorder
- Avoid aggravating factors
- Splinting of wrists in extension
- Surgical decompression of the carpal tunnel with release of the transverse carpal ligament and debridement

PHARMACOLOGIC MANAGEMENT

- Nonsteroidal anti-inflammatory agents in doses sufficient for anti-inflammatory effect
- Local anesthetic and hydrocortisone injection provides temporary relief (40 mg Medrol and 1% lidocaine)

PREGNANCY/LACTATION CONSIDERATIONS

- Pregnancy is a risk factor due to edema
- Local injection of anesthetic and hydrocortisone useful during pregnancy

CONSULTATION/REFERRAL

- Surgeon if severe or persistent despite conservative therapy

FOLLOW-UP

- Evaluate effect of conservative therapy (i.e., splints, NSAIDs and cortisone injections)
- Postoperative evaluation by surgeon

EXPECTED COURSE

- If untreated, there is a risk of permanent loss of function of affected hand
- Recurrence likely with nonsurgical interventions
- Recurrence is unusual following surgery

POSSIBLE COMPLICATIONS

- Postoperative infection
- Surgical complications
- Permanent damage from prolonged median nerve compression

References

Adelman, A.A. (2005). Initial evaluation of the patient with suspected dementia. *American Family Physician, 71*, 1745-1750.

Bell, R. T. (1996). Dementia in the elderly: Is it Alzheimer's? *Patient Care, 30*(18), 18-38.

Bickley, L.S., & Szilagyi, P.G. (2003). *Bates' guide to physical examination and history taking* (8th ed.). Philadelphia: Lippincott Williams & Wilkins.

Branch, W.T. (2003). *Office practice of medicine* (4th ed.). Philadelphia: Saunders.

Burns, C.E., Brady, M.A., Blosser, C., Starr, N.B., & Dunn, A.M. (2004). *Pediatric primary care: A handbook for nurse practitioners* (3rd ed.). Philadelphia: W.B. Saunders.

Champi, C., & Gaffrey-Yocum, P. A. (1999). Managing febrile seizures in children. *The Nurse Practitioner, 24*(10), 28-43.

Craig, C. (1996). Clinical recognition and management of adult attention deficit and hyperactivity disorder. *The Nurse Practitioner, 21*(11), 101-108.

Dambro, M.R. (2005). *Griffith's 5 minute clinical consult.* Philadelphia: Lippincott Williams & Wilkins.

DeNisco, S., Tiago, C., Kravitz, C. (2005). Evaluation and treatment of pediatric ADHD. *The Nurse Practitioner, 30*(8), 14-23.

D'Epiro, N. W. (1996). Treating Alzheimer's disease: Today and tomorrow. *Patient Care, 30*(18), 62-83.

Gilber, D.N., Moellering, R.C., Eliopoulos, G.M., & Sande, M.A. (Eds.). (2004). *Sanford Guide to Antimicrobial Therapy* (34th ed.). Hyde Park, VT: Antimicrobial Therapy.

Graber, M.A., & Lanternier, M.L. (Eds.) (2001). *The family practice handbook.* (4th ed.). St. Louis: Mosby.

Hilton, G. (1997). Seizure disorders in adults: Evaluation and management of new onset seizures. *The Nurse Practitioner, 22*(9), 42-59.

Kasper, D.L., Braunwald, E., Fauci, A.S., Hauser, S.L., Longo, D.L., Jameson, J.L., et al. (2004). *Harrison's principles of internal medicine* (16th ed.). New York: McGraw-Hill.

Jackson, S. (1997). Behavioral and pharmacologic treatment of delirium. *American Family Physician, 56*, 2005-2020.

Kliegman, R.M., Greenbaum, L.A., & Lye, P.S. (2004). *Practical strategies in pediatric diagnosis and therapy* (2nd ed.). Philadelphia: W.B. Saunders.

Mangion, S. (2000). *Physical diagnosis secrets.* Philadelphia: Hanley and Belfus.

Mladenovic, J. (Ed.). (2003). *Primary care secrets.* (3rd Ed.). Philadelphia: Hanley and Belfus.

Peskind, E.R., Tangalos, E.G., & Grossberg, G.T. (2005). A case-based approach to Alzheimer's disease. *Clinical Advisor, 8*(6), 32-46.

Radeka, N., Taylor, J., Taylor, S., Wheeler, L. C., & Griffin, H. C. (1996). Parents' opinions concerning possible causes of cerebral palsy. *The Nurse Practitioner, 21*(4), 126-128.

Rakel, R.E. (Ed.). (1998). *Essentials of family practice.* (2nd ed.). Philadelphia: WB Saunders.

Ryan, C. W. (1996). Evaluation of patients with chronic headache. *American Family Physician, 54*, 1051-1057.

Santiago0Rosado, L. (2005). Syncope: Step-by-step through the workup. *Consultant, 45*, 759-768.

Schwartz, M.W. (Ed.). (2002). *The 5 minute pediatric consult.* (2nd ed.) Philadelphia: Lippincott Williams & Wilkins.

Sheftell, F.D., Cady, R.K., Borchert, L.D., Spalding, W., & Hart, C.C. (2005). Optimizing the diagnosis and treatment of migraine. *Journal of the American Academy of Nurse Practitioners, 17(8),* 309-317.

Silberstein, S. D. (1997). Migraine and pregnancy. *Neurologic Clinics, 15*(1), 209-232.

Solomon, S. (1997). Diagnosis of primary headache disorders: Validity of the International headache society criteria in clinical practice. *Neurologic Clinics, 15*(1), 15-26.

Swain, S. E. (1996). Multiple sclerosis: Primary health care implications. *The Nurse Practitioner, 21*(7), 40-54.

Tapper, V. J. (1997). Pathophysiology, assessment, and treatment of Parkinson's disease. *The Nurse Practitioner, 22*(7), 76-95.

Tunkel, A. R., & Scheld, W. M. (1997). Issues in the management of bacterial meningitis. *American Family Physician, 56,* 1355-1364.

Uphold, C.R., & Graham, M.V. (2003). *Clinical guidelines in family practice.* (4th ed.). Gainesville, FL: Barmarrae Books.

U.S. Preventive Services Task Force. (1996). *Guide to clinical preventive services.* (2nd ed.) Washington, D.C.: Office of Disease Prevention and Health Promotion, U.S. Government Printing Office.

Weiss, J. (1999). Assessing and managing the patient with headaches. *The Nurse Practitioner 24*(7), 18-35.

Wheldon, M. (2005). Untangling the confusion: Alzheimer's management today. *Advance for Nurse Practitioners, 13*(7), 47-52.

Zollo, A.J., Jr (Ed.). (2004). *Medical Secrets.* (4th ed.), St. Louis, MO: Mosby-Year Book.

14

OPHTHALMIC DISORDERS

Ophthalmic Disorders

** Denotes pediatric diagnosis*

OCULAR FOREIGN BODY

DESCRIPTION

Presence of substance, material, objects adhering to the eye or imbedded in the eye

INCIDENCE

- Unknown

RISK FACTORS

- Improper use of protective eyewear
- Lack of protective eye wear

ASSESSMENT FINDINGS

- Feeling that "something is in my eye"
- Red eye
- Tearing
- Pain or photophobia
- Frequent eye rubbing
- Appearance of dark specks against the iris
- Corneal "rust ring" indicates steel or iron foreign body
- Fluorescein staining may also indicate corneal abrasion

DIFFERENTIAL DIAGNOSIS

- Corneal abrasion
- Intraocular penetration of foreign body

DIAGNOSTIC STUDIES

- Assessment of visual acuity (e.g., Snellen chart)
- Examination with slit lamp or binocular loupe after Snellen examination
- Fluorescein staining is used to assess for corneal defects (should be done as last part of examination)
- Consider X-ray of orbits if history dictates

PREVENTION

- Use of protective eyewear devices
- Use of protective eyewear during situations where it is reasonable to expect that eye injury might occur

NONPHARMACOLOGIC MANAGEMENT

- Removal of the foreign body/object/material if it is superficial and NOT embedded
- A patch or metal shield to protect the eye if referred to ophthalmologist
- Keep patient NPO if patient is referred to ophthalmologist in case surgery is needed to remove embedded object
- Referral to ophthalmologist for follow-up
- Inspect entire eye for damage/additional foreign bodies

PHARMACOLOGIC MANAGEMENT

- Antibiotic instillation
- Tetanus prophylaxis for penetrating eye injuries

Corticosteroids are CONTRAINDICATED because they may foster bacterial/fungal growth.

CONSULTATION/REFERRAL

- A penetrating injury is a medical emergency and must be referred immediately
- Referral to ophthalmologist for all but simple nonpenetrating injuries
- Referral after any eye injury if changes in visual acuity occur

FOLLOW-UP

- Depends on degree of injury

EXPECTED COURSE

- Depends on extent of injury

POSSIBLE COMPLICATIONS

- Secondary bacterial infection (endophthalmitis)
- Corneal abrasion
- Traumatic cataract due to foreign body induced shock wave or direct puncture of the lenticular capsule
- Glaucoma due to intraocular inflammation

CORNEAL ABRASION

DESCRIPTION

Complete or partial tear of the epithelium of the cornea

ETIOLOGY

- Disruption of the outermost layer of the cornea, the epithelium, by either chemical or mechanical means

INCIDENCE

- More common in young, active patients
- Common in contact lens wearers
- Uncommon in the elderly

ASSESSMENT FINDINGS

- Complaint of "gritty" feeling or "something" in eye
- Eye pain usually proportional to degree of epithelial damage
- Photophobia
- Red eye
- May identify foreign body embedded in eye
- Lacrimation

DIFFERENTIAL DIAGNOSIS

- Presence of foreign body
- Keratitis, uveitis, iritis
- Corneal ulceration
- Contact lens induced roughing
- Damaged contact lens

DIAGNOSTIC STUDIES

- *Fluorescein staining* to assess corneal integrity: fluorescein is instilled in the eye and areas of epithelial disruption will fluoresce green when exposed to a Wood's lamp
- Assess visual acuity: should be normal unless abrasion is large

PREVENTION

- Protective eye wear for potentially dangerous activities
- Contact lenses may provide some minor protection
- Tetanus prophylaxis

NONPHARMACOLOGIC MANAGEMENT

- Eye patch to protect eye not found to decrease pain or speed healing
- Evaluate for presence of foreign body
- Use normal saline to irrigate eye

PHARMACOLOGIC MANAGEMENT

- Antibiotic ointment or drops 5-7 days to prevent bacterial infection
- Analgesics for pain
- Topical anesthetic for evaluation but warn patient not to rub or touch eye until anesthetic effect resolves

CONSULTATION/REFERRAL

- Ophthalmologist if injury involved thermal or chemical materials; blunt or sharp objects, or penetration into the eye by any object
- Referral for any distortion of vision
- Refer any injury which does not improve in 24 hours

FOLLOW-UP

- 24 hours to assess healing and status
- Dependent on patient condition

EXPECTED COURSE

- Dependent on severity of injury

POSSIBLE COMPLICATIONS

- Loss of vision
- Widespread corneal roughing due to patient's attempts to remove
- Corneal erosion (recurrent roughness at site of original corneal injury)

OCULAR CHEMICAL BURN

DESCRIPTION

Introduction of an acidic or alkaline agent into the eye which results in damage to the eye or its outer structures

ETIOLOGY

- Acidic and alkaline agents can both cause injury, but alkaline agents may be more destructive

INCIDENCE

- Unknown

RISK FACTORS

- Improper eye protection when handling potentially injurious products

ASSESSMENT FINDINGS

- Eye pain, burning, and distorted vision
- Decreased vision due to corneal roughing
- Photophobia
- Eyelid skin burns may be present

DIFFERENTIAL DIAGNOSIS

- Foreign object embedded in eye

DIAGNOSTIC STUDIES

- Defer pending ophthalmology evaluation

PREVENTION

- Protective eye equipment
- Tetanus prophylaxis

NONPHARMACOLOGIC MANAGEMENT

- Flush affected eye with 0.9% sodium chloride for 30 minutes; always irrigate away from unaffected eye
- Always inquire whether contact lenses are in use
- Immediate referral to ophthalmologist

PHARMACOLOGIC MANAGEMENT

- Consider analgesic for eye pain

CONSULTATION/REFERRAL

- Immediate referral to ophthalmologist

EXPECTED COURSE

- Depends on extent of injury

POSSIBLE COMPLICATIONS

- Loss of vision due to scarring
- Traumatic cataract formation
- Chronic ocular discomfort
- Symblepharon: adhesion between the conjunctiva of lid and the eyeball

HYPHEMA

DESCRIPTION

Hemorrhage into the anterior chamber of the eye as a result of iris or ciliary body rupture; may be spontaneous, but usually a result of trauma

ETIOLOGY

- Usually results from a blunt or penetrating trauma to the eye

INCIDENCE

- Unknown

RISK FACTORS

- Blunt trauma to the eye
- Penetrating injury to the eye
- Hemophilia
- Diabetes
- Anticoagulant therapy

ASSESSMENT FINDINGS

- Blood in the anterior chamber
- Visible fluid line in the pupil

DIFFERENTIAL DIAGNOSIS

- Globe trauma
- Eye contusion
- Systemic disease (e.g., hemophilia, diabetes)

DIAGNOSTIC STUDIES

- Consider hematology studies (e.g., clotting factors) based on history and exam

PREVENTION

- Protective eye devices
- Control of diabetes and hemophilia

NONPHARMACOLOGIC MANAGEMENT

- Binocular bandaging
- Head elevated 30-40°
- Complete bedrest

PHARMACOLOGIC MANAGEMENT

- Do not administer any aspirin products, miotics, or mydriatics in the acute setting, however, mydriatics are commonly used by ophthalmologists

CONSULTATION/REFERRAL

- Immediate referral to ophthalmologist

EXPECTED COURSE

- Hospitalization often not necessary
- Hospitalization based on additional injuries (e.g., head trauma).
- Possible evacuation of blood by ophthalmologist

POSSIBLE COMPLICATIONS

- Recurrent bleeding and development of glaucoma
- Loss of vision possible due to corneal staining. This potential complication is more likely in a total hyphema (complete filling of the anterior chamber, also referred to as an "8-ball hyphema").

CONJUNCTIVITIS
(Pink Eye)

DESCRIPTION

An inflammation or irritation of the conjunctiva.

ETIOLOGY

Causes of Conjunctivitis	
Bacterial	*Staphylococcus aureus* *Streptococcus pneumoniae* *Haemophilus influenza* *Pseudomonas sp.* (common in contact lens wearers) *Neisseria gonorrhoeae* *Neisseria meningitidis*
Viral	Adenovirus Coxsackie virus Herpes simplex
Chlamydial	*Chlamydia trachomatis*
Allergic	Environmental (trees, weeds, spores, pollen) Cosmetics
Chemical	Thimerosal Erythromycin Silver nitrate

INCIDENCE

- Very common

RISK FACTORS

- Bacterial or viral: contact lens use, rubbing eyes, contact with the infecting organism, trauma
- Allergic: wind exposure, contact with allergic substance
- Chemical: exposure to irritating chemical substance

ASSESSMENT FINDINGS

- Conjunctival erythema
- Burning
- Profuse exudate
- Itching
- Sensation of foreign body
- Ocular exudate with matting, especially upon awakening
- Preauricular adenopathy
- Tearing
- Normal visual acuity

Assessment Findings	
Bacterial	Exudates, initially unilateral, then often bilateral
Viral	Profuse tearing, burning, concurrent URI
Chlamydial	Profuse exudate, associated GU symptoms *Onset of symptoms:* 1-2 weeks after birth
Gonococcal	Profuse exudate, associated GU symptoms *Onset of symptoms:* 2-4 days after birth
Allergic	Severe itching, tearing, sneezing & rhinitis
Chemical	Conjunctival erythema, conjunctival discharge *Onset of symptoms:* 30 minutes after prophylactic antibiotic drops; usually resolves by 48 hours

DIFFERENTIAL DIAGNOSIS

- Foreign body
- Uveitis, iritis
- Corneal abrasion
- Dacryocystitis

DIAGNOSTIC STUDIES

- Usually none

- Consider culture of exudates, but rarely indicated
- Immunofluorescence test for herpes simplex or chlamydia

PREVENTION

- *See* Risk Factors

NONPHARMACOLOGIC MANAGEMENT

- Good hand-eye hygiene (wash hands frequently to prevent spread to other eye)
- Use clean wash cloths each time face is washed
- Change pillowcase on bed daily until resolved (if bacterial or viral)
- Warm compresses if origin is infectious
- Cool compresses if origin is allergic or chemical
- Irrigation if chemical or allergic etiology
- Teach patient how to instill eye drops/ointment
- Do not wear contact lenses until conjunctival inflammation resolved
- Discard or disinfect contact lenses prior to reusing
- Assess visual acuity
- Consider fluorescein staining

PHARMACOLOGIC MANAGEMENT

Agent	Treatment
Bacterial	Eyedrops or ointment: Tobramycin, gentamicin, sodium sulfacetamide, or ciprofloxacin
Viral	Trifluridine
Chlamydial	Oral doxycycline (Vibramycin®) (tetracyclines increase photosensitivity)
Allergic	Topical antihistamine, oral antihistamine, or topical vasoconstrictor (vasoconstrictors may mask severity), topical steroid*
Chemical	Avoid contact Usually none, but consider steroid use

**Cautious use of topical steroids*

PREGNANCY/LACTATION CONSIDERATIONS

- Tetracycline should not be used in pregnant or lactating patients

CONSULTATION/REFERRAL

- Refer to ophthalmologist if herpes, hemorrhagic conjunctivitis, or ulcerations present
- Refer to ophthalmologist if worse in 24 hours

FOLLOW-UP

- Telephone or office follow up in 24 hours to assess effectiveness of treatment

EXPECTED COURSE

- Bacterial or viral: improvement in 2-4 days
- Viral conjunctivitis associated with pharyngitis: improvement in 5-10 days
- Herpes simplex: improvement in 2-3 weeks

POSSIBLE COMPLICATIONS

- Blepharitis
- Corneal ulcerations
- Scarring (herpes simplex)
- Bacterial superinfection (allergic or chemical)

NEONATAL CONJUNCTIVITIS
(Ophthalmia Neonatorum)

DESCRIPTION

Inflammation (aseptic) or infectious (septic) process of the mucous membrane of the eye (conjunctiva) in the newborn (<40-60 days of age). A significant cause of worldwide blindness.

ETIOLOGY

- Chemical conjunctivitis due to silver nitrate/erythromycin administration; aseptic
- Chlamydial conjunctivitis due to *Chlamydia trachomatis* from perinatal transmission at birth
- Gonococcal conjunctivitis due to *Neisseria gonorrhoeae* from perinatal transmission at birth
- Other pathogens: adenovirus, herpes simplex, *Staphylococcus, Streptococcus, Pseudomonas*

INCIDENCE

- Unknown

RISK FACTORS

- Maternal infection with causative agent
- Silver nitrate/erythromycin/tetracycline prophylaxis

ASSESSMENT FINDINGS

Chemical	*Onset of symptoms:* 30 minutes after prophylactic antibiotic drops; usually resolves by 48 hrs. *Characteristics:* Red eyes, usually bilateral
Chlamydial	*Onset of symptoms:* 1-2 weeks after birth *Characteristics:* Mild mucopurulent discharge, lid erythema and edema, conjunctival erythema, possible pneumonia
Gonococcal	*Onset of symptoms:* 2-4 days after birth *Characteristics:* Mucopurulent discharge, lid edema, possible CNS symptoms

DIFFERENTIAL DIAGNOSIS

- Birth trauma
- Forceps delivery
- Preseptal cellulitis
- Nasolacrimal duct obstruction
- Bacterial vs. viral vs. chemical conjunctivitis
- Congenital glaucoma

DIAGNOSTIC STUDIES

- Gram stain of discharge
- Culture
- Immunofluorescence may be helpful to identify *Chlamydia trachomatis*

PREVENTION

- Treat maternal infection prior to pregnancy and birth
- Instillation of antibiotic drops after birth for prophylaxis

NONPHARMACOLOGIC MANAGEMENT

- Explanation to parents of condition
- Warm compresses
- Good hand washing
- Passage of time for chemical conjunctivitis

PHARMACOLOGIC MANAGEMENT

- Chlamydia: oral erythromycin for 14 days, plus topical erythromycin or tetracycline/ointment
- Gonococcal: intravenous ceftriaxone (Rocephin®), one-time dose, plus topical erythromycin or tetracycline ointment QID for 14 days

CONSULTATION/REFERRAL

- Refer to ophthalmologist for chlamydial infection which may lead to corneal scarring and opacification
- Refer to ophthalmologist for HSV which may lead to loss of vision and corneal scarring
- Refer to ophthalmologist for gonococcal
- Refer any which is slow to respond to treatment

FOLLOW-UP

- Dependent on etiology, but daily for gonorrhea, chlamydia and HSV

EXPECTED COURSE

- Chlamydia and HSV have highest incidence of corneal scarring
- Gonorrhea, if treated early, has relatively benign course, but can be devastating if not recognized or is undertreated

POSSIBLE COMPLICATIONS

- Loss of vision
- Corneal scarring

STRABISMUS
("Crossed Eyes")

DESCRIPTION

Non parallelism of the visual axis of the eyes so that they do not focus on the same object at the same time

ETIOLOGY

- Due to a disorder of the intraocular muscles or their cranial nerves
- Due to an arrest or delay in normal ocular development
- Can be caused by ocular tumors (retinoblastoma)
- 66% of patients with strabismus are affected as children

INCIDENCE

- 4% of population has some form of strabismus

RISK FACTORS

- Positive family history (30% have a family member with strabismus)
- Ocular tumors
- History of forceps delivery
- Presence of cerebral palsy
- Diabetics in poor control due to lateral rectus paralysis. This impairs abduction of one or both eyes.

ASSESSMENT FINDINGS

- Disconjugate gaze
- Possible diminished visual acuity; legal blindness (20/200) not uncommon
- Displaced corneal light reflexes (Hirschberg test)
- Inability to focus on an object without tilting head possible
- Nystagmus may be present
- Abnormal cover/uncover test

- Positive red reflex unless cataracts, retinoblastoma

Esotropia	Eye drifts inward
Exotropia	Eye drifts outward
Hypertropia	Eye drifts upward
Hypotropia	Eye drifts downward

DIFFERENTIAL DIAGNOSIS

- *Pseudostrabismus*: false impression that eyes are malaligned when they really are aligned properly; may be due to craniofacial features such as prominent epicanthal folds
- Neurological abnormalities (e.g., cerebral palsy)

DIAGNOSTIC STUDIES

- Hirschberg test
- Cover/uncover test
- CT/MRI to rule out ocular tumors
- Vision assessment to determine amblyopia

PREVENTION

- Careful monitoring and evaluation of patients with a family history of strabismus
- Referral for patients with true strabismus to ophthalmologist

NONPHARMACOLOGIC MANAGEMENT

- Patching (by ophthalmologist) of strong eye to allow weak eye to work and become stronger
- Visual training exercises are of limited help and can prolong amblyopia if surgical realignment is delayed
- Surgical interventions helpful to physically move the eyes into closer alignment

PHARMACOLOGIC MANAGEMENT

- None

CONSULTATION/REFERRAL

- Immediate referral to ophthalmologist when strabismus is suspected (normal eye alignment usually established by 3 months of age)

FOLLOW-UP

- By ophthalmologist

EXPECTED COURSE

- Goal is improving vision, then correcting alignment
- Most patients will need long-term ophthalmologic care because of recurrence of ocular deviation

POSSIBLE COMPLICATIONS

- Severe visual impairment if not diagnosed and treated early

REFRACTIVE ERRORS/COLOR BLINDNESS

DESCRIPTION

An inability to see near, far, peripherally, certain colors, or a combination of any of these

TERMS

Nearsightedness *(myopia)*	Light is focused anterior to the retina, often hereditary, may also be due to prematurity, progressive with age
Farsightedness *(hyperopia)*	Light is focused behind the retina, often hereditary, normal in young children less than age 6 years
Astigmatism	Due to an irregularly shaped cornea or lens, often hereditary; may prohibit use of contact lenses
Color blindness	Due to an inherited disorder
Presbyopia	Age-related decline in focusing ability due to the loss of elasticity of the lens

INCIDENCE

- Very common
- Color blindness: Males > Females

RISK FACTORS

- Family history
- Eye trauma (refractive errors)

ASSESSMENT FINDINGS

- Nearsightedness: poor distant vision
- Farsightedness: poor near vision
- Astigmatism: poor vision, headache, eye pain, nighttime "blindness" common
- Color blindness: inability to see certain combinations of colors, or in rare cases, inability to see any colors

DIFFERENTIAL DIAGNOSIS

- Other refractive disorders
- Ocular tumors
- Cataract growth may alter refractive error
- Diabetes, if uncontrolled, may significantly impact refractive error

DIAGNOSTIC STUDIES

- Test each eye separately, then together
- Record values with and without correction
- Visual acuity of <u>near</u> vision (reading card)
- Visual acuity of <u>distant</u> vision (Snellen test)
- Color recognition testing (Ishihara test)

CONSULTATION/REFERRAL

- Optometrist or ophthalmologist

FOLLOW-UP

- Lifelong

CATARACT

DESCRIPTION

An opacification of the lens of the eye; and the leading cause of blindness in the U.S.

ETIOLOGY

Age related	**Most common > 90%**
Congenital	1 per 250 newborns
Secondary to: **Trama**	Heat, penetration of eye by foreign object, electricity
Other eye Diseases	Wilson's disease, hypocalcemia
Medications	Long-term steroid use (e.g., arthritis, asthma)

INCIDENCE

- Age-related (most common): about 90%
- Congenital: 0.4% of live births

RISK FACTORS

- Advancing age
- Diabetes
- Familial disorders
- Ocular trauma
- Presence of retinoblastoma or other ocular tumors
- Maternal malnutrition/infectious disorders
- Maternal use of corticosteroids in congenital cataracts
- Steroid use

ASSESSMENT FINDINGS

- Opacification of the lens
- Diminished red reflex
- Leukocoria (white reflex)
- Blurred vision
- Diminished visual acuity (especially at night or glare)

DIFFERENTIAL DIAGNOSIS

- Ocular tumors
- Retinal detachment
- Macular degeneration
- Other ocular disorders
    - ◊ Pterygium (often mistaken for a cataract)
    - ◊ Corneal scars

DIAGNOSTIC STUDIES

- Ocular exam
- Glare testing

PREVENTION

- Depends on the cause
- Wearing of UV protectant eyewear may help slow development
- Tight control of glycemia in diabetics (also helps discourage progression of diabetic retinopathy)

NONPHARMACOLOGIC MANAGEMENT

- Protection from injury caused by diminished visual acuity
- Surgical removal by ophthalmologist (often with lens implant)

PHARMACOLOGIC MANAGEMENT

- None

CONSULTATION/REFERRAL

- Referral to ophthalmologist

FOLLOW-UP

- Postsurgical removal by ophthalmologist
- Assist family in finding resources if needs exist

EXPECTED COURSE

- Prognosis is good if identified and treated early and if no permanent ocular damage existed prior to removal
- Poor prognosis if presence of nystagmus or amblyopia prior to surgery
- Better prognosis for congenital cataracts if surgery performed prior to 3 months to discourage amblyopia. However, intraocular lens implants are not placed in very young patients, requiring use of contact lenses.

POSSIBLE COMPLICATIONS

- Blindness
- If cataract not removed, hyper maturity of the cataract can result in a leaking lens capsule

GLAUCOMA

DESCRIPTION

A disorder characterized by an elevated intraocular pressure. All can lead to blindness. There are 3 predominant forms:

- Chronic open-angle (wide-angle)
- Acute closed-angle (closed-angle, narrow-angle)
- Congenital (infantile)

ETIOLOGY

- Chronic open-angle: slow rise in intraocular pressure
- Acute closed-angle: sudden increase in intraocular pressure
- Congenital: structural abnormalities in the trabecular network which prevent outflow of aqueous humor

INCIDENCE

- Chronic open-angle: most common, approximately 85%
- Acute closed-angle: approximately 15%
- Congenital: 1-2/10,000 births

RISK FACTORS

- Chronic open-angle: age >35 years, diabetes mellitus, myopia, African-American, family history
- Acute closed-angle: age >30 years, hyperopia (thickened "magnifying" eyeglass lenses)

ASSESSMENT FINDINGS

Chronic open-angle	Usually asymptomatic Increased intraocular pressure (usually bilateral) Frequent prescription lens changes Halos around lights Headaches Impaired dark perception Visual disturbances Notching of the optic cup
Acute closed-angle	Increased intraocular pressure (usually unilateral) Severe throbbing eye pain or headache Rapid loss of vision Poorly reacting pupil Patient may present acutely ill with vomiting and may be misdiagnosed as suffering from appendicitis.
Congenital	Tearing Photophobia Corneal haziness Corneal clouding or enlargement

DIFFERENTIAL DIAGNOSIS

- Conjunctivitis
- Macular degeneration
- Foreign body

DIAGNOSTIC STUDIES

- Tonometry (normal intraocular pressure = 10-23 mm Hg)
- Corneal inspection (hazy cornea)

- Inspection of the optic nerves: unequal cups, or cupping >30, should be referred to ophthalmologist
- Visual field testing

PREVENTION

- Monitor intraocular pressure at regular eye exams (more frequent eye exams for high-risk individuals: positive family history, unequal cups)
- Avoid/limit use of OTC vasoconstrictive (oral and ocular) agents, or anticholinergic medications (e.g., scopolamine), especially in patients with narrow-angle anatomy

NONPHARMACOLOGIC MANAGEMENT

- Surgery or laser treatment to reduce intraocular pressure

PHARMACOLOGIC MANAGEMENT

- Topical β-adrenergic blockers
- Miotics: pilocarpine (Pilocar®)
- Systemic agents: carbonic anhydrase inhibitors

Use topical β-adrenergic blockers with caution in patients already on oral β-adrenergic blockers and in patients with COPD.

CONSULTATION/REFERRAL

- Ophthalmologist for suspected disease
- Emergency department for acute symptoms of glaucoma
- Potential for glaucoma in family, therefore, recommend having family members screened

FOLLOW-UP

- By ophthalmologist

EXPECTED COURSE

- Excellent prognosis if identified early and before optic damage occurs
- Need lifelong treatment and monitoring

POSSIBLE COMPLICATIONS

- Blindness
- Decreased peripheral vision (may be classified as visually disabled if severe)

CHALAZION

DESCRIPTION

Granulomatous inflammation of the meibomian gland. Plural form: chalazia

ETIOLOGY

- Obstruction of the meibomian gland duct with occasional secondary infection

INCIDENCE

- Common

RISK FACTORS

- Hordeolum or any condition which may impede flow through the meibomian gland ducts

ASSESSMENT FINDINGS

- May be indistinguishable from a stye on exam, but is usually painless
- Lid edema or palpable mass: often best seen with the lids closed
- Red or gray mass on the inner aspect of the lid margin
- Possible astigmatism from pressure placed on the eyeball, rare

DIFFERENTIAL DIAGNOSIS

- Hordeolum
- Tumor
- Blepharitis
- Embedded foreign body

DIAGNOSTIC STUDIES

- None usually needed

PREVENTION

- Good eye hygiene

NONPHARMACOLOGIC MANAGEMENT

- Warm, moist compresses on effected lid area 5-6 times per day
- Incision and curettage if no resolution with conservative treatment
- May be spontaneous resolution with time

PHARMACOLOGIC MANAGEMENT

- Sulfacetamide, erythromycin or other topical ophthalmic antibiotic for secondarily infected chalazion
- Oral antibiotics (dicloxacillin) may be used for larger/persistent lesions or for multiple chalazia

CONSULTATION/REFERRAL

- Ophthalmologist if no response to treatment after 6 weeks

FOLLOW-UP

- 2-4 weeks if small and uncomplicated
- If infected, depends on severity

EXPECTED COURSE

- Prognosis excellent
- Small chalazia usually resolve spontaneously

POSSIBLE COMPLICATIONS

- Some chalazia may become secondarily infected and cause cellulitis of the lid
- Loss of eyelashes
- Deformity of the eyelid

BLEPHARITIS

DESCRIPTION

Inflammation/infection of the lid margins which is often a chronic problem. There are two basic types:

- Seborrheic (non-ulcerative)
- Ulcerative (usually staphylococcal)

ETIOLOGY

- Seborrheic: irritants (e.g., smoke, eye make-up, chemicals), secondary to scalp or facial seborrhea, or infection (usually *Staphylococcus* or *Streptococcus*)
- Ulcerative: infection with *Staphylococcus* or *Streptococcus*

INCIDENCE

- Common (most frequent ocular disease)

RISK FACTORS

- Frequent hordeola or chalazia
- Facial or scalp seborrhea
- Immunocompromised state
- Acne rosacea
- Diabetes mellitus

ASSESSMENT FINDINGS

Ulcerative	Itching Tearing Recurrent styes Chalazia Photophobia Small ulcerations at eyelid margin Broken or absence of eyelashes
Seborrheic	Chronic inflammation of the eyelid Erythema Scaling, loss of eyelashes

DIFFERENTIAL DIAGNOSIS

- Sebaceous cell/basal cell, squamous cell carcinoma
- Chalazion
- Lice infestation

DIAGNOSTIC STUDIES

- Usually none

PREVENTION

- Good eye hygiene
- Discourage eye rubbing

NONPHARMACOLOGIC MANAGEMENT

- Clean eyelid margins 2-4 times per day with baby shampoo depending on severity
- Warm, moist compresses several times per day
- Remove contact lenses and disinfect

PHARMACOLOGIC MANAGEMENT

- For infected eyelids, antibiotic ointment (bacitracin, erythromycin ointment)
- For infections resistant to topical treatment, consider oral tetracycline for several weeks

CONSULTATION/REFERRAL

- Ophthalmologist for severe infections
- Ophthalmologist for conditions which do not improve after treatment

FOLLOW-UP

- None usually needed for simple cases
- Reevaluate depending on severity

EXPECTED COURSE

- Frequent recurrences expected for seborrheic blepharitis

POSSIBLE COMPLICATIONS

- Corneal infection
- Hordeolum
- Scarring of lids
- Trichiasis: misdirection of eye lashes

DACRYOSTENOSIS

DESCRIPTION

Obstruction in the nasolacrimal duct

ETIOLOGY

- Congenital: due to failure of the nasolacrimal duct to canalize
- Infection: chronic inflammation of the duct caused by staphylococci or streptococci infection may lead to obstruction

INCIDENCE

- Common in neonates (usually resolves by 6 months of age due to maturing facial anatomy)

RISK FACTORS

- Chronic nasal infection in adults

ASSESSMENT FINDINGS

- Epiphora: persistent overflow of tears over the lower lid margin
- Mild crusting of lashes
- Red eye due to conjunctivitis
- Mucus reflux through the punctum when pressure is applied

DIFFERENTIAL DIAGNOSIS

- Dacryocystitis
- Conjunctivitis

DIAGNOSTIC STUDIES

- None usually indicated

PREVENTION

- Maintain patency by applying pressure/massaging nasolacrimal duct several times daily

NONPHARMACOLOGIC MANAGEMENT

- Maintain patency by applying pressure/massaging nasolacrimal duct at least twice daily if chronic

- Surgery to probe the tear duct and facilitate permanent drainage

PHARMACOLOGIC MANAGEMENT

- None needed unless there is purulent drainage from the duct or evidence of conjunctivitis
- Symptoms often subside while antibiotic eyedrops in use

CONSULTATION/REFERRAL

- Ophthalmologist for dacryostenosis beyond 6 months of age
- Ophthalmologist for severe obstruction prior to 6 months of age

FOLLOW-UP

- As needed depending on severity

EXPECTED COURSE

- Excellent prognosis

POSSIBLE COMPLICATIONS

- Conjunctivitis

References

Berman, S., Byrns, P.J., Bondy, J., Smith, P.J., & Lezotte, D. (1997). Otitis media-related antibiotic prescribing patterns, outcomes, and expenditures in a pediatric medicaid population. *Pediatrics, 100*, 585-592.

Bickley, L.S., & Szilagyi, P.G. (2003). *Bates' guide to physical examination and history taking* (8th ed.). Philadelphia: Lippincott Williams & Wilkins.

Branch, W.T. (2003). *Office practice of medicine* (4th ed.). Philadelphia: Saunders.

Brown, C.S., Parker, N.G., & Stegbauer, C.C. (1999). Managing allergic rhinitis. *The Nurse Practitioner*, 24(6): 107-120.

Burns, C.E., Brady, M.A., Blosser, C., Starr, N.B., & Dunn, A.M. (2004). *Pediatric primary care: A handbook for nurse practitioners* (3rd ed.). Philadelphia: W.B. Saunders.

Cozad, J. (1996). Infectious mononucleosis. *The Nurse Practitioner, 21*(3), 14-28.

Daly, K.A., Selvius, R.E., & Lindgren, B. (1997). Knowledge and attitudes about otitis media risk: Implications for prevention. *Pediatrics 100,* 931-936.

Dambro, M.R. (2005). *Griffith's 5 minute clinical consult.* Philadelphia: Lippincott Williams & Wilkins.

Duffy, L.C., Faden, H., Wasielewski, R., Wolf, J., & Krystofik, D. (1997). Exclusive breastfeeding protects against bacterial colonization and daycare exposure to otitis media. *Pediatrics Electronic Pages.* [On-line serial]. Available:www.pediatrics.com e7.

Fell, E. (2000). An update on lyme disease and other tick-borne illnesses. *The Nurse Practitioner*, 25(10): 38-55.

Graber, M.A., & Lanternier, M.L. (Eds.) (2001). *The family practice handbook.* (4th ed.). St. Louis: Mosby.

Hanson, M.J. (1996). Acute otitis media in children. *The Nurse Practitioner, 21*(5), 72-81.

Hara, J.H. (1996). The red eye: Diagnosis and treatment. *American Family Physician, 54*, 2423-2436.

Kasper, D.L., Braunwald, E., Fauci, A.S., Hauser, S.L., Longo, D.L., Jameson, J.L., et al. (2004). *Harrison's principles of internal medicine* (16th ed.). New York: McGraw-Hill.

Kliegman, R.M. (1996). *Practical strategies in pediatric diagnosis and therapy*. Philadelphia: W.B. Saunders.

Lucente, F. & Grady, H.E. (1999). *Essentials of Otolaryngology.* (4th ed.). Philadelphia: Lippincott Williams & Wilkins.

Mangion, S. (2000). *Physical diagnosis secrets.* Philadelphia: Hanley and Belfus.

Mladenovic, J. (Ed.). (2003). *Primary care secrets.* (3rd Ed.). Philadelphia: Hanley and Belfus.

Morrow, G.L., & Abbott, R.L. (1998). Conjunctivitis. *American Family Physician, 57*, 735-746.

Osguthorpe, J.D. (2001). Adult rhinosinusitis: diagnosis and management. *American Family Physician, 63*, 69-76.

Perkins, A. (1997). An approach to diagnosing the acute sore throat. *American Family Physician, 55*(1), 131-140.

Pryor, M.P. (1997). Noisy breathing in children. *Postgraduate Medicine 101*(2), 103-112.

Rabinowitz, P.M. (2000). Noise-induced hearing loss. *American Family Physician, 61*, 2749-2756, 2759-2760.

Rakel, R.E. (Ed.). (1998). *Essentials of family practice.* (2nd ed.). Philadelphia: WB Saunders.

Ruppert, S.D. (1996). Differential diagnosis of common causes of pediatric pharyngitis. *The Nurse Practitioner, 21*(4), 38-49.

Ruppert, S.D. (1996). Differential diagnosis of pediatric conjunctivitis. *The Nurse Practitioner, 21*(7), 12-26.

Schwartz, M.W. (Ed.). (2002). *The 5 minute pediatric consult.* (2nd ed.) Philadelphia: Lippincott Williams & Wilkins.

Scott, P.T., Clark, J.B., & Miser, W.F. (1997). Pertussis: An update on primary prevention and outbreak control. *American Family Physician, 56*, 1121-1130.

Shaw, L. (1997). Protocol for detection and follow-up of hearing loss. *Clinical Nurse Specialist: The Journal for Advanced Nursing Practice, 11*, 240-245.

Tasman, W., & Jaeger, E.A. (2005). *Duane's Clinical Ophthalmology on CD-ROM.* Philadelphia: J.B. Lippincott Co.

Uphold, C.R., & Graham, M.V. (2003). *Clinical guidelines in family practice.* (4th ed.). Gainesville, FL: Barmarrae Books.

U.S. Preventive Services Task Force. (1996). *Guide to clinical preventive services.* (2nd ed.) Washington, D.C.: Office of Disease Prevention and Health Promotion, U.S. Government Printing Office.

Ward, M. R. (1997). Reye's syndrome: An update. *The Nurse Practitioner, 22*(12), 45-53.

Wingate, S. (1999). Treating corneal abrasions. *The Nurse Practitioner, 24*(6): 53-68.

Zollo, A.J., Jr. (Ed.). (2004). *Medical Secrets.* (4th ed.), St. Louis, MO: Mosby-Year Book.

15

ORTHOPEDIC DISORDERS

Orthopedic Disorders

** Denotes pediatric diagnosis*

OSTEOARTHRITIS (OA)

DESCRIPTION

Progressive destruction of the articular cartilage and subchondral bone accompanied by osteophyte formation and sclerosis. OA is confined to the joints. There is an absence of constitutional symptoms.

Osteoarthritis is the most common joint disease in the US.

ETIOLOGY

- Primary OA is a disease with no known cause
- Secondary OA is associated with trauma, infection, or metabolic disorders

INCIDENCE

- Males = Females
- Predominantly >age 40 years
- Common

RISK FACTORS

- Obesity
- Age
- Trauma
- Prolonged use or overuse of joints related to occupation or activity
- Family history
- History of developmental dysplasia of the hip or slipped femoral epiphysis
- Hemophilia
- Paget's disease

ASSESSMENT FINDINGS

- Joint pain, usually asymmetrical, develops insidiously and accompanies or follows physical activity
- Morning stiffness lasting <1 hour
- Joints are cool with possible crepitus and limited range of motion
- Overgrowth of osteophytes results in bony enlargement, especially bunions (MTP joint), Heberden's nodes (DIP joints), and Bouchard's nodes (PIP joints)

Commonly involved joints: distal interphalangeal (DIP), and proximal interphalangeal (PIP) joints, first carpometacarpal (CMC) joint, hips, knees, cervical and lumbar spine, and first metatarsophalangeal (MTP) joint.

DIFFERENTIAL DIAGNOSIS

- Gout, pseudogout
- Infective arthritis
- Rheumatoid arthritis
- Joint injury
- Soft tissue injury
- Peripheral vascular disease
- Giant cell arteritis

DIAGNOSTIC STUDIES

- No diagnostic laboratory tests are available for osteoarthritis; diagnosis is based on history, physical, and x-ray findings
- X-rays: osteophytes, joint space narrowing
- Inflammation markers: negative
  - ◊ Erythrocyte sedimentation rate (ESR)
  - ◊ Rheumatoid factor (RF)
  - ◊ Antinuclear antibodies (ANA)

PREVENTION

- Weight control
- Management of underlying causes of secondary disease

NONPHARMACOLOGIC MANAGEMENT

- Emphasis must be given to nonpharmacologic management to delay or minimize use of medications which have adverse effects
- Weight loss, if indicated
- Education that OA is a chronic disorder requiring patient participation in therapy
- Organized program of supervised exercise
- Rest
- Knee or elbow braces to stabilize joints during exercise
- Orthotic shoes, cane, collar, sling, corset, wedged insoles

- Apply heat and/or cold to affected joints
- Wedge osteotomy, arthroplasty
- Acupuncture may be beneficial

PHARMACOLOGIC MANAGEMENT

- Drugs are usually needed long-term and their use is associated with many possible side effects
- Acetaminophen recommended as first-line therapy by the American College of Rheumatology
- Add NSAID for pain that persists despite acetaminophen at adequate doses
- Short-acting NSAIDs are associated with fewer side effects
- Concomitant use of misoprostol (Cytotec®) to prevent gastric ulcer development caused by NSAIDs
- Consider COX-2 inhibitors for GI protection (risk of GI bleeds decreased but still present)
- Narcotic analgesics indicated briefly for severe exacerbation
- Intraarticular corticosteroid injections, limited to 4 times a year, and not recommended for the hip

AGENT	ACTION	COMMENTS
NSAIDs *Example:* ibuprofen (Advil®) ketoprofen (Orudis®) etodolac (Lodine®) diclofenac (Voltaren®) meloxicam (Mobic®) celecoxib (Celebrex®)	Inhibit cyclooxygenase (COX-1 and COX-2) activity and prostaglandin synthesis. COX-1 inhibition is associated with GI toxicity.	Most NSAIDs are COX-1 selective. Celebrex is mostly COX-2 selective. Do not administer to patients who are ASA allergic because of cross-sensitivity. Serious GI bleeding can occur at any time without warning. Always use the lowest dose possible. NSAIDs are primarily eliminated by the kidneys, do not use in renal patients. Monitor BP while on NSAIDs. Do not use NSAIDs in 3rd trimester, Category D. NSAIDs inhibit platelet aggregation. Monitor peripheral edema and fluid retention (contraindicated in CHF). Do not use concomitantly with salicylates.

CONSULTATION/REFERRAL

- Orthopedist
- Physical therapist
- Supervised exercise program
- Nutritionist for weight loss

FOLLOW-UP

- Regularly scheduled return visits for evaluation, support and education
- NSAID therapy requirements (includes COX-2): periodic CBC, renal function studies, and stool for occult blood

EXPECTED COURSE

- Usually progressive with more pain at rest, joint effusions, and bony enlargement

POSSIBLE COMPLICATIONS

- Adverse effects from NSAIDs
- Corticosteroid adverse effects
- Depression associated with chronic illness

RHEUMATOID ARTHRITIS (RA)

DESCRIPTION

A systemic, frequently progressive illness characterized by joint inflammation and constitutional symptoms. There is inflammation and thickening of the synovial membrane and vascular damage which causes increased metabolic needs.

ETIOLOGY

- Unknown
- Possible genetic predisposition coupled with an environmental trigger
- Antigen-antibody reaction results in inflammatory response

INCIDENCE

- 1% of U.S. population
- Females > Males
- Common in Caucasians, Native Americans; rare in African Americans
- Occurs between ages 30 and 50 years; peak onset is age 40 years

RISK FACTORS

- Family history

ASSESSMENT FINDINGS

- May be acute onset over 24 hours, or gradual and insidious
- Constitutional symptoms:
  - ◊ Weakness, malaise, fatigue, anorexia, weight loss, depression
  - ◊ Lymphadenopathy, aches, low-grade fever
- Joint pain/stiffness at rest and with movement; can disturb sleep and lasts >1 hour in morning upon arising
  - ◊ Polyarticular: proximal interphalangeal (PIP), metacarpophalangeal (MCP), wrist, elbow, knee, ankle
  - ◊ Symmetrical
- Rheumatoid nodules may occur on extensor surfaces of elbows and fingers

Symptoms are usually present for 9 months prior to diagnosis.

DIFFERENTIAL DIAGNOSIS

- Septic arthritis
- Gout
- Trauma
- Bursitis
- Systemic lupus erythematosus: multisystem inflammatory illness with positive antinuclear antibody (ANA)
- Osteoarthritis

DIAGNOSTIC CRITERIA

- Five of the 7 criteria must be present; and the first 4 must be present for at least 6 weeks:
  - ◊ Morning stiffness >1 hour
  - ◊ Soft tissue swelling of 3 or more joints (PIP, MCP, wrist, elbow, knee, ankle, metatarsophalangeal (MTP)
  - ◊ Swelling of at least 1 joint in the hand or wrist
  - ◊ Symmetrical joint swelling
  - ◊ Rheumatoid nodules
  - ◊ Serum rheumatoid factor (RF)
  - ◊ Bony erosions demonstrable by x-ray

DIAGNOSTIC STUDIES

- X-ray studies: joint space narrowing, bony erosion in joints, reduced bone density surrounding joints
- Rheumatoid factor (RF): elevated (20% of patients are negative despite having other symptoms of RA)
- Erythrocyte sedimentation rate (ESR): elevated, nonspecific for RA
- Antinuclear antibodies (ANA): usually negative, but can be positive in 20-30% of patients)
- C-reactive protein: if positive, indicates acute nonspecific inflammation, nonspecific
- Joint aspiration to rule out infectious arthritis and gout

SED rate is a good measure of the disease's activity.

PREVENTION

- Prompt diagnosis and treatment will minimize harmful sequelae

Goals are to prevent damage to joints if possible and to maintain mobility.

NONPHARMACOLOGIC MANAGEMENT

- Exercise program
  - ◊ Increase in pain or swelling indicates excessive exercise
  - ◊ Should not involve joints that are acutely inflamed
- Splinting reduces inflammation and deformities
- Orthotics can relieve pain and prevent deformities
- Cold therapy for analgesic, antiinflammatory effect
- Heat therapy for relaxation and circulatory stimulation
- Weight loss, if indicated, reduces joint pain; avoidance of allergens that precipitate symptoms
- Surgery: arthroscopy with synovectomy, arthroplasty
- Education regarding illness and therapies improves patient's ability to form appropriate goals and participate in treatment plan

PHARMACOLOGIC MANAGEMENT

- Disease-modifying antirheumatic drugs (DMARDs) first line in patients with acute presentation
  - ◊ Methotrexate (Rheumatrex®)
  - ◊ Hydroxychloroquine (Plaquenil®)
  - ◊ Sulfasalazine delayed-release (Azulfidine EN-tabs®)
  - ◊ Gold (Solganal®, Aurolate®)
  - ◊ Enbrel®
  - ◊ Cyclosporine®
  - ◊ Arava®
  - ◊ Remicade®
  - ◊ Azathioprine (Imuran®)
  - ◊ D-penicillamine (Cuprimine®, Depen®)
- Nonsteroidal anti-inflammatory drugs (NSAIDs) indicated for mild symptoms
- Oral and intraarticular steroids and narcotic analgesics are indicated to treat severe pain while waiting for other drugs to become therapeutic

Methotrexate has the most predictable effect. Always prescribe folate with methotrexate to reduce risk of liver toxicity.

PREGNANCY/LACTATION CONSIDERATIONS

- Methotrexate has teratogenic potential. Pregnancy should be avoided if either the male or the female partner is taking the drug. Women should wait at least one ovulatory cycle after stopping methotrexate before conceiving; men should wait at least 3 months.

CONSULTATION/REFERRAL

- Rheumatologist for confirmation of diagnosis, treatment plan, and before initiation of DMARDs
- Occupational therapist, physical therapist
- Nutritionist
- Supervised exercise program
- Arthritis Foundation
- Social services due to personal, social, and financial implications
- Surgeon, if indicated

FOLLOW-UP

- CBC, chemistry profile, renal and liver functions as baseline before initiating anti-inflammatory or antirheumatic therapy
- Eye exam if on Plaquenil®
- Appropriate monitoring of laboratory values depending on therapeutic agents used
- Ongoing assessment of disease symptoms, ESR, CRP

Ongoing laboratory follow up is critical for patients on DMARDs because of potential toxicity of these drugs.

EXPECTED COURSE

- Persistent swelling of PIP joints, early onset (young age) with involvement of >20 joints, high RF, and high ESR have poorest prognosis
- Course may be insidious or acute

- Complete remission is rare, but with appropriate therapy, pain and disability may be minimized
- Average life expectancy is decreased by 7 years for men and 3 years for women

POSSIBLE COMPLICATIONS

- Depression
- Drug toxicity
- Joint destruction
- Sjögren syndrome
- Social and occupational disability

GOUT

DESCRIPTION

Deposition of monosodium urate (MSU) crystals in joints and other connective tissue causing acute or chronic inflammation manifested as acute or chronic arthritis, tophi, nephropathy, and/or renal stones.

ETIOLOGY

- Elevated serum and total body uric acid is a result of either its overproduction or underexcretion
- Underexcretion may be due to renal insufficiency, acidosis, or use of diuretics, aspirin, or cyclosporine
- Overproduction may be due to enzyme deficiencies, psoriasis, or hematologic malignancies
- Dietary excess of purines
- Alcoholism is a contributing factor in both overproduction and underexcretion of urate

INCIDENCE

- Increasing in U.S.
- Males > Females (20:1)
- More common in age > 45 years

RISK FACTORS

- Alcohol abuse
- Medication use
    - ◊ Aspirin
    - ◊ Nicotinic acid
    - ◊ Diuretics
    - ◊ Cyclosporine
- Renal insufficiency
- Acidosis
- Enzyme deficiencies
- Psoriasis
- Hematologic malignancies
- Family history
- Obesity
- Hypertension

ASSESSMENT FINDINGS

- Acute joint pain and swelling, with warmth and erythema, beginning abruptly, usually involving a single joint (75% of time)
    - ◊ Metatarsophalangeal joint of first toe is involved most often
    - ◊ Ankle, tarsal area, knee, wrist or finger joint may be involved
- Acute attacks usually subside without treatment in approximately 1-2 weeks
- Skin may desquamate over the affected joint after the inflammation subsides
- Subsequent episodes may involve several joints, and persist longer
- There may be a history of a stressful event that triggered the first attack
    - ◊ Trauma
    - ◊ Alcohol
    - ◊ Drugs
    - ◊ Surgery
    - ◊ Acute medical illness
- Tophi, MSU crystal-containing deposits in subcutaneous tissue of antihelix of ears and extensor aspect of elbow, occur in fairly advanced gout
- Fever
- Kidney stones

DIFFERENTIAL DIAGNOSIS

- Arterial insufficiency
- Muscular or ligamentous strain
- Traumatic arthritis

- Rheumatoid arthritis
- Septic arthritis
- Pseudogout
- Cellulitis

DIAGNOSTIC STUDIES

- WBC: usually elevated during acute attack
- ESR: usually elevated during acute attack
- X-ray studies of joints: soft tissue swelling, otherwise, normal initially; after multiple episodes, may see tophi and joint changes
- Serum uric acid levels not helpful in diagnosis, but are important in following treatment
- Synovial fluid aspiration (not usually performed):
  - ◊ Presence of monosodium urate crystals is diagnostic
  - ◊ Elevated white blood cells

Normal uric acid levels are common during an acute attack. Elevated uric acid levels are not diagnostic of gout. Therefore, always look at the clinical presentation in conjunction with diagnostic studies.

PREVENTION

- Avoid contributing substances (e.g., alcohol, medications)
- Good hydration
- Maintain ideal body weight

NONPHARMACOLOGIC MEASURES

- Rest acutely inflamed joint
- Educate patient about avoidance of contributing substances
- Weight reduction if indicated
- Fluid intake of 3 liters/day

PHARMACOLOGIC MANAGEMENT

Acute attacks:

- High dose NSAIDs for 2-5 days and reduce dose as soon as symptoms allow
- Corticosteroids may be effective if patient cannot tolerate NSAIDs
- Intraarticular injection of corticosteroids

Infection in joint must be ruled out before intraarticular injection of corticosteroids.

Preventive therapy:

- Used for recurrent attacks or if tophi present
- Urate-lowering agents taken long term
  - ◊ Uricosurics increase excretion of uric acid: probenecid (Benemid®), sulfinpyrazone (Anturane®)
  - ◊ Allopurinol (Zyloprim®): decreases the production of uric acid
- Monitor CBC renal and hepatic function at 1 week, 6 weeks, and every 3 months while on allopurinol. Bone marrow suppression, as well as, renal and hepatic impairment can occur.

CONSULTATION/REFERRAL

- Patients with complications requiring nephrologist, hematologist, oncologist, or urologist

FOLLOW-UP

- Evaluate response to therapy for acute attack within several days
- Assess serum uric acid levels monthly until desirable level (<7 mg/dL) is reached, then annually

EXPECTED COURSE

- Good control can be achieved with early detection and treatment and patient compliance with lifestyle changes
- Recurrent attacks require long-term use of preventive medications and monitoring of laboratory values
- Over half of patients develop chronic disease within 20 years of initial attack

POSSIBLE COMPLICATIONS

- Nephropathy
- Kidney stones
- Joint destruction
- Infection

LOW BACK PAIN
(Secondary to Disc Disorders)

DESCRIPTION

Activity intolerance due to lumbar pain that involves an intervertebral disc; frequently there is referral of pain to the buttocks and posterior thighs, and/or down one or both legs.
Radiculopathy describes a disorder of the roots of the spinal nerves due to compression, inflammation, or tearing of nerve roots at the site of entry into the vertebral canal.

ETIOLOGY

- Often unclear; stretching or tearing of nerves, muscles, tendons, ligaments, or fascia of back secondary to trauma or chronic mechanical stress
- Compression or irritation of a nerve root is a common cause.

The discs most commonly affected are L5-S1 and L4-L5.

INCIDENCE

- >80% of U.S. population affected at some time in their lives
- 31 million people affected in U.S.
- Males = Females

RISK FACTORS

- Obesity
- Sedentary lifestyle, inadequate conditioning, cigarette smoking
- Chronic occupational strain, improper lifting techniques
- Exaggerated lumbar lordosis, chronic poor posture
- Leg length discrepancy

ASSESSMENT FINDINGS

- Pain in back, buttocks, and/or one or both thighs, aggravated by movement, rising from sitting position, standing, and flexion, and may relieved by rest, repositioning, or reclining
- Muscle spasm may be present over lumbosacral area because of soft tissue involvement (ligaments, muscles)
- Pain usually radiates down leg and below the knee

***Sciatic stretch test*: elevation of affected leg in supine position will elicit pain at 15-30 degrees for severe disease; 30-60 degrees for moderate disease**

***Crossed leg raise*: elevating unaffected leg produces pain in affected leg**

- Bowel and bladder function preserved
- Motor, sensory, and reflex examination
- Deep tendon reflexes (DTR)
    * Biceps: test nerves at roots C5-C6
    * Brachioradialis: tests nerves at roots C5-C6
    * Triceps: tests nerves at roots T2-T4
    * Patellar: tests nerves at roots L2-L4
    * Achilles: tests nerves at roots S1-S2
  - ◊ DTR responses are graded as follows:
    * 0: no response
    * +1: diminished response
    * +2: normal response
    * +3: increased response
    * +4: hyperactive response
  - ◊ Responses below normal may imply myopathies, decreased muscle mass, nerve root impairment
  - ◊ Responses above normal are characteristic of pyramidal tract disease, electrolyte imbalance, hyperthyroidism, or other endocrine abnormalities
  - Observe gait, assess lower extremity strength and bulk of muscles, pulses
  - Listen for abdominal bruits and assess rectal sphincter tone

New onset radicular pain in older patients is frequently spinal stenosis.

DIFFERENTIAL DIAGNOSIS

- Low back strain
- Herniated intervertebral disc

- Prostatitis, pyelonephritis
- Vascular occlusion at level of bifurcation, abdominal aneurysm
- Carcinoma if bony metastasis occurs
- Endometriosis, fibromyoma
- Depression, hysteria
- Malingering
- Compression fracture, osteoporosis
- Osteoarthritis
- Ankylosing spondylitis
- Cauda equina syndrome

DIAGNOSTIC STUDIES

- X-rays may identify tumor or a structural abnormality. Consider imaging in the following situations with a complaint of low back pain:
    - ◊ Age over 50 years
    - ◊ Neurologic deficits
    - ◊ History of cancer
    - ◊ Accompanying unexplained weight loss
    - ◊ Substance abuse: steroids, alcohol, drugs
    - ◊ Recurrent or chronic backpain, or unresponsive to treatment after 1 month
    - ◊ History of significant trauma
    - ◊ Patient involved in litigation, desiring compensation
- Studies that may be done to exclude disc disease and tumors:
    - ◊ CT, MRI (study of choice for evaluation of disc disease), bone scan
    - ◊ CBC, ESR, serum calcium, alkaline phosphatase, serum immunoelectrophoresis
    - ◊ Urinalysis

Many asymptomatic patients have bulging discs.

PREVENTION

- Education regarding proper lifting techniques, body mechanics
- Conditioning exercises
- Maintenance of appropriate weight for height
- Avoid cigarette smoking

NONPHARMACOLOGIC MANAGEMENT

- Modify activities for 3 to 6 weeks
    - ◊ Limit bedrest to 2-4 days, then restrict activities to avoid heavy lifting and aggravating activities
    - ◊ Assume position that maximizes comfort
    - ◊ Gradually resume activities as tolerated and include gradually increasing low-stress aerobic exercises
- Physical modalities
    - ◊ Cryotherapy for 20-30 minutes several times up to 48 hours after onset
    - ◊ Apply heat for 20-30 minutes several times a day after the first 48 hours
    - ◊ Exercise: isometric tightening of abdominal and gluteal muscles after acute pain subsides; lumbar hyperextension exercises
    - ◊ Spinal manipulation may be helpful during the first month of back pain, but neurologic involvement must first be ruled out
- Education regarding preventive measures
- Shoe insoles, shoe lifts recommended for leg length discrepancies >2 cm

Conservative measures are usually recommended for the first 6 weeks unless there are neurological deficits or severe pain.

PHARMACOLOGIC MANAGEMENT

- NSAIDs reduce pain and inflammation and promote healing
- Acetaminophen reduces pain but is more effective in combination with a narcotic analgesic or NSAID
- Muscle relaxants have not been proven more effective than NSAIDs, either alone, or used concomitantly but are helpful for spastic conditions
- Short term use of opioid analgesics for pain relief, but have not been proven more effective than NSAIDs and have potential for physical dependence
- Epidural steroid injections to reduce inflammation and pain if more conservative treatments fail

AGENT	ACTION	COMMENTS
NSAIDs *Example:* ibuprofen (Advil®) ketoprofen (Orudis®) etodolac (Lodine®) diclofenac (Voltaren®) meloxicam (Mobic®) celecoxib (Celebrex®)	Inhibit cyclooxygenase (COX-1 and COX-2) activity and prostaglandin synthesis. COX-1 inhibition is associated with GI toxicity.	Most NSAIDs are COX-1 selective. Celebrex is mostly COX-2 selective. Do not administer to patients who are ASA allergic because of cross-sensitivity. Serious GI bleeding can occur at any time without warning. Always use the lowest dose possible. NSAIDs are primarily eliminated by the kidneys, do not use in renal patients. Monitor BP while on NSAIDs. Do not use NSAIDs in 3rd trimester, Category D. NSAIDs inhibit platelet aggregation. Monitor peripheral edema and fluid retention (contraindicated in CHF). Do not use concomitantly with salicylates.
Muscle relaxants *Example:* cyclobenzaprine (Flexeril®) metaxalone (Skelaxin®) tizanidine (Zanaflex®)	Varying mechanisms of action but act on the central nervous system to decrease input to the alpha neurons	Synergistic effect when taken with pain medications, anti-anxiety medications and alcohol. Extremely cautious use in elderly due to risk of falls, disorientation, hypotension Careful use in patients with renal or hepatic abnormalities. May cause profound drowsiness and patient should not drive or engage in activities which require attention. Monitor for drug interactions, especially with Flexeril® and Zanaflex®. Cautious use in patients with rhythm disturbances, conduction defects. Anticholinergic effects can be profound so avoid use in patients with urinary retention and glaucoma.

CONSULTATION/REFERRAL

- Findings that indicate neurological involvement
- Recurrent or chronic pain unresponsive to therapy
- Physical therapy especially initially if pain is moderate and conservative treatment has not provided relief

FOLLOW-UP

- Return for repeat evaluation in 24-48 hours if pain is severe, and in 7-10 days if pain is moderate; follow every 2-4 weeks until able to resume lifestyle
- Ongoing education and support regarding lifestyle changes
- If there is inability to tolerate activities in the face of no serious underlying pathology, explore psychosocial factors

EXPECTED COURSE

- In 80% of cases, symptoms resolve in 4-6 weeks

POSSIBLE COMPLICATIONS

- Prolonged disability associated with physical, psychologic, social, and economic factors

BURSITIS

DESCRIPTION

Inflammation of a bursa, a flattened sac of synovial membrane which contains synovial fluid. These are found in areas where friction is likely to occur, such as, where a tendon overrides bony structures. They may be deep, (e.g., hip, ischial tuberosity), or superficial (e.g., shoulder, knee, heel, elbow).

ETIOLOGY

- Bursitis is often secondary to calcific tendinitis. An acutely inflamed tendon irritates the overlying bursa.
- Contributing factors are overuse and structural and functional abnormalities
- May also be a result of bacterial infection

INCIDENCE

- Common
- Males > Females

RISK FACTORS

- Local trauma
- Repetitive motion
- Sudden increase in level of activity
- Gout
- Rheumatoid arthritis
- Aging
- Obesity
- Leg length discrepancy
- Osteoarthritis
- Penetrating injury

ASSESSMENT FINDINGS

Types of Bursitis	
Infective bursitis	Elevated temperature, red, exquisitely tender overlying tissue
Anserine bursitis	Painful knee, worse with stair climbing
Achilles bursitis	Painful heel, subcutaneous swelling at back of Achilles tendon ("pump bump")
Calcaneal bursitis	Painful plantar surface of heel
Infrapatellar bursitis	Swelling and tenderness below patella
Iliopsoas bursitis	Painful groin and anterior thigh
Ischial bursitis	Pain with sitting or lying, may radiate down back of thigh, point tenderness over ischium
Olecranon bursitis	Elbow pain with subcutaneous swelling, no loss of motion to elbow
Prepatellar bursitis	Pain over medial aspect of knee
Subdeltoid bursitis	Shoulder pain with subcutaneous swelling
Trochanteric bursitis	Gradual onset of lateral hip and thigh pain

DIFFERENTIAL DIAGNOSIS

- Sprain, strain
- Tendinitis
- Osteoarthritis, rheumatoid arthritis
- Gout

DIAGNOSTIC STUDIES

- Aspiration and culture of synovial fluid if infective bursitis suspected

- Bursitis seldom shown on x-ray, but may see calcium deposits
- MRI,CT (not initially done)
- ESR to differentiate soft tissue disease from connective tissue disease
- Blood culture indicated for multiple systemic features: methicillin-resistant *Staphylococcus aureus* is frequent finding
- CBC
- Consider RPR to rule out syphilis

PREVENTION

- Avoid overuse of joints without adequate rest periods
- Maintain physical fitness

NONPHARMACOLOGIC MANAGEMENT

- Identify and avoid aggravating factors
- Slings, shoe lifts, splints, or canes to correct biomechanical disruption
- Physical therapy program of stretching and strengthening
- Ice to inflamed area
- Rest, immobility of affected extremity
- Weight loss if indicated
- Application of ice/heat

PHARMACOLOGIC MANAGEMENT

Inflammatory bursitis:

- Administer NSAIDs at full anti-inflammatory dose (*see* NSAID table in Osteoarthritis)
- Intrabursal aspiration and injection of an anesthetic and a corticosteroid
  - ◊ Avoid injecting Achilles bursitis due to risk of Achilles tendon rupture

Infective bursitis:

- Antibiotic therapy (systemic antibiotics required for septic bursitis)

CONSULTATION/REFERRAL

- Orthopedist for surgical excision of involved area if chronic bursitis develops or for incision and drainage if infected

FOLLOW-UP

- Use NSAID until symptoms have subsided for 1 week
- Up to 3 corticosteroid injections may be given 4-6 weeks apart
- Recurrence of bursitis within 7 days of injection should raise suspicion of septic bursitis and indicate a need for re-aspiration

EXPECTED COURSE

- Once aggravating factors are removed, bursitis usually heals without complications or progression to chronic condition

POSSIBLE COMPLICATIONS

- Progression to chronic bursitis with limitation of range of motion

EPICONDYLITIS
(Tennis Elbow, Golfer's Elbow)

DESCRIPTION

Lateral epicondylitis or "tennis elbow" is inflammation of the common tendinous origin of the extensor muscles of the forearm on the humeral lateral epicondyle.
Medial epicondylitis or "golfer's elbow" is inflammation of the common tendinous origin of the extensor muscles of the forearm at the humeral medial epicondyle.
The principles outlined in epicondylitis apply to other types of tendinitis.

ETIOLOGY

- Repetitive overuse of the involved muscle without sufficient rest to allow rebuilding of muscle tissue

INCIDENCE

- Common over age 40 years

RISK FACTORS

Lateral epicondylitis:

- Overuse activities requiring a strong grasp during wrist extension
  - ◊ Typing
  - ◊ Weight lifting
  - ◊ Knitting
  - ◊ Backhand tennis stroke
  - ◊ Carpentry
  - ◊ Factory work

Medial epicondylitis:

- Activities which require forcefully extending the elbow against resistance with the forearm supinated and the wrist dorsiflexed
- Golf
- Pitching

ASSESSMENT FINDINGS

Lateral epicondylitis:

- Gradual onset of dull, aching pain over a period of weeks or months on the lateral aspect of the elbow; may be present at rest, but usually worse with activity
- Pain may radiate down the back of the forearm
- Shaking hands, lifting a cup, or turning a door knob may elicit sharp pain
- Point tenderness over lateral epicondyle; full range of motion; no swelling, and no erythema
- Pain to the lateral aspect of the elbow when resistance is applied against wrist extension

Medial epicondylitis:

- Pain to the region of the medial epicondyle, reproducible by forcefully extending the elbow against resistance with the forearm supinated and the wrist dorsiflexed
- Pain may radiate down the flexor surface of the forearm
- Point tenderness over medial epicondyle; no swelling or erythema

DIFFERENTIAL DIAGNOSIS

- Olecranon bursitis (may coexist)
- Tendon avulsion or rupture
- Osteoarthritis
- Radial nerve entrapment syndrome
- Radial head dislocation
- Synovitis of the elbow
- Interarticular loose bodies
- Cervical spine disorder
- Carpal tunnel syndrome
- Radial tunnel syndrome
- Fracture

Tendinitis and arthritis may be difficult to differentiate clinically. Arthritis produces pain in the joint. Tendinitis produces pain at the insertion point of the affected tendon (not in the joint).

DIAGNOSTIC STUDIES

- X-rays of the elbow are usually normal and are unnecessary unless there is a history of trauma, or therapy failure
- Diagnosis is made on basis of characteristic presentation
- MRI is preferred diagnostic tool when conservative measures have failed (will identify tears, ruptures)

PREVENTION

- Educate about need to balance repetitive movement with rest
- Educate that all changes in intensity, duration, or frequency of physical activity should be gradual to allow for conditioning
- Ergonomic evaluation if contributory

NONPHARMACOLOGIC MANAGEMENT

- Rest, cessation of exacerbating activity for 2 weeks, with gradual return to full activity
- Ice massage to area: apply ice, with pressure, directly to the skin over the epicondyle and surrounding area for 20 minutes three times a day
- Once acute symptoms have abated, patient should begin forearm strengthening and muscle stretching exercises
- Tennis elbow counterforce brace may help to relieve pain while playing
- Changing size of grip or string tension of tennis racket may be helpful
- Deep massage of the tendinous insertions of the epicondyle is theorized to help regenerate damaged tendons
- Surgical intervention is an option if unresponsive to 6-12 months of therapy

PHARMACOLOGIC MANAGEMENT

- Nonsteroidal anti-inflammatory (NSAID) medication (*see* NSAID table in Osteoarthritis)
- Intraarticular corticosteroid injection, best reserved for cases unresponsive to more conservative therapies

CONSULTATION/REFERRAL

- Orthopedist if unresponsive to therapy
- Physical therapist for instruction on strengthening and stretching exercise
- Occupational therapist for work-related etiology and ergonomic evaluation

FOLLOW-UP

- At 2 weeks to evaluate effect of therapy
- Once acute pain abates, a conditioning program should be initiated

EXPECTED COURSE

- Acute symptoms usually resolve in 2 weeks with conservative treatment
- Return to previous activities without sufficient conditioning may result in recurrence

POSSIBLE COMPLICATIONS

- Reduction in occupational productivity (lost work days)

LITTLE LEAGUE ELBOW

DESCRIPTION

An overuse injury of the elbow that occurs in children

ETIOLOGY

- Repeated forceful pulls of the flexor/pronator muscle group results in post traumatic changes in the medial condylar apophysis

INCIDENCE

- Occurs predominantly in children ages 9-15 years

RISK FACTORS

- Playing baseball, particularly pitching
- Previous elbow trauma

ASSESSMENT FINDINGS

- Pain about the elbow, worse after throwing
- Loss of motion, especially supination and full extension of the elbow
- Pain with passive wrist extension
- Weak grip
- Ulnar nerve paresthesia

DIFFERENTIAL DIAGNOSIS

- Ulnar collateral ligament sprain
- Cervical radiculopathy
- Ulnar neuritis

DIAGNOSTIC STUDIES

- AP, lateral, medial, and lateral oblique x-ray of the elbow: widening of the apophyseal plate, medial epicondylar apophyseal avulsion

PREVENTION

- Education regarding conditioning, proper
- technique
- Avoid repetitious throwing (limit number of games pitched)

NONPHARMACOLOGIC MANAGEMENT

- Rest
- Children who are heavily emotionally involved in sports may tolerate playing in other positions
- Avoid pitching until symptoms are resolved and range of motion is normal
- Counsel overzealous parents or coaches
- Application of ice for 15 minutes three times a day and after activity

PHARMACOLOGIC MANAGEMENT

- NSAIDs (ibuprofen most commonly used in children)

CONSULTATION/REFERRAL

- Orthopedist if not resolved with rest, ice, and therapy
- Physical therapist for conditioning and strengthening

FOLLOW-UP

- Gradual program of increased activity is necessary to prevent recurrence

EXPECTED COURSE

- May return to full activity once free of pain and full range of motion has returned

POSSIBLE COMPLICATIONS

- Avulsion-fragmentation of the apophysis

SUBLUXATION OF THE RADIAL HEAD
(Nursemaid's Elbow, Pulled Elbow)

DESCRIPTION

A radial head subluxation is a partial dislocation but contact between joints remains intact

ETIOLOGY

- Infants and young children's radial heads are not as bulbous as that of an older child or adult
- Subluxation of the annular ligament can be initiated if longitudinal traction is applied to the arm while the elbow is extended
- A jerk of the arm while a child's hand is being held by an adult is a common cause
- Another cause is the child being forcibly lifted by the hand

INCIDENCE

- Occurs in children <4 years of age usually

RISK FACTORS

- History of previous subluxation

ASSESSMENT FINDINGS

- Child holds hand in a pronated position, may refuse to use the hand, and cries when the elbow is moved

As long as pronated position is maintained, child usually does not complain of pain.

DIFFERENTIAL DIAGNOSIS

- Fracture

DIAGNOSTIC STUDIES

- X-rays are not usually necessary for diagnosis

PREVENTION

- Educate parents to avoid lifting or pulling child (especially forcefully) by the hands/arms

MANAGEMENT

- Apply pressure over the radial head while rotating the hand and forearm to a supinated position until a palpable click is felt along the elbow's lateral aspect

EXPECTED COURSE

- Once a subluxation has occurred, there is an increased likelihood of recurrence until age 4 years at which time the radial head is sufficiently developed

SPRAIN

DESCRIPTION

Stretching or partial tearing of ligaments. Ligaments are dense connective tissue arranged in a parallel fashion that connects one bone to another.

Sprains Graded According To Severity	
Grade I	Minimally torn ligament, stable joint
Grade II	More severely torn ligament, stable joint
Grade III	Completely torn ligament, unstable joint

A strain is an injury to a muscle or tendon usually associated with improper use or overuse.

ETIOLOGY

- The relative weakness of the ligament, along with the bony characteristics of the joint, result in susceptibility to injury
- Eversion ankle sprains, resulting from tears in the deltoid ligament, are less common, but tend to be more severe

INCIDENCE

- A common musculoskeletal injury, often sports-related
- 85% of ankle injuries are sprains
- Prevalent in all ages in which patient engages in physical activity
- Males > Females

RISK FACTORS

- Sports participation, especially volleyball, football, and basketball
- Prior sprain
- Trauma, falls
- Excessive exercise
- Inadequate warmup
- Poor strength, flexibility, or proprioception
- Wearing inappropriate shoes for activity

ASSESSMENT FINDINGS

- Pain and edema over and around injured joint
- Erythema
- Ecchymosis
- Audible pop heard at time of injury
- Discomfort upon weight-bearing
- Abnormal gait if affects lower extremity (ankle, knee)
- Decreased range of motion (Grade 1 and 2 sprains)
- No focal point of exquisite tenderness

If increased range of motion occurs at any injured joint, suspect severe tear or rupture of ligament.

DIFFERENTIAL DIAGNOSIS

- Fracture
- Ruptured tendon
- Tendinitis
- Bursitis

Often difficult clinically to distinguish between strain and sprain and so a common diagnosis is strain/sprain.

DIAGNOSTIC STUDIES

- X-rays indicated if there is suspicion of fracture:
  - ◊ Point of exquisite tenderness
  - ◊ Pain near medial or lateral malleolus, pain at base of 5th MT, or mid-foot pain
  - ◊ Inability to bear weight immediately after injury or at time of exam

PREVENTION

- During pre-participation sports examination, discuss importance of training and flexibility
- Consider external supports for patients with poor flexibility, weakness, or decreased proprioception
- Ankle/knee training programs to improve strength, flexibility, and proprioception, and for those with previous history of ankle/knee injury
- Taping or bracing the ankle/knee of those participating in high-risk activities
- Appropriate conditioning and maintenance of physical conditioning

NONPHARMACOLOGIC MANAGEMENT

RICE Therapy
Rest, stop all weight-bearing immediately after injury
Ice applied to injured area for 20 minutes as frequently as possible for the first 24 hours
Compression of injured area, accomplished by wrapping with an elastic bandage
Elevation of injured joint above heart level

- Apply heat for 20 minute periods 4 times a day after the first 48 hours
- Crutches while unable to bear weight
- Air casts provide pain relief and usually allow patient to resume mobility and weight bearing

PHARMACOLOGIC MANAGEMENT

- *Children*: acetaminophen as needed to relieve pain
- *Adults*: nonsteroidal anti-inflammatory (NSAID) agents used to relieve pain and reduce inflammation (*see* NSAID table in Osteoarthritis)
- Short course narcotic analgesics for pain

CONSULTATION/REFERRAL

- Orthopedist if Grade III sprain or eversion sprain
- Orthopedist if not significantly improved in 3 weeks
- Orthotist for support devices

FOLLOW-UP

- Return in 2 weeks:
  - ◊ Educate regarding preventive measures (e.g., ankle strengthening exercises and supportive footwear)
  - ◊ Evaluate for pain, swelling, and weight-bearing ability

EXPECTED COURSE

- Recovery expected in 2-6 weeks, depending on severity of sprain/strain

POSSIBLE COMPLICATIONS

- Arthritis
- Recurrence due to joint instability

FRACTURES

DESCRIPTION

A complete or incomplete break in the continuity of a bone

ETIOLOGY

- Usually associated with a direct blow, fall, crushing injury, snapping force, or twisting motion

INCIDENCE

- Common
- Age of prevalence dependent on fracture location
- 75% of fractures in children occur in the upper extremities

RISK FACTORS

- Osteoporosis, alcohol use, cigarette smoking
- Use of sedatives in the elderly
- Neurological impairment, impaired vision,
- Malignancy
- Frequent falls, frailty
- Participation in contact sports, deconditioning

ASSESSMENT FINDINGS

- Swelling
- Point tenderness at fracture site
- Decreased or abnormal mobility of affected extremity; pain with motion
- Open wound
- Asymmetry of extremities
- Gross deformity of extremity

A hip fracture may be present in the absence of hip pain. The pain may be referred to the knee. This may be the patient's only complaint after trauma or a fall.

DIFFERENTIAL DIAGNOSIS

- Fracture with associated neurovascular damage
- Fracture with associated injuries to joints above and below
- Open fracture vs. closed fracture
- Growth center vs. avulsion fracture
- Nursemaid's elbow
- Sprain, strain, soft tissue injury
- Dislocation of joint
- Presence of malignancy

DIAGNOSTIC STUDIES

- Neurovascular examination to rule out damage to nerves or blood vessels
  - ◊ A cool, pulseless extremity signals an emergency
- AP and lateral x-ray of affected extremity, but consider x-ray above and below affected joint
  - ◊ With inclusion of joints above and below suspected fracture site
  - ◊ Comparison views if growth plate involvement is suspected
- Assessment of underlying organs, e.g., heart, lungs
- Skeletal survey if child abuse suspected

PREVENTION

- Prophylaxis for osteoporosis
- Avoidance of long-acting sedatives in elderly
- Encourage use of walkers, and other devices that assist with mobility for the neurologically impaired or elderly
- Proper protective gear for athletes

NONPHARMACOLOGIC MANAGEMENT

- Splinting for immobilization should precede x-ray evaluation in order to prevent damage due to sharp bony ends
  - ◊ Adequate padding should precede splint
  - ◊ Joint above and below suspected fracture site should be included
- Application of ice for 48-72 hours
- Elevation of extremity if possible

PHARMACOLOGIC MANAGEMENT

- Analgesia
  - ◊ NSAIDs (use is controversial because the inflammatory process is thought to speed healing)
  - ◊ Acetaminophen
  - ◊ Narcotic analgesics (avoid if head injury is suspected)
- Tetanus toxoid for open wounds, if indicated
- Antibiotics if infection is a likely complication

CONSULTATION/REFERRAL

- Orthopedist for casting of nondisplaced fracture or surgical reduction and pinning as needed
- Neurosurgeon for head, spinal injuries, or neurological injuries
- Otorhinolaryngologist/oral surgeon for facial injuries
- Orthotist
- Physical therapist
- Occupational therapist

FOLLOW-UP

- Cast care
  - ◊ Keep dry
  - ◊ Seek attention for pain or severe pressure within cast, or color change (blue), temperature change (cold), tingling, swelling, or decreased motion to fingers or toes
  - ◊ Obvious malodor should be evaluated by healthcare provider
  - ◊ Avoid sticking objects into cast, often used for scratching
- X-ray studies should be obtained after reduction
- Long-term monitoring of growth if growth plate affected

EXPECTED COURSE

- Callus formation expected by 6 weeks
- Remodeling occurs in 1 year
- Growth is likely to be affected if the fracture extends through the epiphysis

POSSIBLE COMPLICATIONS

- Untreated compartment syndrome resulting in ischemic contracture
- Phlebitis
- Deformities related to malreduction or loss of reduction
- Permanent nerve injury
- Infection
- Posttraumatic arthritis
- Growth arrest due to involvement of growth plate

STRESS FRACTURE

DESCRIPTION

Fractures that occur in the tibia, fibula, metatarsals, and femoral neck

ETIOLOGY

- Repetitive force applied to the lower leg during strenuous activity

INCIDENCE

- Females > Males
- Incidence increases with age

RISK FACTORS

- Long-distance running
- Sudden increase in intensity or level of activity
- Age
- Female gender
- Osteoporosis
- Malalignment of the leg

ASSESSMENT FINDINGS

- Vague hip or leg pain, in early stages present only with activity, in later stages present even at rest
- Full range of motion on examination

DIFFERENTIAL DIAGNOSIS

- Bursitis
- Lumbosacral radiculopathy
- Slipped capital femoral epiphysis
- Tibial stress syndrome (shin splints)
- Abdominal or pelvic mass
- Abdominal aortic aneurysm

DIAGNOSTIC STUDIES

- X-ray: may be negative, hairline radiolucency or periosteal callus
- Triple phase bone scan: increased uptake at fracture site

PREVENTION

- Cross-training (engagement in a different type of activity)
- Prevention of osteoporosis
- Education regarding foot gear, technique, and terrain

MANAGEMENT

- Cross-train for 3-6 weeks (e.g., swimming, cycling, running in water)
- Use cane, crutches, or apply air cast, if weight-bearing causes pain

CONSULTATION/REFERRAL

- Orthopedist for fractures at increased risk of nonunion:
  - ◊ Anterior medial third of tibia
  - ◊ Tarsal navicular and diaphyseal-metaphyseal junction of the fifth metatarsal (Jones's fracture)
  - ◊ Fracture in hypovascular area

FOLLOW-UP

- Perform x-ray after 3-6 weeks, prior to returning to running: should demonstrate callus formation and alignment
- Runner should be free of pain with walking for 1-2 weeks before beginning to run
- If symptoms recur, decrease activity for 1 week to a level that is pain-free

EXPECTED COURSE

- Full recovery is expected in 2 months

POSSIBLE COMPLICATIONS

- Avascular necrosis
- Refracture
- Pseudoarthrosis

CLAVICULAR FRACTURE

DESCRIPTION

Disruption of the junction of the middle and lateral aspects of the clavicle. Fractures are differentiated by location and severity:

- *Type I*: distal third of clavicle; supporting ligaments remain intact
- *Type II*: distal third of clavicle; coracoclavicular ligaments remain attached to the distal fragment and the proximal fragment is displaced upward
- *Type III*: intraarticular fracture through the acromioclavicular joint; no displacement

ETIOLOGY

- Trauma: can result from birth injury, a fall on an extended arm, or a blow to the shoulder or chest

INCIDENCE

- The clavicle is the bone most frequently fractured at birth
- Common in childhood secondary to trauma

RISK FACTORS

- Macrosomic infant
- Falls

ASSESSMENT FINDINGS

- Fracture of the distal clavicle may present with no deformity
- Pain with shoulder movement; holding arm against chest to prevent motion
- Edema, crepitus, and/or point tenderness over fracture site
- Ecchymosis or tenting of the skin over the fracture site
- History of difficult delivery, especially if there was shoulder dystocia

DIFFERENTIAL DIAGNOSIS

- Sternoclavicular ligamentous tear
- Acromioclavicular separation
- Brachial palsy

DIAGNOSTIC STUDIES

- X-rays are usually not necessary in infants
- Standard clavicle x-ray series, which includes anteroposterior and apical lordotic views
- If there is strong clinical suspicion in light of negative x-rays, MRI may be indicated

PREVENTION

- Include palpation of clavicles in all newborn examinations for early detection
- Seatbelt use

NONPHARMACOLOGIC MANAGEMENT

- Neonate usually requires only gentle movement until formation of callus, by 2-3 weeks
- Apply ice first 24 hours after injury
- Sling for 3-6 weeks is usually adequate for nondisplaced fracture; figure-8 clavicle strap for 4 to 8 weeks may be preferable for adults
- Instruct patient to use arm as pain permits; avoid contact sports for 2-3 months, and gradually increase activity as symptoms allow
- Open reduction internal fixation (ORIF) for Type II distal clavicle fracture with significant displacement, or for neurovascular or intrathoracic injury

PHARMACOLOGIC MANAGEMENT

- Analgesics as needed during acute stage

CONSULTATION/REFERRAL

- Orthopedist
  - ◊ Neurovascular compromise
  - ◊ Severe tenting of skin
  - ◊ Open fracture
  - ◊ Multiple injuries
  - ◊ If improved cosmetic results are needed
  - ◊ Symptoms of nonunion after 3-4 months
  - ◊ Significant posterior displacement with risk of intrathoracic injury
  - ◊ Type II fracture for possible ORIF

FOLLOW-UP

- 1-2 weeks after injury, then every 2-3 weeks until asymptomatic
- Repeat x-rays may be performed once patient is asymptomatic to assess callus formation

EXPECTED COURSE

- Clinical union occurs by 12 weeks in adults and by 6 weeks in children
- Callus can be felt over site of fracture in neonate within a few days
- Remodeling occurs by 6-12 months

POSSIBLE COMPLICATIONS

- Malunion, resulting in angulation, shortening, and poor cosmetic appearance
- Degenerative arthritis of the acromioclavicular joint
- Underlying intrathoracic injury

OSTEOPOROSIS

DESCRIPTION

Deterioration of bone tissue results in low bone density, bone fragility, and consequent increased risk of fractures

Post menopausal fractures occur because of resorption of bone due to lack of estrogen secretion.

ETIOLOGY

- Genetics influences bone mass by 50%
- Estrogen deficiency
- Calcium deficiency
- Use of alcohol and nicotine
- Immobilization
- Certain medications

INCIDENCE

- 1.2 million fractures each year in the U.S. are attributable to osteoporosis
- 1/3 of women >age 65 years sustain vertebral fractures
- Females > Males
- Common in Caucasians and Orientals
- Uncommon in African-Americans and Latinos

After age 75, osteoporotic fractures occur at the same rate in men and women.

RISK FACTORS

- Age (bone loss is a consequence of aging)
- Medication use: corticosteroids, anticonvulsants, thyroid supplements
- Estrogen deficiency related to menopause
- Testosterone deficiency related to hypogonadism
- Eating disorder patients
- Calcium/Vitamin D deficiency
- Excessive phosphate, protein intake
- Immobilization, sedentary lifestyle
- Cigarette smoking, chronic alcohol use, caffeine intake
- Family history

ASSESSMENT FINDINGS

- Often asymptomatic until present with fractures of the hip, vertebra, proximal humerus, proximal tibia, or pelvis
- Painless dorsal kyphosis (dowager's hump)
- Back pain
- Loss of height

DIFFERENTIAL DIAGNOSIS

- Primary osteoporosis: idiopathic or postmenopausal
- Secondary osteoporosis related to:
  - ◊ Chronic endocrine (hyperthyroidism especially), rheumatic, neurologic, or malabsorptive disease
  - ◊ Chronic renal failure
  - ◊ Liver disease
  - ◊ Anticonvulsant therapy
  - ◊ Malignancy (multiple myeloma and others)

DIAGNOSTIC STUDIES

- Bone mineral density (BMD) of both the spine and proximal femur
- T scores indicative of severity of bone loss:
  - ◊ Normal: $\pm$ 1 SD
  - ◊ Osteopenia: 1-2 SD
  - ◊ Osteoporosis: > 2 SD
- Z scores indicate number of SD compared to age matched controls
- Biochemical profile and CBC to exclude causes of secondary osteoporosis
- TSH to determine presence of hyperthyroidism or excessive thyroid supplementation
- 24-hour urine collection for calcium excretion: hypercalcuria indicates need to change calcium supplementation; low calcium excretion indicates vitamin D deficiency

PREVENTION

- Weight-bearing exercise daily
- Diet and supplements to achieve sufficient calcium and vitamin D
  - ◊ Young adults: calcium 800 mg/day and vitamin D 400 IU/day
  - ◊ Pregnant or lactating women: calcium 1500 mg/day and vitamin D 400 IU/day
  - ◊ Postmenopausal women: calcium 1500 mg/day and vitamin D 800 IU/day
  - ◊ Older male adults: calcium 1000 mg/day and vitamin D 800 IU/day
- Parenteral testosterone for hypogonadal men (benefit may be offset by testosterone's hypertrophic effect on prostate and by its adverse effect on lipoproteins)
- Avoidance of nicotine, alcohol in excess, and if possible, medications known to contribute to bone loss
- Avoid falls and medications which may increase risk of falls

NONPHARMACOLOGIC MANAGEMENT

- Diet, exercise and avoidance of contributing risk factors
- Education regarding appropriate foot wear and lighting for fall prevention

PHARMACOLOGIC MANAGEMENT

- Daily calcium supplementation of 1500 mg/day and vitamin D 800 IU/day
- Humans are only able to absorb about 500 mg of calcium at one time. Therefore, 1500 mg/d must be divided into 3 doses.
- Testosterone replacement, if indicated, in hypogonadal men

AGENT	ACTION	COMMENTS
Calcium supplement *Example:* calcium carbonate (Tums®) calcium citrate (Citracal®)	Increase availability of calcium for absorption	Vitamin D is required for calcium absorption. Absorption is enhanced when taken with food. Calcium may be irritating to the GI tract and may cause constipation. Calcium citrate is more easily absorbed by the human body than calcium carbonate.
SERMS (selective estrogen receptor modulators) *Examples:* raloxifene (Evista®)	Reduce resorption of bone and decrease overall bone turnover	Taken without regard to meals. Increased risk of DVT especially during first 4 months of treatment. Lowers total cholesterol and LDL Drug interaction with ampicillin. Indicated for prevention and treatment of osteoporosis.
Oral biphosphates *Example:* alendronate (Fosamax®) risedronate (Actonel®) ibandronate (Boniva®)	Inhibit bone resorption which leads to an indirect increase in bone mineral density	Must be taken on an empty stomach and must be able to sit upright for 30 minutes after taking. Esophageal erosion can occur. May cause dysphagia, chest pain, new or worsening heartburn. Indicated for treatment and prevention of osteoporosis.

CONSULTATION/REFERRAL

- Appropriate specialist for management of underlying disease
- Exercise program to improve strength, balance, and flexibility
- Occupational therapist for assistance with activities of daily living
- Physical therapist for gait training and transfer skills

FOLLOW-UP

- Evaluate effects of medication at 1 month, then periodically thereafter
- Ongoing education and support regarding lifestyle changes
- Annual bone mineral density assessment
- X-rays as indicated for acute pain (to rule out fractures)
- Consider serum biochemical markers to monitor bone formation response to therapy at 3 months
    - ◊ Serum osteocalcin
    - ◊ Serum bone-specific alkaline phosphatase

EXPECTED COURSE

- In >50% of cases, compliance with treatment will at least stabilize bone mass, and in some cases will increase it to a small degree, resulting in improved mobility and reduced pain
- In <50% of cases, fractures occur despite treatment

POSSIBLE COMPLICATIONS

- Fractures resulting in musculoskeletal and sometimes neurologic deficits
- Disabling pain

OSGOOD-SCHLATTER DISEASE
(Apophysitis of the Tibial Tuberosity)

DESCRIPTION

An abnormality of the epiphyseal ossification of the tibial tubercle

ETIOLOGY

- During periods of rapid bone growth increased traction is placed upon the insertion of the patellar tendon at the tibial tubercle

INCIDENCE

- A common cause of knee pain in children ages 10-18 years
- Males > Females

RISK FACTORS

- Periods of rapid growth
- Repetitive jumping

ASSESSMENT FINDINGS

- Painful swelling of the tibial tubercle at the insertion of the patellar tendon, exacerbated by activity, squatting, or crouching, and relieved by rest
- Pain worsens with contraction of the quadriceps against resistance
- Unilateral or bilateral

DIFFERENTIAL DIAGNOSIS

- Fracture of the tibial plateau or proximal tibia
- Avulsion of the quadriceps tendon
- Patellofemoral syndrome
- Bursitis, synovitis
- Neoplasm of the proximal tibia

DIAGNOSTIC STUDIES

- None usually needed
- X-ray of the proximal tibia and knee: calcified thickening of tibial tuberosity
- Bone scan is not a good choice because there will be increased uptake because of age

NONPHARMACOLOGIC MANAGEMENT

- Rest, avoid activities that increase pain or swelling
- Quadriceps strengthening and stretching
- Application of ice
- Educate that participation in activities is reasonable as long as pain is minimal

PHARMACOLOGIC MANAGEMENT

- Analgesics (acetaminophen)

CONSULTATION/REFERRAL

- Usually none

FOLLOW-UP

- As needed

EXPECTED COURSE

- Self-limiting condition resolves with skeletal maturation

POSSIBLE COMPLICATIONS

- Avulsion injury of the anterior tibial spine
- Chondromalacia
- Patellofemoral degenerative arthritis

DEVELOPMENTAL DYSPLASIA OF THE HIP (DDH)

Congenital Dislocation of the Hip

DESCRIPTION

Partial or complete subluxation/dislocation of the femoral head from the pelvic acetabulum. Originally named congenital hip dislocation, but is now known to occur postnatally rather than congenitally.

ETIOLOGY

- Multifactorial
- Generalized laxity of ligaments
- Maternal estrogen and relaxin contribute to pelvic relaxation
- Breech position results in exaggerated hip flexion with limited hip motion and stretching of the ligaments. The limited motion of the hips leads to underdevelopment of the cartilaginous acetabulum
- Postnatal maintenance of the infant in an adducted, extended position rather than the natural abducted, flexed position

INCIDENCE

- Uncertain, ranges from 1/60 to 1/1000 births
- Females > Males
- 30-50% develop in breech positions
- 20% positive family history

RISK FACTORS

- Breech position, especially frank breech
- Use of swaddling or cradle board maintaining extended adducted position
- Underlying neuromuscular disorders
    - ◊ Myelodysplasia
    - ◊ Arthrogryposis multiplex congenita
- Positive family history
- Congenital muscular torticollis
- Metatarsus adductus
- Down syndrome

ASSESSMENT FINDINGS

- Limited abduction of the affected hip (<60%)
- Asymmetric gluteal or inguinal folds
- Unequal leg length (shorter on affected side)
- Positive Barlow's sign (ability to dislocate an unstable hip)
    - ◊ Stabilize the pelvis with one hand and flex and adduct the opposite hip while applying a posterior force
    - ◊ The unstable hip will easily dislocate, then will relocate once the posterior force is removed
- Positive Ortolani's sign (useful between age 1 month and 3 months only)
    - ◊ Flex and abduct the thigh with the infant in the supine position
    - ◊ Lift the femoral head into the acetabulum
    - ◊ If reduction occurs, there is a palpable "clunk"
- Positive Galeazzi's sign: unequal knee heights when infant is placed in supine position with the hips and knees flexed and feet placed side by side on the table
- Limping, waddling, lumbar lordosis, toe-walking and leg length discrepancy are indications in older children

DIFFERENTIAL DIAGNOSIS

- Nonpathologic hip clicks

DIAGNOSTIC STUDIES

- Pelvic ultrasound is especially useful in neonates: unstable hip with limited acetabular development
- Anteroposterior and frog lateral x-rays are helpful after age 3 months. The newborn hip joint is too cartilaginous for x-ray to be reliable.
- Arthrography, MRI and tomography are useful in cases that are difficult to diagnose

PREVENTION

- Educate about possible deleterious effect of maintaining the infant in the hip adducted and extended position (e.g., in swaddling or cradle board)

- Include hip examination in all infant and child assessments up to two years of age for early detection

MANAGEMENT

- Early treatment is crucial for good prognosis
- The earlier the therapy is begun, the less likely surgical reduction will be necessary
- Abduction orthoses hold the hip in the flexed abducted position for 1-2 months
  - ◊ Pavlik harness
  - ◊ Frejka splint
- Surgical closed reduction is primary treatment after age 6 months
- After age 18 months, open reduction with osteotomy is the only effective treatment

CONSULTATION/REFERRAL

- Immediate referral to orthopedist for orthosis or surgery

FOLLOW-UP

- Therapy is continued until there is clinical hip stability and radiographic evidence of resolution
- After surgical reduction, a spica cast is worn for 6-8 weeks
- Child and family require frequent support and education regarding cast care, skin care, car safety, and developmental stimulation while immobilized

EXPECTED COURSE

- Best outcomes achieved with early detection and treatment

POSSIBLE COMPLICATIONS

- Permanent dislocation of the femoral head with consequent limited mobility is the result of
- failure to treat
- Aseptic and avascular necrosis of the capital femoral epiphysis
- Redislocation or persistent dysplasia
- Postoperative complications (e.g., infection)

LEGG-CALVE-PERTHES DISEASE

Legg-Perthes Disease

DESCRIPTION

Osteonecrosis of the capital femoral epiphysis due to interrupted vascular supply results in ischemia and alteration in cartilage growth. The area eventually revascularizes and new bone begins to grow, but there is the likelihood of fracture due to fragility of bone. If a fracture occurs, the shape of the femoral head changes, causing interruption in articulation of the femoral head in the hip joint.

ETIOLOGY

- Pathology of the compromised blood flow to the femoral head is unclear
- Familial tendency

INCIDENCE

- Predominant age is 7 years; occurs from age 3-12 years
- Males > Females (4:1)

RISK FACTORS

- Slipped capital femoral epiphysis
- Developmental dysplasia of the hip
- Corticosteroid use
- Sickle cell disease
- Family history

ASSESSMENT FINDINGS

- Pain to the hip or referral to the medial aspect of the knee (pain has usually been present or 2-3 weeks before child complains)
- Limp
- Limited internal rotation and abduction of femur
- Unequal leg lengths, antalgic gait
- Atrophy of thigh muscles, muscle spasm
- History of hip trauma
- Positive Trendelenburg's sign:
  - ◊ Child stands and raises one leg off the ground
  - ◊ The pelvis drops on the raised leg side

DIFFERENTIAL DIAGNOSIS

- Toxic synovitis
- Lymphoma
- Osteomyelitis
- Juvenile rheumatoid arthritis
- Spondyloepiphyseal dysplasia
- Slipped capital femoral epiphysis

DIAGNOSTIC STUDIES

- CBC: normal
- ESR: normal
- AP and frog lateral x-rays: altered epiphysis, subluxation
- MRI: necrosis
- Aspiration of synovial fluid: normal

The goal of treatment is to avoid severe arthritis.

NONPHARMACOLOGIC MANAGEMENT

- Initially, bedrest with possible femoral traction for 1-2 weeks
- Maintain range of motion
- Education regarding disease process

PHARMACOLOGIC MANAGEMENT

- Nonsteroidal anti-inflammatory agents

CONSULTATION/REFERRAL

- Immediate orthopedic surgeon referral
- Physical therapist

FOLLOW-UP

- Serial AP and frog lateral x-rays to determine progression

EXPECTED COURSE

- Self-limiting, revascularization occurs in 2-3 years
- Older children have a poorer prognosis; less growth period allows for decreased remodeling time

POSSIBLE COMPLICATIONS

- Osteoarthritis
- Decreased use of hip joint due to femoral head distortion

SLIPPED CAPITAL FEMORAL EPIPHYSIS (SCFE)

DESCRIPTION

A fracture through the proximal femoral physis. Shear force placed on the growth plate can cause osteonecrosis as the bone moves because at this age, blood supply to this part of the bone is tenuous.

ETIOLOGY

- Unknown
- Basis is believed to be endocrine due to the fact that it is often accompanied by growth abnormalities

INCIDENCE

- The most common adolescent hip disorder
- 1 per 100,000 children
- Seen in adolescents
- Males > Females
- More common in African American boys

RISK FACTORS

- Obese adolescents with delayed skeletal maturation
- Tall, thin adolescents with a recent growth spurt
- Hypothyroidism
- Pituitary disorder
- Pseudohypoparathyroidism

ASSESSMENT FINDINGS

- Pre slip: mild discomfort of the hip, frequently noticed in the opposite hip of a previous SCFE
- Acute: mild pain or limp lasting <3 weeks followed by sudden hip pain so severe that the child is unable to bear weight, even with support; severe pain with any attempted hip motion
- Acute or chronic: child has had moderate pain, limp, and externally rotated gait lasting several months, then the epiphysis slips acutely, resulting in severe pain and inability to bear weight
- Chronic: several months of progressively worsening hip pain that is not severe enough to keep the child from walking with an antalgic, externally rotated gait; lack of internal rotation and increased external rotation noted on examination

This diagnosis is often misdiagnosed because only 50% of patients have hip pain and 25% have knee pain.

DIFFERENTIAL DIAGNOSIS

- Osgood Schlatter disease
- Patellofemoral stress syndrome
- Legg-Calve-Perthes disease
- Transient synovitis of the hip
- Toxic synovitis
- Femoral neck stress fracture
- Septic arthritis
- Osteomyelitis

DIAGNOSTIC STUDIES

- AP x-ray of the pelvis
- Lateral frog leg x-ray
- MRI and CT are rarely needed for diagnosis

CONSULTATION/REFERRAL

- Urgent orthopedic referral for pinning (epiphysiodesis)

FOLLOW-UP

- By orthopedist; screw removal following closure of the capital femoral epiphysis (CFE) is controversial

EXPECTED COURSE

- Pinning prevents progression

POSSIBLE COMPLICATIONS

- Long-term disability from progression of the slip if pinning is not performed
- Osteonecrosis
- Chondrolysis

TRANSIENT SYNOVITIS OF THE HIP

DESCRIPTION

A self-limited, usually benign condition causing acute onset of limp and hip pain in children; it occurs rarely in adults

ETIOLOGY

- Uncertain
- Possibly related to a recent virus, trauma, or hypersensitivity reaction

INCIDENCE

- The most common cause of hip pain in children 3-10 years of age
- Mean age of onset is 6 years, but can occur at any age
- Males > Females

RISK FACTORS

- History of upper respiratory infection 7-14 days before onset of symptoms in 70% of affected children
- History of trauma

ASSESSMENT FINDINGS

- Acute onset of groin, anterior thigh, or knee pain
- Child remains ambulatory but walks with a limp to avoid pain (antalgic gait)
- May have low grade temperature
- Does not hold hip flexed or abducted; abduction and internal rotation are restricted
- Hip may be tender to palpation
- Most sensitive test is log roll: with child supine, roll affected hip from side to side: may see guarding or decreased range of motion
- May have decreased range of motion in knee on affected side
- Usually unilateral

In young children, the only symptom may be crying at nighttime.

DIFFERENTIAL DIAGNOSIS

- Legg-Calve-Perthes disease
- Septic arthritis
- Osteomyelitis
- Slipped capital femoral epiphysis
- Femoral neck stress fracture

DIAGNOSTIC STUDIES

- ESR: mildly elevated
- CBC: normal
- Fluoroscopic arthrocentesis: negative except for possibly a 1-3 ml synovial effusion
- AP & Lauenstein (frog) lateral x-rays of the pelvis: normal
- Ultrasound of the hip: effusion
- Bone scan or MRI to rule out infection or Legg-Calve-Perthes disease

NONPHARMACOLOGIC MANAGEMENT

- Bedrest and non-weight-bearing until pain resolves, usually 7 days
- Limited activities for 2 weeks thereafter
- Check temperature regularly to exclude possibility of septic arthritis

PHARMACOLOGIC MANAGEMENT

- Nonsteroidal anti-inflammatory agents

CONSULTATION/REFERRAL

- Orthopedist if not resolved in 2 weeks with appropriate rest

POSSIBLE COMPLICATIONS

- Recurrence if activities are not sufficiently limited
- Coxa magna: enlargement and deformity of the femoral head and neck
- Legg-Calve-Perthes disease

SCOLIOSIS

DESCRIPTION

Lateral curvature of the spine

- *Idiopathic:* curve is >10° and occurs in an otherwise healthy child > 10 years of age
- *Functional scoliosis:* appearance of a lateral curvature without structural changes in the vertebral column
- *Structural scoliosis:* true deformity of the vertebrae rather than a postural problem

ETIOLOGY

- Usually idiopathic
- Can be associated with anomalies of the spinal column, neuromuscular disease, or genetic disease
- Sometimes related to infection, tumor, or metabolic disease

INCIDENCE

- Females > Males (4-5:1)

- 3% of U.S. population affected

RISK FACTORS

- Legs of unequal length
- Anomalies of spinal column
- Cerebral palsy
- Neurofibromatosis
- Marfan syndrome
- Poliomyelitis
- Muscular dystrophy
- Friedreich's ataxia
- Charcot-Marie-Tooth disease
- Family history of scoliosis

ASSESSMENT FINDINGS

- Nonpainful, insidious onset of lateral curvature of the spine
- Unequal shoulder heights
- Unequal scapula prominences and heights
- Unequal waist angles
- Unequal rib prominences
- Chest asymmetry

DIFFERENTIAL DIAGNOSIS

- Neurofibromatosis
- Cerebral palsy
- Juvenile idiopathic scoliosis
- Multiple sclerosis
- Rett syndrome
- Rickets
- Tuberculosis
- Tumor
- Functional scoliosis disappears when child is placed in Adam's position (bending forward at the waist); structural scoliosis is accentuated

DIAGNOSTIC STUDIES

- Posteroanterior and standing x-rays of the entire spine identify the degree of curvature
- MRI to rule out tumor if there is associated back pain

Diagnosis is made when lateral curvature is 10° or more.

PREVENTION

- Screening and early identification helps prevent need for more invasive treatment

Scoliosis is seen most often at the beginning of growth spurts and during adolescence and so screening should take place PRIOR to this time (around age 10 years).

MANAGEMENT

- Infants with curve >25° usually require casting followed by a brace
- Spinal fusion may be necessary in adolescence (usually recommended once curve is 40°)
- Curves up to 25° are observed for 4-6 months
- Curves >25 °: refer
- Patient and family support

CONSULTATION/REFERRAL

- Orthopedic or neurosurgeon for surgical evaluation

FOLLOW-UP

- Monitoring and treatment continues until growth is complete

EXPECTED COURSE

- Depends on degree of curvature and how quickly treatment is initiated
- Full correction of deformity is not usually expected

POSSIBLE COMPLICATIONS

- Severe deformity may limit physical activities
- Cardiovascular and respiratory impairment
- Psychological sequelae: anger, low self-esteem

TALIPES EQUINOVARUS
(Club Foot)

DESCRIPTION

A congenital deformity of the foot, involves plantar flexion of the foot at the ankle joint, inversion deformity of the heel, and adduction of the forefoot. Unlike positioning deformities, correction requires active treatment. The foot cannot be manually corrected with the heel down. The condition can range from mild to severe.

ETIOLOGY

- Congenital
- Usually idiopathic
- May be associated with neurological problems or muscular disease
- Uterine positioning may also be a factor

INCIDENCE

- Occurs in 1/1000 births
- Males > Females (2:1)

RISK FACTORS

- Myelomeningocele
- Cerebral palsy
- Family history

ASSESSMENT FINDINGS

- Present at birth, ranging from mild to severe
- Foot in pointed toe position, plantar flexed
- Sole of foot is inverted
- Convex shape to foot, markedly adducted
- Position cannot be manually corrected with the heel down, heel cord not flexible
- Unilateral or bilateral
- In the older child, there is foot and calf atrophy

DIFFERENTIAL DIAGNOSIS

- Metatarsus adductus

DIAGNOSTIC STUDIES

- AP and lateral standing or simulated weight-bearing x-rays with line measurements to determine the navicular bone position and overall foot alignment

PREVENTION

- Early intervention results in easier correction due to greater flexibility of joints of the newborn

MANAGEMENT

- Orthopedist may attempt casting, but surgery (soft tissue release, naviculectomy, or arthrodesis) is usually required for correction

CONSULTATION/REFERRAL

- Urgent orthopedic referral

FOLLOW-UP

- Prolonged orthopedic follow-up is necessary

EXPECTED COURSE

- Possible recurrence
- Goal is a pain-free foot and ability to wear shoes
- Lifelong orthosis is frequently necessary

POSSIBLE COMPLICATIONS

- Surgery complications

METATARSUS ADDUCTUS

DESCRIPTION

A condition which occurs at birth and is characterized by a straight hindfoot and an adducted forefoot. The result is a curved, intoeing shape to the foot.

ETIOLOGY

- Intrauterine positioning

INCIDENCE

- Commonly occurs at birth

RISK FACTORS

- Family history

ASSESSMENT FINDINGS

- Convexity of the lateral border of the foot in contrast to the normal straight appearance
- If a line drawn from the center of the heel through the center of the metatarsal-tarsal line bisects lateral to the space between the second and third toes, the forefoot is adducted in relation to the hindfoot.
- If the foot is flexible, the forefoot can be abducted past midline; in rigid metatarsus adductus, the forefoot cannot be abducted past midline
- Foot turns inward whether or not the child is weight-bearing

DIFFERENTIAL DIAGNOSIS

- Congenital vertical talus
- Talipes equinovarus

DIAGNOSTIC STUDIES

- X-rays of the foot are indicated in rigid metatarsus adductus

MANAGEMENT

- Flexible foot: teach parent to perform passive stretching of the forefoot into the straight position several times a day
- Rigid foot: may require serial casting or surgery for correction

CONSULTATION/REFERRAL

- Rigid foot: orthopedist at time condition is identified
- Condition unresponsive after 4-6 months: orthopedist
- Following casting, orthotist for out flaring or reverse last shoes

FOLLOW-UP

- Evaluate response to passive exercise every 2 months

EXPECTED COURSE

- 85% of cases resolve spontaneously
- Resolution occurs most rapidly with a flexible foot
- Children older than 2-3 years of age are more likely to require corrective surgery

POSSIBLE COMPLICATIONS

- Surgery complications

References

Anderson, B.C. (1995). *Office orthopedics for primary care.* Philadelphia: WB Saunders.

Ballas, M., Tytko, J., & Mannarino, F. (1998). Commonly missed orthopedic problems. *American Family Physician, 57*, 267-274.

Barkin, R.M., & Rosen, P. (Eds.). (2003). *Emergency pediatrics* (6th ed.). St. Louis, MO: Mosby.

Behrman, R. E., Kliegman, R. M., A. M., & Nelson, W. E. (Eds.). (1996). *Nelson textbook of pediatrics* (15th ed.). Philadelphia: Saunders.

Bellantoni, M. (1996). Osteoporosis prevention and treatment. *American Family Physician, 54*(3), 986-995.

Bigos, S., Bowyer, O., Braen, G., et al. (1994). *Acute low back problems in adults.* Clinical Practice Guideline No. 14. AHCPR Publication No. 95-0642. Rockville, MD: Agency for Health Care Policy and Research, Public Health Service, U.S. Department of Health and Human Services.

Bickley, L.S., & Szilagyi, P.G. (2003). *Bates' guide to physical examination and history taking* (8th ed.). Philadelphia: Lippincott Williams & Wilkins.

Branch, W.T. (2003). *Office practice of medicine* (4th ed.). Philadelphia: Saunders.

Brooks, E., & Bermas, B. (1997). Elbow pain: Olecranon bursitis and epicondylitis. *Hospital Medicine, 33*(4), 47-60.

Bruce, M.L., & Peck, B. (2005). New rheumatoid arthritis treatments. *The Nurse Practitioner, 30*(4), 28-39.

Burns, C.E., Brady, M.A., Blosser, C., Starr, N.B., & Dunn, A.M. (2004). *Pediatric primary care: A handbook for nurse practitioners* (3rd ed.). Philadelphia: W.B. Saunders.

Carr, A.J., & Hamilton, W. (2005). *Orthopedics in primary care.* St. Louis, MO: Elsevier.

Clough, J., Lambert, T., & Miller, D. (1996). The new thinking on osteoarthritis. *Patient Care, 30*(14),110-137.

Crowther, C.L.(2003). *Primary orthopedic care* (2nd ed.). St. Louis, MO: Mosby.

Dambro, M.R. (2005). *Griffith's 5 minute clinical consult.* Philadelphia: Lippincott Williams & Wilkins.

Downs, D. (1997). Nonspecific work-related upper extremity disorders. *American Family Physician, 55*, 1296-1301.

Eiff, M. (1997). Clavicle fracture. *American Family Physician, 55*(1), 121-128.

Gates, S.J., & Mooar, P.A. (Eds.). (1999). *Musculoskeletal primary care.* Philadelphia: Lippincott Williams & Wilkins.

Goroll, A. H., & Mulley, A. G., Jr. (Eds.). (2000). *Primary care medicine: Office evaluation and management of the adult patient* (4th ed.). Philadelphia: Lippincott Williams Wilkins.

Graber, M.A., & Lanternier, M.L. (Eds.) (2001). *The family practice handbook.* (4th ed.). St. Louis: Mosby.

Hart, J. (1996). Transient synovitis of the hip. *American Family Physician, 54*(5), 1587-1591.

Helms, C., & Pearson, J. (1996). Radiology in primary care: Part 3, knee, ankle, and foot. *Patient Care, 30*(19), 31-47.

Helms, C. & Pearson, J. (1996). Radiology in primary care: Part 4, shoulder and elbow. *Patient Care, 30*(20), 115-130.

Kasper, D.L., Braunwald, E., Fauci, A.S., Hauser, S.L., Longo, D.L., Jameson, J.L., et al. (2004). *Harrison's principles of internal medicine* (16th ed.). New York: McGraw-Hill.

Jones, J., Davidson, C. & Sevier, T. (1996). Managing sports-related overuse injuries. *Patient Care, 30*(7), 55-71.

Mangion, S. (2000). *Physical diagnosis secrets.* Philadelphia: Hanley and Belfus.

McCance, K.L., & Huether, S.E. (Eds.). (2001). *Pathophysiology: The biologic basis for disease in adults and children* (4th ed.). St. Louis, MO: Mosby.

Mellion, M.B., Putukian, M., & Madden, C.C. (2002). *Sports medicine secrets.* (3rd Ed.). Philadelphia: Hanley and Belfus.

Mochan, E. (2005) Rheumatoid arthritis: Clues to early diagnosis. *Consultant, 45*, 545-552.

O'Dell, J., Pischel, K., & Weinblatt, M. (1997). Rheumatoid arthritis: What's new in treatment. *Patient Care, 31*(5), 81-96.

Pincus, T. (2005). Managing the patient with musculoskeletal pain. *Clinical Advisor, 8*(5) (Suppl.) 3-19.

Rakel, R.E. (Ed.). (1998). *Essentials of family practice.* (2nd ed.). Philadelphia: WB Saunders.

Rifat, S., & McKeag, D. (1996). Practical methods of preventing ankle injuries. *American Family Physician, 53*, 2491-2497.

Ross, C. (1997). A comparison of osteoarthritis and rheumatoid arthritis: Diagnosis and treatment. *The Nurse Practitioner, 22*(9), 20-39.

Saguil, A. (2005). Evaluation of the patient with muscle weakness. *American Family Physician, 71*, 1327-1336.

Seller, R. (2000). *Differential diagnosis of common complaints* (4th ed.). Philadelphia: W.B. Saunders.

Steinberg, G.G., Akins, C. M., & Baran, D.T. (1999). *Orthopedics in primary care.* (3rd ed.). Philadelphia: Lippincott Williams & Wilkins.

Sutter, C., & Shelton, D. (1996). Three phase bone scan in osteomyelitis and other musculoskeletal disorders. *American Family Physician, 54*, 1639-1647.

Schwartz, M.W. (Ed.). (2002). *The 5 minute pediatric consult.* (2nd ed.) Philadelphia: Lippincott Williams & Wilkins.

Uphold, C.R., & Graham, M.V. (2003). *Clinical guidelines in family practice* (4th ed.). Gainesville, FL: Barmarrae Books.

Wegener, S.T., Belza, B.L., & Gall, E.P. (2001). *Clinical care in the rheumatic diseases* (2nd ed.).Atlanta, GA: American College of Rheumatology.

Wofle, M. W. (2001). Management of ankle sprains. *American Family Physician, 63,* 93-104.

Whyte, J. (2005). Stress fractures of the pelvis and lower extremities. *Advance for Nurse Practitioners, 13*(7), 55-59.

Zollo, A.J., Jr (Ed.). (2004). *Medical Secrets.* (4th ed.), St. Louis, MO: Mosby-Year Book.

Zoltan, T.B., Taylor, K.S., & Achar, S.A. (2005). Health issues for surfers. *American Academy of Family Physicians, 71,* 2313-2317.

16

PREGNANCY

Pregnancy

PRECONCEPTUAL CARE

DEFINITION

Interventions aimed at promoting the health and well-being of a woman before pregnancy

TERMS

Nulligravida	a woman who has never been pregnant
Primigravida	a woman during her first pregnancy
Primipara	a woman who has had or who is giving birth to her first child
Multigravida	a woman who has been pregnant two or more times
Multipara	a woman who has borne more than one offspring

HEALTH ASSESSMENT

- Complete physical examination
- Past medical history
- Obstetric history
  - ◊ Menstrual history
  - ◊ Contraceptive history
  - ◊ Sexual history
  - ◊ Reproductive history
  - ◊ Complications during previous pregnancies

Assessment of risk factors
◊ Maternal age (increased risk at age extremes) ◊ Ethnic origin ◊ Presence of chronic disease (e.g., diabetes mellitus, essential hypertension, heart disease, renal disease, seizure disorder, thyroid abnormality, asthma, rheumatoid arthritis, and tuberculosis) may affect pregnancy through pathophysiological mechanisms or as a result of medications used in their treatment ◊ In utero exposure to DES ◊ Previous preterm labor and/or delivery ◊ Repeated early miscarriages ◊ Presence of infectious disease or exposure to infectious disease ◊ Domestic violence risk ◊ Substance abuse ◊ Tobacco use

- Nutrition assessment
- Cultural history
- Support systems

DISCONTINUATION OF CONTRACEPTION

- Oral contraceptives should be stopped 2-3 months before attempting pregnancy
- Intrauterine devices should be removed and pregnancy delayed one month after removal
- Barrier methods of contraception may be used (e.g., condoms, diaphragm) in the interim

GENETIC ISSUES

- Complete genetic history should be taken including genogram
- Couple should be referred for genetic counseling if history of genetic disorders in family, especially Tay-Sachs, thalassemia, hemophilia, phenylketonuria, cystic fibrosis, sickle cell disease or trait, birth defects, and mental retardation

IMMUNIZATIONS

- Bring all immunizations up to date
- Rubella vaccine if not immune

Pregnancy should not be attempted for 28 days after rubella vaccine.

DIAGNOSTIC STUDIES

- Hematocrit and hemoglobin
- Blood type and Rh factor
- Coombs' test
- Urinalysis
- Pap smear
- HIV screening
- Screening for sexually transmitted diseases (e.g., syphilis, gonorrhea, chlamydia)
- Rubella titer
- Screening for hepatitis B

NUTRITION

- Maintain or attain average body weight for height
- Folic acid 0.4 mg/day to decrease risk of neural tube defects
- Assess for cultural nutrition practices which may affect pregnancy

EXERCISE

- Establish a regular exercise program at least 3 months before attempting to become pregnant. Should include aerobic and toning exercises.

Even if no exercise was engaged in prior to pregnancy, walking can be safely encouraged during pregnancy.

SMOKING CESSATION

- Assist couples with smoking cessation before pregnancy
- Educate about risk of cigarette smoking during pregnancy
    - ◊ Lower birth weight
    - ◊ Stillbirth
    - ◊ Spontaneous abortion
    - ◊ Sudden infant death syndrome

Second hand smoke has adverse effects on the fetus.

ALCOHOL

- Educate about risk of alcohol use in pregnancy
    - ◊ Decreased birth weight
    - ◊ Stillbirth
    - ◊ Spontaneous abortion
    - ◊ Fetal alcohol syndrome
- Safety level for alcohol use during pregnancy has not been established
- Total avoidance is recommended

MEDICATIONS

- Avoidance of medications which could have negative effect on pregnancy

Categories of Medications According to their Risk in Pregnancy

Category	Explanation	Drug Examples
A	Controlled studies show no human risk	Folic acid, thyroid supplement
B	Animal studies show no risk, but no good human studies have been done	Penicillin, cephalosporins
C	No adequate studies exist in either animals or humans	Pseudoephedrine, SSRI
D	Evidence of fetal risk is clear-cut, but the benefits may outweigh the risks	Phenytoin Lithium Tetracycline
X	Proven fetal risks clearly outweigh any benefit	Alcohol Warfarin Diethylstilbestrol Isotretinoin Methotrexate Valproic acid

Note: FDA

OCCUPATIONAL ISSUES

- Assess potential teratogenic occupational environment of the woman and her partner

SEXUAL ACTIVITY

- Safe sex practices

PHYSIOLOGIC AND PSYCHOLOGIC CHANGES OF PREGNANCY

BREASTS

- Increased in size
- Darkening and enlargement of areola and nipples occurs
- Prominent superficial veins
- Hypertrophy of Montgomery's glands
- Striae may develop
- Leakage of colostrum can occur

CARDIOVASCULAR SYSTEM

- Heart is pushed upward, to the left and rotated forward
- Decreased peripheral and pulmonary vascular resistance
- Cardiac output increased
- Pulse rate increased 10-15 beats per minute
- Blood pressure decreased slightly

Blood pressure is lowest in the second trimester.

ENDOCRINE SYSTEM

- Thyroid
  - ◊ TSH decreases; T_4 level increases
  - ◊ Basal metabolic rate increases
- Parathyroid
  - ◊ Increased size
  - ◊ Increased parathormone levels
- Pituitary
  - ◊ Enlarges
- Adrenals
  - ◊ Increased cortisol levels
  - ◊ Increased aldosterone
- Pancreas
  - ◊ Increased insulin needs

EYES

- Decreased intraocular pressure
- Increased corneal thickness
- Transient loss of accommodation

GASTROINTESTINAL SYSTEM

- Increased human chorionic gonadotropin (HCG) is associated with nausea and vomiting of first trimester
- Hyperemic gum tissue
- Increased salivation
- Increased acidity of gastric contents
- Intestines are displaced as the uterus grows
- Relaxation of lower esophageal sphincter
- Gastric emptying and intestinal motility are delayed
- Decreased plasma albumin
- Prolonged emptying time of the gallbladder

Elevated estrogen levels make gallstones more likely during pregnancy.

HEMATOLOGICAL SYSTEM

- Blood volume progressively increased secondary to increased plasma volume and erythrocytes
- Hemoglobin and hematocrit decrease slightly
- Increased leukocyte production
- Increased fibrin level, fibrinogen, blood factors VII, VIII, IX, and X
- Increased erythrocyte sedimentation rate (ESR)
- Physiologic anemia occurs in response to the increased plasma volume

INTEGUMENTARY SYSTEM

- Hyperpigmentation of areola, nipples, vulva, perianal area
- Linea nigra
- Facial chloasma (mask of pregnancy)
- Striae gravidarum (stretch marks) of abdomen, breasts, thighs
- Vascular spider nevi
- Decreased rate of hair growth

MUSCULOSKELETAL SYSTEM

- Relaxation of sacroiliac, sacrococcygeal, and pubic joints of the pelvis due to the effects of the hormones progesterone and relaxin
- Progressive lordosis

REPRODUCTIVE SYSTEM

Uterus Increase in size to accommodate growing fetus	
10-12 weeks	Fundus slightly above symphysis pubis
16 weeks	fundus midway between symphysis pubis and umbilicus
20-22 weeks	fundus at level of umbilicus
28 weeks	fundus three finger breadths above umbilicus
36 weeks	fundus just below xiphoid

- Cervix
  - ◊ Production of thick, tenacious mucus plug in the endocervical canal
  - ◊ Softening (Goodell's sign)
  - ◊ Increased vascularity causing the cervix to appear blue
- Ovaries
  - ◊ Ovulation ceases
  - ◊ Corpus luteum produces progesterone and other hormones in early pregnancy
- Vagina
  - ◊ Hypertrophy
  - ◊ Increased vascularity and hyperemia causing the vagina to appear bluish-purple (Chadwick's sign)
  - ◊ Increased vaginal secretion
  - ◊ Vaginal pH becomes more acidic

RESPIRATORY SYSTEM

- Increased tidal volume
- Increased oxygen consumption
- Decreased functional residual capacity and residual volume
- Decreased airway resistance
- Elevation of diaphragm as pregnancy progresses
- Increased subcostal angle
- Increased AP: lateral diameter
- Increased vascular congestion and edema of nasal mucosa

URINARY TRACT

- Decreased capacity of bladder due to uterine pressure
- Dilation of kidney and ureter due to pressure of uterus
- Increased glomerular filtration rate and renal plasma flow

PSYCHOLOGICAL ADJUSTMENT

- Developmental tasks of each trimester
  - ◊ First: accept biologic fact of pregnancy; ambivalence common
  - ◊ Second: accept fetus as distinct entity
  - ◊ Third: preparation for separation from baby, labor, and parenthood

PRENATAL CARE

INITIAL PRENATAL VISIT

DIAGNOSIS OF PREGNANCY

Subjective (*Presumptive*) signs:
* Amenorrhea * Nausea and vomiting * Urinary frequency * Breast tenderness * Perception of fetal movement (quickening: usually felt between 16-18 weeks gestation) * Fatigue

Objective (*Probable*) signs:
* *Goodell's sign*: softening of the cervix * *Chadwick's sign*: dark blue to purplish-red color of vaginal mucosa * *Hegar's sign*: softening of the isthmus of the uterus * Uterine enlargement * *Braxton-Hicks contractions*: painless uterine contractions that occur every 10-20 minutes after the third month of pregnancy and do not represent true labor * Uterine souffle * Hyperpigmentation of skin * Abdominal striae * Ballottement * Positive pregnancy test * Palpation of fetal outline

Diagnostic (*Positive*) signs:
* Auscultation of fetal heartbeat * Fetal movements palpated by examiner * Ultrasound recognition of pregnancy

DETERMINATION OF ESTIMATED DATE OF CONFINEMENT (EDC)

- *Naegele's Rule* (Due Date)
  - ◊ Subtract 3 months from last menstrual period then add 7 days and one year

HISTORY

- Menstrual history
- Previous pregnancy history
- Current and past health problems
- Current medications
- Contraception used prior to pregnancy
- Assessment of risk factors which may complicate pregnancy

PHYSICAL EXAMINATION

- Blood Pressure
- Height
- Weight
- Uterus: uterine fundal height.

Between 18 and 32 weeks there is good correlation between fundal height and gestational age of the fetus. (*McDonald's rule*)

- Vagina: anomalies, lesions
- Cervix: consistency, length, and dilation; lesions
- Pelvis: clinical measurement of pelvis and its general configuration
- Breast: presence of nipple abnormalities, masses
- Extremities: varicosities
- Fetal heart sounds

DIAGNOSTIC STUDIES

- Pregnancy test if not previously done
- CBC
- Urinalysis
- Urine culture
- Blood group and Rh type
- Rubella titer
- Syphilis serology
- HIV screen
- Hepatitis B screen
- Sickle cell screen for African-American women and others at risk
- Screen for gonorrhea if high-risk
- Chlamydia testing

- Wet prep for *Trichomonas vaginalis* and *Candida albicans*
- Cervical cytology screen

NUTRITION

- Recommended weight gain for normal weight women: 25-35 lbs; more for women who are underweight and less for women who are overweight
- Recommended nutrition during pregnancy
  - ◊ Calories: increase of 300 kcal/day over prepregnancy requirement
  - ◊ Folic acid: 0.4 mg/day
  - ◊ Iron: 30 mg/day
  - ◊ Calcium: 1200 mg/day
- Avoid raw or undercooked foods, especially seafood, unpasteurized dairy products, etc.
- Pica may be a problem, especially in some cultures

ACTIVITIES

- Not necessary for pregnant woman to limit activity if she does not become excessively fatigued or risk injury to herself or fetus
- Women who are accustomed to aerobic exercise may continue, but new aerobic exercise program (except walking) should not be started
- Scuba diving, roller coasters, and bungee jumping are contraindicated

SEXUAL ACTIVITY

- Generally accepted that in healthy pregnant women sexual intercourse causes no harm
- Sexual intercourse should be avoided in the presence of threatening abortion or preterm labor

DANGER SIGNS OF PREGNANCY

- Any vaginal bleeding
- Swelling of face or fingers
- Severe or continuous headache
- Dimness or blurring of vision
- Abdominal pain
- Persistent vomiting
- Chills or fever
- Dysuria
- Escape of fluid from the vagina
- Marked changes in frequency or intensity of fetal movements

OCCUPATIONAL ISSUES

- Avoidance of potential teratogens in workplace (e.g., radiation, chemotherapy, anesthesia, chemicals)
- Frequent rest periods during the work day

TRAVEL

- Travel in properly pressurized aircraft offers no unusual risk to the pregnant woman and her fetus
- While traveling, the woman should walk at least every 2 hours
- Lap and shoulder belts should be used at all times. The lap belt should be placed under the abdomen and across the upper thighs. The shoulder belt should be placed snugly across the abdomen and between the breasts.

Pregnancy produces a state of hypercoagulability, so, pregnant women should walk at least every 2 hours after having been immobile to help prevent DVT.

AVOIDANCE OF POTENTIAL TERATOGENS

- Teach women to avoid medications unless specifically prescribed by health care provider
- Avoid hot tubs
- Avoid douching
- Avoid working with chemicals, paint, etc., especially in poorly ventilated area

CHILDBIRTH PREPARATION

- Introduce subject of childbirth preparation and childbirth options

SUBSEQUENT PRENATAL VISITS

TRADITIONAL SCHEDULE OF VISITS IN UNCOMPLICATED PREGNANCY

- Every 4 weeks until 28 weeks gestation
- Every 2 weeks between 28 and 36 weeks gestation
- Every week after 36 weeks of gestation

ASSESSMENT

- Blood pressure
- Weight
- Urinalysis as indicated
- Review of symptoms indicating danger signs of pregnancy
- Fundal height
- Later in pregnancy: vaginal examination to determine cervical dilatation and effacement, station of presenting part
- Fetal heart sounds: normal is 120-160 beats/minute
- Presenting fetal part (later in pregnancy)
- Fetal activity

DIAGNOSTIC STUDIES

8-18 weeks:
- Ultrasound
- Amniocentesis if indicated

16-18 weeks:
- Maternal serum α-fetoprotein (AFP)

24-28 weeks:
- Diabetes screening (If plasma glucose measured one hour after 50 gram oral glucose challenge is >140 mg/dL, additional testing should be performed on a different day. A 100 g glucose load is administered and glucose values are measured at 1 hour, 2 hours, and 3 hours. If 2 of the 3 values are abnormal, a diagnosis of gestational diabetes is made.
- Repeat hemoglobin or hematocrit

28 weeks:
- Repeat antibody test for non-sensitized Rh-negative women

28-32 weeks:
- Syphilis serology repeated if high-risk
- Gonorrhea and chlamydia test if high-risk or if previously positive

32-36 weeks:
- Ultrasound
- Testing for sexually transmitted diseases
- Repeat hemoglobin or hematocrit

LEOPOLD'S MANEUVERS

- Used to palpate fetal presentation and position
- Composed of four maneuvers by examiner
  - ◊ Palpate fundus
  - ◊ Palpate to identify fetal back and extremities
  - ◊ Palpate presenting part
  - ◊ Palpate down sides of abdomen to locate cephalic prominence or brow

Differentiation of True vs. False Labor

True Labor	False Labor
Contractions occur at regular intervals	Contractions are irregular
Intervals between contractions gradually shorten	Usually no change
Contractions increase in duration and intensity	Usually no change
Discomfort begins in back and radiates around to abdomen	Discomfort usually in abdomen
Intensity usually increases with walking	Walking has no effect on or lessens contractions
Progressive cervical dilatation and effacement	No cervical changes

EDUCATION

- Reinforce previous teaching
- Follow-up on plans for childbirth and breastfeeding
- Signs and symptoms of labor
  - ◊ Lower back pain
  - ◊ Passage of "bloody show"
  - ◊ Regular contractions
  - ◊ Rupture of membranes

COMMON DISCOMFORTS OF PREGNANCY

ANKLE EDEMA

CAUSES

- Prolonged standing or sitting
- Increased sodium levels due to hormonal influences
- Increased capillary permeability
- Varicose veins

USUAL TIMING IN PREGNANCY

- Second and third trimesters

DIFFERENTIAL DIAGNOSIS

- Thrombophlebitis
- Preeclampsia

MANAGEMENT

- Frequent dorsiflexion of feet when sitting or standing
- Elevate legs when sitting or resting
- Avoid tight garters or restrictive bands around legs

NAUSEA AND VOMITING

CAUSE

- Chorionic gonadotropin (hCG) is likely cause of nausea and vomiting during pregnancy
- Changes in carbohydrate metabolism
- Emotional factors
- Fatigue

USUAL TIMING IN PREGNANCY

- First trimester of pregnancy

DIFFERENTIAL DIAGNOSIS

- Hyperemesis gravidarum
- Gastroenteritis

MANAGEMENT

- Reassurance and support
- Avoidance of medications if possible
- Eat small frequent meals
- Avoid foods with strong odor
- Eat dry crackers or toast before arising in morning
- Increase carbohydrate percentage in diet
- Decrease fat in diet
- Eating ginger in soda, tea, or ginger snaps
- Supplemental vitamin B_6 (pyridoxine)
- If severe, hospitalization may be considered for rehydration and parenteral nutrition

BACKACHE

CAUSES

- Increased curvature of the lumbosacral vertebrae as the uterus enlarges
- Increased weight
- General relaxation of pelvic ligaments and motion of the symphysis pubis and lumbosacral joints
- Fatigue
- Poor body mechanics

USUAL TIMING IN PREGNANCY

- Second and third trimesters

DIFFERENTIAL DIAGNOSIS

- Herniated disc
- Sciatica
- Muscle strain

MANAGEMENT

- Rest
- Lumbar support
- Avoidance of straining and lifting
- Proper body mechanics
- Pelvic tilt exercises
- Avoid uncomfortable working heights, high-heeled shoes, and fatigue

CONSTIPATION

CAUSES

- Generalized relaxation of smooth muscle and decreased motility of the gastrointestinal tract in response to increased level of progesterone
- Compression of the lower bowel by the enlarging uterus and presenting part
- May be exacerbated by iron and calcium supplementation
- Lack of exercise
- Decreased fluid intake

USUAL TIMING IN PREGNANCY

- Any time during pregnancy

MANAGEMENT

- Increase daily fiber intake
- Increase fluid intake
- Daily exercise
- Mild laxative (e.g., prune juice, milk of magnesia), bulk-producing agents, or stool-softening agents
- Harsh laxatives and enemas are not recommended
- Regular bowel habits

HEARTBURN

CAUSE

- Reflux of gastric contents into the lower esophagus due to:
    - ◊ Increased production of progesterone decreasing gastrointestinal motility and increasing relaxation of cardiac sphincter
    - ◊ Displacement of stomach by enlarging uterus

USUAL TIMING IN PREGNANCY

- Second and third trimesters

MANAGEMENT

- Small frequent meals
- Avoidance of bending over
- Elevation of head of bed
- Avoidance of tight and binding clothing
- Antacid preparations (avoid sodium containing products)
- Avoid overeating, fatty foods

HEMORRHOIDS

CAUSE

- Increased pressure in the rectal veins due to obstruction of venous return
- Constipation

USUAL TIMING IN PREGNANCY

- Second and third trimesters

MANAGEMENT

- Increased fiber and fluids in diet to keep stool soft
- Stool softeners may be needed to soften stool
- Topical ointments
- Warm sitz baths
- Ice packs

LEG CRAMPS

CAUSE

- Imbalance of calcium/phosphorous ratio
- Increased pressure of uterus on nerves
- Fatigue
- Decreased venous circulation in legs

USUAL TIMING IN PREGNANCY

- Second and third trimesters

DIFFERENTIAL DIAGNOSIS

- Thrombophlebitis
- Electrolyte imbalance

MANAGEMENT

- Avoid pointing toes

Pregnancy

- Dorsiflexion of foot to stretch affected muscles
- Apply heat to affected muscles

LEUKORRHEA

CAUSE

- Increased mucus formation by the cervix in response to elevated estrogen levels

USUAL TIMING IN PREGNANCY

- First trimester

DIFFERENTIAL DIAGNOSIS

- Trichomoniasis
- Candidal vaginitis
- Bacterial vaginosis
- Gonorrhea
- Chlamydia

MANAGEMENT

- Wearing of perineal pad with frequent change
- Daily bathing
- Good perineal hygiene
- Avoid douching
- Wear cotton underwear
- Avoid panty hose

NASAL CONGESTION AND EPISTAXIS

CAUSE

- Elevated estrogen levels

USUAL TIMING IN PREGNANCY

- First trimester

DIFFERENTIAL DIAGNOSIS

- Allergic rhinitis
- Upper respiratory infection

MANAGEMENT

- Cool air vaporizer
- Avoid use of nasal sprays and decongestants
- Consider topical nasal steroid for nasal congestion

ROUND LIGAMENT PAIN

CAUSE

- Stretching of the round ligaments as the uterus enlarges

USUAL TIMING IN PREGNANCY

- Second and third trimesters

DIFFERENTIAL DIAGNOSIS

- Appendicitis
- Cholecystitis
- Labor

MANAGEMENT

- Heating pad to abdomen
- Position with knees into chest
- Acetaminophen

URINARY FREQUENCY

CAUSE

- Pressure of uterus resting on bladder

USUAL TIMING IN PREGNANCY

- First and third trimester

DIFFERENTIAL DIAGNOSIS

- Urinary tract infection

MANAGEMENT

- Void when urge is felt
- Increase fluid intake during day
- Decrease fluid intake in evenings to decrease nocturia

VARICOSE VEINS

CAUSE

- Increased pressure in femoral veins due to obstruction of venous return
- Hereditary factors
- Weight gain
- Increased age

USUAL TIMING IN PREGNANCY

- Second and third trimesters

MANAGEMENT

- Avoid prolonged standing or sitting
- Elevate legs frequently
- Support stockings
- Avoid crossing legs at the knees or wearing knee-hi stockings which restrict venous return

ASSESSMENT OF FETAL WELL-BEING

AMNIOCENTESIS

DESCRIPTION

Involves inserting a needle through the maternal abdomen into the uterine cavity to withdraw a sample of amniotic fluid

INDICATIONS

16-18 weeks gestation:

- Pregnancies in women aged 35 or older
- Previous pregnancy resulting in the birth of a child with a chromosomal abnormality
- Down syndrome or other chromosome abnormality in either parent or a close family member
- Mother who is a carrier of any X-linked disease
- Neural tube defect in either parent or a first-degree relative
- Previous child born with a neural tube defect
- Abnormal serum maternal α-fetoprotein level
- Either parent being a carrier of a genetically transmitted metabolic disease
- Pregnancy after three or more spontaneous abortions

Late pregnancy:

- Determine fetal lung maturity based on phospholipids
- Detect isoimmunization

PROCEDURE

- Woman positioned with left lateral tilt to prevent vena cava compression
- Done under ultrasound guidance for location of fetus and placenta
- Needle is inserted into an adequate pocket of fluid under sterile conditions
- Fetal heart rate is monitored for 15 minutes after procedure
- Rh-negative women should be given Rh immune globulin (RhoGAM®) after procedure

AMNIOTIC FLUID TESTS

- α-fetoprotein: elevated in open neural tube defect, abdominal wall defect, congenital nephrosis, cystic hygroma, multiple gestation, fetal death (only done after a positive α-fetoprotein screen of the serum)
- Lecithin-to-sphingomyelin (L/S) ratio: If L/S is greater than 2.0, there is a low risk of respiratory distress secondary to prematurity
- Phosphatidylglycerol (PG): PG first appears at 35 weeks gestation and increases in concentration until 40 weeks; if present, it provides reassurance of fetal lung maturity
- Identification of meconium staining

POSSIBLE COMPLICATIONS

- Complications occur in <1% of cases

- Fetus, umbilical cord, or placenta may be punctured inadvertently
- Hemorrhage
- Fetal anemia
- Intraamniotic infection
- Induction of preterm labor

BIOPHYSICAL PROFILE

DESCRIPTION

Ultrasonographic assessment and nonstress test to evaluate five fetal biophysical variables:

- Fetal heart rate reactivity
- Amniotic fluid volume measurement
- Fetal breathing movements
- Fetal body movements
- Fetal tone

INDICATIONS

- Hypertension
- Diabetes mellitus
- Multiple gestation
- Suspected oligohydramnios/intrauterine growth restriction (IUGR)
- Known placental abnormality
- Maternal heart or renal disease
- Hemoglobinopathy
- Postdate pregnancies
- Previous unexplained fetal demise
- Maternal perceptions of decreased fetal movement
- Assessment of fetus at risk for intrauterine compromise

FINDINGS

- Each component is worth 2 points, with a maximum possible score of 10
- 8-10: reassuring
- 6: suspicious and indicates need for further evaluation and possible intervention
- 4 or less: ominous and indicates need for immediate intervention

MATERNAL ASSESSMENT OF FETAL ACTIVITY

DESCRIPTION

Maternal perception of fetal activity; has been shown to be an effective screening method of fetal well-being

INDICATION

- All pregnant patients should monitor fetal activity daily

PROCEDURE

- Patient lies on her left side 30 minutes after eating
- She records the time she starts the test and notes each time the baby moves or kicks

FINDINGS

- A healthy fetus should move 3-5 times within one hour.

NONSTRESS TESTING (NST)

DESCRIPTION

Indirect measurement of uteroplacental function

INDICATIONS

- Hypertension
- Diabetes mellitus
- Multiple gestation
- Suspected oligohydramnios/IUGR
- Known placental abnormality
- Maternal heart or renal disease
- Hemoglobinopathy
- Postdate pregnancies
- Previous unexplained fetal demise
- Maternal perceptions of decreased fetal movement
- Assessment of fetus at risk for intrauterine compromise

PROCEDURE

- Patient should either sit or lie on her left side
- Electronic fetal monitor is used to monitor fetal heart rate and uterine activity
- The patient presses a button on the monitor that marks the tracing every time she feels fetal movement

FINDINGS

- Reassuring or reactive test: shows at least two 15 beats/minute accelerations in fetal heart rate lasting at least 15 seconds in a 20 minute period
- Nonreassuring or nonreactive test: does not meet the above criteria; suggests that fetus may be compromised
- Unsatisfactory test: inadequate tracing of fetal heart rate
- 65% of healthy fetuses will have a reactive nonstress test at 28 weeks gestation; 85% at 32 weeks and 95% at 34 weeks.

CONTRACTION STRESS TEST
(Oxytocin Challenge Test)

DESCRIPTION

Method used to evaluate respiratory function (oxygen and carbon dioxide exchange) of the placenta

INDICATIONS

- Identifies the fetus at risk for intrauterine asphyxia
- Intrauterine growth restriction
- Diabetes mellitus
- Postdates ($\geq$42 weeks gestation)
- Abnormal or suspicious biophysical profile

CONTRAINDICATIONS

- Patients at high risk for premature labor
- Patients who have a classic uterine scar from uterine surgery or cesarean section
- Patients with a placenta previa or marginal abruptio placentae

PROCEDURE

- The goal of the test is for the patient to have three uterine contractions during a 10 minute time period
- The contractions may occur spontaneously, with nipple stimulation, or with oxytocin infusion
- An electronic fetal monitor is used to monitor fetal heart rate and uterine activity
- Woman assumes semi-Fowler's or side-lying position to avoid vena cava compression

FINDINGS

- Negative: no late decelerations observed
- Positive: late decelerations detected with more than 50% of contractions

POSSIBLE COMPLICATIONS

- Uterine hyperstimulation

ULTRASOUND

INDICATIONS

- Determine the presence or absence of an intrauterine pregnancy
- Determine the gestational age
- Measure fetal growth and identify intrauterine growth restriction
- Identify multiple gestation pregnancies
- Detect fetal anomalies (nearly 100% sensitive for the detection of neural tube defects)
- Detect oligohydramnios or polyhydramnios
- Demonstrate placental abnormalities
- Identify maternal uterine and pelvic anomalies

PROCEDURE

- May be done transabdominally or endo vaginally
- Woman should have partially full or full bladder

FINDINGS

- The following data may be obtained from ultrasound:
  - ◊ Cardiac activity
  - ◊ Crown-rump length of fetus for accurate dating of pregnancy before 12 weeks of gestation
  - ◊ Fetal biparietal diameter (BPD)
  - ◊ Femur length
  - ◊ Abdominal and head circumference

COMPLICATIONS ASSOCIATED WITH PREGNANCY

ABRUPTIO PLACENTAE

DESCRIPTION

Premature separation of the placenta from the uterine wall

TERMS

Marginal	Separation at the periphery of the placenta; vaginal bleeding present
Central	Placenta separates centrally and blood is trapped between placenta and uterine wall; vaginal bleeding absent
Complete	Total separation of the placenta from the uterine wall with resultant massive vaginal bleeding

ETIOLOGY

- Primary cause unknown

INCIDENCE

- Occurs in 10% of all births, but severe abruptio is rare
- Accounts for 15% of fetal deaths
- More common in African-American women

RISK FACTORS

- Maternal age >35 years
- Grand multiparity
- Pregnancy-induced hypertension
- Essential hypertension
- Prematurely ruptured membranes
- Abdominal trauma
- Cigarette smoking
- Cocaine use
- Uterine fibroids
- Maternal coagulopathies
- Malnutrition or severe folate deficiency
- Abdominal trauma
- Short umbilical cord

ASSESSMENT FINDINGS

- Profuse to absent vaginal bleeding
- Amount of bleeding has no correlation with degree of separation
- Uterine tenderness
- Board-like uterus on palpation
- Abdominal pain
- Back pain
- Fetal distress
- Hypertonus
- Preterm labor
- Shock

DIFFERENTIAL DIAGNOSIS

- Placenta previa

DIAGNOSTIC STUDIES

- Ultrasound
- Fetal monitoring
- Fibrinogen level: decreased
- Platelet count: decreased
- Prothrombin time and partial thromboplastin time: normal to prolonged
- Fibrin degradation products: increased
- Hematocrit and hemoglobin

MANAGEMENT

- Prompt delivery. If separation mild, labor induction may be attempted; if severe separation, immediate cesarean section is indicated.
- Blood transfusions if bleeding severe
- Fluid replacement therapy
- Correction of coagulation defects with cryoprecipitate or plasma
- Hysterectomy may be needed in extreme cases

EXPECTED COURSE

- Risk of recurrence in subsequent pregnancy is high
- Fetal/neonatal mortality 20-35% overall; is near 100% in complete separations

POSSIBLE COMPLICATIONS

Fetal risks:
- Fetal demise
- Fetal hypoxia
- Preterm birth
- Anemia
- Neurological damage

Maternal risks:
- Disseminated intravascular coagulation
- Couvelaire uterus (infiltration of blood into uterine musculature)
- Renal failure
- Shock

ECTOPIC PREGNANCY

DESCRIPTION

Pregnancy which implants outside the uterus; most common site is the ampulla of the fallopian tube

ETIOLOGY

- Tubal damage secondary to PID
- Previous pelvic or tubal surgery
- Presence of an IUD
- High levels of estrogen and progesterone which alter the motility of the egg in the fallopian tube
- Congenital anomalies of the tube
- Blighted ovum

INCIDENCE

- >1/100 pregnancies
- 85% of these occur in the fallopian tubes

RISK FACTORS

- History of pelvic inflammatory disease
- Multiple sexual partners
- History of endometriosis
- Previous ectopic pregnancy
- Present or past use of intrauterine device
- History of pelvic or tubal surgery
- Cigarette smoking
- In vitro fertilization

ASSESSMENT FINDINGS

- Initially may have normal signs of pregnancy
- Vaginal bleeding
- Fainting or dizziness
- Lower abdominal pain
- Palpable adnexal mass
- If tube has ruptured, has acute onset of a sharp lower abdominal pain
- Right-sided shoulder pain due to irritation of the subdiaphragmatic phrenic nerve by blood
- Shock if bleeding profuse and rapid
- Abdomen may gradually become rigid and very tender
- Abdominal tenderness
- Cervical motion pain

DIFFERENTIAL DIAGNOSIS

- Intrauterine pregnancy
- Appendicitis
- Cholecystitis
- Pelvic inflammatory disease
- Spontaneous abortion
- Ruptured ovarian cyst
- Torsion of the ovary
- Urinary tract infection

DIAGNOSTIC STUDIES

- Serial quantitative β-hCG determinations
- Pelvic ultrasound
- Serum progesterone: <5 ng/ml exclude viable pregnancy; <25 ng/ml exclude ectopic pregnancy
- Culdocentesis: presence of nonclotting blood
- Laparoscopy

MANAGEMENT

- Refer immediately to ER or obstetrician/gynecologist
- Laparotomy and surgical removal of fallopian tube
- If tube has not ruptured: methotrexate or microsurgery may save the tube
- If woman is Rh-negative: Rh immune globulin (RhoGAM®) should be administered
- Intravenous fluids
- Blood transfusion may be needed
- Anticipatory guidance regarding reaction to loss of pregnancy
- Assess support systems

POSSIBLE COMPLICATIONS

- Second leading cause of maternal mortality
- Loss of fertility

GENETIC DISORDERS

CATEGORIES OF GENETIC DISORDERS

Chromosomal Abnormalities:

- Numerical autosomal abnormalities: result of uneven distribution of chromosomes during cell division. Most common are trisomy (presence of an extra chromosome)
  - ◊ Examples: trisomy 21 (Down syndrome), trisomy 13, trisomy 18
- Structural autosomal abnormalities: variety of structural chromosomal alterations including deletions and rearrangements (e.g., rings, inversions, and translocations).
  - ◊ Examples: *Cri du chat* syndrome, Robertsonian translocations
- Mosaicism: presence of two or more distinct cell lines in the same individual
- Sex chromosome abnormalities: involve abnormalities in number of X and Y chromosomes
  - ◊ Examples: Turner's syndrome, Klinefelter's syndrome

Single Gene Defects:

- Autosomal dominant inheritance: expressed when only one copy of a mutant gene is inherited. Nearly 1200 have been identified.
  - ◊ Examples: Huntington's chorea, Marfan's syndrome, neurofibromatosis, von Willebrand disease
- Autosomal recessive inheritance: expressed when two copies of a mutant gene are inherited. More than 600 have been identified.
  - ◊ Examples: cystic fibrosis, sickle cell anemia, thalassemia, PKU, Tay-Sachs
- Sex-linked or X-linked inheritance: classified as dominant, recessive, or fragile with the majority being recessive. X-linked recessive disorders are carried by females and only males are affected. One half of male offspring of a carrier mother will be affected and half of the daughters will be carriers.
  - ◊ Examples: color blindness, hemophilia A, Duchenne muscular dystrophy

Multifactorial Inheritance:

- Multifactorial inheritance: characteristic inherited patterns are not found, but there is an increased frequency of the disorder in families. Thought to involve multiple genes and environmental factors.
  - ◊ Examples: neural tube defects, congenital heart disease, orthopedic anomalies, cleft lip and palate, pyloric stenosis

Unknown:

- The etiology of a number of congenital anomalies is unknown
  - ◊ Examples: hydrocephaly, urinary tract anomalies, diaphragmatic hernia

INCIDENCE

- 5% of all newborns have a recognizable birth defect, 20-25% of these are caused by a genetic disorder
- 1 in 170 newborns are affected by some type of chromosomal abnormality
- 1% have a single gene defect

RISK FACTORS

- Family history of genetic disorder
- Preterm infant
- Increased maternal age (over 35 years)
- Recurrent spontaneous abortion
- Infertility
- Exposure to ionizing radiation

DIAGNOSTIC STUDIES

- Maternal α-fetoprotein
- Ultrasound
- Amniocentesis
- Chromosomal analysis

MANAGEMENT

- Preconceptual counseling for couples with a family history of genetic disorders
- Refer for genetic counseling and testing
- Surgical repair of structural defects
- Dietary modifications necessary in some disorders

DOWN SYNDROME
(Trisomy 21)

DESCRIPTION

Chromosomal abnormality in which there is an extra chromosome 21, resulting in a characteristic combination of birth defects

ETIOLOGY

- Unknown

INCIDENCE

- Incidence of 1/1000 births
- 20 year old woman: 1 in 1200 chance
- 40 year old woman: 1 in 70 chance
- Occurs slightly more in Caucasians than African-Americans, Asians, Hispanics

RISK FACTORS

- Mother older than 35 years of age
- Previous child with Down syndrome

ASSESSMENT FINDINGS

- Simian crease on one or both palms
- Fingers short and stubby
- Fifth fingers are often incurved (clinodactyly)
- Epicanthal folds
- Flattened nasal bridge
- Head relatively small with flattened occiput
- Loose skin at nape of neck
- Poor muscle tone
- Protruding tongue
- Low-set ears
- Mental retardation of varying severity

ASSOCIATED MAJOR MALFORMATIONS

- Congenital heart defects
- Gastrointestinal atresias

DIAGNOSTIC STUDIES

- In utero diagnosis by amniocentesis
- Chromosomal analysis

MANAGEMENT

- Immunizations according to schedule
- Genetic counseling
- Surgical correction of anomalies
- Educate parents regarding syndrome
- Refer to support groups and community resources

EXPECTED COURSE

- Life expectancy 50 years of age

POSSIBLE COMPLICATIONS

- Frequent respiratory infections
- Increased risk of leukemia

- Feeding problems related to protruding tongue and hypotonia

GESTATIONAL TROPHOBLASTIC DISEASE
(Hydatidiform Mole, Molar Pregnancy)

DESCRIPTION

Includes hydatidiform mole, invasive mole (chorioadenoma destruens), and choriocarcinoma. Hydatidiform mole is the most common form; there is abnormal development of the placenta, resulting in fluid-filled, grapelike clusters with trophoblastic tissue proliferation. There is a risk of development of choriocarcinoma from the trophoblastic tissue.

ETIOLOGY

- Develops from ovum which has lost its genetic material
- Reason for this loss is unknown

INCIDENCE

- 1/2000 pregnancies in the U.S.

RISK FACTORS

- Extremes of maternal age
- Familial tendency
- Previous molar pregnancy

ASSESSMENT FINDINGS

- Severe nausea and vomiting at 12-16 weeks gestation
- Continuous or intermittent brown discharge for several weeks
- Heavy vaginal bleeding
- Uterus may be soft
- Uterine size greater than expected for gestational age
- Absent fetal heart tones
- Anemia
- Hydropic vesicles may be passed vaginally
- Pregnancy-induced hypertension may be present in the first half of the pregnancy

DIFFERENTIAL DIAGNOSIS

- Multiple gestation
- Spontaneous abortion

DIAGNOSTIC STUDIES

- Quantitative β-hCG levels higher than expected for gestational age
- Ultrasound: characteristic "starburst" pattern

MANAGEMENT

- Immediate evacuation of uterus
- Hysterectomy may be the treatment of choice in an older woman who has completed her childbearing
- Biweekly serum β-hCG until values return to normal, then monthly for 6 months, then every other month for 6 months for a total of one year
- Pregnancy should be avoided for at least one year
- If woman is Rh-negative: Rh immune globulin (RhoGAM®) should be administered

CONSULTATION/REFERRAL

- Treatment at a center specializing in gestational trophoblastic disease is recommended if hCG levels remain high or continue to rise

POSSIBLE COMPLICATIONS

- Choriocarcinoma develops following evacuation of a molar pregnancy in 20% of women
- Anemia
- Hyperthyroidism
- Infection
- Disseminated intravascular coagulation (DIC)
- Trophoblastic embolization of the lung
- Ovarian cysts

HYPEREMESIS GRAVIDARUM

DESCRIPTION

Persistent, intractable vomiting during pregnancy

ETIOLOGY

- Not completely known
- Multifactorial: hormonal, neurologic, metabolic, psychosomatic factors
- May be related to increased levels of human chorionic gonadotropin (hCG) and estradiol

INCIDENCE

- Relatively rare condition

RISK FACTORS

- Multiple gestation
- Hydatidiform mole

ASSESSMENT FINDINGS

- Weight loss
- Persistent nausea and vomiting
- Signs of dehydration
- Jaundice
- Hemorrhage
- Peripheral neuropathy

DIFFERENTIAL DIAGNOSIS

- Gastroenteritis
- Appendicitis
- Cholecystitis
- Viral hepatitis
- Hydatidiform mole
- Peptic ulcer disease
- Intestinal obstruction

DIAGNOSTIC STUDIES

- Electrolytes: hypokalemia
- Urinalysis: ketonuria
- Hematocrit: elevated
- BUN: elevated
- Total protein: decreased

DIAGNOSTIC CRITERIA

- Intractable vomiting in the first half of pregnancy
- Dehydration
- Ketonuria
- Weight loss of 5% of prepregnancy weight

MANAGEMENT

- Hospitalization may be necessary with intravenous fluids and parenteral nutrition
- Conservative management as with nausea and vomiting
- Medications may be needed
- Antiemetics
    - ◊ Doxylamine (Unisom®)
    - ◊ Promethazine (Phenergan®) intramuscular or suppository
    - ◊ Trimethobenzamide (Tigan®) suppository

POSSIBLE COMPLICATIONS

- Starvation
- Ketosis
- Electrolyte imbalance
- Dehydration
- Embryonal or fetal death

INCOMPETENT CERVIX

DESCRIPTION

Premature dilatation of the cervix, usually in the fourth or fifth month of pregnancy; is associated with repeated second trimester spontaneous abortion

ETIOLOGY

Congenital causes:
- Cervical structural defects
- Uterine anomalies
- Abnormal cervical development secondary to in utero exposure to DES

Acquired causes:
- Previous traumatic birth

- Trauma to cervix during dilation and curettage
- Cervical conization
- Cervical cauterization

INCIDENCE

- Occurs in 0.5-1.0% of pregnancies
- Responsible for 15-20% of second trimester pregnancy losses

RISK FACTORS

- History of repeated second trimester spontaneous abortions

ASSESSMENT FINDINGS

- Progressive effacement and dilation of the cervix
- Bulging of membranes through cervical os
- Uterine contractions absent until late in process

DIFFERENTIAL DIAGNOSIS

- Spontaneous abortion

DIAGNOSTIC STUDIES

- Serial ultrasound
- Cervical cultures for gonorrhea and group B *Streptococcus* before placement of cerclage

MANAGEMENT

- Cervical cerclage placed at 14-18 weeks gestation in women with history of incompetent cervix
- Bedrest
- Abstinence of coitus
- Education regarding rupture of membranes

EXPECTED COURSE

- Success rate for carrying a pregnancy to term is 80-90% with appropriate treatment

POSSIBLE COMPLICATIONS

- Premature rupture of membranes
- Failure to stop fetal loss
- Tearing of cervix

MULTIPLE GESTATION

DEFINITION

Pregnancy with multiple fetuses

ETIOLOGY

- Results from fertilization of separate ova (fraternal) or from a single fertilized ovum that divides into separate structures (identical)

INCIDENCE

- Incidence of twins in U.S. is 1/80 pregnancies

RISK FACTORS

- African-American
- Women who were twins are more likely to have twins
- Increased maternal age
- Increased parity
- More common in large and tall women than in small women
- Use of fertility agents
- In vitro fertilization

ASSESSMENT FINDINGS

- Uterus size is larger than expected for gestational age
- Auscultation of two separate fetal heart sounds

DIAGNOSTIC STUDIES

- Serial ultrasound to determine growth of each fetus
- Maternal α-fetoprotein: elevated
- Chorionic gonadotropin: elevated
- Biophysical profile and nonstress testing beginning at 30-34 weeks gestation

DIFFERENTIAL DIAGNOSIS

- Inaccurate menstrual history
- Hydramnios

- Hydatidiform mole
- Uterine fibroids
- Adenomyosis
- Adnexal mass
- Fetal macrosomia

MANAGEMENT

- More frequent prenatal visits
- Dietary intake increased an additional 300 kcal/day
- Iron intake increased to 60-100 mg/day
- Folic acid intake increased to 1 mg/day
- Bedrest may be necessary toward end of pregnancy or at any time if preterm labor threatens
- Cesarean section indicated for birth of three or more fetuses

EXPECTED COURSE

- Morbidity and mortality are considerably increased in pregnancy with multiple fetuses

POSSIBLE COMPLICATIONS

Maternal risks:

- Anemia
- Pregnancy-induced hypertension
- Placenta previa
- Abruptio placenta
- Uterine dysfunction
- Preterm labor
- Increased physical discomfort

Fetal risks:

- Spontaneous abortion
- Increased perinatal mortality
- Low birthweight
- Congenital anomalies
- Fetal-fetal hemorrhage
- Cord accidents
- Hydramnios
- Abnormal fetal presentation
- The more fetuses conceived, the smaller they tend to be at birth
- Death of one or more fetuses

PLACENTA PREVIA

DESCRIPTION

Improper implantation of the placenta in the lower uterine segment. Four common classifications:

- *Complete*: placental tissue completely covers cervical os
- *Partial*: only a portion of os is covered
- *Marginal*: the edge of the placenta is at the margin of the os
- *Low-lying*: placenta does not cover os, but is low in the uterine segment

ETIOLOGY

- Unknown

INCIDENCE

- 1/250 births

RISK FACTORS

- History of previous placenta previa
- Grand multiparity
- Maternal age over 35 years
- Previous cesarean section
- Previous induced abortion
- Cigarette smoking
- Multiple gestation
- History of dilatation and curettage
- History of myomectomy
- Large placenta

ASSESSMENT FINDINGS

- Painless vaginal bleeding usually beginning at the end of the second trimester
- A vaginal examination should not be performed if placenta previa is suspected

DIFFERENTIAL DIAGNOSIS

- Abruptio placentae
- Coagulation defects
- Bloody show
- Vaginal/cervical lesion
- Trauma
- Trophoblastic disease

DIAGNOSTIC STUDIES

- Ultrasound

MANAGEMENT

- Dependent on gestational age of fetus and degree of bleeding
- Expectant management if pregnancy <37 weeks gestation and bleeding not severe
  - ◊ Bedrest
  - ◊ No rectal or vaginal examinations
  - ◊ Electronic fetal monitoring
  - ◊ Intravenous fluids
- Cesarean section before 37 weeks is required if frequent, recurrent, or profuse bleeding persists or if fetal well-being jeopardized
- Refer for physician management

POSSIBLE COMPLICATIONS

- Shock
- Preterm delivery
- Placenta accreta

ADOLESCENT PREGNANCY

INCIDENCE

- 1 in 10 adolescent girls (approximately 1 million) become pregnant each year in the U.S.

RISK FACTORS

- Early dating
- Early onset of sexual activity
- Dating male 5-6 years older
- Low self-esteem
- Daughter of an adolescent mother
- Daughter of a single parent
- Poverty
- Minority
- Poor academic achievement
- Substance abuse
- Depression

PREVENTION

- Counseling about pregnancy prevention (e.g., abstinence, contraception)
- Early identification of at-risk children

FACTORS WHICH INCREASE RISKS TO ADOLESCENTS DURING PREGNANCY

- <15 years of age
- Failure to seek prenatal care
- Inadequate nutrition
- Poor health before pregnancy
- Sexually transmitted diseases
- Smoking
- Alcohol and drug abuse

MANAGEMENT

- Increased attention to nutrition counseling
- Smoking cessation counseling
- Assess for alcohol and substance abuse
- Counseling regarding pregnancy options
- Education regarding importance of prenatal care
- Screening for sexually transmitted diseases
- Assessment of support systems
- Education regarding physiology of pregnancy in terms adolescent can understand

RISKS TO ADOLESCENT MOTHER

- Increased death rate
- Increased rate of premature labor, prolonged labor, pregnancy-induced hypertension, cephalopelvic disproportion, and anemia
- Increased elective abortion rates
- Fewer adolescent mothers receive prenatal care
- Adolescents may have poor eating habits, and are more likely to smoke and take drugs during pregnancy
- Slowed linear growth
- Less likely to complete high school
- Chronic unemployment
- Limited job opportunities
- Social isolation
- Depression

RISKS TO INFANT OF ADOLESCENT MOTHER

- Low birth weight
- Premature delivery
- Increased neonatal death rate
- Increased risk of child abuse and neglect
- Increased rates of birth defects
- Increased risk of being raised in poverty
- Sudden infant death syndrome

PREGNANCY-INDUCED HYPERTENSION (PIH)

(Toxemia of Pregnancy, Preeclampsia)

DESCRIPTION

Hypertensive condition that occurs during pregnancy and resolves after pregnancy; occurs after 20 weeks

TERMS

Preeclampsia	Pregnancy-induced hypertension which may progress to eclampsia if untreated
Eclampsia	Stage of pregnancy-induced hypertension in which seizures occur; today PIH rarely progresses to this stage

ETIOLOGY

- Unknown

INCIDENCE

- Most common hypertensive disorder in pregnancy
- Occurs in 6-8% of all pregnancies
- Among African-American primigravidas the incidence is 15-20%
- In young primigravidas with twin pregnancy, the incidence is 30%

RISK FACTORS

- Primigravida
- Family history of preeclampsia
- History of preeclampsia in a previous pregnancy
- Adolescents of lower socioeconomic status
- Women over 35 years
- Multiple gestation
- Polyhydramnios
- Malnutrition
- Preexisting hypertension or renal disease
- Hydatidiform mole
- Rh incompatibility
- Diabetes mellitus

DIAGNOSTIC CRITERIA

- Increase in systolic blood pressure of 30 mm Hg over baseline obtained before 20 weeks gestation (need 2 readings 6 hours apart) *OR*
- Increase in diastolic blood pressure of 15 mm Hg over baseline obtained before 20 weeks gestation (need 2 readings 6 hours apart) *OR*
- Blood pressure of 140/90 mm Hg if baseline pressures not known
- Excretion of >300 mg/dL of protein over 24 hours; dipstick reading of 1+ (30 mg/dL) or greater
- Pedal edema 1+ or greater that does not resolve with overnight rest, edema of the face and hands, and edema associated with more than a 2 kg weight gain in one week

ASSESSMENT FINDINGS

- Hypertension, tachycardia
- Hyperreflexia
- Oliguria or anuria in severe preeclampsia
- Proteinuria, hematuria, edema
- Dizziness, headache
- Blurred vision, diplopia
- Scotomata (spots before the eyes)
- Retinal edema
- Dyspnea
- Crackles in lung fields
- Epigastric pain
- Hepatomegaly

DIFFERENTIAL DIAGNOSIS

- Essential hypertension
- Renal disease

DIAGNOSTIC STUDIES

- Hematocrit: increased
- Platelet counts: decreased
- Prothrombin time and activated partial thromboplastin time: prolonged
- BUN and serum creatinine: increased in worsening disease
- Urinalysis: high specific gravity, proteinuria
- Liver enzymes: increased if HELLP syndrome present
- 24-hour urine specimen for creatinine clearance and total protein
- Uric acid: increased
- Total protein: decreased
- Lactate dehydrogenase: increased
- Nonstress testing
- Ultrasound for determination of fetal growth
- Biophysical profile
- Amniocentesis to determine fetal lung maturity

MANAGEMENT

- Hospitalization recommended if proteinuria present and/or outpatient management has not been successful
- Bed rest in left lateral recumbent position to decrease pressure on vena cava
- Quiet, low stimulus environment
- Seizure precautions
- Well-balanced diet with moderate to high intake of protein
- Excessive salt intake should be avoided, but strict sodium restriction not recommended
- Diuretics not recommended for treatment
- Magnesium sulfate intravenous for prevention or treatment of seizures
- Antihypertensives
    - ◊ Methyldopa (Aldomet®) is the drug of choice
    - ◊ Hydralazine (Apresoline®)
- Education regarding signs and symptoms or worsening preeclampsia
- Delivery of infant is definitive treatment

CONSULTATION/REFERRAL

- Obstetrician consultation or referral
- Women with HELLP syndrome should be referred to tertiary care center
- Refer to hospital if BP $\geq$160/110

EXPECTED COURSE

- Perinatal mortality associated with preeclampsia is 10%; with eclampsia 20%
- Risk for eclampsia continues until 48 hours postpartum

POSSIBLE COMPLICATIONS

- Cerebral edema
- Cerebral hemorrhage
- Seizures
- Coma
- Intrauterine growth restriction of fetus
- Chronic fetal hypoxia
- Fetal distress
- Premature delivery
- Increased intraocular pressure leading to retinal detachment
- *HELLP* syndrome: involves **H**emolysis, **E**levated **L**iver enzymes, and **L**ow **P**latelet count; associated with severe preeclampsia

PRETERM LABOR

DESCRIPTION

Onset of regular uterine contractions which effect cervical change occurring between 20 and 37 weeks of pregnancy

ETIOLOGY

- Actual cause unknown

Maternal factors:

- Cardiovascular disease
- Renal disease
- Diabetes
- Pregnancy-induced hypertension
- Abdominal surgery

- Uterine anomalies
- Incompetent cervix
- In utero DES exposure
- Infection
- Retained IUD

Fetal factors:
- Multiple gestation
- Hydramnios
- Fetal or amniotic fluid infection
- Fetal death
- Premature rupture of membranes
- Fetal or placental anomaly

Placental factors:
- Placenta previa
- Abruptio placentae

INCIDENCE

- 7-10% of all live births occur prematurely in the U.S.

RISK FACTORS

- Low socioeconomic status
- History of preterm births
- Poor prenatal care
- Maternal smoking
- *See* ETIOLOGY

ASSESSMENT FINDINGS

- Painful or painless uterine contractions at least every 10 minutes with a duration of 30 seconds
- Pelvic pressure
- Menstrual-like cramping
- Watery or bloody vaginal discharge
- Low back pain
- Cervical effacement and dilatation

DIFFERENTIAL DIAGNOSIS

- Braxton-Hicks contractions
- Leukorrhea

DIAGNOSTIC STUDIES

- Biophysical profile to assist with determination of gestational age of fetus

PREVENTION

- Early identification of women at risk using risk-scoring system
- Education of high-risk women regarding signs and symptoms of preterm labor
- Appropriate prenatal care

MANAGEMENT

- Fetal heart monitoring
- Uterine contraction monitoring
- Bedrest
- Hydration
- Sedation
- Tocolytics
  - ◊ Magnesium sulfate or β-adrenergic agonists (e.g., ritodrine, terbutaline) administered intravenously
  - ◊ Oral tocolytics once contractions stop
  - ◊ Subcutaneous terbutaline via infusion pump may be used if needed for long-term maintenance
- Administration of corticosteroids (e.g., betamethasone, dexamethasone) to accelerate fetal lung maturation
- Care of the woman at home may be accomplished once stable utilizing home monitoring
- Contraindications of interrupting labor: severe PIH, eclampsia, maternal hemodynamic instability, fetal anomalies incompatible with life, chorioamnionitis, fetal maturity, severe abruptio placentae, acute fetal distress

POSSIBLE COMPLICATIONS

- Delivery of premature infant
- Complications from tocolytics (e.g., magnesium and β-adrenergic agonists)

POSTTERM PREGNANCY

DESCRIPTION

Pregnancy that persists beyond 42 weeks gestation and is associated with placental changes that causes a decrease in the uterine-placental-fetal circulation. This reduces the blood supply, oxygen, and nutrition for the fetus.

ETIOLOGY

- Not completely understood
- Associated with lack of usually high estrogen level in normal pregnancy
- Extrauterine pregnancy

INCIDENCE

- 7-12% of all pregnancies

RISK FACTORS

- Nullipara between 15 and 20 years of age
- Multipara over age 35 years
- Fetal adrenal hypoplasia
- Anencephalic fetus

ASSESSMENT FINDINGS

- Oligohydramnios
- Macrosomic infant
- High incidence of fetal heart rate baseline changes (e.g., tachycardia, variable decelerations)
- Meconium stained amniotic fluid
- Neonatal depression

DIFFERENTIAL DIAGNOSIS

- Inaccurate assessment of gestational age

DIAGNOSTIC STUDIES

- Biophysical profile
- Nonstress testing 2-3 times/week after 40 weeks of gestation

MANAGEMENT

- Electronic fetal monitoring during labor
- Induction of labor after 42 weeks of gestation if cervix favorable (soft, with some effacement)
- Birth accomplished at 43 weeks by induction or cesarean section if vaginal delivery not possible

EXPECTED COURSE

- Induction of labor is usually 95% successful at delivery
- Perinatal mortality doubles by 43 weeks gestation and triples by 44 weeks

POSSIBLE COMPLICATIONS

- Macrosomia (large for gestation age infant)
- Shoulder dystocia
- Postmature infant
  - ◊ Long, thin infant with loss of subcutaneous tissue
  - ◊ Desquamation present
  - ◊ Meconium stained skin and nails
  - ◊ Long nails
  - ◊ Wrinkled hands and feet
- Fetal distress
- Oligohydramnios
- Asphyxia
- Birth trauma
- Umbilical cord compression
- Infant hypoglycemia

PROLAPSED UMBILICAL CORD

DESCRIPTION

The umbilical cord precedes the fetal presenting part causing pressure on the cord and vessels as it is trapped between the maternal pelvis and the presenting part

ETIOLOGY

- The cord can fall or be washed through the cervix into the vagina anytime the pelvic inlet is not completely filled by the fetus

INCIDENCE

- 0.2-0.6% of births

RISK FACTORS

- Malpresentation of fetus
- Low birth weight
- Multipara with more than 5 previous births
- Multiple gestation

- Presence of a long cord
- Premature rupture of membranes
- Amniotomy

ASSESSMENT FINDINGS

- Visualization of cord protruding from vagina
- Palpation of cord in vagina or protruding through cervical os
- Fetal bradycardia
- Persistent variable decelerations

DIFFERENTIAL DIAGNOSIS

- Fetal distress from another cause

MANAGEMENT

- Relief of pressure on cord by positioning patient in knee-chest or Trendelenburg position and pushing presenting part upward off of cord
- Electronic fetal monitoring
- Oxygen to mother
- Immediate cesarean section

POSSIBLE COMPLICATIONS

- Fetal hypoxia
- Neurological damage
- Fetal death

SPONTANEOUS ABORTION

DESCRIPTION

Involuntary expulsion of the products of conception during the first 20 weeks of gestation

ETIOLOGY

- Incompetent cervix
- Fetal chromosomal abnormalities
- Cigarette smoking
- Immunologic rejection
- Uterine structural abnormalities
- Teratogenic drugs
- Endocrine imbalance
- Maternal infections

TERMS

Threatened Abortion	Unexplained bleeding, cramping, or backache; cervix is closed; may be followed by partial or complete expulsion of pregnancy or continuance of viable pregnancy; 50% progress to inevitable abortion
Imminent or inevitable abortion	Bleeding and cramping increase; internal cervical os dilates; membranes may rupture
Complete abortion	Complete abortion: complete products of conception are expelled
Incomplete abortion	Part of the products of conception are retained, usually the placenta
Missed abortion	Fetus dies in utero, but is not expelled
Habitual abortion	Abortion occurs in three or more consecutive pregnancies with no apparent cause
Septic	Any of the above scenarios plus a temperature >100.4° F (38° C) without another source of fever may be septic abortion. Associated with IUD or instrumentation in attempted induced abortion.

INCIDENCE

- May be as high as 31%, including recognized and unrecognized pregnancy

RISK FACTORS

- Previous spontaneous abortion

ASSESSMENT FINDINGS

- Vaginal bleeding
- Lower abdominal cramping
- Backache
- Dilation of cervix

DIFFERENTIAL DIAGNOSIS

- Spontaneous abortion
- Ectopic pregnancy

Pregnancy

- Abruptio placentae
- Placenta previa
- Vaginal and/or cervical lesions
- Trauma
- Trophoblastic disease

DIAGNOSTIC STUDIES

- Ultrasound: absence of fetal cardiac activity
- Quantitative β-human chorionic gonadotropin (β-hCG): levels fall shortly after fetal death
- Serum progesterone level: <5 ng/ml is indicative of a nonviable pregnancy
- Hemoglobin and hematocrit to assess blood loss

MANAGEMENT

- Bedrest
- Abstinence from coitus
- Hospitalization may be required if bleeding persists
- Intravenous fluids and blood replacement may be required
- Evacuation of the uterus once fetal death has occurred, usually by dilation and curettage or suction evacuation
- If woman is Rh-negative: Rh immune globulin (RhoGAM®) should be administered
- Anticipatory guidance regarding reaction to loss of pregnancy
- Educate regarding support groups and other available resources

POSSIBLE COMPLICATIONS

- Disseminated intravascular coagulation
- Endometritis
- Sepsis
- Retained products of conception
- Hemorrhage
- Shock

SUBSTANCE ABUSE IN PREGNANCY

INCIDENCE

- 12-14% of pregnant women consume some alcohol during pregnancy with binge drinking reported by 1-2%
- 5.5% of pregnant women use illicit drugs during pregnancy with the most common being cocaine and marijuana

SUBSTANCES COMMONLY ABUSED DURING PREGNANCY

- Alcohol
- Cocaine
- Marijuana
- Amphetamines
- Barbiturates
- Hallucinogens
- Heroin and other narcotics

DIAGNOSTIC STUDIES

- Urine drug screening throughout pregnancy
- Screening for sexually transmitted diseases

MANAGEMENT

- Emphasis on adequate nutrition: high protein, high caloric diet; supplemental vitamins
- Assess support systems
- Referral to treatment program
- Referral to social services
- Hospitalization may be needed
- Detoxification
- Counseling regarding risk of substance abuse to self and developing fetus
- Breastfeeding is not recommended if woman continues using drugs
- Plan for frequent follow-up after delivery including home visits

POSSIBLE CONSEQUENCES

Alcohol:

- Fetal alcohol syndrome: small eyes, short, upturned nose, small, flat cheeks, heart anomalies, mental retardation, short

attention span, behavioral problems, poor coordination
- Intrauterine growth restriction
- Morphologic anomalies
- Neurologic, behavior, and cognitive defects
- Folic acid and thiamine deficiencies in mother
- Increased infections in mother
- Withdrawal syndrome in mother and infant

Cocaine:
- Abruptio placentae
- Decreased blood flow to fetus
- Withdrawal syndrome in mother and infant: seizures, hallucinations, pulmonary edema, respiratory failure, cardiac problems
- Increased incidence of first trimester spontaneous abortion
- Intrauterine growth restriction
- Preterm birth
- Stillbirth
- Malformations of fetal genitourinary tract
- Lowered Apgar scores
- Increased risk of sudden infant death syndrome (SIDS)
- Neurobehavioral disturbances in infant

Marijuana:
- Decreased sperm counts in men
- Infants exposed to marijuana may have fine tremors, prolonged startles, and irritability

Heroin:
- Hepatitis
- AIDS
- Increased incidence of pregnancy-induced hypertension
- Abruptio placentae
- Preterm labor
- Premature rupture of membranes
- Meconium staining
- Intrauterine growth restriction
- Fetal hypoxia
- Withdrawal syndrome: irritability, poor consolability, high-pitched cry, vomiting, seizures

References

Benson-Soros, J., & Glazer, G.L. (2005). The forgotten component of postpartum assessment. *Advance for Nurse Practitioner, 13*(6), 47-49, 76.

Bickley, L.S., & Szilagyi, P.G. (2003). *Bates' guide to physical examination and history taking* (8th ed.). Philadelphia: Lippincott Williams & Wilkins.

Branch, W.T. (2003). *Office practice of medicine* (4th ed.). Philadelphia: Saunders.

Briscoe, D., Nguyen, H., Mencer, M., Gautam, N., Kalb, D.B. (2005). Management of pregnancy beyond 40 weeks gestation. *American Family Physician, 71,* 1935-1941.

Burns, C.E., Brady, M.A., Blosser, C., Starr, N.B., & Dunn, A.M. (2004). *Pediatric primary care: A handbook for nurse practitioners* (3rd ed.). Philadelphia: W.B. Saunders.

Centers for Disease Control and Prevention. (2003). Surveillance for selected maternal behaviors and experiences before, during, and after pregnancy. *MMWR, 52*, (SS-11). Added these 2

Centers for Disease Control and Prevention. (2003). Pregnancy-related mortality surveillance. *MMWR, 52*, (SS-02).

Centers for Disease Control and Prevention. (1998). Sexually transmitted diseases treatment guidelines. *MMWR, 47*, (RR-1).

Centers for Disease Control and Prevention. (1995). U.S. public health service recommendations for human immunodeficiency virus counseling and voluntary testing for pregnant women. *MMWR, 44*(RR-7).

Cunningham, F.G., Leveno, K.J., Bloom, S.L., Hauth, J.C., Gilstrap, L.C., & Wenstrom, K.D. (2005). *Williams Obstetrics.* (22nd ed.). New York: McGraw-Hill.

Goroll, A. H., & Mulley, A. G., Jr. (Eds.). (2000). *Primary care medicine: Office evaluation and management of the adult patient* (4th ed.). Philadelphia: Lippincott Williams Wilkins.

Guyette, L. (1997). Bleeding in pregnancy: Deciphering this danger sign. *Advance for Nurse Practitioners, 5*(9), 35-40.

Hungerford, D.W., Hymbaugh, K.J., & Floyd, R.L. (1994). Alcohol abuse during pregnancy: Identification and management. *The Female Patient, 19*(10), 27-49.

Lerner, H.M. (1997). Prepregnancy counseling. *Hospital Medicine, 33*(6), 28-40.

Kolasa, K.M., & Weismiller, D.G. (1995). Nutrition during pregnancy. *American Family Physician, 56*, 205-212.

Kirkham, C., Harris, S., & Grzybowski, S. (2005). Evidence-based prenatal care: Part 1. General prenatal care and counseling issues. *American Family Physician, 71*, 1307-1316.

Kong, A.P., & Stamos, M.J. (2005). Anorectal complaints: Office diagnosis and treatment. *Consultant, 45,* 731-738.

McKennett, M., & Fullerton, J.T. (1995). Vaginal bleeding in pregnancy. *American Family Physician, 51*, 639-646.

Olds, S.B., London, M.L., & Ladewig, P.W. (1999). *Maternal-newborn nursing: A family-centered approach* (5th ed.). Menlo Park, CA: Addison Wesley.

Olds, S.B., London, M.L., Ladewig, P.W., Davidson, M.R. (2003). *Maternal-newborn nursing and women's health care.* (7th ed.). Upper Saddle River, NJ: Prentice Hall.

Perry, L.E. (1996). Preconception care: A health promotion opportunity. *The Nurse Practitioner, 21*(11), 24-41.

Ransom, S.B., & McNeeley, S.G. (Eds.). (1997). *Gynecology for the primary care provider.* Philadelphia: W.B. Saunders.

Simpson, C.C., Pruitt, R.H., Blackwell, D., & Swearingen, G.S. (1997). Preventing pregnancy in early adolescence. *Advance for Nurse Practitioners, 5*(4), 22-29, 96.

Smith-Levitin, M., Petrikovsky, B., & Schneider, E.P. (1997). Practical guidelines for antepartum fetal surveillance. *American Family Physician, 56*, 1981-1988.

Swan, L.L., & Apgar, B.S. (1995). Preconceptual obstetric risk assessment and health promotion. *American Family Physician, 51*, 1875-1885.

U.S. Preventive Services Task Force. (1996). *Guide to clinical preventive services.* (2nd ed.) Washington, D.C.: Office of Disease Prevention and Health Promotion, U.S. Government Printing Office.

Zamorski, M.A., & Green, L.A. (1996). Preeclampsia and hypertensive disorders of pregnancy. *American Family Physician, 53*, 1595-1604.

17

PROFESSIONALISM IN ADVANCED PRACTICE NURSING

Professionalism
in Advanced Practice Nursing

HISTORY OF THE NURSE PRACTITIONER ROLE

- The first nurse practitioner program started at the University of Colorado in response to the need for accessible, affordable, and humane health care for children. Loretta Ford and Henry Silver, MD developed the program, interpreting the shortage of primary care physicians as an opportunity for this new role for nurses. The program focused on health promotion, disease prevention, and growth and development.

SCOPE OF PRACTICE

- **Assessment** of health status of adults, children, and pregnant women
  - ◊ Obtain history, identify health risks and medical needs
  - ◊ Perform screening procedures and physical examinations, considering age and history of patient
- **Diagnosis**, based on history, physical examination, and diagnostic studies, and analysis of data
- Development and **implementation** of a plan of care, including patient and family education, pharmacologic and nonpharmacologic therapies, and follow-up care
  - ◊ Goal is promotion of wellness, and maintenance or restoration of health
  - ◊ Collaboration with other health care professionals and/or referral to other health care professionals in order to meet patient and family needs
- **Evaluation** of patient status to determine appropriateness and effectiveness of care
  - ◊ Modification of plan of care to achieve goals
- Promotion of self-care
  - ◊ Provide information regarding utilization of health care personnel and health resources
  - ◊ Provide information regarding health promotion, health maintenance, and health restoration
  - ◊ Facilitate entry into the health care system and encourage appropriate follow-up
- Contribute to the definition of the role of nurse practitioner; identify and implement strategies that positively affect the processes regulating the role of nurse practitioner and the health care system in general

STANDARDS OF PRACTICE

- The American Academy of Nurse Practitioners and the American Nurses Association (ANA) are professional organizations of registered nurses:
  - ◊ Set standards of practice for advanced practice nursing
    - * The objective of standards of practice is to provide the public with a basis for determining the quality of the advanced practice nursing care they receive
    - * www.aanp.org
    - * www.nursingworld.org
  - ◊ Recognize excellence in each area of clinical practice through the certification process
- Standards of practice are based on scope of practice
- Standards of practice describe, measure, and guide nurse practitioners in achievement of excellence

  - ◊ Outcome criteria, listed for each standard, allow for measurement of attainment of patient outcomes
- Standards of practice are divided into two categories: practice and performance
  - ◊ Practice category deals with provision of care
  - ◊ Performance category deals with advancement of nursing as a profession

LEGAL AUTHORITY FOR PRACTICE

- State legislative decisions determine the legal authority for advanced practice nurses' scope of practice
- Scope of practice is specific to each state
- In most states, the state board of nursing has sole authority over the scope of practice
- In a few states, scope of practice is authorized by the board of nursing along with the board of medicine

CREDENTIALING

- Professional levels restricting nursing practice
  - ◊ Recognition
    - * Least restrictive
    - * Informs public regarding titles
    - * Provides no guarantee of practitioner's competence
  - ◊ Registration
    - * Lists names and titles of individuals
    - * Does not define practice
    - * Provides no guarantee of practitioner's competence
  - ◊ Certification
    - * Requires candidates to attain specific educational requirements
    - * Requires demonstration of competence prior to practice
  - ◊ Licensure
    - * Occupational licensure is the responsibility of each state
    - * Scope of practice is defined by each state Board of Nursing
    - * Allows states to impose disciplinary actions against licensees practicing outside scope of practice
    - * Provides highest level of guarantee of practitioner's competence
- Mechanisms used by states to facilitate advanced nursing practice
  - ◊ Legislation specifically addressing advanced nursing practice
  - ◊ Expansion of the definition of "nursing" to encompass advanced nursing practice
  - ◊ Extension of the definition of medical practice to enable physicians to delegate medical acts to non-physicians
  - ◊ Second licensure: a separate and additional license to practice advanced practice nursing

CERTIFICATION

- Nurse practitioner certifying agencies
  - ◊ American Nurses Credentialing Center (ANCC): a subsidiary of American Nurses Association (ANA)
  - ◊ AANP (American Academy of Nurse Practitioners)
- Eligibility requirements for national nurse practitioner certification
  - ◊ Applicant must hold an active RN license in the U.S. or its territories
  - ◊ Hold a masters or higher degree in nursing (unless grandfathered in by specific states)
  - ◊ Have been prepared as a nurse practitioner in either a master's program or a formal postgraduate nurse practitioner program in a school of nursing granting graduate-level academic credit
  - ◊ The educational program must include both didactic and clinical components
- Practice requirements
  - ◊ Majority of states require certification by either ANCC or AANP to practice as a nurse practitioner
  - ◊ Minority of states do not require certification to practice
- Maintenance of certification
  - ◊ Continuing Education Units (CEUs)
    - * The individual state Boards of Nursing may have additional requirements for practice eligibility than those of the certifying agency
    - * Requirements by the certifying agency (ANCC, AANP) are necessary to maintain certification and recertify
  - ◊ Hours of practice: must have designated number of hours of practice as a nurse practitioner in order to maintain certification
  - ◊ Maintenance of license(s): must remain in good standing with state Board of Nursing

PRESCRIPTIVE AUTHORITY

- *Definition*: the legal right to direct, order, or designate the preparation of drugs or to order therapeutic devices for patients; this may be done in writing or by verbal order
- *Purpose*: to enable the nurse practitioner to efficiently function within the scope of practice
- Levels of prescriptive authority
  - ◊ Right to prescribe medications *including* controlled substances independent of physician involvement
  - ◊ Right to prescribe medications *including* controlled substances with some degree of physician involvement (term used to describe this relationship between a NP and a physician is "collaboration". Some states use the term "supervision".)
  - ◊ Right to prescribe medications *excluding* controlled substances independent of physician involvement
  - ◊ Right to prescribe medications *excluding* controlled substances with some degree of physician involvement
- No universal legislation for prescriptive authority
  - ◊ Power to authorize prescriptive authority lies with each state
  - ◊ Authority may be under sole supervision of Board of Nursing, Board of Medicine, or joint supervision
- The usual course for nurse practitioners (or other advanced practice nurses) to acquire prescriptive authority is via state statute. This implies that a bill authorizing such activity has passed through the state's legislature and has been signed by the

state's governor. In many states the actual rules are promulgated by the state Board of Nursing, state Board of Medicine, and/or the state Board of Pharmacy. Specific language indicates whether prescriptive authority may occur independent of physician relationship, in collaboration with a physician, or under the supervision of a physician. As of 2005 all 50 states allow some degree of prescriptive authority by nurse practitioners.

FISCAL ISSUES

Third-Party Payers

- Medicare: patient may or may not be enrolled with a managed care organization (MCO)
  - ◊ If patient not enrolled with an MCO, Medicare reimburses the health care provider on a fee-for-service basis
    - * The nurse practitioner must apply for a Medicare provider number in order to bill Medicare if the patient is not part of an MCO
    - * Nurse practitioners receive 85% of the physician's rate of payment if self-employed
    - * If the nurse practitioner is employed by a physician, the physician practice can receive 100% of payment under "incident to" rules
  - ◊ If patient enrolled in an MCO, Medicare pays the plan on a capitated basis. The MCO then reimburses the provider on either a fee-for-service basis or on a capitated basis
    - * A nurse practitioner must apply for admission to the MCO provider panel in order to be reimbursed through the MCO
- Medicaid patients may or may not be enrolled with an MCO
  - ◊ If the patient is not enrolled in an MCO, the nurse practitioner is reimbursed on a fee-for-service basis
    - * The nurse practitioner must apply to the state to be a Medicaid provider
    - * Medicaid pays 70-100% of physician's fee-for-service payment rate, depending on the individual policies of each state
  - ◊ If the patient is enrolled in an MCO, the nurse practitioner must apply for admission to the MCO provider panel. The nurse practitioner receives reimbursement from the MCO.
- Managed Care Organizations sell a health service package to their patients, who are agencies, or individuals
  - ◊ To provide care to a patient in an MCO, the nurse practitioner must apply to become a primary care provider (PCP)
    - * The nurse practitioner agrees to comply with the MCOs standards
    - * The MCO reimburses the PCP on either a fee-for-service, capitated, or combination fee-for-service/capitation basis
  - ◊ Credentialing is part of qualifying as a provider in an MCO
    - * The MCO collects information regarding education, certification, licensure, employment, and malpractice, then decides whether that provider is qualified to provide care to its members
  - ◊ The group-model MCO pays the provider a salary to provide health care for a group of patients
  - ◊ The practice-model MCO contracts with providers for services
- Indemnity insurers pay providers on a fee-for-service basis
  - ◊ Nurse practitioner submits a bill to the insurance company and is reimbursed according to the company's "usual and customary" charge for the particular service rather than the actual amount billed

  * Usual and customary charges are based on the average for that geographic area
  * Providers may collect (from the patient) the difference between the amount billed and the amount reimbursed by the insurer

RISK MANAGEMENT

- The concept of risk management is based on the assumption that injuries to patients and consequent litigation are preventable
  ◊ **Negligence** is the failure of an individual to do something that a reasonable person would do, and this results in injury to another
  ◊ **Malpractice** is professional negligence (i.e., the failure of a professional to perform his duty with the diligence, precaution, and degree of care that another professional in similar circumstances would display)
    * The failure to maintain standards of care results in a compensable injury

MALPRACTICE INSURANCE

- Recommended for all nurse practitioners
- Two types of malpractice policies:
  ◊ **Claims made**: only those claims made during the policy's period of coverage are honored
    * *Tail coverage* can be purchased to extend insurance coverage for claims made
  ◊ **Occurrence**: covers events occurring during the policy period, regardless of when the claim is filed

QUALITY IMPROVEMENT

- Definition: a system used to evaluate the quality of patient care
- Purpose
  ◊ To improve the quality of care delivered by the nurse practitioner or healthcare provider
  ◊ To evaluate, identify, and monitor quality of care delivered
  ◊ Provide a mechanism to evaluate overall practice, particular aspects of care delivered, and effectiveness of delivery
  ◊ To identify areas of improvement and excellence
  ◊ Provide a means of comparing delivery of care with others
- Methods of Review
  ◊ *Peer Review*: comparison of care provided with that (which would be) provided by a similar nurse practitioner in a similar region of the country
  ◊ *Auditing*: examination of medical documentation and other medical records for the purpose of evaluation
  ◊ *Patient satisfaction questionnaires*: evaluation of patient's health care experience

- ◊ *Outcomes Review*: evaluation of patient outcomes for the purpose of improving quality of care provided

PROFESSIONAL ORGANIZATIONS

- Examples of Nurse Practitioner Professional Organizations
  - ◊ National Association of Pediatric Nurse Practitioners (NAPNAP): the first NP organization
  - ◊ National Organization of Nurse Practitioner Faculties (NONPF)
  - ◊ American Association of Nurse Practitioners (AANP)
  - ◊ State specific nurse practitioner organizations (LANP: Louisiana Association of Nurse Practitioners)
- Importance to Profession and Individuals
  - ◊ Information source
  - ◊ Peer support
  - ◊ Advancement of the profession
  - ◊ Shape/determine/participate in development of legislative policies
  - ◊ Influence and develop goals and objectives
  - ◊ Continuing education

HEALTHY PEOPLE 2010

- A prevention agenda for the U.S. with 2 main goals:
  - ◊ Increase quality and years of healthy life
  - ◊ Eliminate Health Disparities
- Indicators used to measure the nation's health are:
  - ◊ Physical activity
  - ◊ Overweight and obesity
  - ◊ Tobacco use
  - ◊ Substance abuse
  - ◊ Responsible sexual behavior
  - ◊ Mental health
  - ◊ Injury and violence
  - ◊ Environmental quality
  - ◊ Immunization
  - ◊ Access to health care
- For more information see www.health.gov/healthypeople

References

Buppert, C. (1998). Reimbursement for nurse practitioner services. *The Nurse Practitioner, 23*(1), 67-81.

Buppert, C. (2001). Avoiding Medicare fraud part 2. *The Nurse Practitioner, 26*(2), 34-41.

Buppert, C. (2001). Avoiding Medicare fraud part 1. *The Nurse Practitioner, 26*(1), 70-75.

Buppert, C. (2003). Nurse practitioner's business practice and legal guide (2nd ed.). Houston, TX: Jones and Bartlet.

Burke, D., Pohl, J. M., & Franck, C. E. (2000). APN prescriptive authority and policy making: It's about more than winning. *The Nurse Practitioner, 25*(12), 8-11.

Joel, L.A. (2003). *Advanced practice nursing: Essentials for role development.* Philadelphia: F.A. Davis.

Hamric, A., Spross, J., & Hanson, C.M. (2004). *Advanced practice nursing: An integrative approach* (3rd ed.). St. Louis, MO: W.B. Saunders.

Mezey, M., & McGivern, D. (1993). *Nurses, Nurse Practitioners.* New York: Springer Publishing.

Price, L. (2005). Fright of passage. *Advance for Nurse Practitioners, 13*(6), 35-38.

Rustia, J., & Bartek, J. K. (1997). Managed care credentialing of advanced practice nurses. *The Nurse Practitioner, 22*(9), 90-103.

Shay, L. E. (2001). Provider and physician: title use in HMO provider panels. *The Nurse Practitioner 26*(3), 71-74.

Smolenski, M.C. (2005). Credentialing, certification, and competence: Issues for new and seasoned nurse practitioners. *Journal of the American Academy of Nurse Practitioners, 16,* 201-212.

Tumolo, J. (2005). Controversial, confident and committed: How a close-knit group of believers launched the NP profession. *Advance for Nurse Practitioners, 13*(7), 53-54.

Wetmore, B. (2005). Make your message work. *Advance for Nurse Practitioners, 13*(6), 39-42.

Zaumeyer, C. (1995). *The Nurse Practitioner as Entrepreneur: How to Establish and Operate an Independent Practice.* Fort Lauderdale: Women's Health Watch, Inc.

Zaumeyer, C. (2003). *How to start an independent practice: The nurse practitioner's guide to success.* Philadelphia: F.A. Davis.

18

RESPIRATORY DISORDERS

Respiratory Disorders

**Denotes pediatric diagnosis*

ACUTE BRONCHITIS

DESCRIPTION

Inflammation of the bronchioles, bronchi, and trachea; usually follows an upper respiratory infection or exposure to a chemical irritant.

ETIOLOGY

- Adenovirus
- Rhinovirus
- Influenza A and B
- Parainfluenza
- RSV
- Coxsackie virus
- Other viral agents
- Secondary bacterial infection from *Streptococcus pneumoniae, Haemophilus influenzae*, *Moraxella catarrhalis, Chlamydia pneumoniae, Bordetella pertussis,* or other bacteria

INCIDENCE

- Common

RISK FACTORS

- Upper respiratory infection
- Air pollutants
- Smoking and/or secondary exposure
- Reflux esophagitis
- Allergy
- Chronic obstructive pulmonary disease
- Acute and chronic sinusitis

ASSESSMENT FINDINGS

- Cough: dry and nonproductive, then productive, may be purulent
- Fatigue
- Fever due to infection with pathogens; more common in smokers and patients with COPD
- Burning chest
- Crackles, wheezes

DIFFERENTIAL DIAGNOSIS

- Pneumonia
- Tuberculosis
- Asthma
- Pertussis
- Influenza
- Sinusitis

DIAGNOSTIC STUDIES

- Consider chest x-ray: only if high index of suspicion of pneumonia or superimposed CHF
- Consider PPD: expect negative results
- Consider sputum culture: usually not diagnostic; often contains mixed flora
- CBC

PREVENTION

- Smoking cessation
- Avoid known respiratory irritants
- Treat underlying conditions which contribute to risk (asthma, gastroesophageal reflux disease, etc.)
- Influenza immunization in high-risk population

NONPHARMACOLOGIC MANAGEMENT

- Increase fluid intake
- Use humidifier
- Rest
- Smoking cessation
- Patient education regarding disease, treatment, and emergency actions

PHARMACOLOGIC MANAGEMENT

- Cough suppressants for nighttime
- Avoid antihistamines
- Antibiotics if organism is bacterial
- Decongestants and antihistamines are ineffective unless sinusitis or allergy are underlying
- Bronchodilators if wheezing

Antibiotics are commonly prescribed, but are not recommended.

AGENT	ACTION	COMMENTS
Cough suppressants *Examples:* dextromethorphan (Robitussin® DM, Delsym) Codeine (Robitussin® AC)	Suppresses cough in the medullary center of the brain	Avoid narcotic cough suppressants in COPDers and asthmatics. Potential drug intervention with MAOI and some SSRIs.
benzonatate (Tessalon®)	Topical anesthetic effect on the respiratory stretch receptors	Do not break or chew capsule – may reduce patient's gag reflex. Monitor for dizziness, drowsiness, and visual changes.

CONSULTATION/REFERRAL

- Refer to pulmonologist if not improved after 14-21 days

FOLLOW-UP

- 7 days if not improved or if condition worsens
- High-risk groups (i.e., those with co-existing disease) are usually followed up sooner

EXPECTED COURSE

- Symptoms of shorter duration if causative agent is rhinovirus or coronavirus
- Symptoms may persist up to 3-4 weeks

POSSIBLE COMPLICATIONS

- Pneumonia
- Chronic cough
- Chronic bronchitis
- Secondary bacterial infection

CHRONIC BRONCHITIS

DESCRIPTION

The production of sputum for at least 3 months annually for 2 consecutive years accompanied by cough. Chronic mucus production results from hyperplasia of the mucous membranes (hallmark) lining the bronchial walls. This is usually an **irreversible and progressive** airway disease. The majority of patients has coexisting emphysema and is classified as having chronic obstructive pulmonary disease (COPD), an irreversible airway disease (*see* Emphysema).

ETIOLOGY

- Prolonged exposure to bronchial irritants

INCIDENCE

- Common (14.2 million people have COPD)
- 12.5 million have chronic bronchitis
- Fourth leading cause of death in US
- Typical patient is male smoker in his fifties

RISK FACTORS

- Cigarette smoking (90% attributable to smoking)
- Chronic respiratory infections
- Chronic, poorly controlled respiratory allergies

ASSESSMENT FINDINGS

- Symptoms usually begin in 50s age group
- Chronic, productive cough – worse in a.m.
- Sputum production
- Dyspnea on exertion
- Increased respiratory rate
- Crackles and wheezes
- Barrel chest
- Prolonged expiratory phase

- Secondary polycythemia (HCT > 52% in males, HCT > 47% in females)
- Tobacco staining of fingers and/or teeth
- Signs of right-sided heart failure

DIFFERENTIAL DIAGNOSIS

- Asthma
- Congestive heart failure
- Pneumonia
- Asbestosis

DIAGNOSTIC STUDIES

- Spirometry defines severity and response to therapy
- FEV_1/FVC ratio (<70% constitutes diagnosis)

FEV_1 (forced expiratory volume in one second) **FVC (forced vital capacity)**

- Chest x-ray (may see hyperinflation and/or flattened diaphragm)
- Consider CBC, PPD, ABGs, pulse oximetry, ECG
- For patients 45-50 years, consider testing for α-1-protease inhibitor deficiency

Classification of Severity		
Stage 0	*At risk*	Normal spirometry; cough, sputum production
Stage 1	*Mild COPD*	FEV_1 ≥80% predicted
Stage 2	*Moderate*	FEV_1 <80% and ≥ 50% predicted
Stage 3	*Moderately severe*	FEV_1 <50% and ≥30% predicted
Stage 4	*Severe*	FEV_1 <30% predicted

Note: From Global Strategy for Diagnosis, Management, and Prevention of Chronic Obstructive Pulmonary Disease, 2004.

PREVENTION

- Avoid cigarette smoking
- Minimize exposure to known respiratory irritants
- Once diagnosed: Pneumococcal immunization, influenza immunization annually, minimize exposure to persons with known respiratory infections

NONPHARMACOLOGIC MANAGEMENT

- Adequate fluid intake
- Postural drainage
- Smoking cessation
- Regular exercise training
- Pursed-lip breathing
- Diaphragmatic exercises
- Consider pulmonary rehabilitation
- Patient education regarding disease, treatment, early signs and symptoms of infection, pursed lip breathing, emergency treatment for respiratory distress
- Avoid travel at high altitudes

PHARMACOLOGIC MANAGEMENT

Stage 1	Bronchodilator (BD) PRN
Stage 2	Long-acting anticholinergic plus albuterol (as rescue med); or long-acting BD plus anticholinergic, albuterol or combo
Stage 3	Long-acting anticholinergic plus long-acting BD; short-acting BD as rescue med; inhaled corticosteroid for recurrent exacerbations
Stage 4	Long-acting BD plus long-acting anticholinergic; inhaled corticosteroid; consider theophylline for insufficient response; short-acting BD for rescue

Note: From Global Strategy for Diagnosis, Management, and Prevention of Chronic Obstructive Pulmonary Disease, 2004.

AGENT	ACTION	COMMENTS
Bronchodilators ***Short-acting*** *Examples:* albuterol (Ventolin®) *(may be inhaled or nebulized)*	Stimulate beta 2 receptors in the lungs causing bronchodilation	Can increase heart rate, blood pressure, and cause QT prolongation and ST segment depression.
Long-acting *Examples:* Salmeterol (Serevent®) Formoterol (Foradil®)	Stimulate beta 2 receptors in the lungs causing bronchodilation	Do not use long-acting agents for immediate relief of acute symptoms. These agents take 15-20 min to produce bronchodilation. Albuterol produces bronchodilation rapidly and should be used for rapid symptom relief. Tolerance develops with prolonged use.
Xanthine *Examples:* theophylline (Slo-Phyllin®, Theo®-24, Theo-Dur®) aminophylline (Phyllocontin®)	Cause bronchodilation by relaxing smooth muscle of the bronchi and pulmonary blood vessels. The xanthines are central respiratory stimulants and reduce fatigability in COPDers	Must monitor levels (10-20 mcg/ml is desirable). Elevated levels predispose patient to ventricular arrhythmias, seizures. Monitor for tremors, anxiety, and jitteriness. Many food-drug interactions involving CYP 450 system.
Anticholinergics ***Short-acting*** *Example:* ipratropium(Atrovent®) ***Long-acting*** *Example:* tiotropium (Spiriva®)	Blocks action of acetylcholine and thus, causes mild bronchodilation and prevents bronchoconstrictions.	Not indicated for relief of acute bronchospasm. Works well in conjunction with a bronchodilator.
Inhaled corticosteroids *Examples:* triamcinolone (Azmacort®) fluticasone (Flovent®) budesonide (Pulmicort®)	Glucocorticoids decrease activity of inflammatory cells and mediators. Steroid activity is local (in the lungs) and is associated with minimal systemic absorption	Slowly wean patients who are on oral steroids to inhaled steroids. Abrupt withdrawal can cause symptoms of adrenal insufficiency (fatigue, weakness, and hypotension). Monitor for symptoms of fungal infection in the mouth and pharynx.

CONSULTATION/REFERRAL

- Consult specialist for patients with signs/symptoms of right-sided heart failure and/or respiratory distress/failure

FOLLOW-UP

- Follow-up visits every 3-6 months for stable disease
- Maintain close follow-up with patients with acute respiratory infections
- Review treatment program with patient at each visit

EXPECTED COURSE

- Irreversible, chronic disease with frequent exacerbations and remissions

POSSIBLE COMPLICATIONS

- Frequent serious pulmonary infections
- Acute bronchospasm
- Congestive heart failure
- Acute respiratory failure

EMPHYSEMA

DESCRIPTION

Lung disease characterized by enlargement of the alveolar ducts and air spaces distal to the terminal bronchioles. The mechanism by which alveolar walls are destroyed is incompletely understood, but these results in air trapping and loss of elastic recoil of the lungs. This is usually an **irreversible and progressive** airway disease. The majority of patients have coexisting chronic bronchitis and are classified as having chronic obstructive pulmonary disease (COPD), an irreversible airway disease (*see* Chronic Bronchitis).

ETIOLOGY

- 14.2 million people have COPD
- 1.7 million have emphysema
- 4th leading cause of death in US
- < 1% of cases due to α-1-antitrypsin deficiency (contributes to premature emphysema); consider if patient is nonsmoker and < 45-50 years old
- Remainder of cases due to alveolar wall destruction from known and unknown causes

INCIDENCE

- Major cause of disability in the U.S.
- Males > Females
- Age > 40 years

RISK FACTORS

- Cigarette smoking most common cause
- Passive smoke
- Chronic pulmonary infections, allergies
- Chronic exposure to lung irritants (e.g., asbestos)
- α-1-antitrypsin deficiency

ASSESSMENT FINDINGS

- Disease begins early in adult life, but symptoms usually appear in the fifties
- Smoker's cough often present
- Dyspnea on exertion most common complaint
- Cough, wheezes
- Inability to take a deep breath
- Slowed, prolonged expiration
- Barrel chest
- Diminished breath sounds
- Clubbing of fingers
- Varying degrees of respiratory distress
- Diffuse pulmonary fibrosis
- Often significant weight loss

DIFFERENTIAL DIAGNOSIS

- Congestive heart failure
- Asthma
- Combination of chronic bronchitis/emphysema
- Chronic sinusitis
- Tuberculosis
- Mesothelioma (asbestos exposure)

DIAGNOSTIC STUDIES

- Spirometry defines severity and response to therapy
- FEV_1/FVC ratio (<70% constitutes diagnosis)
- FEV_1 (forced expiratory volume in one second)
- FVC (forced vital capacity)
- Consider CBC, PPD, ABGs, pulse oximetry, ECG
- α-1-antitrypsin level: positive in 1% of patients
- Chest x-ray: emphysematous changes, hyperinflation, flattened diaphragm
- Hematocrit and hemoglobin to determine severity of chronic hypoxemia
- Electrocardiogram: to exclude cardiac disease

PREVENTION

- Avoid cigarette smoking
- Avoid inhaling known respiratory irritants

- Once diagnosed: Pneumococcal immunization, influenza immunization annually, minimize exposure to persons with known respiratory infections

NONPHARMACOLOGIC MANAGEMENT

- Adequate fluid intake
- Postural drainage
- Smoking cessation
- Regular exercise training
- Pursed-lip breathing
- Diaphragmatic exercises
- Consider pulmonary rehabilitation
- Teach patients early signs and symptoms of infection
- Avoid travel at high altitude

PHARMACOLOGIC MANAGEMENT

Stage 1	Bronchodilator (BD) PRN
Stage 2	Long-acting anticholinergic plus albuterol (as rescue med); or long-acting BD plus anticholinergic, albuterol or combo
Stage 3	Long-acting anticholinergic plus long-acting BD; short-acting BD as rescue med; inhaled corticosteroid for recurrent exacerbations
Stage 4	Long-acting BD plus long-acting anticholinergic; inhaled corticosteroid; consider theophylline for insufficient response; short-acting BD for rescue

Note: From Global Strategy for Diagnosis, Management, and Prevention of Chronic Obstructive Pulmonary Disease, 2004.

AGENT	ACTION	COMMENTS
Bronchodilators ***Short-acting*** *Examples:* albuterol (Ventolin®) *(may be inhaled or nebulized)*	Stimulates beta 2 receptors in the lungs causing bronchodilation	Can increase heart rate, blood pressure, and cause QT prolongation and ST segment depression.
Long-acting *Examples:* Salmeterol (Serevent®) Formoterol (Foradil®)	Stimulate beta 2 receptors in the lungs causing bronchodilation	Do not use long-acting agents for immediate relief of acute symptoms. These agents take 15-20 min to produce bronchodilation. Albuterol produces bronchodilation rapidly and should be used for rapid symptom relief. Tolerance develops with prolonged use.
Xanthine *Examples:* theophylline (Slo-Phyllin®, Theo®-24, Theo-Dur®) aminophylline (Phyllocontin®)	Cause bronchodilation by relaxing smooth muscle of the bronchi and pulmonary blood vessels. The xanthines are central respiratory stimulants and reduce fatigability in COPDers	Must monitor levels (10-20 mcg/ml is desirable). Elevated levels predispose patient to ventricular arrhythmias, seizures. Monitor for tremors, anxiety, and jitteriness. Many food-drug interactions involving CYP 450 system.
Anticholinergics ***Short-acting*** *Example:* ipratropium(Atrovent®) ***Long-acting*** *Example:* tiotropium (Spiriva®)	Blocks action of acetylcholine and thus, causes mild bronchodilation and prevents bronchoconstriction	Not indicated for relief of acute bronchospasm. Works well in conjunction with a bronchodilator.
Inhaled corticosteroids *Examples:* triamcinolone (Azmacort®) fluticasone (Flovent®) budesonide (Pulmicort®)	Glucocorticoids decrease activity of inflammatory cells and mediators. Steroid activity is local (in the lungs) and is associated with minimal systemic absorption	Slowly wean patients who are on oral steroids to inhaled steroids. Abrupt withdrawal can cause symptoms of adrenal insufficiency (fatigue, weakness, and hypotension). Monitor for symptoms of fungal infection in the mouth and pharynx.

CONSULTATION/REFERRAL

- Consult specialist for any patient with signs/symptoms of right-sided heart failure and/or respiratory distress/failure

FOLLOW-UP

- Follow-up visits every 3-6 months for stable disease
- Monthly follow-up for unstable patients
- Maintain close follow-up with patients with acute respiratory infections
- Review treatment program with patient at each visit

EXPECTED COURSE

- A irreversible, chronic disease with frequent exacerbations and remissions

POSSIBLE COMPLICATIONS

- Frequent serious pulmonary infections
- Congestive heart failure
- Acute respiratory failure

ASTHMA

DESCRIPTION

A chronic, respiratory disease characterized by **reversible** airway obstruction, inflammation, and airway hyperresponsiveness. Symptoms range from occasional and mild to severe and debilitating.

ETIOLOGY

- Inflammation of the bronchial mucosa and spasm of the bronchial smooth muscle leads to narrowing of the small and occasionally large airways
- Produces characteristic cough and wheezing

INCIDENCE

- About 15 million Americans have asthma
- Most common disease of early childhood
- Leading cause of missed school days

RISK FACTORS

- History of allergies
- Family history
- Cigarette smoke exposure
- Cockroaches and dust
- Gastroesophageal reflux disease (GERD)
- Viral respiratory infection in susceptible individuals (RSV)
- Exercise
- Cold air intolerance
- Chronic sinusitis

ASSESSMENT FINDINGS

- Cough is the earliest symptom
- Wheezes
- Hyperresonance
- Prolonged expiration
- Accessory muscle use
- Sudden nocturnal dyspnea
- Decreased exercise tolerance
- Normal growth and development in children even with frequent steroid use

Classification of Severity	
Mild intermittent	Symptoms $\leq$ 2 days per week ***or*** $\leq$2 nights per month Exacerbations brief
Mild persistent	Symptoms $\geq$ 2 times per week, but < 1 time per day ***or*** < 2 nights per month
Moderate persistent	Daily symptoms ***or*** more than 1 night per week
Severe persistent	Continual symptoms ***or*** frequent nighttime symptoms

Note: From National Heart, Lung, and Blood Institute, *National Asthma Education and Prevention Program Expert Panel Report 2: Guidelines for the diagnosis and Management of Asthma*, 2004.

DIFFERENTIAL DIAGNOSIS

- Respiratory infections

- Congestive heart failure
- GERD
- Habitual cough
- Tuberculosis
- Foreign body aspiration, especially in children

DIAGNOSTIC STUDIES

- Spirometry
- Pulmonary function tests
- Consider allergy testing
- Peak flow monitoring
- Methacholine challenge test

PREVENTION

- Learn early signs and symptoms of asthma exacerbation
- Influenza and pneumococcal pneumonia immunizations
- Monitor peak flow values
- Learn correct use of inhalers, spacers, and other medications
- Implement prearranged action plan for asthma exacerbations

NONPHARMACOLOGIC MANAGEMENT

- Peak flow monitoring
- Avoidance of asthma triggers if possible
- Patient and family education regarding disease, treatment, avoidance of triggers, asthma management plan, and emergency actions

PHARMACOLOGIC MANAGEMENT

Mild intermittent	Short-acting bronchodilator for exacerbations
Mild persistent	**Preferred treatment**: low dose inhaled corticosteroids **Alternative treatment**: cromolyn, leukotriene , OR sustained-release theophylline (serum concentration 5-15 mcg/mL) Short-acting bronchodilator for exacerbations Consider leukotriene blocker (Singulair®, Accolate®)
Moderate persistent	**Preferred treatment**: low to medium dose inhaled corticosteroid and long-acting inhaled bronchodilator **Alternative treatment**: low to medium dose inhaled corticosteroid and either leukotriene blocker or theophylline Short-acting bronchodilator for exacerbations
Severe persistent	**Preferred treatment:** high dose inhaled corticosteroids and long acting inhaled bronchodilators ***AND*** if needed, oral corticosteroids (2mg/kg/day not to exceed 60mg/day) Short-acting bronchodilator for exacerbations

Note: From National Heart, Lung, and Blood Institute, *National Asthma Education and Prevention Program Expert Panel Report 2: Guidelines for the diagnosis and Management of Asthma*, 2004.

For infants and children <5 years of age:	
Mild intermittent	Short-acting bronchodilator for exacerbations
Mild persistent	**Preferred treatment**: low dose inhaled corticosteroids **Alternative treatment**: cromolyn, leukotriene Short-acting bronchodilator for exacerbations Consider leukotriene blocker (Singulair®)
Moderate persistent	**Preferred treatment:** low dose inhaled corticosteroid and long-acting inhaled bronchodilator OR medium dose inhaled corticosteroid **Alternative treatment:** low dose inhaled corticosteroid and either leukotriene blocker or theophylline Short-acting bronchodilator for exacerbations

Severe persistent	**Preferred treatment:** high dose inhaled corticosteroids and long acting inhaled bronchodilators ***AND*** if needed, oral corticosteroids (2mg/kg/day not to exceed 60mg/day) Short-acting bronchodilator for exacerbations Cromolyn (Intal®) preferred over steroids if provides adequate symptom management Nebulized bronchodilator preferred over metered dose inhaler Use spacer/holding chamber and face mask

Note: From National Heart, Lung, and Blood Institute, *National Asthma Education and Prevention Program Expert Panel Report 2: Guidelines for the diagnosis and Management of Asthma*, 2004.

AGENT	ACTION	COMMENTS
Bronchodilators ***Short-acting*** *Examples:* albuterol (Ventolin®) *(may be inhaled or nebulized)*	Stimulate beta 2 receptors in the lungs causing bronchodilation	Can increase heart rate, blood pressure, and cause QT prolongation and ST segment depression.
Long-acting *Examples:* Salmeterol (Serevent®) Formoterol (Foradil®)	Stimulate beta 2 receptors in the lungs causing bronchodilation	Do not use long-acting agents for immediate relief of acute symptoms. These agents take 15-20 min to produce bronchodilation. Albuterol produces bronchodilation rapidly and should be used for rapid symptom relief. Tolerance develops with prolonged use.
Xanthines *Examples:* theophylline (Slo-Phyllin®, Theo®-24, Theo-Dur®) aminophylline (Phyllocontin®)	Cause bronchodilation by relaxing smooth muscle of the bronchi and pulmonary blood vessels. The xanthines are central respiratory stimulants and reduce fatigability in COPDers	Must monitor levels (10-20 mcg/ml is desirable). Elevated levels predispose patient to ventricular arrhythmias, seizures. Monitor for tremors, anxiety, and jitteriness. Many food drug interactions involving CYP 450 system.
Anticholinergic ***Short-acting*** *Example:* ipratropium(Atrovent®) ***Long-acting*** *Example:* Tiotropium (Spiriva®)	Blocks action of acetylcholine and thus causes mild bronchodilation and prevents bronchoconstrictions	Not indicated for relief of acute bronchospasm. Works well in conjunction with a bronchodilator.
Inhaled corticosteroids *Examples:* triamcinolone (Azmacort®) fluticasone (Flovent®) budesonide (Pulmicort®)	Glucocorticoids decrease activity of inflammatory cells and mediators Steroid activity is local (in the lungs) and is associated with minimal systemic absorption	Slowly wean patients who are on oral steroids to inhaled steroids. Abrupt withdrawal can cause symptoms of adrenal insufficiency (fatigue, weakness, and hypotension). Monitor for symptoms of fungal infection in the mouth and pharynx.

AGENT	ACTION	COMMENTS
Leukotriene blockers *Examples:* zafirlukast (Accolate®) montelukast (Singulair®)	Leukotriene blockers inhibit the action of leukotrienes which are released from mast cells and eosinophils and are associated with airway edema, increased inflammatory activity, and smooth muscle contraction	These agents are not substitutes for bronchodilators or inhaled steroids. Take daily. Monitor for drug interactions with zafirlukast.

PREGNANCY/LACTATION CONSIDERATIONS

- Stress importance of prevention
- Poor control can result in low birth weight infants, premature labor/delivery, increased risk of fetal mortality
- Aggressive treatment of symptoms with steroids, bronchodilators, and theophylline if needed

CONSULTATION/REFERRAL

- Allergist/pulmonologist for patients with severe persistent asthma

FOLLOW-UP

- As needed to educate patient, parent, caregiver about disease and management
- Every 3-6 months for stable disease

EXPECTED COURSE

- Excellent with proper use of medications and patient education
- Small percentage of patients have poor control even with proper medication use
- Risk of mortality increased by: nocturnal symptoms, history of intubation for asthma, history of hospitalization/ICU admission for asthma, >3 emergency department visits annually for asthma, and oral steroid dependence.

POSSIBLE COMPLICATIONS

- Respiratory failure/death from unrelieved bronchospasms
- Steroid dependence

PNEUMONIA

DESCRIPTION

Infection of the lung which may include the parenchyma, alveolar spaces, and/or interstitial tissue. It can be confined to a lobe (*lobar pneumonia*), a segment of a lobe (*segmental pneumonia*), the interstitial tissue (*interstitial pneumonia*), or alveolar/bronchi (*bronchopneumonia*). Pneumonia is commonly classified as community acquired (CAP) or nosocomial.

ETIOLOGY

Adults:

- Viruses
- Bacteria are most common cause
    - ◊ *Streptococcus pneumoniae* (accounts for 30-50%)
    - ◊ *Haemophilus influenzae* (common in smokers)
    - ◊ *Chlamydia pneumoniae*
    - ◊ *Moraxella catarrhalis*
    - ◊ *Legionella pneumophila*
    - ◊ *Klebsiella pneumoniae*
    - ◊ Anaerobic bacteria (common with aspiration)

Young adults and older children:

- *Mycoplasma pneumoniae* (most common cause)
- Viruses
- *Chlamydia pneumoniae* (NOT the same agent that causes chlamydial pneumonia in

newborns at 3-8 weeks which is *Chlamydia trachomatis*)

Children and infants:

- Viral agents are most common cause
- Respiratory syncytial virus
- Adenovirus
- Parainfluenza
- Influenza A and B
- Bacteria
  - ◊ *Streptococcus pneumoniae*
  - ◊ *Haemophilus influenzae*

Immunocompromised individuals:

- *Pneumocystis carinii*

INCIDENCE

- 2-3 million people in the U.S. get pneumonia annually
- 6th leading cause of death
- Most common cause of death from infectious disease

RISK FACTORS

- Age extremes (very young, very old)
- Other respiratory viral infections
- Cigarette smoking
- Chronic diseases (e.g., diabetes, renal disease, COPD, CAD, CHF)
- Alcoholism
- Institutionalization
- Poor cough effort
- GERD

ASSESSMENT FINDINGS

- Cough (often productive)
- Fever
- Malaise/fatigue
- Sudden chills
- Chest pain (pleuritic)
- Sputum production
- Increased respirations and pulse
- Diminished breath sounds
- Consolidation on percussion
- Egophony (*e* to *a* changes)
- Bronchophony: voice sounds are louder and clearer than normal
- Whispered pectoriloquy: whispered sounds are louder and clearer than normal
- Tactile fremitus

SPECIFIC ASSESSMENT FINDINGS/PATIENT PROFILES/ SYMPTOMATOLOGY

Pneumococcal pneumonia:

- Preceded by a URI
- Chills, fever
- Chest pain
- Dry cough becoming productive of rusty-colored sputum
- Myalgias
- GI symptoms

Klebsiella pneumoniae pneumonia:

- Upper lobe involvement
- Currant jelly sputum
- Tissue necrosis
- Mortality rate is 25-50%

Haemophilus influenzae pneumonia:

- Younger age group if not vaccinated
- Coryza as prodrome
- Underlying lung disease present in adults or other pre-existing disease

Legionella pneumophila pneumonia:

- Common in middle-aged males
- Smokers
- Alcohol abusers
- Immunosuppressed patients
- Prodrome resembles influenza
- Fever
- Headache
- Neurological manifestations
- Nonproductive cough becomes productive of mucoid sputum
- Relative bradycardia

Mycoplasma pneumonia *(primary atypical pneumonia):*

- Typically in <35 year old age group
- Malaise
- Sore throat
- Dry cough
- Paroxysmal coughing
- Disease generally mild and resolution is spontaneous (though may take 6 weeks with treatment)
- Maculopapular rash (10-20% of the time)

Chlamydial pneumonia:

- Cough
- Fever
- Sputum production
- Not seriously ill

Viral pneumonia:

- Headache
- Fever
- Myalgia
- Cough productive of mucopurulent sputum
- Overall milder symptoms than bacterial pneumonias

DIFFERENTIAL DIAGNOSIS

- Acute bronchitis
- Bronchiolitis
- Asthma
- Croup
- Congestive heart failure
- Bronchogenic carcinoma
- Tuberculosis

DIAGNOSTIC STUDIES

- PA and lateral chest x-ray (infiltrates present)
- CBC with differential
- Gram stain and sputum specimen (no test for an etiologic agent recommended if outpatient)

PREVENTION

- Influenza and pneumococcal pneumonia immunizations
- Smoking cessation
- High-risk individuals should avoid crowds

NONPHARMACOLOGIC MANAGEMENT

- Hydration with increased fluids
- Analgesia for pain
- Reduced activity during acute phase
- Patient education regarding disease, treatment, emergency actions

PHARMACOLOGIC MANAGEMENT

- Treatment based on immunocompetent patients
- Empiric antibiotic treatment based on patient age, comorbidity, immunization status, risk factors etc.

Outpatient, previously health, no recent antibiotic (AB)	Macrolide (erythromycin, azithromycin, or clarithromycin) ***OR*** doxycycline
Outpatient, previously healthy, recent AB:	Respiratory fluoroquinolone (FQ); ***OR*** advanced macrolide (azithromycin or clarithromycin) plus high dose amoxicillin; ***OR*** advanced macrolide plus high dose amoxicillin/clavulanate
Outpatient, co-morbidities (COPD, diabetes, renal or CHF, or malignancy), *no recent AB*:	advanced macrolide; ***OR*** respiratory FQ
Outpatient, co-morbidities, recent AB:	respiratory FQ ***OR*** advanced macrolide plus a beta-lactam (high dose amoxicillin, high dose amoxicillin/ clavulanate, cefpodoxime, cefprozil, or cefuroxime)

Note: From Infectious Disease Society of America, *Practice guidelines for management of community acquired pneumonia*, 2003.

AGENT	ACTION	COMMENTS
Macrolides *Examples:* erythromycin (E-mycin®) azithromycin (Zithromax®) clarithromycin (Biaxin®)	Antibiotic binds to the 50S subunit of susceptible organisms and prevents protein synthesis	Erythromycin is not active against *H. influenza* infections. Erythromycin commonly causes GI upset. Macrolides are particularly effective with Staph and Strep infections as well as lower respiratory tract pathogens and atypical organisms (*Chlamydia pneumoniae, Mycoplasma pneumoniae, Legionella species*) Monitor for drug interactions especially with erythromycin.
Fluoroquinolones *Examples:* levofloxacin (Levaquin®) moxifloxacin (Avelox®) gatifloxacin (Tequin®)	Antibiotic inhibits the action of DNA gyrase which is essential for the organism to be able to replicate itself	Broad-spectrum antibacterial agents. Monitor for QT prolongation and photosensitivity. Avoid in children < 18 years old and in pregnant women due to potential adverse effects on bone and cartilage formation. Monitor for hypoglycemic reactions. Absorption significantly affected by dairy product consumption and multivitamins, especially containing calcium and iron.
Tetracyclines *Examples:* Tetracycline (Sumycin®) doxycycline (Doryx®, Vibramycin®)	Tetracyclines inhibit protein synthesis	Tetracyclines are active against many species of *Mycoplasma pneumoniae, Haemophilus influenzae, Klebsiella* (respiratory species) and *Strep pneumoniae.* Monitor for photosensitivity. Avoid in pregnant and lactating women and children < 8 years old due to discoloration of teeth. Never take expired tetracyclines since they are highly nephrotoxic. Absorption is diminished if taken with food or dairy products.
Penicillins *Examples:* amoxicillin (Amoxil®, Trimox®) amoxicillin and potassium clavulanate (Augmentin® XR, Augmentin®) ampicillin (Principen®)	Penicillins inhibit cell wall synthesis. They are most effective during active multiplication of pathogenic bacteria	Monitor for hypersensitivity reactions (1-10% of patients taking PCN products will report allergy). Safe use during pregnancy and in children. Penicillin (given in high enough concentrations) is effective against Strep species in the lower respiratory tract. In species that produce beta-lactamase, amoxicillin, and ampicillin are ineffective. Amoxicillin/potassium clavulanate is effective against organisms that produce beta-lactamase.
Cephalosporins ***Second generation*** *Examples:* cefprozil (Cefzil®) cefuroxime (Ceftin®) cefaclor (Ceclor®)	Inhibit cell wall synthesis of bacteria. Contains beta lactam ring like PCN. Provides coverage of many Gram positive and Gram negative bacteria but NOT those organisms that produce beta lactamase.	Well tolerated Cross sensitivity (≈2-10%) with PCN. Do NOT administer if patient has had anaphylactic response to PCN.
Third generation *Examples:* cefdinir (Omnicef®) cefixime (Suprax®) ceftibuten (Cedax®) cefpodoxime (Vantin®)	Exactly as for second generation cephalosporins but covers many more Gram negative organisms and is protected, if the organism produces beta-lactamase	Same as for second generation cephalosporins. Good choice if patient is PCN allergic and needs beta lactamase coverage.

PREGNANCY/LACTATION CONSIDERATIONS

- Doxycycline should not be used (pregnancy category D)
- Doxycycline is excreted in breast milk
- Influenza immunization may be used in pregnancy during 2nd or 3rd trimester
- Quinolones contraindicated in pregnant patients

CONSULTATION/REFERRAL

- Consider referral for patients who appear toxic, have severe shortness of breath, have worsening symptoms despite treatment

FOLLOW-UP

- Depends on severity of illness and patient's general state of health
- Within 24-72 hours as condition warrants
- Consider follow-up chest x-ray 4-6 weeks after treatment completed in patients over 40 years and smokers (bronchogenic carcinoma often presents as pneumonia)

EXPECTED COURSE

- Excellent prognosis with proper treatment
- Improvement should take place 48-72 hours after treatment initiation
- Poor prognosis for patients at age extremes, presence of comorbidities, immunocompromised states, poorly controlled diabetics

POSSIBLE COMPLICATIONS

- Empyema
- Respiratory failure
- Adult respiratory distress syndrome
- Death

TUBERCULOSIS (TB)
(Consumption)

DESCRIPTION

Chronic, recurrent infection which primarily affects the lungs (effected organ in 85% of cases) but which can affect any organ in the human body; 90-95% of primary infections go unrecognized. There are 3 stages:

- Primary or initial infection
- Latent or dormant infection
- Recrudescent

ETIOLOGY

- *Mycobacterium tuberculosis*
- *Mycobacterium bovis*
- *Mycobacterium africanum*

INCIDENCE

- U.S. rates vary according to risk factors (age, race, gender, socioeconomic status)
- Rates range from 10-200/100,000 in the U.S. (higher rates among those with risk factors)
- Incidence decreasing in U.S.

RISK FACTORS

- Homelessness
- Closes contact with an infected individual
- Asian, African, Latin American immigrants (within 5 years)
- Institutionalization (e.g., prisons, nursing homes, mental hospitals)
- Health care workers (particularly those working with HIV-positive populations)
- Immunocompromised (particularly HIV-positive patients, steroid use, cancer patients)
- Chronic disease (HIV, DM, renal failure)

ASSESSMENT FINDINGS

- Cough
- Night sweats
- Fever
- Hemoptysis
- Weight loss

DIFFERENTIAL DIAGNOSIS

- Pneumonia
- Bronchitis
- Pulmonary fungal infections
- Tumor

DIAGNOSTIC STUDIES

- Mantoux skin testing using purified protein derivative (PPD) is the primary screening tool: induration as described below
- False positive skin test if BCG vaccine used
- False negative skin test: steroid use, HIV infection, new-onset TB infection, anergy, age < 6 months
- Chest x-ray: may show infiltrates, cavitary lesions and/or hilar adenopathy
- Sputum culture/sensitivity (obtain at least 3 early morning specimens): positive for organism (takes 2-6 weeks for results)
- Acid-fast bacillus (AFB) stain: red rods

TB SKIN TESTS CONSIDERED POSITIVE IF at 48-72 hours:
Induration ≥ 5 mm and:
◊ Recent close contact with person with active TB ◊ HIV patient or someone immunocompromised ◊ Clinical evidence of disease
Induration ≥ 10 mm and:
◊ Injecting drug user ◊ Contact with high-risk groups (e.g., health care workers) ◊ Immigrants from countries where TB is prevalent ◊ Children <4 years, children, and adolescents exposed to adults at high risk ◊ Members of high-risk populations
Induration ≥ 15 mm and:
◊ Anyone who is not a member of the above populations

Note: From U.S. Department of Health and Human Services, *Core curriculum on tuberculosis*, 2000.

Anyone with a positive PPD is considered infected until proven otherwise. Anyone with a positive PPD AND signs and symptoms is defined as having active disease.

PREVENTION

- Avoid contact with known infected persons
- Reporting by health care providers
- Careful tracking of known patients to insure proper treatment
- PPD screening annually for persons with risk factors
- Complete course of therapy once initiated

NONPHARMACOLOGIC MANAGEMENT

- Notification of local health department
- Identification of contacts
- Respiratory precautions as long as patient is contagious
- Activity as tolerated for patient
- Patient education regarding disease, treatment, importance of completion of drug regimen, treatment of contacts, etc.

PHARMACOLOGIC MANAGEMENT

- Drugs commonly used to treat TB:
  - ◊ Isoniazid (INH)
  - ◊ Rifampin (RIF)
  - ◊ Pyrazinamide (PZA)
  - ◊ Streptomycin (SM)
  - ◊ Ethambutol (EMB)
- For active disease, multi-drug regimens are recommended
- HIV-positive patients: treat with minimum of 3 drugs
- For severe disease: use of 4 drugs for first 2-3 months is indicated

Multi-drug regimens change frequently as resistance develops.

IMPORTANT NOTES ABOUT MEDICATIONS

- Pyridoxine for patients taking isoniazid to
- prevent peripheral neuritis, especially in children, adolescents, and pregnant women
- Alternative drug for regimen is ethambutol
  - ◊ Optic neuritis possible (only use in patients who can cooperate for vision and color checks)

- Streptomycin should NOT be prescribed longer than 12 weeks due to possible ototoxicity
- Rifampin colors tears, urine, perspiration orange, can stain contact lenses; may decrease effectiveness of oral contraceptives

PREGNANCY/LACTATION CONSIDERATIONS

- Drugs considered safe to use during pregnancy are: isoniazid, ethambutol (add pyridoxine) and rifampin
- Avoid streptomycin (ototoxicity, nephrotoxicity)
- Breast-feeding OK during TB treatment

CONSULTATION/REFERRAL

- Refer patients to local health department for treatment. Close contacts should be screened as well.

FOLLOW-UP

- Liver function studies for patients taking INH, PZA, RIF and in HIV positive patients, pregnant patients or anyone with liver disease
- Monthly sputum cultures until 2 consecutive negative cultures
- If cultures positive after 2 months of treatment, consider poor compliance and re-assess sensitivity
- Chest x-ray every 2-3 months during treatment
- Chest x-ray for any changes in symptomatology

EXPECTED COURSE

- Good prognosis if drug treatment regimen followed
- Poor prognosis for severely infected patients or HIV patients with multi drug resistant organisms

POSSIBLE COMPLICATIONS

- Cavitary lesions
- Drug resistance
- Spread to other body organs

PERTUSSIS

DESCRIPTION

A respiratory disease which has 3 stages:

- Catarrhal stage: upper respiratory symptoms and mild cough (1-2 weeks)
- Paroxysmal stage: cough (2-4 weeks)
- Convalescent stage: cough is still present (1-2 weeks)

ETIOLOGY

- *Bordetella pertussis* spread by respiratory droplets, direct or indirect contact with secretions (highly communicable)

INCIDENCE

- Common in infants unimmunized or partially immunized
- 10-20% of adults who cough >14 days have pertussis
- 2.7 cases per 100,000 in US
- 80% of cases occur in ages < 18 years
- Incidence among adolescents and adults has increased 60% since late 1990's
- Pertussis immunization may lose effectiveness as one ages

RISK FACTORS

- Incomplete immunizations, no immunizations
- Contact with an infected person

ASSESSMENT FINDINGS

- Depends on stage of disease
- Fever may or may not be present
- Rhinorrhea

- Characteristic paroxysmal, high-pitched "whooping" cough
- In adolescents and adults, hallmark symptom is long-standing cough

DIFFERENTIAL DIAGNOSIS

- Upper respiratory infection
- Bronchitis
- Pneumonia
- Asthma
- Cystic fibrosis
- Foreign body aspiration
- Tuberculosis

DIAGNOSTIC STUDIES

- Nasopharyngeal culture to isolate organism
- PCR detection of *B. pertussis* DNA
- Chest x-ray: focal atelectasis
- CBC: >20,000 WBC with lymphocytic predominance

PREVENTION

- Immunizations for pertussis
- Avoid exposure to patients with known pertussis before immunization complete
- Erythromycin prophylaxis for exposed patients (cultures usually negative 5 days after prophylaxis, but continue for 14 days)

NONPHARMACOLOGIC MANAGEMENT

- Respiratory isolation for 5 days after antibiotic initiated
- Identify household and other close contacts
- Patient education regarding disease, treatment, emergency actions, importance of immunizations

PHARMACOLOGIC MANAGEMENT

- Erythromycin for 14 days; azithromycin or clarithromycin (5-7 days)
- Prophylactic antibiotics for close household contacts regardless of immunization status
- Antibiotics do not alter course of disease, only prevent transmission

AGENT	ACTION	COMMENTS
Macrolides *Examples:* erythromycin (E-mycin®) azithromycin (Zithromax®) clarithromycin (Biaxin®)	Antibiotic binds to the 50S subunit of susceptible organisms and prevents protein synthesis	Azithromycin and clarithromycin may be substituted for erythromycin. Erythromycin often poorly tolerated because of GI symptoms. Macrolide may abort or eliminate pertussis in catarrhal stage but does not shorten paroxysmal stage. Monitor for drug interactions especially with erythromycin.

CONSULTATION/REFERRAL

- Consider referral for infants <6 months of age because of severity of symptoms and increased morbidity and mortality
- Report to local health department

FOLLOW-UP

- Depends on severity of illness and age of patient

EXPECTED COURSE

- Catarrhal stage lasts 1-2 weeks
- Paroxysmal stage lasts 2-4 weeks
- Convalescent stage can last for several months accompanied by cough
- Prognosis worse in infants < 6 months
- Early treatment with antibiotics can shorten illness

POSSIBLE COMPLICATIONS

- Pneumonia with secondary bacterial infection (responsible for 90% of deaths due to pertussis)
- Encephalopathy
- Seizures may be due to high fever or hyperventilation

BRONCHIOLITIS

DESCRIPTION

Inflammation or infection of the small airways which leads to an impedance to airflow

ETIOLOGY

- Respiratory syncytial virus (RSV): most common cause
- Parainfluenza virus
- Adenovirus
- Influenza A virus
- *Mycoplasma pneumoniae* (more common in older children)
- Rhinovirus
- Respiratory irritants

INCIDENCE

- Common in infants and young children under age 2 years
- Many adult cases
- More common in winter and spring

RISK FACTORS

- Contact with infected person
- Daycare attendance
- In adults: exposure to respiratory irritants (cigarette smoke exposure, toxic inhalants)

ASSESSMENT FINDINGS

- Upper respiratory infection for 1-3 days which progresses to lower respiratory tract infection
- Fever
- Cough: may be hoarse before becoming very productive
- Inspiratory crackles; expiratory wheezes
- Tachypnea
- Thick, purulent nasal secretions
- Evidence of respiratory distress (i.e., use of accessory muscles, tachypnea, cyanosis)

DIFFERENTIAL DIAGNOSIS

- Asthma
- Pneumonia
- Emphysema
- GERD

DIAGNOSTIC STUDIES

- CBC
- Chest x-ray (hyperinflation, infiltrates, or atelectasis)
- ELISA of nasopharyngeal washings (80-90% sensitivity and specificity)
- Oxygenation assessment (ABGs, pulse oximetry)

PREVENTION

- Avoid direct contact with others known to be infected with RSV

NONPHARMACOLOGIC MANAGEMENT

- Maintain adequate hydration
- Patient education regarding disease, treatment, emergency actions

PHARMACOLOGIC MANAGEMENT

- Oxygen for hypoxic patients
- Nebulized bronchodilators for wheezing
- Steroids for patients with reactive airway disease and adults (rarely alters course in infants)
- Antiviral agents ribavirin (Virazole®) for high-risk patients (inconsistent demonstration of clinical efficacy)

AGENT	ACTION	COMMENTS
Bronchodilators ***Short-acting*** *Examples:* albuterol (Ventolin®) *(may be inhaled or nebulized)*	Stimulates beta 2 receptors in the lungs causing bronchodilation	Can increase heart rate, blood pressure, and cause QT prolongation and ST segment depression.

PREGNANCY/LACTATION CONSIDERATIONS

- Ribavirin is considered a pregnancy category X drug

CONSULTATION/REFERRAL

- Consider referral for infants who were premature, <3 months of age, or have underlying disease
- Refer to nearest emergency department for airway management and possible need for mechanical ventilation

FOLLOW-UP

- Depends on patient age, underlying disease, severity, but, daily telephone calls until clinical condition dictates improvement

EXPECTED COURSE

- Should begin to improve in 3-5 days
- Complete recovery 5-10 days

POSSIBLE COMPLICATIONS

- Respiratory failure requiring mechanical ventilation
- Increased incidence of asthma, reactive airway disease in children
- Apnea

CROUP
(Laryngotracheobronchitis)

DESCRIPTION

An acute viral illness characterized by stridor, barking cough, and hoarseness. Infection of the nasopharynx, larynx, and trachea produces swelling and subglottic obstruction.

ETIOLOGY

- Parainfluenza types 1 (most frequent causes)
- Adenovirus
- Influenza virus Type A
- *Mycoplasma pneumoniae*
- Respiratory syncytial virus

INCIDENCE

- Common; especially in fall and winter
- 80% occur in children <5 years
- Most common age of occurrence is 6 months to 3 years

RISK FACTORS

- Age (6 months to 3 years)
- Exposure (spread by respiratory droplet)
- Infection with one of the causative agents

ASSESSMENT FINDINGS

- Prodrome of coryza, fever, barking cough
- Symptoms worse at night
- Usually low grade fever
- Rarely, hypoxia as characterized by lethargy, irritability, anxiety
- Respiratory distress: nasal flaring, drooling, abdominal breathing, use of accessory muscles

- Possible stridor (most common cause in children is croup)
- Supraglottic area with normal appearance

Do NOT attempt to visualize the pharynx if severe respiratory distress. This may precipitate laryngeal spasms.

DIFFERENTIAL DIAGNOSIS

- Epiglottitis
- Tracheitis
- Retropharyngeal abscess
- Foreign body aspiration
- Diphtheria
- Neck trauma
- Tumor

DIAGNOSTIC STUDIES

- Usually none
- Lateral neck radiograph: "steeple" sign due to subglottic swelling is diagnostic
- Pulse oximetry

NONPHARMACOLOGIC MANAGEMENT

- Cool mist humidifier
- Patient educations regarding disease, treatment, signs and symptoms of respiratory distress and appropriate actions (i.e., go to nearest emergency department)

PHARMACOLOGIC MANAGEMENT

- Usually no pharmacologic treatment needed, but nebulized racemic epinephrine may be necessary for severe respiratory distress (watch for rebound dyspnea 2-3 hours after treatment)
- Steroids (oral or nebulized)
- Fever management

CONSULTATION/REFERRAL

- Refer to nearest emergency department for airway distress or if pulse oximetry < 92%

FOLLOW-UP

- Depends on patient's condition and age but 24-48 hours usually

EXPECTED COURSE

- General improvement seen by day 2-3 with resolution by day 5-7
- Good prognosis, usually no need for hospitalization

POSSIBLE COMPLICATIONS

- Need for intubation due to severe respiratory distress (occurs <1% of time)
- Bacterial superinfection

FOREIGN BODY ASPIRATION

DESCRIPTION

The inhalation or swallowing of a foreign object which becomes lodged in some part of the respiratory system.

ETIOLOGY

- Any object, substance, or part of an object which is small enough to enter the oral or nasal orifices
- Most common objects are foods (e.g., nuts, hot dog pieces, popcorn, hard candy)

INCIDENCE

- Common in infants, toddlers, and preschoolers

RISK FACTORS

- Poorly supervised or unsupervised children
- Curious toddlers
- Households with children of varied ages (older siblings leave unsafe objects lying around play area)

ASSESSMENT FINDINGS

- Abrupt onset of wheezing in otherwise healthy child
- Fixed, localized, or unilateral wheezing
- Cough
- Chronic cough
- Possible acute stridor
- Unilateral coryza (for nasal objects)
- Halitosis (for nasally lodged objects)

DIFFERENTIAL DIAGNOSIS

- Asthma
- Allergic rhinitis
- Sinusitis
- Upper respiratory illness
- Epiglottitis
- Tracheitis

DIAGNOSTIC STUDIES

- Chest, neck, or facial x-ray
- Bronchoscopy

PREVENTION

- Create safe play environment for toddlers and preschoolers
- Provide adequate supervision for children

NONPHARMACOLOGIC MANAGEMENT

- Provide oxygen supplementation if needed until transfer to emergency department
- Remove obstruction if possible
- Heimlich maneuver if appropriate
- Patient and family education regarding infant/toddler food safety, actions to take during emergency

PHARMACOLOGIC MANAGEMENT

- None usually needed unless secondary infection is present

CONSULTATION/REFERRAL

- Referral depending on where item is lodged (ENT physician, surgeon, pulmonologist, gastroenterologist)

FOLLOW-UP

- Depends on patient status, age, type of object aspirated, length of time before object discovered

EXPECTED COURSE

- Prognosis usually good

POSSIBLE COMPLICATIONS

- Respiratory distress
- Infection
- Death

CYSTIC FIBROSIS (CF)

DESCRIPTION

An autosomal recessive disease characterized by COPD, pancreatic exocrine deficiency, and elevated chloride concentration in sweat. Pancreas becomes atrophied, cirrhosis of the liver occurs, and the gallbladder becomes hypoplastic.

ETIOLOGY

- An abnormal variation in the cystic fibrosis transmembrane regulator blocks transport of chloride ions. Cell surface becomes inadequately hydrated, organs are damaged, and secretions become extremely viscous.

INCIDENCE

- 1/2500 in Caucasian population (most common chromosomal disorder in Caucasians)
- Rarely seen in African-Americans

RISK FACTORS

- Family history
- Parents who are carriers of the gene

ASSESSMENT FINDINGS

- Early symptoms may be gastrointestinal problems (e.g., failure to thrive, foul smelling stools, steatorrhea, meconium ileus)
- Fat malabsorption
- Barrel chest
- Clubbing of fingers
- Cough with mucopurulent sputum
- Crackles and wheezes with recurrent respiratory infections
- Electrolyte imbalances
- Delayed growth and development
- Hepatosplenomegaly in patients with cirrhosis
- Elevated blood glucose

DIFFERENTIAL DIAGNOSIS

- Asthma
- Recurrent respiratory infections
- Failure to thrive
- Immunodeficiency problems

DIAGNOSTIC STUDIES

- Gold standard: Sweat test (chloride >60 mEq/L considered abnormal)
- Genetic testing
- Stool: increased fat
- Pulmonary function tests 3-4 times annually
- Chest x-ray: hyperaeration
- Pancreatic function tests

PREVENTION

- Genetic counseling for parents with family history
- Immunizations to help prevent childhood respiratory illnesses
- Influenza and pneumococcal immunizations to prevent respiratory infections
- Avoid persons who have acute respiratory illnesses

NONPHARMACOLOGIC MANAGEMENT

- Chest physiotherapy with postural drainage to optimize mucus clearance (thick mucus precipitates respiratory distress)
- High calorie, sodium, protein, fat diet
- Extensive family and patient education
- Supportive care depending on patient and family needs

PHARMACOLOGIC MANAGEMENT

- Mucolytic agents (acetylcysteine,
- Aerosolized bronchodilators
- Antibiotic therapy for pulmonary infections especially *Pseudomonas* and Staph
- Pancreatic enzymes for patients who have insufficient production
- Vitamin supplements (fat soluble replacement)

CONSULTATION/REFERRAL

- Refer to cystic fibrosis center if available
- Refer to cystic fibrosis support group if appropriate
- Referral to specialist for newly diagnosed patients

FOLLOW-UP

- Depends on stage of disease
- Depends on severity of illness

EXPECTED COURSE

- Poor prognosis, average age at death is 25 years
- Babies born in the 1990's expect to live 40+ years
- Frequent pulmonary infections

POSSIBLE COMPLICATIONS

- Failure to thrive
- Poor growth
- Recurrent pneumonias and respiratory infections
- Respiratory failure requiring mechanical ventilation
- Pancreatic insufficiency necessitating replacement
- Diabetes mellitus

- Cirrhosis and organomegaly

SUDDEN INFANT DEATH SYNDROME (SIDS)

DESCRIPTION

The sudden and unexpected death of an infant less than one year of age for which there is no explanation even after a complete autopsy and investigation.

ETIOLOGY

- Unknown
- Possible respiratory control abnormality

INCIDENCE

- 1 per 2000 births; more common in males
- 90% occur before 6 months of age
- Highest rate in Native Americans (1.46/1000 births)
- Peaks at 2 - 4 months of age

RISK FACTORS

- Low-birth weight
- Small for gestational age
- Maternal cigarette smoking or drug use
- Poverty
- Young maternal age during pregnancy
- Males > Females
- Infants who sleep in the prone position
- Drug addicted mothers
- Family history

ASSESSMENT FINDINGS

- Well-developed, well-nourished infant
- No evidence of abuse or trauma
- Possible previous apparent life-threatening event (ALTE) including apnea, cyanosis, choking

DIFFERENTIAL DIAGNOSIS

- Trauma or accidental death
- Child abuse
- Congenital heart disease
- Arrhythmias

DIAGNOSTIC STUDIES

- Autopsy

PREVENTION

- Avoid placement in prone position for sleeping
- Apnea monitor for prior ALTE patients

CONSULTATION/REFERRAL

- Notification of coroner's office or medical examiner

- Counseling for family if needed

PRIMARY LUNG MALIGNANCIES

DESCRIPTION

The most common primary lung malignancies are of two types: small cell and non-small cell. They may be a primary malignancy or secondary metastasis.

ETIOLOGY

- Small cell malignancies
- Non-small cell malignancies include squamous cell (most common), adenocarcinoma, and large cell carcinoma

INCIDENCE

- Leading cause of cancer mortality
- 70/100,000 cases in the U.S.
- Males > Females

- Usually discovered in fifties, sixties, or seventies

RISK FACTORS

- Smoking (greater than 90% of patients smoke or have smoked)
- Asbestos exposure (pleural mesothelioma)
- COPD
- Exposure to heavy metals, gases
- Secondary smoke

ASSESSMENT FINDINGS

- Usually asymptomatic until an advanced stage
- Cough
- Palpable supraclavicular nodes
- Hemoptysis
- Dyspnea
- Weight loss
- Fatigue

DIFFERENTIAL DIAGNOSIS

- Primary lesion vs. metastatic lesion (50% are metastatic at diagnosis)
- Tuberculosis

DIAGNOSTIC STUDIES

- Chest x-ray
- CT scan
- Bronchoscopy
- Biopsy

PREVENTION

- Avoid tobacco use, especially cigarettes
- Avoid exposure to asbestos, other potentially carcinogenic agents
- Research indicates that screening provides no decrease in mortality, therefore, routine screening of asymptomatic patients is not recommended

NONPHARMACOLOGIC MANAGEMENT

- Radiation if indicated
- Surgical resection

PHARMACOLOGIC MANAGEMENT

- Chemotherapy if indicated
- Pain medication as needed
- Oxygen supplementation as needed

CONSULTATION/REFERRAL

- Surgeon, oncologist, pulmonologist
- Consider hospice if consistent with patient's advance directives

FOLLOW-UP

- Depends on patient status, advance directives, and staging

EXPECTED COURSE

- Depends on staging at time of diagnosis, whether surgically resectable, and tumor type
- 5-year survival for all stages is 15%

POSSIBLE COMPLICATIONS

- Metastasis-brain, bones, liver common
- Death

References

Berlow, B. A. (1997). Eight key questions to ask when your patient with asthma doesn't get better. *American Family Physician, 55*, 183-191.

Bickley, L.S., & Szilagyi, P.G. (2003). *Bates' guide to physical examination and history taking* (8th ed.). Philadelphia: Lippincott Williams & Wilkins.

Branch, W.T. (2003). *Office practice of medicine* (4th ed.). Philadelphia: Saunders.

Burns, C.E., Brady, M.A., Blosser, C., Starr, N.B., & Dunn, A.M. (2004). *Pediatric primary care: A handbook for nurse practitioners* (3rd ed.). Philadelphia: W.B. Saunders.

Craig, T. J. (1996). Drugs to be used with caution in patients with asthma. *American Family Physician, 54*, 947-956.

Centers for Disease Control, and Infectious Disease Society of America. (2003). Treatment of Tuberculosis: American Thoracic Society, CDC, and Infectious Diseases Society of America, *MMWR,* vol. 52, RR-11.

Center for Disease Control (2000). *Core curriculum on tuberculosis*, (4th ed.). Atlanta, GA: U.S. Department of Health and Human Services, U.S. Government Printing Office.

Codina, R., & Lockey, R.F. (2005) Environmental asthma: 9 questions physicians often ask. *Consultant, 45*, 685-693.

Courtney, A.U., McCarter, D.F., Pollart, S.M. (2005). Childhood asthma: Treatment update. *American Family Physician, 71,* 1959-1967.

Dambro, M.R. (2005). *Griffith's 5 minute clinical consult.* Philadelphia: Lippincott Williams & Wilkins.

Fowler, C. (2001). Preventing and managing exercise-induced asthma. *The Nurse Practitioner, 26*(3), 25-33.

Global Initiative for Chronic Obstructive Lung Disease (2004). *Global strategy for diagnosis, management, and prevention of chronic obstructive pulmonary disease.* Bethesda, MD: Agency for Healthcare Research and Quality.

Graber, M.A., & Lanternier, M.L. (Eds.) (2001). *The family practice handbook.* (4th ed.). St. Louis: Mosby.

Hall, K.L., & Zalman, B. (2005). Evaluation and management of apparent life-threatening events in children. *American Academy of Family Physicians, 71,* 2301-2308.

Kasper, D.L., Braunwald, E., Fauci, A.S., Hauser, S.L., Longo, D.L., Jameson, J.L., et al. (2004). *Harrison's principles of internal medicine* (16th ed.). New York: McGraw-Hill.

Kemp, J. P., & Kemp, J. A. (2001). Management of asthma in children. *American Family Physician, 63*, 1341-1348, 1353-1354.

Kliegman, R.M., Greenbaum, L.A., & Lye, P.S. (2004). *Practical strategies in pediatric diagnosis and therapy* (2nd ed.). Philadelphia: W.B. Saunders.

Leiner, D. S. (1997). Acute bronchitis in adults: Commonly diagnosed but poorly defined. *The Nurse Practitioner, 22*, 104-114.

Lozano, P., Fishman, P., VanKorff, M., & Hecht, J. (1997). Health care utilization and cost among children with asthma who were enrolled in a health maintenance organization. *Pediatrics, 99*, 757-764.

Madell, L. A., Bartlett, J. G., Dowell, S.F., File, Jr., F. M., Musher, D. M. and Whitney, C. (2003). Update of practice guidelines for the management of community-acquired pneumonia in immunocompetent adults. *Clinical Infectious Diseases, 37*, 1405-1433.

Madell, L. A., Bartlett, J. G., Dowell, S.F., File, Jr., F. M., Musher, D. M. and Whitney, C. (2000). Practice guidelines for the management of community-acquired pneumonia in adults. *Clinical Infectious Diseases, 31*, 347-382.

Mangion, S. (2000). *Physical diagnosis secrets.* Philadelphia: Hanley and Belfus.

Mladenovic, J. (Ed.). (2003). *Primary care secrets.* (3rd Ed.). Philadelphia: Hanley and Belfus.

Morgan, W. C., & Hodge, H. L. (1998). Diagnostic evaluation of dyspnea. *American Family Physician, 57*, 711-716.

National Institutes of Health, National Heart, Lung, and Blood Institute. (2004). *National asthma education program expert panel report 2: Guidelines for diagnosis and management of asthma.* NIH Publication No. 97-4051. Bethesda, MD: National Institutes of Health.

Niederman, M. S., Mandell, L. A., Anzueto, A., et al. (2001). Guidelines for the management of adults with community-acquired pneumonia. *American Journal of Respiratory Critical Care Medicine, 163*, 1730-1754.

Oyen, N., Markestad, T., Skjaerven, R., Irgens, L. M., Helweg-Larson, K., Alm, B., Norvenius, G., & Wennergren, G. (1997). Combined effects of sleeping position and prenatal risk factors in sudden infant death syndrome: The Nordic epidemiological SIDS study. *Pediatrics, 100*, 613-621.

Patrick, H., and Patrick, F. (1995). Chronic cough. *The Medical Clinics of North America, 79*, 361-372.

Pryor, M. P. (1997). Noisy breathing in children. *Postgraduate Medicine, 101*, 103-112.

Rakel, R.E. (Ed.). (1998). *Essentials of family practice.* (2nd ed.). Philadelphia: WB Saunders.

Schwartz, M.W. (Ed.). (2002). *The 5 minute pediatric consult.* (2nd ed.) Philadelphia: Lippincott Williams & Wilkins.

Scott, P. T., Clark, J. B., & Miser, W. F. (1997). Pertussis: An update on primary prevention and outbreak control. *American Family Physician, 56*, 1121-1130.

Uphold, C.R., & Graham, M.V. (2003). *Clinical guidelines in family practice.* (4th ed.). Gainesville, FL: Barmarrae Books.

U.S. Preventive Services Task Force. (1996). *Guide to clinical preventive services.* (2nd ed.) Washington, D.C.: Office of Disease Prevention and Health Promotion, U.S. Government Printing Office.

Ward, M. R. (1997). Reye's syndrome: An update. *The Nurse Practitioner, 22*(12), 45-53.

Whyte, J.J. (2005) Glycemic index: How useful is it? *Consultant, 45*, 558-560.

Zollo, A.J., Jr. (Ed.). (2004). *Medical Secrets.* (4th ed.), St. Louis, MO: Mosby-Year Book.

19

SEXUALLY TRANSMITTED DISEASES

Sexually Transmitted Diseases

HUMAN IMMUNODEFICIENCY VIRUS (HIV) INFECTION

DESCRIPTION

Viral infection that causes cell death and gradual decline in immune function resulting in opportunistic infections, malignancies, and neurologic lesions. CD4 cell count <200 is classified as AIDS.

ETIOLOGY

- Retrovirus (human immunodeficiency virus) that infects cells, most notably the CD4 lymphocytes (T helper cells)
- Is transmitted through sexual intercourse, transfusion of blood or blood products, and perinatally from mother to infant

INCIDENCE

- >500,000 AIDS cases
- 40,000-80,000 new cases annually
- Occurs mostly among young adults ages 25-44 years
- Males > Females

RISK FACTORS

- Sexual activity
- Prostitution
- Multiple sexual partners or sexual partner has multiple partners
- Engaging in sex for money
- Sexual partner of injecting drug user
- Men who have sex with men
- Injecting drug use and sharing of contaminated needles
- Recipient of blood products, especially from 1975 to March 1985
- Hemophiliacs who have received pooled plasma products
- Infants born to HIV-infected women
- Infants breast fed by HIV-infected mother
- Health care workers

ASSESSMENT FINDINGS

Initial infection:

- Fever
- Pharyngitis
- Nonpruritic maculopapular skin rash
- Myalgia/arthralgia
- Malaise
- Diarrhea
- Headache
- Lymphadenopathy
- Hepatosplenomegaly
- Self-limiting viral-type syndrome occurring about 6-8 weeks postinfection; often goes unnoticed by patient
- An asymptomatic period of variable length follows the initial infection.
- The time between infection and development of AIDS ranges from a few months to 17 years with the median time being 10 years.

Established HIV:

- Anemia
- Leukopenia
- Thrombocytopenia
- Involuntary weight loss
- Diarrhea
- Dementia
- *Pneumocystis carinii* pneumonia (PCP), which is characterized by nonproductive cough, dyspnea, and fever that persists for days or weeks.
- Candidal infections: esophageal, bronchial, pulmonary, oral, vaginal
- Other opportunistic infections
- Herpes zoster, may be disseminated
- Pulmonary tuberculosis
- Kaposi's sarcoma: nodule or papule that appears purple or dark brown, found on skin, mucous membranes, and/or viscera

DIAGNOSTIC STUDIES

- ELISA for screening
- Western blot or immunofluorescence assay (IFA) for confirmation
- May be negative in first 6-12 weeks after initial infection
- Informed consent must be obtained before HIV testing is performed

- In infants born to HIV-infected mothers, maternally acquired HIV IgG antibodies and infant-derived IgG antibodies cannot be differentiated. A positive ELISA or Western blot, therefore, does not confirm an infection in the child <18 months of age.

Consider early referral to an HIV care specialist.

PREVENTION

- Avoid unprotected sexual intercourse
- Use of condoms
- Avoid contact with intravenous products and fluids
- HIV screening for all persons at risk of infection
- Screening recommended for all pregnant women and newborn infants at risk for HIV infection

POSTEXPOSURE PROPHYLAXIS:

- CDC recommends postexposure prophylaxis with zidovudine, lamivudine, and indinavir for health care workers with a significant exposure

NONPHARMACOLOGIC MANAGEMENT

- Counseling regarding behavioral, psychosocial, and medical implications of HIV infection
- Encourage regular exercise and good nutrition
- Avoid raw eggs, raw seafood, unpasteurized milk, and other potentially contaminated foods
- Review immunization status and bring up to date (Pneumococcal, influenza, Td, Hepatitis A & B)
- Education regarding methods of transmission
- Teach how to minimize risk to others
- Partner notification (sexual partners and those who share needles or other injected drug equipment)
- Notification of local health department
- Polymerase chain reaction (PCR) RNA assays detect presence of virus and are used to monitor progression and response to therapy
- Once HIV is confirmed:
  - ◊ CBC with differential and platelets
  - ◊ Chemistry profile
  - ◊ Syphilis serology
  - ◊ Baseline CD4 count
  - ◊ Viral load (HIV RNA) tests are increasingly being used to monitor progression of disease and determining when to initiate treatment
  - ◊ Hepatitis profile
  - ◊ Chest x-ray
  - ◊ PPD with controls
  - ◊ Toxoplasmosis antibody test
  - ◊ Serology for cytomegalovirus and toxoplasmosis
  - ◊ Pap smear every 6 months
  - ◊ Cervical culture for gonorrhea and chlamydia
  - ◊ Wet prep

CD4 counts should be checked at least every 3-6 months.

PHARMACOLOGIC MANAGEMENT

- Vitamin supplement
- Antiretroviral therapy – current standard: requires multidrug therapy to prevent emergence of resistance
- Consider antiretroviral therapy if CD4 <350
- PCP prophylaxis (indicated if CD4 count <200/mm^3 and for infants born to HIV-infected mothers):
  - ◊ Trimethoprim-sulfamethoxazole (Bactrim DS®)
- Toxoplasmosis prophylaxis (indicated if CD4 count <100):
  - ◊ Same as PCP prophylaxis
- *Mycobacterium avium* complex prophylaxis if CD4 count <50:
  - ◊ Clarithromycin (Biaxin®) or azithromycin (Zithromax®)
- Pneumococcal vaccine every 6 years
- Influenza vaccine in fall annually
- Td booster if >5 years since last dose
- Hepatitis B vaccine if not immune

Commonly used drugs:

- Nucleoside reverse transcriptase inhibitors: abacavir (ABC®, Ziagen®), didanosine (ddI

or Videx®), lamivudine (3TC or Epivir®), stavudine (Zerit®), zalcitabine (Hivid®), zidovudine (AZT or Retrovir®)
- Protease inhibitors: indinavir (Crixivan®), ritonavir (Norvir®), saquinavir (Fortovase®), nelfinavir (Viracept®)
- Nonnucleoside reverse transcriptase inhibitors: nevirapine (Viramune®), delavirdine (Rescriptor®), efavirenz (Sustiva®)

At least 3 different drugs from different classes are recommended to decrease viral load and delay onset of AIDs.

PREGNANCY/LACTATION CONSIDERATIONS

- Approximately 15-25% of infants born to untreated HIV-infected mothers will be infected
- Antiretroviral therapy during pregnancy and the first 6 weeks of an infant's life has been shown to decrease incidence of transmission to infant from 25% to 8%
- CDC recommends all women be offered HIV counseling and testing
- Breastfeeding is contraindicated in women who are HIV-infected due to the risk of transmission
- Trimethoprim-sulfamethoxazole DS (Bactrim DS®) is indicated for PCP prophylaxis in all HIV-infected women who are pregnant. Dapsone may be substituted in first trimester.
- Azithromycin (Zithromax®) is the drug of choice in pregnancy for *Mycobacterium avium* complex (MAC) prophylaxis

CONSULTATION/REFERRAL

- Refer to health care professional experienced in management of HIV infection

FOLLOW-UP

- Patients on antiretroviral therapy need close monitoring due to significant drug toxicities

Close follow up needed for evaluation of neurological symptoms which could indicate CNS infection.

EXPECTED COURSE

- Life expectancy after HIV progresses to AIDS is two to three years. With development of better treatment life expectancy is increasing.
- Opportunistic infections usually begin to develop when CD4 count are <200
- The majority of children who are infected have a gradual course and do not meet criteria for case definition until about age 3 years. A smaller number of children become symptomatic early and die before age 1 year.

POSSIBLE COMPLICATIONS

- Immunodeficiency
  - ◊ Candidal infections
  - ◊ Staphylococcal infections
  - ◊ *Salmonella* bacteremia
  - ◊ Genital warts
  - ◊ Herpes simplex and zoster
- Depression
- Suicide

BACTERIAL VAGINOSIS (BV)

(Gardnerella Vaginosis, Nonspecific Vaginosis)

DESCRIPTION

Clinical syndrome resulting from replacement of the normal vaginal flora, *Lactobacillus* sp., with high concentrations of anaerobic bacteria (e.g., *Prevotella* sp. and *Mobiluncus* sp., *Gardnerella. vaginalis,* and *Mycoplasma hominis).*

BV is associated with having multiple sex partners. Women who have never been sexually active are less affected.

ETIOLOGY

- Cause of the microbacterial overgrowth not completely understood

INCIDENCE

- 4-33% of women affected depending on setting
- Most prevalent vaginal infection of women of reproductive age in the U.S.

RISK FACTORS

- Multiple sexual partners
- Use of an IUD

ASSESSMENT FINDINGS

- Asymptomatic in about 50% of women
- Grayish-white malodorous vaginal discharge
- Unpleasant, fishy, or musty vaginal odor
- Profuse discharge
- Pruritus and burning of vulvovaginal area

Suspect BV in patients who complain of malodorous discharge after sexual intercourse.

DIFFERENTIAL DIAGNOSIS

- Candidiasis
- *Chlamydia trachomatis* infection
- Gonorrhea
- Trichomoniasis
- *Staphylococci* infection
- Foreign body

DIAGNOSTIC STUDIES

- Clinical criteria for diagnosis requires three of the following symptoms or signs be present:
  - ◊ A homogeneous, white, noninflammatory discharge that smoothly coats the vaginal walls
  - ◊ The presence of clue cells on microscopic examination
  - ◊ A pH of vaginal fluid >4.5
  - ◊ A fishy odor of vaginal discharge before or after addition of 10% KOH ("positive whiff test")
- Gram stain: absence or decreased lactobacilli

PREVENTION

- Good hygiene
- Use of condoms
- Avoid douching
- Screen for STDs

NONPHARMACOLOGIC MANAGEMENT

- Consider screening for sexually transmitted disease
- Avoid sexual intercourse until treatment completed
- No alcohol if on metronidazole due to a disulfiram-type reaction
- Stress good personal hygiene
- Avoid douching to prevent recurrences
- Treatment of the male sex partner has not been beneficial in reducing recurrence of BV

PHARMACOLOGIC MANAGEMENT

- Metronidazole (Flagyl®) *OR*
- clindamycin (Cleocin®) *OR*
- clindamycin 2% vaginal cream *OR*
- metronidazole vaginal gel 0.75%
- Consider treating partner, especially if infection recurrent

Patient must refrain from use of alcohol while taking metronidazole.

PREGNANCY/LACTATION CONSIDERATIONS

- CDC recommends use of metronidazole orally in symptomatic women
- Clindamycin cream should not be used in pregnancy because of its association with preterm labor
- BV during pregnancy is associated with adverse pregnancy outcomes (e.g., preterm labor, premature rupture of membranes, and premature birth)
- Screen in second trimester if woman at high risk for preterm labor (e.g., has had previous preterm delivery or labor)

CONSULTATION/REFERRAL

- Not usually indicated

FOLLOW-UP

- Not usually indicated
- One month follow-up during pregnancy recommended

EXPECTED COURSE

- Recurrences common

POSSIBLE COMPLICATIONS

- May be a factor in premature rupture of membranes and preterm delivery
- Associated with postpartal endometritis
- PID
- Postoperative infections

CHLAMYDIA

DESCRIPTION

Sexually transmitted disease with an often asymptomatic clinical course with serious sequelae.

ETIOLOGY

- *Chlamydia trachomatis*

INCIDENCE

- Most prevalent STD in United States
- Over 4 million cases diagnosed annually
- Highest incidence among adolescents and young adults

RISK FACTORS

- Sexually active
- New sexual partner
- Multiple sexual partners or partner of person with multiple partners
- Use of oral contraceptives
- Lower socioeconomic groups
- Women at greater risk for contraction of chlamydia than are men
- Age <21 years

ASSESSMENT FINDINGS

- Often asymptomatic
- Mucopurulent cervicitis
- Edematous, congested friable cervix
- Vaginal discharge
- Discharge from Bartholin's gland when milked
- Cervical motion tenderness
- Dysuria
- Urethritis
- Salpingitis
- Proctitis
- Epididymitis
- Abnormal vaginal bleeding
- Pelvic pain
- Prostatitis

Infants:
- Afebrile
- Pneumonia
- Conjunctivitis

DIFFERENTIAL DIAGNOSIS

- Gonorrhea
- Vaginitis
- Pelvic inflammatory disease
- Salpingitis
- Urinary tract infection

DIAGNOSTIC STUDIES

- Urinalysis: positive for WBCs
- Wet prep: >20 WBC/high-powered field
- Ligase chain reaction (LCP) or polymerase chain reaction (PCR) are newer tests
- DNA probe
- Culture: not usually used, however it is the gold standard for diagnosis
- Gonorrhea culture or DNA probe

PREVENTION

- Use of condoms
- Screening should be done for target populations:
  - ◊ Sexually active females
  - ◊ Women 20-24 years old who meet either of two following criteria:
    - * Inconsistent use of barrier contraception
    - * New or more than one sex partner during the past three months
    - * In the third trimester of pregnancy
- Screen for other STDs

NONPHARMACOLOGIC MANAGEMENT

- Education regarding serious sequelae of chlamydia infection
- Abstinence until treatment completed
- Evaluate and treat sexual partners
- Sexual abuse should be considered for any child with confirmed chlamydia after the neonatal period
- Report to local health department

PHARMACOLOGIC MANAGEMENT

- Doxycycline (Vibramycin®) *OR*
- Azithromycin (Zithromax®) *OR*
- Erythromycin *OR*
- Ofloxacin (Floxin®)
- Use doxycycline for 10-14 days if epididymis involved

Children:
- <45 kg: erythromycin base
- >45 kg and <9 years old: azithromycin
- >8 years old: azithromycin *OR* doxycycline

PREGNANCY/LACTATION CONSIDERATIONS

- Prevalence among pregnant women in U.S. is 5%
- Treat with erythromycin base *OR* amoxicillin
- Safety of azithromycin in pregnancy not established
- Doxycycline and ofloxacin contraindicated in pregnancy
- Screen in third trimester in women at risk (e.g., <25 years old, recent new sexual partner, more than one sexual partner)

FOLLOW-UP

- Test of cure is not needed unless symptoms persist or reinfection suspected
- Screen for HIV and syphilis in persons with chlamydia infection

EXPECTED COURSE

- Complete resolution with early and compliant therapy
- Due to asymptomatic nature of disease, many persons develop complications

POSSIBLE COMPLICATIONS

- Transient oligospermia
- Post epididymitis urethral stricture
- PID
- Infertility
- Ectopic pregnancy
- Chronic pelvic pain
- Acute or chronic salpingitis
- Fitz-Hugh-Curtis syndrome (perihepatitis)
- Conjunctivitis in infants born to infected mothers
- Pneumonia in infants born to infected mothers

GONORRHEA

DESCRIPTION

A sexually transmitted disease that produces a purulent inflammation of mucous membranes.

ETIOLOGY

- *Neisseria gonorrhoeae* infection transmitted by sexual contact and from infected mother to infant during childbirth

INCIDENCE

- 800,000 new cases in U.S. annually
- Incidence highest among females aged 15-19 years

RISK FACTORS

- Sexual exposure to an infected individual without barrier protection
- Multiple sexual partners
- Infant born to infected mother
- Sexually abused children
- Use of IUD increases risk of PID

ASSESSMENT FINDINGS

Males:
- Purulent urethral discharge
- Dysuria
- Testicular pain
- Asymptomatic

Females:
- Often asymptomatic
- Endocervical discharge
- Vaginal discharge
- Dysuria
- Bartholin's gland abscess
- Abnormal vaginal bleeding
- Abdominal/pelvic pain
- Adnexal tenderness
- Cervical motion tenderness

Males & Females:
- Rectal discharge
- Tenesmus
- Rectal burning or itching
- Exudative pharyngitis
- Purulent discharge from eye

Infants:
- Most common:
    - ◊ Eye infection (ophthalmia neonatorum)
- Less common:
    - ◊ Sepsis
    - ◊ Serious systemic disease

Disseminated disease:
- Fever
- Chills
- Arthralgias of small joints
- Pustular, red, and tender skin lesions
- Septic arthritis, usually symmetric, polyarticular, especially seen in elbow, knee and distal joints

DIFFERENTIAL DIAGNOSIS

- Chlamydia
- Urinary tract infection
- Vaginitis from another etiologic agent
- Pelvic inflammatory disease

DIAGNOSTIC STUDIES

- Gram stain of exudate
- DNA probe
- Culture of exudate or joint aspirate on Thayer-Martin agar (also called chocolate agar)
- Cervical culture or DNA probe for *C. trachomatis*
- Syphilis serology
- HIV testing if appropriate

PREVENTION

- Use of condoms
- Neonatal ocular prophylaxis: silver nitrate, erythromycin, or tetracycline eye drops
- Screening during pregnancy if high-risk
- Screen for other STDs

NONPHARMACOLOGIC MANAGEMENT

- Avoid sexual intercourse until treatment completed
- Treatment of sexual contacts
- Sexual abuse should be considered for any child with confirmed gonorrhea after neonatal period
- Report all cases to local health department

PHARMACOLOGIC MANAGEMENT

- Ceftriaxone (Rocephin®) *OR*
- Cefixime (Suprax®) *OR*
- Ofloxacin (Floxin®) *OR*
- Ciprofloxacin (Cipro®) *PLUS*
- Doxycycline (Vibramycin®) or azithromycin (Zithromax®) for treatment of chlamydia because of frequent coinfection
- Persons allergic to cephalosporins and quinolones may be treated with spectinomycin intramuscular, but is not as effective

Children:
- Quinolones are contraindicated
- <45 kg: ceftriaxone
- If allergic to cephalosporins, spectinomycin intramuscular may be used

PREGNANCY/LACTATION CONSIDERATIONS

- All pregnant women should be screened at first prenatal visit
- For high-risk women an additional screen should be done in third trimester
- Cephalosporin is treatment of choice
- If allergic to cephalosporins, spectinomycin intramuscular may be used
- Quinolones and tetracycline are contraindicated

CONSULTATION/REFERRAL

- Not usually needed unless dissemination occurs or resistance to treatment

FOLLOW-UP

- Test of cure not necessary unless symptoms persist or noncompliance is an issue
- If spectinomycin used, follow-up testing is necessary

EXPECTED COURSE

- Complete resolution

POSSIBLE COMPLICATIONS

- Urethral stricture in men
- Infertility in women
- PID
- Destruction of joints and cardiac valves
- Meningitis
- Endocarditis
- Pneumonia
- Endometritis

Infants:
- Corneal scarring in infants
- Disseminated disease in infants
- Ophthalmia neonatorum

SYPHILIS

DESCRIPTION

Sexually transmitted disease characterized by sequential stages and involving multiple systems. Syphilis has the following stages:
- Primary
- Secondary
- Latent (infection present at least 12 months)
- Tertiary

Also transmitted from an infected mother to her infant in congenital syphilis

ETIOLOGY

- Spirochete *Treponema pallidum* penetrates intact skin or mucous membrane during sexual intercourse enters the bloodstream and is transported to other tissues

- Congenital syphilis is acquired transplacentally from an infected mother

INCIDENCE

- Over 110,000 new cases annually
- More prevalent among persons 15-25 years of age

RISK FACTORS

- Multiple sexual partners
- Injecting drug use
- Male homosexuality
- HIV infection
- Presence of another sexually transmitted disease

ASSESSMENT FINDINGS

Primary syphilis:
- Chancre at site of inoculation begins as papule then ulcerates with a hard edge and clean, yellow base; indurated and painless; usually located on genitalia; may be solitary or multiple; persists for 1-5 weeks and heals spontaneously
- Chancre may go unnoticed in females
- Regional lymphadenopathy

Secondary syphilis:
- Rash that is bilaterally symmetrical, polymorphic, nonpruritic, frequently on soles and palms, and usually persists for 2-6 weeks then spontaneously resolves
- Condyloma lata which are moist, pink, peripheral warty lesions. These may be present on glans, perianal, vulval areas, and intertriginous areas
- Mucous patches in mouth, throat, cervix
- Generalized lymphadenopathy
- Flu-like symptoms
- Mild hepatosplenomegaly

Latent syphilis:
- Asymptomatic

Tertiary syphilis:
- Cardiovascular manifestations: aortic valve disease, aneurysms
- Neurological manifestations: meningitis, encephalitis, tabes dorsalis, dementia
- Integumentary manifestations: gummas
- Orthopedic manifestations: Charcot joints, osteomyelitis

Congenital syphilis:
- Early
  - ◊ Failure to thrive
  - ◊ Stillbirths
  - ◊ Hydrops fetalis
  - ◊ Prematurity
  - ◊ Rhinitis
  - ◊ Lymphadenopathy
  - ◊ Jaundice
  - ◊ Anemia
  - ◊ Hepatosplenomegaly
  - ◊ Nephrosis
  - ◊ Hallmark rash similar to secondary syphilis in adult, may be bullous or vesicular
- Late (due to chronic inflammation or hypersensitivity)
  - ◊ CNS changes
  - ◊ Bony abnormalities
  - ◊ Dental deformities
  - ◊ Cataracts, blindness
  - ◊ Stage of congenital syphilis is dependent on the maternal stage of syphilis

DIFFERENTIAL DIAGNOSIS

Primary syphilis:
- Chancroid
- Lymphogranuloma venereum
- Granuloma inguinale
- Herpes simplex
- Behçet's syndrome
- Trauma

Secondary syphilis:
- Pityriasis rosea
- Guttate psoriasis
- Drug eruption

DIAGNOSTIC STUDIES

- Nontreponemal tests
  - ◊ Rapid plasma reagin (RPR)
  - ◊ Venereal Disease Research Laboratory (VDRL)

- Treponemal tests (usually positive for life after treatment):
  - ◊ Fluorescent treponemal antibody absorbed (FTA-ABS)
  - ◊ Microhemagglutination assay for antibody to *T. Pallidum* (MHA-TP)
- Lumbar puncture for CSF serologies when neurologic symptoms are present and in all children diagnosed after the newborn period
- Darkfield microscopy or direct fluorescent antibody test of exudate or tissue

PREVENTION

- Use of condoms
- Screening for syphilis in asymptomatic persons
- Screening for HIV in persons with syphilis infection

NONPHARMACOLOGIC MANAGEMENT

- Avoid sexual intercourse until treatment complete
- Sexual abuse should be considered for any child with confirmed syphilis
- Treatment of all sexual partners
- Evaluate for other STDs

PHARMACOLOGIC MANAGEMENT

- Benzathine penicillin G (Bicillin®) intramuscular in adults and children
- Neurosyphilis:
  - ◊ aqueous crystalline penicillin G intravenous *OR*
  - ◊ procaine penicillin with probenecid intramuscular
- Congenital:
  - ◊ aqueous crystalline penicillin G intravenous *OR*
  - ◊ procaine penicillin intramuscular
- Patients with penicillin allergy:
  - ◊ doxycycline (Vibramycin®) *OR*
  - ◊ tetracycline *OR*
  - ◊ erythromycin
- Desensitization is recommended for penicillin-allergic persons in the following cases:
  - ◊ HIV-positive
  - ◊ Children
  - ◊ Pregnancy

PREGNANCY/LACTATION CONSIDERATIONS

- If penicillin allergic, desensitization is recommended
- All pregnant women should be screened for syphilis at the first prenatal visit
- Those at high risk should be screened again in the third trimester and at delivery

CONSULTATION/REFERRAL

- Consultation with or referral to obstetrician in pregnant women
- Report to local health department

FOLLOW-UP

- Repeat syphilis serology for 3 months, then annually to confirm treatment
- HIV-positive patients: repeat serology at 3 month intervals
- Infants: repeat syphilis serology at 3, 6, and 12 months or until nonreactive

EXPECTED COURSE

- Excellent prognosis except in late syphilis complications and in HIV-infected patients

POSSIBLE COMPLICATIONS

- Cardiovascular disease
- Central nervous system disease
- Membranous glomerulonephritis
- Paroxysmal cold hemoglobinemia
- Organ damage that cannot be reversed
- Multiple disorders
- Jarisch-Herxheimer reaction often occurs among person being treated for early syphilis. Antipyretics may be used, but there is no proven method to prevent this reaction. May induce early labor in pregnant women, but this concern should not prevent treatment in pregnancy.

GENITAL HERPES
(Herpes Simplex II, Herpes Genitalis)

DESCRIPTION

Recurrent, incurable cutaneous or mucous membrane infection

ETIOLOGY

- Herpes simplex virus type 1 or 2 (usually HSV-2)
- Transmitted by direct contact with active lesions or by virus-containing fluid
- An asymptomatic patient can be infective while shedding virus
- Incubation period is 2-12 days

INCIDENCE

- 300,000-700,000 cases annually in the U.S.
- 31 million persons in U.S. currently infected

RISK FACTORS

- Sexual activity

The incubation period after exposure is 1-45 days.

ASSESSMENT FINDINGS

Primary infection:
- Asymptomatic
- Painful papules followed by vesicles on an erythematous base that ulcerate, crust, and resolve within 21 days
- Hyperesthesia
- Fever
- Headache
- Malaise
- Myalgia
- Dysuria
- Lymphadenopathy

Recurrent infections:
- Prodrome of pain, burning, and/or paresthesia over area of eruption
- Burning genital pain
- Lesions as above that resolve within 7-10 days

DIFFERENTIAL DIAGNOSIS

- Primary syphilis
- Atypical genital warts
- Candidiasis
- Herpes zoster

DIAGNOSTIC STUDIES

- Viral tissue culture
- DNA prep has the highest sensitivity
- Serologic assays (usually positive 4-6 weeks after onset of symptoms)
- Tzanck prep
- ELISA
- Syphilis serology

Varicella zoster will give same results as Tzanck prep.

PREVENTION

- Use of condoms
- Cesarean section indicated in women with lesions to prevent infection in newborn
- Screen for other STDs

NONPHARMACOLOGIC MANAGEMENT

- Counseling
  - ◊ Natural course of disease
  - ◊ Asymptomatic viral shedding
  - ◊ Potential for recurrent episodes
  - ◊ Sexual transmission
  - ◊ Implications for pregnancy
- Cool compresses with Burow's solution
- Ice packs to lesion area
- Good hygiene
- Avoid sexual contact during symptomatic periods, for 48 hours after symptoms resolve, and during prodromal symptoms

- Use of condoms during all sexual exposures to decrease risk of transmission when asymptomatic
- Avoidance of triggers to recurrent infection when possible (e.g., genital trauma, emotional stress, concurrent infection)
- Sexual abuse should be considered for any child with confirmed herpes infection

PHARMACOLOGIC MANAGEMENT

Primary infection:

- Treatment for 7-10 days or until clinical resolution attained
  - ◊ acyclovir (Zovirax®) *OR*
  - ◊ famciclovir (Famvir®) *OR*
  - ◊ valacyclovir (Valtrex®)

Recurrent episodes:

- Should be started during prodrome or within one day of onset of lesion:
  - ◊ acyclovir (Zovirax®) *OR*
  - ◊ famciclovir (Famvir®) *OR*
  - ◊ valacyclovir (Valtrex®) for 5 days

Suppressive therapy:

- Use in persons with 6 or more recurrences annually:
  - ◊ acyclovir (Zovirax®) *OR*
  - ◊ famciclovir (Famvir®) *OR*
  - ◊ valacyclovir (Valtrex®) for 1 year

Reassess after one year of daily suppressant therapy.

PREGNANCY/LACTATION CONSIDERATIONS

- Acyclovir may be used during pregnancy for treatment of an initial episode
- Cesarean section is indicated if genital herpetic lesions are present during labor

CONSULTATION/REFERRAL

- If symptoms persist or frequent recurrences
- Immunocompromised persons

FOLLOW-UP

- Reevaluate in one week if no improvement
- Screen for other STDs
- Annual Pap smear

EXPECTED COURSE

- Resolution of primary lesions in 14-21 days
- Resolution of recurrent lesions 7-10 days
- Recurrences occur in 50% of persons within 6 months of primary infection

POSSIBLE COMPLICATIONS

- Prolonged severe local disease
- Disseminated disease
- Secondary bacterial infection
- Increased risk for HIV infection

HUMAN PAPILLOMA VIRUS
(Condyloma Acuminata, Genital Warts)

DESCRIPTION

Viral infection transmitted sexually through an epidermal defect that produces warts on genital area. Generally benign and produce no symptoms except the cosmetic appearance.

High degree of cervical dysplasia associated with HVP 16, 18, 31, and 33.

ETIOLOGY

- Human papilloma virus Types 6 and 11 most commonly cause genital warts. These have very low oncogenic potential and usually do not cause cancer.
- Types 16, 18, 31, and 33 have the highest oncogenic potential and are usually associated with subclinical infections, but may be found in warts
- Is transmitted sexually and through fomites, is highly contagious

INCIDENCE

- 24 million persons in U.S. currently infected
- 0.5-1 million new cases annually
- Approximately 50% of all sexually active college women may be infected

RISK FACTORS

- Sexual activity
- Multiple sexual partners
- Exposure without barrier protection

ASSESSMENT FINDINGS

- Soft, flesh-colored warts
- Warts are usually painless
- Surface smooth to very rough
- Multiple finger-like projections
- May be confluent
- Perianal warts usually rough and cauliflower-like
- Penile lesions often smooth and papular
- Pruritus
- Irritation
- Bleeding secondary to trauma
- Asymptomatic in subclinical infections
- Common sites of male infection: penile glans and shaft, anus, buttocks; scrotal involvement uncommon
- Common sites of female infection: labia, clitoris, periurethral area, perineum, vagina, cervix, anus, buttocks

DIFFERENTIAL DIAGNOSIS

- Condyloma lata (syphilitic wart)
- Molluscum contagiosum
- Herpes simplex

DIAGNOSTIC STUDIES

- Acetowhitening can make subclinical lesions visible
- Biopsy for persistent warts or if diagnosis uncertain
- Pap smear
- Colposcopy with biopsy when Pap smear positive

PREVENTION

- Use of condoms provides limited protection
- Screen for other STDs

NONPHARMACOLOGIC MANAGEMENT

- Use of condoms
- Abstinence until therapy completed
- CO_2 laser for external genital warts

Sexual abuse should be considered for any child with confirmed papilloma infection.

PHARMACOLOGIC MANAGEMENT

- Podophyllin resin 10-25%
- Trichloroacetic acid (TCA) 80-90%
- Topical 5-fluorouracil is not recommended by CDC

Self-treatment options for external warts:
- Podofilox 0.5% gel or cream (Condylox®)
- Imiquimod 5% cream (Aldara®)

PREGNANCY/LACTATION CONSIDERATIONS

- Often grow larger during pregnancy and regress spontaneously after delivery
- May need cesarean section if large and obstruct vagina, otherwise not indicated
- Cryotherapy is treatment of choice
- Podofilox and podophyllin contraindicated during pregnancy
- Imiquimod safety not established in pregnancy

CONSULTATION/REFERRAL

- Refer patients with extensive or refractory disease and intraurethral warts, to gynecologist or dermatologist

FOLLOW-UP

- Every 1-2 weeks for treatment until resolved
- Screen for syphilis
- Pap smear annually
- Monitor sexual partners

EXPECTED COURSE

- Warts clear with treatment or spontaneously regress
- Recurrence is common with all forms of therapy
- Growth may be stimulated by oral contraceptives, immunosuppression, and local trauma

POSSIBLE COMPLICATIONS

- Male urethral obstruction
- Secondary infection
- Aspiration of secretions from infected mothers at delivery may result in laryngeal papillomas in 2-5% of infants

PELVIC INFLAMMATORY DISEASE (PID)

(Salpingitis, Salpingo-oophoritis)

DESCRIPTION

Sexually transmitted disease caused by ascent of microorganisms from vagina and endocervix to uterus, fallopian tubes, ovaries, and contiguous structures.

ETIOLOGY

- Can be caused by *N. gonorrhea, C. trachomatis, Bacteroides, Peptostreptococcus, Peptococcus, E. coli,* Diphtheroids, *Gardnerella vaginalis*, and other microorganisms

Most infections are polymicrobial.

INCIDENCE

- 1 million women annually are treated for PID

RISK FACTORS

- Intrauterine device
- Sexual activity
- Age <25 years
- Adolescence
- Multiple sexual partners
- Previous history of PID

ASSESSMENT FINDINGS

- Asymptomatic
- Symptoms often begin during or within one week of menses
- Lower abdominal pain
- Fever, malaise
- Vaginal discharge or lesion
- Urinary discomfort
- Nausea and vomiting
- Abdominal tenderness
- Cervical motion tenderness
- Adnexal tenderness

DIFFERENTIAL DIAGNOSIS

- Appendicitis
- Ectopic pregnancy
- Ruptured ovarian cyst
- Endometriosis

DIAGNOSTIC STUDIES

- Pregnancy test
- CBC
- WBC: >10,000
- Wet prep
- Pelvic ultrasound
- Culture for gonorrhea
- Culture or antigen test for chlamydia
- Hepatitis serology
- Syphilis serology
- HIV screen

Diagnosis of PID is often difficult to make because symptoms can be ambiguous.

DIAGNOSTIC CRITERIA

- Suggested criteria for diagnosis (sufficient for empiric therapy)
    - ◊ Lower abdominal tenderness
    - ◊ Cervical motion tenderness
    - ◊ Adnexal tenderness

- Additional criteria
  - ◊ Temperature ≥101°F (38.3°C)
  - ◊ WBC ≥10,500
  - ◊ Purulent material obtained with culdocentesis
  - ◊ Abnormal cervical or vaginal discharge
  - ◊ Elevated C-reactive protein
  - ◊ Adnexal mass
  - ◊ Laboratory evidence of gonorrhea or chlamydia
- Elaborate criteria
  - ◊ Histopathologic endometritis on biopsy
  - ◊ Transvaginal sonography or other imaging techniques showing thickened fluid-filled tubes with or without free pelvic fluid or tubo-ovarian complex
  - ◊ Laparoscopic evidence of PID

PREVENTION

- Use of condoms and spermicide
- Use of oral contraceptives has been shown to decrease incidence of PID
- Screen for STDs

NONPHARMACOLOGIC MANAGEMENT

- Abstinence until treatment completed
- Evaluation and treatment of sexual partners

PHARMACOLOGIC MANAGEMENT

Outpatient management: CDC recommends several different regimens

No specific regimen is considered superior because treatment is empiric until cultures confirm organisms present. However, antibiotic coverage should include chlamydia, gonorrhea, anaerobes, gram negative rods, and streptococcus.

- Cefoxitin (Mefoxin®) intramuscular plus oral probenecid and doxycycline (Vibramycin®) *OR*
- Ceftriaxone (Rocephin®) intramuscular with oral doxycycline *OR*
- Ofloxacin 400 mg orally
- *PLUS* metronidazole (Flagyl®)

PREGNANCY/LACTATION CONSIDERATIONS

- Hospitalization required during pregnancy

CONSULTATION/REFERRAL

- Hospitalization for the following:
  - ◊ Presence of pelvic abscess
  - ◊ Severe illness
  - ◊ Failed response to outpatient management
  - ◊ Noncompliance with therapy
  - ◊ Comorbid HIV infection
  - ◊ Adolescent
  - ◊ Pregnancy
  - ◊ Failure of medical treatment

FOLLOW-UP

- Close observation of clinical course with reevaluation in 72 hours; sooner if symptoms worsen
- Test of cure in 7-10 days and at 4-6 weeks posttreatment
- Use of intrauterine device is contraindicated in women with a previous episode of PID

Patient should feel better within 72 hours if empiric selection of antibiotics was appropriate.

EXPECTED COURSE

- Good prognosis if treated early with effective treatment
- Poor prognosis related to poor compliance and repeated infections

POSSIBLE COMPLICATIONS

- Recurrent infection
- Increased risk of ectopic pregnancy
- Infertility
- Sepsis

TRICHOMONIASIS

DESCRIPTION

Sexually transmitted disease which can infect vagina, Skene's ducts, and lower genitourinary tract in women and lower genitourinary tract in men

ETIOLOGY

- *Trichomonas vaginalis*, a single-celled, flagellated protozoan parasite

INCIDENCE

- Account for 10-25% of all vaginal infections

RISK FACTORS

- Multiple sexual partners
- History of previous STDs

ASSESSMENT FINDINGS

Female:
- Asymptomatic (up to 40%)
- Vaginal discharge that is frothy, copious, and pale yellow to gray-green in color
- Vulvovaginal irritation
- Dysuria
- Foul, fishy odor
- Intense erythema of the vaginal mucosa
- Dyspareunia
- Symptoms may worsen during menstruation

Cervical petechiae ("strawberry cervix") can be visible secondary to tiny hemorrhages.

Male:
- Asymptomatic (almost 80% of men are asymptomatic)
- Urethral discharge
- Dysuria
- Epididymitis
- Prostatitis

DIFFERENTIAL DIAGNOSIS

- Vaginal candidiasis
- Bacterial vaginosis
- Gonococcal or chlamydial infections in women
- Chlamydia urethritis in men

Incubation period is 3-28 days.

DIAGNOSTIC STUDIES

- Wet prep:
  - ◊ Visualization of trichomonads as flagellated, motile cells slightly larger than WBCs
  - ◊ Polymorphonuclear cells
- Vaginal secretion pH: >4.5
- Culture rarely needed
- Pap smear

PREVENTION

- Use of condoms
- Screen for other STDs

NONPHARMACOLOGIC MANAGEMENT

- Abstinence until treatment completed
- Treat sexual partner(s)
- Abstain from alcohol if taking metronidazole

PHARMACOLOGIC MANAGEMENT

- Metronidazole (Flagyl®) orally

PREGNANCY/LACTATION CONSIDERATIONS

- Metronidazole 2 gram orally in single dose

CONSULTATION/REFERRAL

- None usually needed
- Consider consult regarding treatment of pregnant women

FOLLOW-UP

- No follow-up needed if symptoms resolve

EXPECTED COURSE

- Complete resolution.
- Recurrent infection raises possibility of noncompliance, reinfection, or infection with resistant organism

POSSIBLE COMPLICATIONS

- Recurrent infections

References

American Academy of Pediatrics. (2003). *Red book: Report of the committee on infectious disease* (26th ed.). Elk Grove Village, IN: American Academy of Pediatrics.

Bickley, L.S., & Szilagyi, P.G. (2003). *Bates' guide to physical examination and history taking* (8th ed.). Philadelphia: Lippincott Williams & Wilkins.

Branch, W.T. (2003). *Office practice of medicine* (4th ed.). Philadelphia: Saunders.

Burns, C.E., Brady, M.A., Blosser, C., Starr, N.B., & Dunn, A.M. (2004). *Pediatric primary care: A handbook for nurse practitioners* (3rd ed.). Philadelphia: W.B. Saunders.

Carmichael, C. (1997). Preventing perinatal HIV transmission: Zidovudine use during pregnancy. *American Family Physician, 55*, 171-174.

Carpenter, C. et al (2000). Antiretroviral therapy in adults: updated recommendations of the International AIDS society-USA Panel. *Journal of the American Medical Society. 283*(3): 381-90.

Carpenter, C. C., Fischl, M. A., Hammers, S. M., et al. (1997). Antiretroviral therapy for HIV infections in 1997. *Journal of the American Medical Association, 277,* 1962.

Carson, S. (1997). Human papillomatous virus infection update: Impact on women's health. *The Nurse Practitioner, 22*(4), 24-37.

Centers for Disease Control and PREVENTION. (1993). Recommendations for the prevention and treatment of *Chlamydia trachomatis* infections, 1993. *MMWR, 42.*

Centers for Disease Control and PREVENTION. (1998). Sexually transmitted diseases treatment guidelines. *MMWR, 47*, (RR-1).

Centers for Disease Control and PREVENTION. (1996). Update: Provisional public health service recommendations for chemoprophylaxis after occupational exposure to HIV. *MMWR, 45*, 468-480.

Centers for Disease Control and PREVENTION. (1997). USPHS/IDSA guidelines for the prevention of opportunistic infections in persons infected with human immunodeficiency virus. *MMWR, 46*, (RR-12).

Centers for Disease Control (2001): Report of the NIH Panel to Define Principles of Therapy of HIV Infection and Guidelines for the Use of Antiretroviral Agents in HIV-infected Adults and Adolescents. *MMWR*, 47, (NO RR-5).

Champion, J.D., Piper, J.M., Holden, A.E., Shain, R.N., Perdue, S., & Korte, J.E. (2005). Relationship of abuse and pelvic inflammatory disease risk behavior in minority adolescents. *American Academy of Nurse Practitioners, 16,* 234-241.

Dambro, M.R. (2005). *Griffith's 5 minute clinical consult.* Philadelphia: Lippincott Williams & Wilkins.

Dykeman, M., Fugate, K., & Lau, S. (1997). Human immunodeficiency virus: Early steps in management. *The Nurse Practitioner, 22*(3), 94-100.

El-Sadr, W., Oleske, J. M., Agins, B. D., et al. (1994). *Evaluation and management of early HIV infection.* Clinical Practice Guideline No. 7. AHCPR Publication No. 94-0572. Rockville, MD: Agency for Health Care Policy and Research, Public Health Service, U.S. Department of Health and Human Services.

Frederickson, H.L., & Wilkins-Haug, L. (1997). *OB/GYN secrets.* (2nd ed.). Philadelphia: Hanley and Belfus.

Gilber, D.N., Moellering, R.C., Eliopoulos, G.M., & Sande, M.A. (Eds.). (2004). *Sanford Guide to Antimicrobial Therapy* (34th ed.). Hyde Park, VT: Antimicrobial Therapy.

Goodman, L., Croke, V., Rodman, A., et al. (1999). Cervical dysplasia in women with HIV. *The Nurse Practitioner, 24*(8),

79-85.

Goroll, A. H., & Mulley, A. G., Jr. (Eds.). (2000). *Primary care medicine: Office evaluation and management of the adult patient* (4th ed.). Philadelphia: Lippincott Williams Wilkins.

Graber, M.A., & Lanternier, M.L. (Eds.) (2001). *The family practice handbook.* (4th ed.). St. Louis: Mosby.

Grimshaw, L.J. (2005). How to recognize and manage HPV infections. *Clinical Advisor, 8*(5) 24-32.

Heath, C. B. (1995). *Chlamydia trachomatis* infection update. *American Family Physician, 51*, 1455-1459.

Mangion, S. (2000). *Physical diagnosis secrets.* Philadelphia: Hanley and Belfus.

Liberatore, J., Schwarze, S., & Silva, C. (2005). HIV aware in primary care: A refresher on assessment and treatment. *Advance for Nurse Practitioners, 13*(7), 49-54.

Miller, D. M., & Brodell, R. T. (1996). Human papillomavirus infection: Treatment options for warts. *American Family Physician, 53*, 135-143.

Rakel, R.E. (Ed.). (1998). *Essentials of family practice.* (2nd ed.). Philadelphia: WB Saunders.

Ransom, S. B., & McNeeley, S. G. (1997). *Gynecology for the primary care provider.* Philadelphia: W.B. Saunders.

Santangelo, J. (2001). Acute seroconversion of HIV infection in the ambulatory care setting. *The Nurse Practitioner, 24*(8), 79-85.

Searight, H. R., & McLaren, L. (1997). Behavioral and psychiatric aspects of HIV infection. *American Family Physician, 55*, 227-1236.

Skolnik, N. S. (1995). Screening for *Chlamydia trachomatis* infection. *American Family Physician, 51*, 821-826.

Uphold, C.R., & Graham, M.V. (2003). *Clinical guidelines in family practice.* (4th ed.). Gainesville, FL: Barmarrae Books.

U.S. Preventive Services Task Force. (1996). *Guide to clinical preventive services.* (2nd ed.) Washington, D.C.: Office of Disease Prevention and Health Promotion, U.S. Government Printing Office.

Verdon, M. E. (1996). Issues in the management of human papillomavirus genital disease. *American Family Physician, 55*, 1813-1819.

Walker, Y. L. (1996). Early manifestations of HIV infections. *Hospital Medicine, 32*(7), 21-26.

Zollo, A.J., Jr (Ed.). (2004). *Medical Secrets.* (4th ed.), St. Louis, MO: Mosby-Year Book.

20

SOCIAL-PSYCHIATRIC PROBLEMS

Social-Psychiatric Problems

ANXIETY

DESCRIPTION

A psychic and physical experience of dread, foreboding, apprehension, or panic in response to emotional or physiologic stimuli; may be acute or chronic

Common types of anxiety: acute situational anxiety, generalized anxiety disorder, panic disorder, post-traumatic stress disorder, obsessive-compulsive disorder, and phobias

ETIOLOGY

- Behavioral theory: anxiety is the conditioned response to specific environmental stimuli
- Biologic theories
  - ◊ Norepinephrine, serotonin, and γ-aminobutyric acid (GABA) are poorly regulated
  - ◊ The autonomic nervous system responds inappropriately to stimuli
  - ◊ Functional cerebral pathology causes anxiety disorder symptoms

INCIDENCE

- 6-25% lifetime prevalence in general population of U.S.
- Females > Males
- Most prevalent in 20-45 year olds
- Separation anxiety is the most common reason given for school refusal (mean age 9 years)

Anxiety is the most common psychiatric disorder in the US.

RISK FACTORS

Organic causes:
- Organic syndromes: endocrinopathies, cardiorespiratory disorders, anemia
- Use of or withdrawal from medications and substances
  - ◊ Alcohol
  - ◊ Antihypertensives
  - ◊ Caffeine, including analgesics containing caffeine
  - ◊ Cocaine, marijuana, hallucinogens
  - ◊ Corticosteroids
  - ◊ Lidocaine
  - ◊ Oral contraceptives
  - ◊ Nonsteroidal anti-inflammatories (NSAIDs)
  - ◊ Withdrawal from selective serotonin reuptake inhibitors (SSRIs)
- Family history

Psychosocial stress:
- Marital discord
- Medical illness
- Job-related stress
- Financial problems

Psychiatric disorders:
- Major depression
- Panic disorders
- Personality disorders
- Schizophrenia

ASSESSMENT FINDINGS

Children:
- Excessive anxiety about separation after preschool age
- Unrealistic worry about harm to self or family
- Somatic complaints in absence of physical illness
- Persistent worry about past behavior, competence, or future events

Adults:
- Complaints of apprehension, restlessness, edginess, distractibility
- Insomnia
- Somatic complaints
  - ◊ Fatigue
  - ◊ Paresthesias, near syncope, derealization, dizziness
  - ◊ Palpitations, tachycardia, chest pain/tightness
  - ◊ Dyspnea, hyperventilation

- ◊ Nausea, vomiting, diarrhea
- Excessive rumination

DIFFERENTIAL DIAGNOSIS

- Any medical condition that involves stimulation of the sympathetic nervous system
  - ◊ Arrhythmias, MI, valvular disease
  - ◊ Endocrinopathies: hyperthyroidism, Cushing's syndrome, hypoglycemia, electrolyte imbalances, menopause
  - ◊ Medication and substance reactions
  - ◊ Medication and substance withdrawal
  - ◊ Anemia
  - ◊ Asthma, COPD, pulmonary embolism, pneumothorax

DIAGNOSTIC STUDIES

- TSH
- CBC, urinalysis
- Urine drug screen
- Focus on medical conditions for which patient is already being treated
- Direct attention toward arrhythmias, hyperthyroidism, drugs
- Evaluate prominent constellation of symptoms
- Psychologic testing
  - ◊ Interview based on DSM-IV criteria
  - ◊ Hamilton Anxiety Scale
  - ◊ Zung Anxiety Self-Assessment

NONPHARMACOLOGIC MANAGEMENT

- Psychotherapy
  - ◊ Education regarding diagnosis, treatment plan, and prognosis
  - ◊ Support and empathic listening
- Behavioral therapy
  - ◊ Relaxation techniques
  - ◊ Reconditioning: exposure to feared stimuli in controlled setting to develop tolerance and eventually eradicate the anxiety response
- General measures
  - ◊ Regular exercise
  - ◊ Serial office visits

PHARMACOLOGIC MANAGEMENT

- Should be of limited duration, with intent of allowing patient to benefit from behavioral treatments
  - ◊ Drugs should play an adjunctive role, except in panic disorder
  - ◊ Drugs reduce, but do not eradicate symptoms

TCA and SSRI may take 2-4 weeks before therapeutic response is realized by patient.

Use of benzodiazepine until TCA or SSRI becomes effective is a commonly employed strategy.

- Situational anxiety
  - ◊ Benzodiazepines (short-term, up to one month)
- Generalized anxiety disorder
  - ◊ BuSpar®
  - ◊ SSRIs
- Panic disorder
  - ◊ SSRIs
  - ◊ TCA
  - ◊ Benzodiazepines
- Obsessive-compulsive disorder
  - ◊ TCA
  - ◊ SSRIs

AGENT	ACTION	COMMENTS
Benzodiazepines (BNZ) *Example:* lorazepam (Ativan®) alprazolam (Xanax®) diazepam (Valium®)	Benzodiazepines increase binding of GABA to the GABA receptors. This promotes a feeling of calm.	Response usually occurs in 30 minutes to 2 hours. Contraindicated in hepatic dysfunction, renal impairment. Cautious use in the elderly to prevent excessive sedation. Monitor for drug interactions. May worsen depression, cause sedation, and slurred speech. Effect is exacerbated by alcohol. Tolerance develops with daily use.
Tricyclic antidepressants (TCA) *Examples:* amitriptyline (Elavil®) nortriptyline (Pamelor®) imipramine (Tofranil®)	Inhibit the re-uptake of norepinephrine and serotonin	Up to 2-4 weeks are required to achieve therapeutic response. TCA lowers the seizure threshold. Can cause dry mouth, sedation. Due to the anticholinergic effects, use cautiously in patients with urinary retention, glaucoma. May cause conduction defects, worsen psychosis, and trigger a manic or depressive episode in a manic depressive patient. May precipitate sexual dysfunction, weight gain. Many drugs can interact with TCA. Do not abruptly stop TCA.
Selective Serotonin Re-uptake Inhibitors (SSRI) *Examples:* citalopram (Celexa®) fluoxetine (Prozac®) paroxetine (Paxil®) sertraline (Zoloft®)	Inhibit the re-uptake of serotonin and have a weak effect on re-uptake of norepinephrine and dopamine	May take 2-4 weeks to achieve therapeutic response. Cautious use in hepatic patients because SSRI are extensively metabolized in the liver. Many drugs can interact with SSRI. May cause mild nausea at onset of use, headache, and/or insomnia. May cause dry mouth, sexual dysfunction, and weight gain. Serotonin syndrome (confusion, hyperthermia, bizarre behavior) is a rare complication. Do not abruptly stop SSRI. Must wean off.

PREGNANCY/LACTATION CONSIDERATIONS

- Benzodiazepines contraindicated in pregnancy and lactation
- TCA contraindicated in pregnancy
- SSRIs contraindicated in first trimester but are often continued by obstetrician

CONSULTATION/REFERRAL

- Parent/child or family intervention
- Evidence of substance abuse
- Disabling symptoms
- Symptoms that worsen despite treatment

FOLLOW-UP

- Regular follow-up visits are important to reinforce education regarding nonpharmacologic management and proper use of medications
- Avoid prescribing anxiolytics by telephone
- Remain alert to signs of medication misuse
- Tricyclic antidepressants require periodic serum levels

EXPECTED COURSE

- Anxiety in children can be a precursor to agoraphobia or panic disorder in adulthood
- Treatment of medical cause usually, but not always, initiates improvement
- Short-term anxiety disorders usually respond well to treatment
- Obsessive compulsive disorder requires long-term pharmacologic therapy along with psychotherapy

POSSIBLE COMPLICATIONS

- Work and school related difficulties
- Self medication leading to alcohol abuse, benzodiazepine dependence
- Social impairment
- Cardiac arrhythmias related to TCA use
- Falls due to sedating effects of medications, especially in the elderly

DEPRESSION AND SUICIDE

DESCRIPTION

- Depression is a constellation of signs and symptoms that is an abnormal reaction to life's difficulties. Disturbances in cognitive, emotional, behavioral, and somatic regulation are involved. Depressed mood, and loss of interest or pleasure are the major symptoms
- Suicide is self-inflicted death. Attempted suicide is a potentially lethal act that does not result in death.

Anhedonia is a loss of pleasure or interest in things which had always given joy or pleasure. Depressed patients exhibit anhedonia.

ETIOLOGY

- Impaired synthesis and/or metabolism of the neurotransmitters norepinephrine, serotonin, and/or dopamine
- Evidence indicates genetic basis

Serotonin produces calmness and relaxed states of being.
Norepinephrine and dopamine enhance productivity, ambition, and ability to concentrate.

INCIDENCE

Depression:

- Will affect 5-20% of the U.S. population at some time
- 1.5-3 times more common among those with an affected first-degree relative
- Affects 2% of preadolescents and 5% of adolescents in the U.S.

Suicide:

- Successful suicide: Males > Females
- Suicide attempts: Females > Males
- Threefold increase in adolescent suicide reports over the last 40 years
- 9-18% of preadolescents with nonpsychiatric diagnoses entertain suicidal ideations

RISK FACTORS

- Female gender
- Psychosocial stressors
- Postpartum period
- Physical or chronic illness, especially migraines and back pain
- Prior episodes of depression
- Family history
- Alcohol or substance abuse
- Children with behavioral disorders, especially hyperactivity
- Retirement, aging, significant losses (death of a spouse, loss of a job, etc.)

ASSESSMENT FINDINGS

Children:

- Anorexia
- Sleep disturbance
- Apathy
- Developmental delay

- Anxiety, irritability, cries easily
- Aggression, hyperactivity
- School problems
- GI or other somatic complaints

Adolescents:
- Similar to adults
- Impulsivity
- Fatigue
- Hopelessness
- Substance abuse

Adults:
- Depressed mood
- Anhedonia
- Decreased or increased appetite
- Sleep disorder
- Psychomotor agitation or retardation
- Fatigue, loss of energy
- Feelings of worthlessness, inappropriate guilt
- Recurrent thoughts of death

In adults, depression is likely if the patient experiences anhedonia or depression and (any 4 or more of the following): change in appetite, sleep pattern, fatigue, psychomotor retardation or agitation, poor self-image, difficulty concentrating, or suicidal ideation.

DIFFERENTIAL DIAGNOSIS

Children:
- Bipolar disorder
- Attention deficit disorder
- Separation anxiety
- Chronic physical illness
- Conduct disorder
- Physical or sexual abuse

Adults:
- Bipolar disorder
- Substance abuse
- Physical illness: organic brain diseases, diabetes, liver, or renal failure
- Grief reaction
- Other psychiatric disorders
- Medication abuse/use
- Medication withdrawal
- Hypothyroidism, B12 deficiency
- Dementia

DIAGNOSTIC STUDIES

Structured interviews/questionnaires:
- The Children's Depression Inventory
- Children's Depression Scale
- Depression Self-Rating Scale
- Center for Epidemiological Studies Depression Scale for Children
- Beck's Depression Inventory
- Child Behavior Checklist for Ages 4-18 Years
- Pediatric Symptom Checklist
- Zung Self-rating Depression Scale
- Halstead-Reitan battery: helps distinguish dementia from depression
- Ye savage's Geriatric Depression scale

Laboratory studies do not diagnose depression, but, are used to rule out other conditions.

Laboratory studies:
- TSH; indicated for women >age 50 years to rule out hypothyroidism
- Laboratory tests specific to depression are under clinical investigation (serotonin, dopamine, norepinephrine levels)
- Urine screen for substance use disorders
- ECG as baseline to rule out arrhythmias or heart block before instituting TCA

TCA may provoke arrhythmias in patients with subclinical sinus node dysfunction.

PREVENTION

- Maintain a high index of suspicion in adolescents and adults with family or personal history of depression, or with chronic illness or recent loss
- Question persons suspected of suicide intent regarding plan and availability of method
- Routine questioning regarding use of alcohol and drugs starting during adolescence

NONPHARMACOLOGIC MANAGEMENT

- Identify suicidal risk, plan, and intent
- Establish safe environment: ensure patient safety in least restrictive environment
    - ◊ Negotiate suicide contract

- Provide community resources, suicide hotline
- Suicide threats should be interpreted as a communication of desperation and are to be taken *seriously*
- Psychoeducation
  - ◊ Ongoing information regarding illness, symptoms, prognosis, and therapy
  - ◊ Include interpersonal relationships, work, other health related needs
  - ◊ Discourage major life changes while in a depressive state
  - ◊ Help set realistic, attainable, concrete goals
  - ◊ Educate regarding importance of avoiding alcohol
- Psychotherapy
  - ◊ Establish and maintain a supportive therapeutic relationship
  - ◊ Remain available during times of crisis
  - ◊ Maintain vigilance for signs of destructive impulses
  - ◊ Strengthen expectations of help and hope for the future
  - ◊ Enlist support of others in patient's social network
- Electroconvulsive therapy (ECT)
  - ◊ Indicated for depression in which a rapid antidepressant response is imperative: depression coupled with psychotic features, catatonic stupor, severe suicidality, or severe nutritional compromise
  - ◊ Indicated for patients who prefer this method of treatment, or who have responded unsatisfactorily to antidepressant medication in the past
  - ◊ High rate of therapeutic success
  - ◊ Chief side effect is transient postictal confusional state, and memory impairment which resolves in a few weeks
- Light therapy
  - ◊ Particularly effective for seasonal affective disorder
  - ◊ Exposure to bright white artificial light for 30 minutes or more in morning and/or evening
  - ◊ May be used along with pharmacotherapy

Psychotherapeutic interventions in conjunction with pharmacologic therapy are superior to either when used alone.

PHARMACOLOGIC MANAGEMENT

- Determine coexisting substance use disorders and general medical conditions
- Cyclic antidepressants (tri and tetracyclics)
- Selective serotonin-reuptake inhibitors
- Monoamine oxidase inhibitors are not used first or second line because of numerous food and drug interactions
- Others
  - ◊ Effexor®
  - ◊ Wellbutrin®

TCA and SSRI are equally efficacious but the SSRIs have a better side effect profile and would not be fatal if a month's supply were taken at once.

CONSULTATION/REFERRAL

- Psychiatrist if patient has suicide plan, or for ECT if severe major depression is coupled with psychosis, nutritional compromise, or suicidality. Make appointment and referral at time of visit
- Indications for inpatient psychiatric treatment
  - ◊ Unable to adequately care for themselves or cooperate with outpatient treatment
  - ◊ Have suicidal or homicidal ideation and plan, particularly if method is violent
  - ◊ Lack of psychosocial support
  - ◊ Complicating psychiatric or medical conditions that make outpatient treatment unsafe

In the elderly, depression often coexists with dementia.

FOLLOW-UP

- Follow-up within 2 weeks after initiating medication or sooner if patient's condition dictates
- Antidepressant medications should be continued for at least 4-6 months after complete remission of symptoms

- Antidepressant medications should be tapered rather than abruptly discontinued
- Patients with multiple prior episodes of depression may require long-term pharmacologic management
- After recovery from a suicide attempt, explore frame of mind to determine whether suicidal thoughts persist
- Educate regarding constructive methods of seeking help for future problems

EXPECTED COURSE

- 60-70% response rates to antidepressants of all classes
- Patients take 4-6 weeks to fully respond to medication management
- High relapse rate during the first 8 weeks after resolution of symptoms

POSSIBLE COMPLICATIONS

- Suicide: overdose of tricyclics is potentially lethal
- Bizarre behavior may endanger social relationships and reputation
- Complicating psychiatric or medical conditions
- Substance abuse resulting from attempts to self medicate

ALCOHOL USE DISORDER

DESCRIPTION

Alcohol *abuse* is a pattern of inappropriate alcohol consumption for one month or more, without the development of physical tolerance. This may include drinking in the presence of a medical condition, or when driving. It may or may not precede alcohol *dependence*. In alcohol dependence, tolerance develops, causing cellular changes, altered metabolism, and the withdrawal symptoms that result when blood alcohol levels drop.

ETIOLOGY

- Combination of social, cultural, biological and emotional factors
- Probable genetic influence

INCIDENCE

- Males > Females (3:1)
- Predominant age is 18-25 years
- Heavy drinking (>5 drinks/day) is reported by 10% of adult men and 2% of women
- 40% of unintentional injuries involving adolescents are alcohol-related
- Alcohol abuse implicated in 50% of traffic fatalities, 67% of drowning and murders, 70-80% of deaths in fires, and 35% of suicides

RISK FACTORS

- Genetic vulnerability: family history
- Use of other psychoactive substances
- Alcohol use in peer group or by parents, cultural acceptance of alcohol abuse
- Recent stressful life events
- Low socioeconomic status
- Unemployment

ASSESSMENT FINDINGS

- Reliability of patient reporting is highly variable
- Medical problems associated with alcohol dependence
  - ◊ Psychosis, dementia, memory impairment, blackouts, insomnia
  - ◊ Nausea, vomiting, peptic ulcer disease, abdominal pain
  - ◊ Hepatitis, cirrhosis, pancreatitis
  - ◊ Thiamine deficiency: anorexia, weight loss, peripheral neuropathy, irritability, tremors
  - ◊ Cardiomyopathy, hypertension, arrhythmias
  - ◊ Aspiration pneumonia, bronchitis
  - ◊ Cancer of oropharynx, larynx, esophagus, and liver
  - ◊ Impotence
  - ◊ Cushingoid appearance, gynecomastia

- ◊ Signs of accidents (e.g., fractures, bruises, burns)
- ◊ Poor hygiene, plethoric facies
- Social consequences of alcohol abuse
  - ◊ Divorce
  - ◊ Depression
  - ◊ Suicide
  - ◊ Domestic violence
  - ◊ Arrests, legal problems
  - ◊ Unemployment, employment problems
  - ◊ Poverty
  - ◊ Unsafe sexual behavior, sexually transmitted diseases
  - ◊ Children may experience abnormal psychosocial development related to parental alcohol abuse

Delays in maturation and sexual development are common in adolescents who abuse alcohol.

DIFFERENTIAL DIAGNOSIS

- Depression, anxiety, bipolar disorder
- Essential hypertension, ischemic heart disease
- Peptic ulcer disease, viral gastroenteritis, cholelithiasis, viral hepatitis, pancreatitis
- Primary endocrine disorder
- Solar skin damage
- Primary seizure disorder

DIAGNOSTIC STUDIES

- Blood alcohol levels may be detected; breath alcohol commonly used
- Liver function tests (γ-glutamyltransferase, ALT, AST) abnormal in 50% of cases
- AST : ALT > 2.0
- Mean corpuscular volume (MCV): elevated
- Uric acid, PT, triglycerides elevated
- Brief screening questionnaires: all have limitations, may be less sensitive and specific in adolescents
  - ◊ CAGE questionnaire: most popular; less sensitive for early or heavy drinking
  - ◊ Michigan Alcoholism Screening Test (MAST): highly sensitive and specific, but too long for routine screening
  - ◊ Alcohol Use Disorders Identification Test (AUDIT): sensitive and specific for hazardous or harmful drinking
- Biopsy of liver diagnostic of alcoholic hepatitis or cirrhosis

PREVENTION

- Screen all adolescents and adults concerning alcohol utilizing patient inquiry or standardized instruments
- Offer counseling to problem drinkers
- Careful discussion with all adolescents regarding alcohol use, including regular advice to abstain from alcohol
- Counsel parents regarding their use of alcohol in the home

NONPHARMACOLOGIC MANAGEMENT

- Substance abuse counseling
  - ◊ Establish a therapeutic relationship
  - ◊ Make medical office off-limits for substance abuse
  - ◊ Present information about negative health consequences
  - ◊ Involve family and other support
  - ◊ Set goals
  - ◊ Involve community treatment services
- Balanced diet: common deficiencies are folate, thiamine, magnesium, phosphate, and zinc
- Provide education about Alcoholics Anonymous
- Treatment for adolescents should be developmentally appropriate, peer oriented, and involve the family

PHARMACOLOGIC MANAGEMENT

- Detoxification: symptoms of withdrawal (e.g., seizures, hallucinations, and delirium) typically begin within 12 hours of cessation of alcohol use and resolve within 5 days
  - ◊ Lorazepam (Ativan®)
  - ◊ Chlordiazepoxide (Librium®)
  - ◊ Oxazepam (Serax®)
  - ◊ Taper according to patient response
  - ◊ Elderly may require higher benzodiazepine doses and a longer detoxification period

- Naltrexone (ReVia®) reduces craving for alcohol
- Disulfiram (Antabuse®)
  - ◊ Produces sensitivity to alcohol which results in a highly unpleasant reaction when alcohol is ingested
  - ◊ Patient must want to remain in a state of enforced sobriety
  - ◊ Should never be administered to a patient who is in a state of denial, or who is intoxicated, or without his full knowledge
- Thiamine (B1) supplementation due to poor thiamine absorption associated with alcohol ingestion (intramuscular or intravenous initially, then oral)
- Folic acid, B6, B12, multivitamin, magnesium sulfate

First dose of benzodiazepine should make patient sleepy. Dose is tapered to control withdrawal symptoms.

PREGNANCY/LACTATION CONSIDERATIONS

- Pregnant women at high risk for sexually transmitted diseases, hepatitis, anemia, tuberculosis, hypertension, and failure to obtain prenatal care
- Alcohol passes through the placenta, resulting in higher risk of birth defects, fetal alcohol syndrome, cardiovascular problems, impaired growth and development, prematurity, low birth weight, and stillbirth
- Neonate may suffer from withdrawal
- Abstinence recommended when planning conception, and throughout pregnancy
- Mothers with alcohol abuse problems often need education in parenting and nutrition

CONSULTATION/REFERRAL

- Indications for inpatient detoxification treatment:
  - ◊ Patients in severe withdrawal or with a prior history of delirium tremens
  - ◊ History of very heavy alcohol use and high tolerance
  - ◊ Severe comorbid medical or psychiatric disorder
  - ◊ History of repeatedly failing to benefit from outpatient detoxification
- Alcoholics Anonymous for support and education
- Family support groups (e.g., Al-Anon, Alateen)
- Addiction specialist

FOLLOW-UP

- Daily visits during detoxification, reduce to weekly, then less frequent
- Involvement in some form of aftercare is a strong predictor of a successful outcome
- Aftercare should include coping skills training to prevent relapse

The first 3 months after withdrawal are the most important in predicting long term success.

EXPECTED COURSE

- Relapses are common and should be expected
- Patients may learn from relapse, resulting in ability to pursue complete recovery
- Long-term sobriety is attainable

POSSIBLE COMPLICATIONS

- Accidents, trauma
- Social problems: financial, marital, occupational, legal
- Psychiatric problems: suicide, depression
- Cirrhosis, GI malignancies
- Cardiovascular disorders
- Respiratory problems
- Neurologic problems
- Hematologic disorders
- Metabolic disorders
- Obstetric problems
- Oropharyngeal and esophageal cancers
- Fetal alcohol syndrome

SUBSTANCE USE DISORDERS

DESCRIPTION

A maladaptive pattern of substance use leading to impairment or distress; substances commonly abused are alcohol, amphetamines, cocaine, hallucinogens, inhalants, marijuana, opioids, sedatives, and steroids. Manifestations of impairment or distress involve school, work, family, legal, physical, or social difficulties.

ETIOLOGY

- Biological factors: the intrinsic addictiveness of a drug coupled with inherited familial biologic markers
- Psychological factors: increased prevalence of certain psychiatric problems (e.g., affective disorders, borderline personality, antisocial personality)
- Social factors: increased prevalence among economically and culturally impoverished

The brain's dopamine system is stimulated when mood altering substances are consumed.

INCIDENCE

- Predominant age is young adult (age 16-25 years)
- Males > Females

RISK FACTORS

- Personal history of substance abuse
- Family history of substance abuse
- Substance abuse among peers
- Psychiatric illness (e.g., depression, anxiety, bipolar disorder)
- Chronic pain
- Health professionals

ASSESSMENT FINDINGS

Results of intoxication or withdrawal:

- Accidents, trauma
- Legal difficulties
- Physical signs
    - ◊ *Opioid intoxication*: somnolence, bradycardia, hypotension, hypoventilation, pupillary constriction
    - ◊ *Opioid withdrawal*: tearing, anxiety, disturbed sleep, nausea, vomiting, diarrhea, pain, restlessness, rhinorrhea
    - ◊ *Inhalant intoxication*: sedation, slurred speech, unsteady gait, irritation of the nasal and ocular tissues, foul odor to breath, paint on the body or clothing, excitation, depression, impulsiveness, exhilaration
    - ◊ *Sedative intoxication*: sedation, somnolence, disinhibition, staggering gait, slurred speech, depressed respirations, slowed pulse, diminished reflexes
    - ◊ *Sedative withdrawal*: insomnia, restlessness, tremor, anxiety, poor sleep, poor appetite, limb twitching, agitation, seizures, fever
    - ◊ *Cannabis reactions* (marijuana or hashish): distortion of time, space, sound, and color, paranoia, disorientation
    - ◊ *Stimulant intoxication* (cocaine or amphetamine): confusion, paranoia, restlessness, irritability, delusions, tremor, anxiety, tachycardia, hypertension, high fever, convulsion, coma
    - ◊ *Stimulant withdrawal*: somnolence, depressed mood, fatigue, strong desire to obtain more stimulants
    - ◊ *Hallucinogen intoxication*: panic reaction, hallucinations, loss of contact with reality, disturbed behavior, increased pulse, elevated blood pressure, perspiration, blurred vision

Results of chronic use:

- Frequent infections: hepatitis B and C, tuberculosis, sexually transmitted diseases, endocarditis
- Regression or retardation of all aspects of personal and psychologic functioning (e.g., family, peers, marital, occupation, school)
- Needle tracks on skin

- Perforated nasal septum with cocaine use

Patients are often malnourished.

DIFFERENTIAL DIAGNOSIS

- Thyroid disorders
- Delirium, depression, anxiety
- Dementia secondary to HIV, syphilis, neurologic disease, alcohol abuse
- Hypo/hyperglycemia
- Hypo/hyperthyroidism
- Bipolar disorder, depression
- Schizophrenia, psychosis
- Stroke
- Head trauma

DIAGNOSTIC STUDIES

- Urine drug screen
  - ◊ Direct supervision of patient voiding helps ensure validity
  - ◊ Sensitive, but not specific; therefore, all positive results should be confirmed by radioimmunoassay
- CBC, glucose, metabolic panel, RPR
- TSH to rule out thyroid dysfunction
- Serum chemistries to rule out physiologic causes for bizarre behavior
- B_{12} and folate levels to rule out deficiencies as cause of memory impairment
- CT scan may be indicated in some cases especially if tumor or head injury is suspected
- Consider lumbar puncture

PREVENTION

- New innovative approaches and research regarding effective methods of prevention are needed. Effective methods of drug use prevention are still unknown.
- Education of patient and parents about risk factors and effects of substance abuse
- Early identification of substance abuse; clinicians should discuss drug use with all children and adolescents during routine visits

NONPHARMACOLOGIC MANAGEMENT

- Consider that denial is often an integral problem and anticipate defenses
- Behavioral therapies
  - ◊ Counseling
  - ◊ Cognitive therapy
  - ◊ Relaxation techniques (e.g., biofeedback and self-hypnosis) to help alleviate detoxification symptoms
- Self-help groups for patient: twelve-step programs (e.g., Narcotics Anonymous, Cocaine Anonymous)
- Self-help groups for families
- Nutritional education
- Detoxification if needed, must be done in appropriate environment
  - ◊ Most basic consideration is acceptance of treatment plan by patient
  - ◊ Consider financial resources
  - ◊ Consider risk of suicide or homicide
  - ◊ Consider patient's general and mental health status and comorbid conditions
  - ◊ Consider support resources
- Fundamental requirement is abstinence from use of mood altering substances
- A caring, nonjudgmental attitude is essential to patient's acceptance of treatment

PHARMACOLOGIC MANAGEMENT

- Opiate withdrawal
  - ◊ Decreasing doses of methadone, a synthetic narcotic analgesic with actions similar to morphine; dispensed only to FDA-approved pharmacies, hospitals, and maintenance programs
  - ◊ Clonidine ameliorates abstinence-related withdrawal symptoms
  - ◊ Naltrexone blocks the subjective and physiologic effects of subsequently administered opioids
- Use of sedatives is discouraged. Short-term use of benzodiazepines may be necessary for physical withdrawal from amphetamines, cocaine, and other stimulant drugs if patient is severely agitated.
- Intravenous diazepam (Valium®) is the drug of choice for treatment of cocaine toxicity characterized by agitation, seizures, and dysrhythmias. β- adrenergic blockers are **not** recommended.
- Sedative withdrawal is accomplished by gradually decreasing the amount of drug

available in order to avoid precipitating CNS rebound, hyperactivity
- Medications to treat comorbid psychiatric conditions

Thiamine is often added to the diet of substance abusing patients.

PREGNANCY/LACTATION CONSIDERATIONS

- Women who substantially reduce cocaine use during pregnancy have outcomes similar to nonusers
- Methadone maintenance is the usual treatment for opiate addiction in pregnancy. Withdrawal during pregnancy is dangerous. Methadone prolongs withdrawal in the infant, but can be done safely.
- The most seriously affected drug users often present late in pregnancy, making treatment very difficult
- The American College of Obstetrics and Gynecology recommends that clinicians take a thorough history of substance abuse in all pregnant women
- Substance abuse in pregnancy increases the risk of spontaneous abortion, preeclampsia, abruptio placentae, early labor, and prolonged labor

Opiates and cocaine are most likely to affect the fetus in the third trimester due to increased maternal blood flow rate and increased placental transport.

- Parenting behavior is likely to be affected by substance abuse

FOLLOW-UP

- Treatment for substance abuse needs to continue on a long-term basis and should include group and individual therapy

Medication intervention in conjunction with counseling yields higher success rates than either alone.

EXPECTED COURSE

- Relapse is common
- Absolute abstinence occurs in a minority of patients, but there is an excellent chance for improvement
- Ongoing encouragement and support is crucial to successful treatment
- When relapse occurs, it is important to identify triggers and modify life to prevent future relapse

POSSIBLE COMPLICATIONS

- Amotivational syndrome
- Depression, suicide
- Spouse battering
- Child abuse
- Hepatitis
- HIV
- Tuberculosis
- Unintentional overdose
- Cocaine poisoning: hyperpyrexia, vasoconstriction, vasospasm, seizures, MI, ischemic stroke, arrhythmias

SMOKING CESSATION

DESCRIPTION

Cigarette smoking is a behavior that involves the continuous use of tobacco and becomes addictive. As physiologic tolerance develops, the smoker increases the number of cigarettes smoked per day. Withdrawal from nicotine produces anxiety, craving, hunger, irritability, drowsiness, tremors, diaphoresis, insomnia, dizziness, and headaches. Successful smoking cessation is defined as abstaining from cigarette smoking for at least one year.

ETIOLOGY

- The two primary reasons people smoke are psychosocial stress and nicotine dependence. A patient's reasons for smoking, as well as motivation to quit, are age-related:

- ◊ Teenagers smoke to appear grown up, due to peer pressure, and are influenced by media and marketing

Teenagers are motivated to quit by recognizing the immediate undesirable effects of cigarette smoking (e.g., bad odor, expense, decreased exercise capacity, relationship between smoking and acute respiratory illness).

- ◊ Adults smoke due to physical dependence, and due to a belief, which is promoted by marketing, that smoking is fashionable and attractive

Adults quit smoking if there is provision of healthy alternatives, if psychosocial issues are addressed, and if recognition of the relationship between smoking and acute illness occurs.

- ◊ Older adults continue to smoke because they feel it is too late to undo damage that is already done

Older adults quit smoking because of immediate benefits (e.g., fewer upper respiratory infections, improved taste sensation, less coughing, and to save money) and the belief that if they quit they can prevent further damage.

INCIDENCE

- Smoking has generally declined in incidence, particularly in higher-educated groups, but children continue to start smoking at the same rate
- 3000 teenagers start smoking every day in the U.S. 60% of current smokers start by age 14 years
- There are 3 million users of smokeless tobacco under age 21 years in the U.S.
- 46 million adults smoke cigarettes
- 1/5 of annual deaths in the U.S. are attributable to smoking-related problems

RISK FACTORS

- Adolescent boys participating in team sports are at increased risk of using smokeless tobacco
- Low education level, low socioeconomic status
- Friends and household members who smoke
- Other substance abuse

ASSESSMENT FINDINGS

- Chronic cough
- Inflammation of oropharynx, sinuses, nose
- Cigarette odor to breath, hair, clothing
- Stained teeth and fingers
- Prematurely aged skin
- Frequent upper respiratory infections
- Chronic obstructive pulmonary disease
- Past attempts at quitting

Smokeless tobacco:
- Erythema of isolated areas of intraoral soft tissue
- Leukoplakia (white patches) on gums

DIAGNOSTIC STUDIES

- Fagerstrom Tolerance Questionnaire: an 8-item tool used to assess level of nicotine addiction
- Spirometry: abnormal indicates damage
- Lipid panel to determine risk factor for heart disease

Chest x-rays are not recommended as screening tools for patients who smoke.

PREVENTION

- Ask all patients and adolescents at each visit whether they use tobacco
- Educate regarding tobacco use and its consequences
- Target prevention programs to the less educated, economically disadvantaged population, and toward adolescents and children
- Provide information about smoking cessation programs
- Link education regarding smoking cessation to the individual's age and to presenting complaints

NONPHARMACOLOGIC MANAGEMENT

- Advise all smokers to quit at each visit
- Suggest replacing smoking with some other activity (e.g., hobbies, exercise, sports)

- Address the patient's personal concerns:
  - ◊ Weight gain: average is an 8 pound weight gain
- Stop-smoking contracts may be helpful
- Identify triggers to smoking by journaling
- Involve friends and family as support system
- Recommend and instruct on relaxation techniques (e.g., deep breathing, guided imagery)
- Educate patients that chewing tobacco or snuff results in nicotine levels equal to that of smokers
- Meticulous oral hygiene and twice a year dental exams for all users of smokeless tobacco

PHARMACOLOGIC MANAGEMENT

- Nicotine replacement therapies
  - ◊ Help relieve the withdrawal symptoms while quitting
  - ◊ Should be used in conjunction with counseling
  - ◊ Patient should quit smoking before using nicotine replacement (do not use concurrently)
  - ◊ Transdermal patch releases a constant dose of nicotine through the skin
  - ◊ Not recommended for those less than 18 years of age, but recent studies indicate can be used safely in adolescents
  - ◊ Nicotine gum helps reduce the urge to smoke
  - ◊ Nicotine nasal spray is highly effective but carries the risk of dependence due to the rapid absorption of nicotine
- Non-nicotine based therapy
  - ◊ Bupropion (Zyban®): theorized to block noradrenergic and dopaminergic pathways, addiction receptors in the brain, resulting in a reduction in the urge to smoke and reduction in withdrawal symptoms
  - ◊ Patients should start taking bupropion before they stop smoking and stop smoking during the second week of therapy. It is continued for 7 to 12 weeks. If used in conjunction with nicotine replacement therapy, the nicotine replacement should be started only after the patient has stopped smoking.

The brain's dopamine system is stimulated when nicotine is consumed.

PREGNANCY/LACTATION CONSIDERATIONS

- Smoking during lactation exposes infant to secondhand smoke and nicotine in breast milk
- Nicotine decreases volume and fat content of breast milk and interferes with production of prolactin and oxytocin
- Premature birth and low birth weight are associated with smoking during pregnancy
- Increased incidence of upper respiratory infections is seen in children exposed to secondhand smoke
- Nicotine replacement therapy products are pregnancy category D drugs and should not be used
- Bupropion is a pregnancy category B drug, but not recommended

CONSULTATION/REFERRAL

- Smoking cessation programs report a cessation rate of 20-30% compared to a 2.5% success rate without participation in a program
- Dentist or ENT physician for any changes in the oral mucosa

Leukoplakia (white patches) on gums may be indicative of pre-malignant or malignant changes. They cannot be diagnosed clinically, but, must be biopsied.

FOLLOW-UP

- If patient is unwilling to quit, provide literature and broach subject again at subsequent visits
- FOLLOW-UP every 2 weeks is recommended (while quitting) to reinforce education and provide encouragement and support
- Weekly supportive phone calls may be helpful

EXPECTED COURSE

- Relapse usually occurs during the first 2 weeks due to withdrawal symptoms
- The use of a nicotine patch doubles the likelihood of abstinence from smoking at 6 months
- Abstinence rates 3 months after use of nicotine nasal spray is 45%
- 12-month abstinence rates with the use of nicotine gum is 18%

POSSIBLE COMPLICATIONS

- Side effects of nicotine replacement therapies and bupropion therapy
- Lung, pancreatic, bladder, esophageal, and head and neck carcinomas
- Chronic obstructive pulmonary disease
- Cardiovascular disease
- Peripheral vascular disease
- Stroke
- Premature aging of the skin
- Otitis media with effusion

Smokeless tobacco:
- Dental caries, gingivitis, discolored teeth, gum recession
- Soft tissue changes, dysplasia, carcinoma
- Elevated cholesterol
- Elevated blood pressure

DOMESTIC VIOLENCE

DESCRIPTION

Use of physical, emotional, economic, or sexual manipulation to control a family member or partner in an intimate relationship. Examples: withholding of money, barring means of transportation, making it difficult to hold a job, routine disparagement and humiliation, forced sexual intercourse, threats of violence, and preventing access to medical treatment.

ETIOLOGY

- Perpetrators generally share low self-esteem and a need for power and control. They presume injustice and the tension culminates in an act of violence.
- In elder abuse, immense responsibilities are often an overwhelming stressor, resulting in neglect
- Children who witness violence learn to use it as adults

INCIDENCE

- 1000 children annually die in the U.S. as a result of abuse or neglect
- 1-4 million women are battered annually by their husband or partner
- 150,000 men are victims each year of assault, robbery, or rape committed by their partner or ex-partner, over half of these result in minor injuries
- 7-18% of pregnant women are abused
- 4% of the elderly in the U.S. are abused by relatives or caretakers
- 90-95% of adult victims of domestic violence are female; 59% of spouse-murder victims are female

RISK FACTORS

- Female gender
- Dependence (physical, financial, or emotional)
- Alcohol or other substance abuse by perpetrator or victim
- Isolation, on part of perpetrator or victim
- Families with poor social support
- Single-parent families
- Unplanned or unwanted pregnancies
- Low socioeconomic status
- Victims of abuse
- Mental retardation or mental illness
- Children with congenital anomalies

ASSESSMENT FINDINGS

- Signs of neglect: poor hygiene, nutritional deficits, lack of dental or medical attention
- Chemical dependency
- Mental illness or mental retardation

- Fear, unwillingness to disclose causes of injuries
- Injuries to abdomen, breasts, genitals, and/or torso
- Burns to back, buttocks, genitals, soles, or palms
- Injuries inconsistent with explanation offered
- Gap between time of injury and presentation for treatment
- Multiple injuries in various stages of healing
- History of multiple pregnancies, spontaneous abortions, preterm labor, or low-birthweight infants
- Unexplained hearing loss
- Children with aggressive behavior, enuresis, excessive masturbation, poor school performance

DIFFERENTIAL DIAGNOSIS

- Burnout as distinguished from bullying, in reference to care of a dependent
- Accidental injuries
- Hypochondriasis

PREVENTION

- Routine patient histories should include questions concerning violence in the home
  - ◊ Has anyone at home ever threatened or hurt you?
  - ◊ Have your children ever been threatened or abused?
  - ◊ Has anyone ever forced you to have sex?
  - ◊ Are you afraid of anyone at home?
  - ◊ Do you feel safe at home?
  - ◊ Have you ever been denied access to medical care?
  - ◊ Have you ever been coerced to sign papers you didn't understand?
  - ◊ How do members of your household get along?
  - ◊ What type of punishment is used at home?
  - ◊ Repeat these questions during patient history updates periodically, but, especially in high risk patients (though, it may be difficult to identify those at high risk)
- Interview patients alone
- Family violence should be part of the differential diagnosis when treating any injury
- Direct questioning may substantially increase reports of episodes of domestic violence

NONPHARMACOLOGIC MANAGEMENT

- Direct victims toward resources to assist in developing survival skills
- Do not recommend joint counseling; abuser may punish victim for exposure
  - ◊ Two independent adults who resolve disagreements with physical fights might benefit from family counseling regarding alternative methods of arbitration
- Maintain a supportive, nonjudgmental attitude
- Assist in development of a safety plan including availability of clothes, keys, documents, and cash
- Reinforce to patients that abuse and violence is never justified. Confirm alliance with the patient.
- Reporting of abuse is mandatory if the victim is a child or an elderly adult
- Some states mandate reporting of suspected domestic violence
- Refrain from attempting to make decisions for competent adults
- Recommend emergency shelter if there seems to be a life-threatening situation
- Assure patient's safety before releasing from care
- Meticulous documentation is crucial in case of future legal action
  - ◊ Include photographs if patient consents
  - ◊ Describe events using patient's own words

PHARMACOLOGIC MANAGEMENT

- Dependent on extent of injuries
- Treat underlying psychiatric illness if appropriate

PREGNANCY/LACTATION CONSIDERATIONS

- Pregnant victims are more likely to defer prenatal care until the third trimester, perhaps in part due to forced isolation by abusers

CONSULTATION/REFERRAL

- National Resource Center on Domestic Violence
  - ◊ Provides information
  - ◊ 1-800-537-2238
- National Domestic Violence Hotline
  - ◊ Immediate crisis intervention
  - ◊ 1-800-799-SAFE (7233)
- Local shelters
- Family therapists, if appropriate
- Nursing home placement

FOLLOW-UP

- Dependent on extent of injuries and needs of patient
- Report of abuse against children and elderly adults is mandatory

EXPECTED COURSE

- Most cases of domestic violence begin early in a relationship and escalate with time
- Battered individuals may eventually resort to violence themselves, against children, or possibly against the batterer

POSSIBLE COMPLICATIONS

- Women with a history of domestic abuse are more likely to abuse alcohol
- Women with a history of domestic abuse are more likely to attempt suicide
- Victims are more likely to be killed when there is escalating violence, substance abuse, death threats, or a weapon in the home
- Adolescents and adults who were abused as children are more likely to abuse tobacco and alcohol, attempt suicide, and exhibit violent or criminal behavior
- Psychological trauma related to child sexual abuse often persists into adulthood
- Sexually transmitted diseases

SEXUAL ASSAULT
(Rape Crisis Syndrome)

DESCRIPTION

Any penetration of a person's intimate parts using force or coercion which occurs against his/her will; forcible carnal knowledge. Includes a range of sexual acts, including rape, incest, sodomy, oral copulation, or penetration of genital or anal opening by a foreign object.

Definitions vary from state to state.

ETIOLOGY

- Pedophiles seem to develop propensity for children during their own adolescence
- Father's need for sexual gratification and a daughter's need for nurturance may lead to incest

INCIDENCE

- 100,000 cases reported annually in U.S.
- Females > Males in both adults and children
- Prevalent age is teens and twenties

Reported rape in children is 1 in 15-20 occurrences.
Reported rape in adults is 1 in 5-10 occurrences.

RISK FACTORS

- Child sexual abuse is often multigenerational
- Alcohol or drug use
- Closely knit, socially isolated family

PHYSICAL ASSESSMENT

Children:

- Sexually transmitted diseases are often the first indication of sexual abuse in children
- Dysuria
- Genital or perianal rash or pain
- Vaginal, penile, or rectal discharge or bleeding
- Presence of sperm and/or semen
- Enuresis, encopresis
- Regressive behaviors (e.g., thumb-sucking, bedwetting, reluctance to sleep alone)
- Compulsive behaviors, unusual fears
- Change in school performance, peer relationships, or behavior
- Inappropriate sexually oriented behavior
- Depression, anger, suicide attempts
- Substance abuse
- Running away
- Recurrent gastrointestinal or gynecological complaints
- Hymenal lacerations
- Gaping anal opening
- Genital or rectal injuries inconsistent with explanation
- Pregnancy

Adults:

- Report of sexual contact without consent
- Evidence of use of forceful sexual contact
- Presence of semen and/or sperm

DIFFERENTIAL DIAGNOSIS

- Consenting sex among adults
- Straddle injury to genital or rectal area
- Perinatally acquired STD
- Lichen sclerosis
- Poor hygiene
- Pinworm infestation

DIAGNOSTIC STUDIES

- Collection of forensic specimens:
  - ◊ Specimens are of limited value if >72 hours since event
  - ◊ All specimens must be handled carefully, maintaining chain of custody
  - ◊ Clothing
  - ◊ Hair specimens obtained by combing pubic hair of victims
  - ◊ Vaginal fluid to test for sperm (motile or nonmotile)
- Rectal, throat, urethral, and/or endocervical cultures for *N. gonorrhoeae* and *C. trachomatis*
- Syphilis serology
- In selected cases as appropriate:
  - ◊ Herpes simplex
  - ◊ Hepatitis B, C
  - ◊ Bacterial vaginosis
  - ◊ Human papillomavirus
  - ◊ *Trichomonas vaginalis*
- Colposcopic examination of genital and rectal area by an expert may be requested by law enforcement agencies
- Pregnancy test, if appropriate
- Initial HIV test, if indicated, should be completed within 7 days

PREVENTION

- Instruct parents and caregivers to educate child about self-defense regarding inappropriate sexual advances
- Early referral of known victims for counseling to prevent future psychological problems
- Educate that children are at risk and unsafe around a pedophile
- Prompt reporting of suspected abuse to child protection authorities
- Assertiveness training, self-defense training

NONPHARMACOLOGIC MANAGEMENT

- Consider SANE (Sexual Assault Nurse Examiner) for exam (shown to be more beneficial for victim)
- Careful documentation of history and physical examination findings for medicolegal purposes
- Supportive and understanding communication, respecting privacy and allowing patient to ventilate feelings
- If emergency contraception is objectionable to patient, inform that fertilization may occur
- All those involved in patient care must be prepared to testify in court
- Inform of need to return at appropriate times for follow-up assessment and/or treatment

A complete genital and rectal exam should be performed with careful attention to documentation.

PHARMACOLOGIC MANAGEMENT

Emergency contraception:
- Failure rate of <2%

Prophylactic antibiotics:
- Ceftriaxone (Rocephin®), cefixime (Suprax®), spectinomycin (Trobicin®), ciprofloxacin (Cipro®), ampicillin/probenecid, *OR* amoxicillin/probenecid for prevention of gonorrhea
- Azithromycin (Zithromax®), doxycycline (Vibramycin®) for prevention of chlamydia
  - ◊ Substitute erythromycin for tetracycline in children <9 years of age
  - ◊ May be given along with pharmacologic treatment for gonorrhea
- Tetanus prophylaxis

PREGNANCY/LACTATION CONSIDERATIONS

- Antibiotic prophylaxis for pregnant women:
  - ◊ Amoxicillin/probenecid, or ceftriaxone (Rocephin®) for prevention of gonorrhea and syphilis
  - ◊ Erythromycin for prevention of chlamydia
- Sedation may be indicated
- Tetanus prophylaxis
- Hepatitis B immune globulin within 14 days, followed by hepatitis B vaccine series

CONSULTATION/REFERRAL

- If possible, victims of sexual assault should be referred to providers who specialize in performing the examination
- Refer to expert in field of sexual abuse for psychosocial interview and crisis counseling

FOLLOW-UP

- Report cases of sexual assault or abuse to law enforcement agency and to social services
- FOLLOW-UP observation and involvement of patient in social support
- 7-10 days: pregnancy testing and counseling
- Repeat cervical culture, VDRL, and pregnancy test in 2 weeks
- 5-6 weeks: tests for syphilis and gonorrhea
- Repeat HIV and hepatitis B in 6 months

EXPECTED COURSE

- Acute phase usually lasts 3 weeks, involves anxiety, fear, pain, mood swings, guilt, shame, grief
- Chronic phase may develop, involving flashbacks, nightmares, fear of intercourse, fear of men, depression, anxiety, and post-traumatic stress syndrome
- Patients who are provided with counseling and are able to express themselves after the event usually recover more quickly

POSSIBLE COMPLICATIONS

- Sexually transmitted disease
- Pregnancy
- Post- traumatic stress disorder
- Emotional trauma
- Physical trauma

ANOREXIA NERVOSA (AN)

DESCRIPTION

Disorder characterized by morbid fear of obesity and nutritionally significant weight loss

ETIOLOGY

- Unknown, but serotonergic dysregulation is thought to play a major role

- May be related to underlying metabolic, psychological, and/or genetic predisposition

INCIDENCE

- Females > Males
- Most common in adolescents and young adults (1-4%)
- Predominantly a disease of white, middle and upper class, but increasing in males, minorities, and women of all ages
- May coexist with depression (50-75%) or obsessive-compulsive disorder (10-13%)

RISK FACTORS

- Meticulous, compulsive personality
- Low self-esteem
- High self-expectations
- Multiple responsibilities
- Early puberty
- Family history

ASSESSMENT FINDINGS

- Insidious initially
- Significant and noticeable weight loss (generally 15% below body weight)
- Preoccupation about weight loss and being fat is primary symptom
- Denial that there is a problem (prominent feature of the disease)
- Disturbance in body image (i.e., complaints of feeling bloated and being fat despite emaciation)
- Strenuous exercise to lose weight
- Resistance to medical treatment
- Possible depression
- Elaborate food rituals
- Amenorrhea (absence of 3 consecutive menstrual cycles) may appear before significant weight loss

The following findings are related to starvation:

- Sparse scalp hair, dry skin
- Growth arrest, arrested sexual maturation
- Lanugo on extremities, face, and trunk
- Cognitive decline
- Bradycardia, hypotension, cardiovascular compromise
- Hypothermia
- Weight loss of 30% in 6 months requires hospitalization

DIFFERENTIAL DIAGNOSIS

- Bulimia
- Severe depression
- Food phobia
- Schizophrenia
- Physical disorder (e.g., malignancy, diabetes mellitus)

Anorexia is commonly accompanied by other psychiatric illnesses like depression, social phobias, or obsessive compulsive disorder.

DIAGNOSTIC STUDIES

- No lab or imaging can diagnose anorexia nervosa
- Tests done to determine level of malnutrition
  - ◊ CBC: anemia
  - ◊ LFTs
  - ◊ LH, FSH, T_3: all are diminished
  - ◊ BUN, total protein: decreased
  - ◊ Fasting blood glucose: low
  - ◊ Potassium level: low

PREVENTION

- Enhance self-esteem
- Encourage healthy attitude about weight and self
- Encourage reasonable self-expectations

NONPHARMACOLOGIC MANAGEMENT

- Usually treated on outpatient basis
- Restoration of weight is primary goal and may result in cessation of obsessive focus on food
- Monitor physical, psychological and nutritional status
- Supportive therapy in an eating disorders clinic or group
- Build trust with patient
- Consider bedrest if physical and nutritional status is severe (inpatient treatment is preferable for patients who are 70% of weight for height)

- Involve patient and family in treatment plan and establishing target weight
- Supervised meals
- Increase calories gradually by about 300 kcal/day as tolerated
- Weigh 3 times weekly, then weekly
- Goal is 1-2 pound weight gain per week until target is reached
- Discuss fear of weight gain as part of program
- Slowly increase patient's activity level as weight is gained
- Goal is weight stabilization and resumption of normal eating pattern

PHARMACOLOGIC MANAGEMENT

- May treat anxiety before meals to lessen anxiety about weight gain
- Careful dosing of medications required because patients may have compromised hepatic and/or renal function
- Consider treatment with antidepressants if depression is persistent

Underweight patients are more sensitive to usual dosages of medications. Dose carefully!

CONSULTATION/REFERRAL

- Refer to psychiatrist for initial treatment plan
- Consult support group or eating disorders clinic
- Refer to psychiatrist for weight less than 75% expected for age and height; compromised physical status (hypothermia, hypotension, bradycardia, etc.)
- Registered dietitian for meal planning

FOLLOW-UP

- Monitor weight weekly until stable, then monthly
- Monitor for depression, possible suicide
- Monitor abnormal lab values
- Participation in long-term maintenance program is recommended to help prevent relapse

EXPECTED COURSES

- Relapses are common
- Fewer than 50% completely recover
- Poor prognosis for failed inpatient hospitalization and for patients with a history of disturbed family relationships
- Possible depression during or after recovery
- Food rituals, low self-esteem, and distorted body image may persist even after treatment and recovery

POSSIBLE COMPLICATIONS

- 5% mortality (often due to suicide)
- Cardiac arrhythmias from electrolyte imbalances
- Osteoporosis
- Congestive heart failure
- Necrotizing colitis
- Seizures

BULIMIA NERVOSA

DESCRIPTION

Disorder characterized by distorted body image, recurrent episodes of overeating and either self-induced vomiting, use of laxatives, diuretics, rigorous exercise, dieting, or any combination of these. Diagnostic criteria according to DSM-IV: 2 binge episodes per week for at least 3 months

ETIOLOGY

- Unknown

INCIDENCE

- Females > Males (5:1)
- Young adults and adolescents are at highest risk

- College females thought to have the highest incidence, however, <2% prevalence rate in this group
- Actual incidence is unknown because of the secretive nature of the disease

RISK FACTORS

- Meticulous, compulsive personality
- Low self-esteem
- High self-expectations
- Multiple responsibilities
- Increased stress levels
- Individuals considered at high risk to develop: ballet dancers, cheerleaders, gymnasts, weightlifters, jockeys, runners
- Obesity
- History of sexual abuse
- Chemical dependency
- Anxiety

ASSESSMENT FINDINGS

- May exist concurrently with anorexia
- Belief that they are fat despite weight that is average or higher
- Frequent weight fluctuations
- Express extreme concern about weight gain; preoccupation with weight
- Expression of feelings of "lack of control" during binge episodes
- May hoard food
- Secret abuse of diet pills, laxatives, diuretics, syrup of ipecac
- Erosion of dental enamel from acid in vomitus
- Abdominal pain, esophagitis, enlargement of the parotid glands, gastric dilation
- Scarring on knuckles from inducing vomiting
- Denial that eating habits are a problem
- Depression may follow recovery initiation
- May feel guilty about behavior when asked about it
- More prone to impulsive behavior than anorexics

DIFFERENTIAL DIAGNOSIS

- Anorexia
- Depression
- Gastrointestinal disorder
- Schizophrenia
- Psychogenic vomiting

DIAGNOSTIC STUDIES

- Electrolyte levels: all may be low, especially potassium, chloride (alkalosis from vomiting), and magnesium from laxative abuse; or maybe normal values
- BUN: elevated
- Other chemistries as patient condition dictates
- Consider ECG if electrolytes are severely decreased
- Consider a urine drug screen

PREVENTION

- Encourage healthy attitudes about weight and self
- Encourage reasonable self-expectations
- Appropriate stress management

NONPHARMACOLOGIC MANAGEMENT

- Most treated on outpatient basis
- Consider inpatient if suicidal, severe concurrent chemical dependency, or if entirely out of control and unresponsive to outpatient treatment
- Monitor physical, psychological and nutritional status
- Supportive therapy in an eating disorders clinic or group
- Build trust with patient. Development of trust is good prognostic indicator.
- Involve patient and family in treatment plan and in establishing goals
- Monitor exercise and eating patterns
- Supervised meals, supervised bathroom privileges for at least 2 hours after meals
- Discuss fear of weight gain and use this challenge as part of recovery
- Slowly increase patient's activity level
- Goal is weight stabilization and resumption of normal eating pattern

Non-compliance with treatment regimen and lack of honesty with counselor, health care provider is common.

PHARMACOLOGIC MANAGEMENT

- Antidepressant medications for depression: fluoxetine (Prozac®), sertraline (Zoloft®), trazodone (Desyrel®), desipramine (Norpramin®)
- Avoid MAO inhibitors due to potential severe reactions induced by food interactions (hypertensive crisis)
- Avoid use of tricyclics and lithium in patients with hypokalemic patients

PREGNANCY/LACTATION CONSIDERATIONS

- Pregnancy may worsen or improve disorder
- Danger to fetus due to poor nutritional status

CONSULTATION/REFERRAL

- Consult physician for all new diagnoses and for development of treatment plan
- Psychologist for behavioral therapy
- Dietitian for meal planning

FOLLOW-UP

- Dictated by severity of patient disorder
- Attendance at eating disorders clinic should be coordinated with routine follow-up
- Monitor potassium as long as patient is purging

EXPECTED COURSES

- Expect noncompliance and frequent relapses
- Expect improvement, but some symptoms often persist over a period of years

POSSIBLE COMPLICATIONS

- Erosion of dental enamel
- Gastric dilation
- Esophagitis
- Life threatening arrhythmias from electrolyte imbalances, cardiomyopathy, and sudden death related to vomiting
- Suicide
- Abuse of drugs or alcohol

References

American Psychiatric Association. (1996). *American Psychiatric Association Practice Guidelines.* Washington, DC: Author.

Baldwin, D., & Landa, H. (1996). Evaluating pediatric gynecologic problems. *Patient Care, 30*(12), 89-111.

Barkin, R.M., & Rosen, P. (Eds.). (2003). *Emergency pediatrics* (6th ed.). St. Louis, MO: Mosby.

Beers, M.H., & Berkow, R. (Eds.). (1999). *The Merck manual of diagnosis and therapy* (17th ed.). Rahway, NJ: Merck & Company.

Bickley, L.S., & Szilagyi, P.G. (2003). *Bates' guide to physical examination and history taking* (8th ed.). Philadelphia: Lippincott Williams & Wilkins.

Branch, W.T. (2003). *Office practice of medicine* (4th ed.). Philadelphia: Saunders.

Brandt, E., Hadley, S., & Holtz, H. (1996). Family violence: A covert health crisis. *Patient Care, 30*(14), 138-165.

Burns, C.E., Brady, M.A., Blosser, C., Starr, N.B., & Dunn, A.M. (2004). *Pediatric primary care: A handbook for nurse practitioners* (3rd ed.). Philadelphia: W.B. Saunders.

Comerci, G., Fuller, P., & Morrison, S. (1997). Cigarettes, drugs, alcohol and teens. *Patient Care, 31*(4), 56-84.

Dambro, M.R. (2005). *Griffith's 5 minute clinical consult.* Philadelphia: Lippincott Williams & Wilkins.

Danis, P., & Seaton, T. (1997). Helping your patients to quit smoking. *American Family Physician, 55*, 1207-1217.

Epperly, T. D., & Moore, K. E. (2000). Health issues in men: Part II. Common psychosocial disorders. *American Family Physician, 62*, 117-24.

Giannini, A. J., (2000). An approach to drug abuse, intoxication and withdrawal. *American Family Physician, 61*, 2763-74.

Goroll, A. H., & Mulley, A. G., Jr. (Eds.). (2000). *Primary care medicine: Office evaluation and management of the adult patient* (4th ed.). Philadelphia: Lippincott Williams Wilkins.

Graber, M.A., & Lanternier, M.L. (Eds.) (2001). *The family practice handbook.* (4th ed.). St. Louis: Mosby.

Hahn, S.R., & Sydney, E. (2005). Detecting depression in the primary-care setting. *Clinical Advisor, 8*(6) (Suppl.), 9-14.

Hentz, P.B. (2005). Depression: Effective management strategies. *Clinical Advisor, 8*(6) (Suppl.), 15-20.

Herrington, R., Jacobson, & G., Benzer, D. (1987). *Alcohol and drug abuse handbook.* St. Louis, MO: Warren H. Green.

Kopcha, J. (2005). Would you recognize a problem drinker? *Clinical Advisor, 8*(6), 49-51.

Martin, A. C., Schaffer, S. D., & Campbell, R. (1999). Managing alcohol related problems in the primary care setting. *The Nurse Practitioner, 24*(8), 14-39.

Merriam, A.E. (2005). The etiology of depression remains elusive. *Clinical Advisor, 8*(6) (Suppl.), 3-8.

Mitchel, A.E., & Thomas, G.P. (2005). Using combination therapy for smoking cessation. *Clinician Reviews, 15*(5), 40-45.

Mladenovic, J. (Ed.). (2003). *Primary care secrets.* (3rd Ed.). Philadelphia: Hanley and Belfus.

Morgan, K., & Deneris, A. (1997). Emergency contraception: Preventing unwanted pregnancy. *The Nurse Practitioner, 22*(11), 34-40.

Rakel, R.E. (Ed.). (1998). *Essentials of family practice.* (2nd ed.). Philadelphia: WB Saunders.

Rush, A. J., Golden, W. E., Hall, G. W., et al. (1993). *Depression in primary care: Volume 1. Detection and Diagnosis.* Clinical Practice Guideline, No. 5. Publication No. 93-0550. Rockville, MD: U.S. Department of Health & Human Services, Public Health Service Agency for Healthcare Policy and Research.

Rush, A. J., Golden, W. E., Hall, G. W., et al. (1993). *Depression in primary care: Volume 2. Treatment of major depression.* Clinical Practice Guideline, No. 5. Publication No. 93-0551. Rockville, MD: U.S. Department of Health & Human Services, Public Health Service Agency for Healthcare Policy and Research.

Shoultz, J., Tanner, B., & Harrigan, R. (2000). Culturally appropriate guidelines for alcohol and drug abuse prevention. *The Nurse Practitioner, 25*(11), 50-56.

Thompson, R. (2005). Intimate partner violence: A culturally sensitive approach. *Advance for Nurse Practitioners, 13*(7), 57-59.

Uphold, C.R., & Graham, M.V. (2003). *Clinical guidelines in family practice.* (4th ed.). Gainesville, FL: Barmarrae Books.

U.S. Preventive Services Task Force. (1996). *Guide to clinical preventive services.* (2nd ed.). Washington, D.C.: Office of Disease Prevention and Health Promotion, U.S. Government Printing Office.

21

UROLOGICAL DISORDERS

Urological Disorders

**Denotes pediatric diagnosis*

ASYMPTOMATIC BACTERIURIA

DESCRIPTION

Significant bacterial count present in the urine of a person without symptoms

ETIOLOGY

- Bacteria (e.g., *E. coli*, *Proteus mirabilis*, *Klebsiella pneumoniae*, and *Staphylococcus saprophyticus*)
- More commonly caused by gram negative bacteria

INCIDENCE

- 20% of elderly women living in the community
- 30-50% of institutionalized elderly women
- 4-7% of pregnancies

RISK FACTORS

- Female
- Perimenopausal
- Increasing age
- Structural abnormalities that impede the flow of urine
- Indwelling urinary catheter

ASSESSMENT FINDINGS

- By definition, none

DIFFERENTIAL DIAGNOSIS

- Contaminated specimen
- Symptomatic bacteriuria

DIAGNOSTIC STUDIES

- Urinalysis: WBCs
- Urine culture may be positive

PHARMACOLOGIC MANAGEMENT

- Pharmacological treatment is controversial. It is generally recommended in persons with diabetes, polycystic renal disease, and AIDS, and before urological procedures.

PREGNANCY/LACTATION CONSIDERATIONS

- Associated with acute pyelonephritis, preterm labor, and low birthweight infants
- Screening of all pregnant women should be done at the initial prenatal visit
- Treatment recommended in pregnancy
- Recommended medications for treatment during pregnancy are nitrofurantoin (Macrodantin®), ampicillin, amoxicillin, *OR* a cephalosporin
- Trimethoprim-sulfamethoxazole (Bactrim®) and quinolones should not be used in pregnancy

CONSULTATION/REFERRAL

- None usually needed

FOLLOW-UP

- None unless patient becomes symptomatic

POSSIBLE COMPLICATIONS

- Development of symptomatic bacteriuria
- Disseminated infection
- Acute pyelonephritis in pregnancy
- Delivery of low birth weight infant

URINARY TRACT INFECTION
(Cystitis, UTI)

DESCRIPTION

Infection and inflammation of the bladder mucosa; presence of bacteria in the urine

ETIOLOGY

- Bacteria (e.g., *E. coli* (most common pathogen), *Proteus mirabilis*, *Klebsiella pneumoniae*, *Enterobacter*, and *Staphylococcus saprophyticus*)
- More commonly caused by gram negative bacteria of colonic origin
- Most UTI in adult women are due to ascending infections from the urethra
- Hematogenous spread is rarely the cause

INCIDENCE

- 43% of women aged 14-61 years have had at least one UTI
- Females > Males
- Uncommon in men < 50 years old
- 4-7% prevalence in pregnant women
- Most common of all bacterial infections in women
- In girls is most common in ages 7-11 years

Females are more likely than men to have urinary tract infections because women have short urethras compared to men.

RISK FACTORS

- Previous urinary tract infection
- Diabetes mellitus in women
- Pregnancy
- Increase in frequency of sexual activity
- Use of spermicides and/or diaphragm, oral contraceptive use
- Urinary tract abnormalities (e.g., tumors, calculi, strictures, anomalies, neuropathic bladder)
- Benign prostatic hyperplasia
- Fecal/urinary incontinence
- Cognitive impairment
- Immunocompromised host
- Infrequent voiding
- Indwelling urinary catheter

ASSESSMENT FINDINGS

- Burning, frequency, and/or urgency during urination
- Pain during or after urination
- Sensation of incomplete bladder emptying
- Fever, chills
- Hematuria: gross or microscopic
- No symptoms (but unusual)
- Lower abdominal and/or back pain
- Dribbling of urine in men
- Small volume voiding
- Foul-smelling urine

DIFFERENTIAL DIAGNOSIS

- Vaginitis
- Sexually transmitted disease
- Hematuria from another cause
- Pregnancy
- Pelvic inflammatory disease
- Prostatitis, epididymitis
- Enuresis

DIAGNOSTIC STUDIES

- Urinalysis: WBCs present, positive leukocyte esterase, positive nitrites
- Bacterial count > 100,000/ ml of urine if midstream catch
- Urine culture with sensitivity for recurrent infections, infection refractory to treatment, and in children

Urine culture results will be altered if patient has taken an antibiotic prior to collection of urine for culture.

PREVENTION

- Good hydration
- Emptying bladder immediately after sexual intercourse
- Estrogen therapy in postmenopausal women

- Good perineal hygiene
- Cranberry juice
- Frequent voiding
- Prophylactic antibiotics

NONPHARMACOLOGIC MANAGEMENT

- Good hydration
- Voiding after intercourse if infection associated with sexual intercourse
- Good perineal hygiene

PHARMACOLOGIC MANAGEMENT

AGENT	ACTION	COMMENTS
Sulfa Agent *Examples:* Trimethoprim (TMP)-sulfamethoxazole (SMZ) (Bactrim®, Septra®)	Block synthesis of folic acid by bacteria and thus inhibit bacterial replication	Do not give to pregnant women. Hypersensitivity reactions like Stevens-Johnson epidermal necrolysis and blood dyscrasias have been associated with sulfa use. Photosensitivity may occur with these drugs.
Fluoroquinolones *Examples:* levofloxacin (Levaquin®) moxifloxacin (Avelox®) gatifloxacin (Tequin®)	Antibiotic inhibits the action of DNA gyrase which is essential for the organism to be able to replicate itself	Broad-spectrum antibacterial agents. Monitor for QT prolongation and photosensitivity. Avoid in children < 18 years old and in pregnant women due to potential adverse effects on bone and cartilage formation. Monitor for hypoglycemic reactions. Absorption significantly affected by dairy product consumption and multivitamins, especially containing calcium and iron.
Penicillins *Examples:* amoxicillin (Amoxil®, Trimox®) amoxicillin and potassium clavulanate (Augmentin® XR, Augmentin®) ampicillin (Principen®)	Penicillins inhibit cell wall synthesis. They are most effective during active multiplication of pathogenic bacteria	Monitor for hypersensitivity reactions (1-10% of patients taking PCN products will report allergy). Safe use during pregnancy and in children. In species that produce beta-lactamase, amoxicillin, and ampicillin are ineffective. Amoxicillin/potassium clavulanate is effective against organisms that produce beta-lactamase.
Cephalosporins ***Second generation*** *Examples:* cefprozil (Cefzil®) cefuroxime (Ceftin®) cefaclor (Ceclor®)	Inhibit cell wall synthesis of bacteria. Contains beta lactam ring like PCN. Provides coverage of many Gram positive and Gram negative bacteria but NOT those organisms that produce beta lactamase.	Well tolerated. Cross sensitivity (≈2-10%) with PCN. Do NOT administer if patient has had anaphylactic response to PCN.
Third generation *Examples:* cefdinir (Omnicef®) cefixime (Suprax®) ceftibuten (Cedax®) cefpodoxime (Vantin®)	Exactly as for second generation cephalosporins but covers many more Gram negative organisms and is protected, if the organism produces beta-lactamase	Same as for second generation cephalosporins. Good choice if patient is PCN allergic and needs beta lactamase coverage.

AGENT	ACTION	COMMENTS
Miscellaneous Nitrofurantoin (Macrobid®)	Interferes with the function of several bacterial enzyme systems which inhibits metabolism and cell wall synthesis	*Pseudomonas* and *Proteus* are often resistant to nitrofurantoin. Category B: good choice in pregnant women but contraindicated at term. Not a good choice in the elderly or if CrCl <60 ml/min. May be used relatively safely in children and adults. Generally well tolerated.
Anti-spasmotic *Example:* flavoxate (Urispas®)	Inhibit smooth muscle spasm of the bladder and urinary tract	Relieves symptoms; burning, urgency, frequency. Must be used in conjunction with an antibiotic for treatment of UTI. Do not use in patients with glaucoma, intestinal obstruction.
phenazopyridine, (Pyridium®)	The dye exerts an analgesic effect on the bladder and urinary tract mucosa via unknown means	Must be used in conjunction with an antibiotic to treat UTI. Discolors urine orange and can stain undergarments. Use with caution in patients with hepatic or renal dysfunction. Maximum of 6 doses per UTI because accumulation of drug can occur and toxicity can result.

- Women: three day treatment usually adequate for uncomplicated UTI; consider 7-14 days if complicated
- Men: treat for 7-10 days

PREGNANCY/LACTATION CONSIDERATIONS

- Urine culture recommended
- Penicillin, cephalosporin, or nitrofurantoin are good first choices usually
- Treat for 10-14 days
- May need prophylactic antibiotics for duration of pregnancy
- Avoid quinolones and sulfa drugs

CONSULTATION/REFERRAL

- Consultation with urologist for recurring infections, infection in child under 4 months, pyelonephritis in children, and in presence of acute illness
- Referral to urologist is indicated if anatomic abnormality is suspected or diagnosed
- Hospitalization may be required in patients with severe symptoms

FOLLOW-UP

- Post treatment culture if patient having frequent or recurrent UTI and in children
- Evaluate children one week after therapy started

EXPECTED COURSE

- Complete resolution without complications within 2-3 days after starting treatment

POSSIBLE COMPLICATIONS

- Pyelonephritis
- Renal abscess

ACUTE PYELONEPHRITIS

DESCRIPTION

Infection of the upper urinary tract and renal parenchyma; if not managed appropriately can lead to bacteremia and death

ETIOLOGY

- 75% caused by *E. coli*
- Other gram negative bacteria (e.g., *Proteus mirabilis, Klebsiella pneumoniae,* and *Enterobacter* sp.) are responsible for 10-15%
- Gram positive bacteria (e.g., *Staphylococcus aureus* and *saprophyticus*) account for another 10-15%
- In older children and adults the most common route of infection is ascension of bacteria from bladder
- In neonates, the most common route is hematogenous spread to the kidneys

INCIDENCE

- 15.7/100,000 persons develop pyelonephritis annually

RISK FACTORS

Adults:
- Urinary tract abnormalities
- Recent untreated or undertreated UTI
- Indwelling urinary catheter
- Urinary tract instrumentation
- Renal calculi
- Diabetes mellitus
- Immunocompromised host
- Elderly
- Institutionalization, especially women
- Recent pyelonephritis
- Obstruction of normal urine flow (e.g., urethral stricture, benign prostatic hyperplasia)
- Fecal incontinence
- Pregnancy

Children:
- Vesicoureteral reflux
- Anatomical abnormalities in the renal system
- Behavioral factors (e.g., deferral of voiding, poor hygiene)
- Lack of circumcision in male infants

ASSESSMENT FINDINGS

Adolescents and adults:
- Fever, chills
- Costovertebral angle tenderness
- Flank pain
- Abdominal tenderness
- Malaise, myalgia
- Hematuria
- Nausea and vomiting
- Headache
- Dysuria, frequency, urgency

Infants and children:
- Fever which can progress to sepsis
- Failure to thrive
- Irritability
- Enuresis
- Nausea and vomiting

DIFFERENTIAL DIAGNOSIS

- Renal calculi
- Prostatitis, epididymitis
- Low back pain secondary to disc disease, aortic aneurysm, strain
- Urinary tract tumors
- Herpes zoster
- Ectopic pregnancy

DIAGNOSTIC STUDIES

- Urinalysis: pyuria, positive leukocyte esterase test, possibly hematuria, proteinuria, alkaline pH, WBC casts
- Urine culture with sensitivity
- CBC: leukocytosis

NONPHARMACOLOGIC MANAGEMENT

- Requires inpatient treatment if patient appears toxic, pregnant, intolerant of oral

medications, fluids, and food, or in young children
- Encourage fluids

PHARMACOLOGIC MANAGEMENT

- Initial treatment is broad spectrum antibiotic until culture and sensitivity available (consider quinolone or third generation cephalosporin, broad spectrum penicillin until culture available): *see* Urinary Tract Infection
- Do not use nitrofurantoin since poor tissue levels are achieved in the renal parenchyma

PREGNANCY/LACTATION CONSIDERATIONS

- Requires hospitalization during pregnancy
- Common reason for hospitalization during pregnancy

CONSULTATION/REFERRAL

- Consult urologist if patient has been febrile > 72 hours (probable invasive/extensive workup: IVP, cysto, spiral CT)
- Refer if no improvement after 48 hours of outpatient treatment
- Refer for inpatient treatment if acutely ill
- Refer to urologist for urologic workup if recurring infections occur

FOLLOW-UP

- Evaluate patient with urine culture 2 weeks after completing treatment

EXPECTED COURSE

- Good prognosis with adequate treatment
- Should see improvement in 48 hours in outpatient setting

POSSIBLE COMPLICATIONS

- Sepsis
- Preterm labor/delivery
- Chronic renal insufficiency
- Chronic pyelonephritis

URETHRITIS

DESCRIPTION

Inflammation of the urethra; generally due to infection with gonorrhea, but maybe non-gonococcal

ETIOLOGY

- Usually a sexually transmitted disease
- Most common organisms: *N. gonorrhoeae, C. trachomatis, Ureaplasma urealyticum, Trichomonas vaginalis*, and viruses
- May be due to foreign bodies, irritating soaps, indwelling urinary catheter

INCIDENCE

- Gonococcal urethritis usually found in males
- Non-gonococcal usually found in females

RISK FACTORS

- Sexual activity
- Multiple sexual partners
- Previous sexually transmitted disease

ASSESSMENT FINDINGS

- Asymptomatic (especially females)
- Fever
- Dysuria
- Frequency
- Urethral discharge
- Suprapubic discomfort
- Urethral tenderness
- Pruritus of urethra
- Dyspareunia
- Tenderness, edema, and inflammation of the urethra, especially in women
- Vaginitis, cystitis, and cervicitis may also be present in women

- Proctitis, pharyngitis, and conjunctivitis may also be present

Males usually report symptoms 3-5 days after exposure to an STD. Females are usually asymptomatic initially.

DIFFERENTIAL DIAGNOSIS

- Cystitis
- Epididymitis, prostatitis
- Trauma
- Atrophic vaginitis
- Intraurethral foreign bodies or growths
- Allergic or sensitivity reaction

DIAGNOSTIC STUDIES

- Diagnosis made if ≥ 5 WBC per high power field (HPF)
- Gram stain and culture of discharge
- Urinalysis not as sensitive as direct culture
- Chlamydia testing
- Wet prep of discharge: WBCs, trichomonads may be visible

Encourage screening for other STDs, hepatitis B & C, and HIV.

PREVENTION

- Use of condoms
- Urinating immediately after sexual intercourse
- Screen for STDs

NONPHARMACOLOGIC MANAGEMENT

- Evaluation and treatment of sexual partners
- Abstinence until treatment completed

- Sexual abuse should be investigated in children with any STD

Treat all known sexual partners in the last 60 days.

PHARMACOLOGIC MANAGEMENT

- Ceftriaxone (Rocephin®) intramuscular plus doxycycline *OR* azithromycin (Zithromax®) orally
- Metronidazole (Flagyl®) orally if cause is *Trichomonas vaginalis*

Do not wait until cultures are available to treat. Treat initially for gonorrhea and chlamydia.

PREGNANCY/LACTATION CONSIDERATIONS

- Avoid use of tetracycline
- Do not use metronidazole (Flagyl®) in first trimester
- Test of cure recommended after treatment complete

FOLLOW-UP

- Test of cure not necessary if course of treatment completed

EXPECTED COURSE

- Improvement of symptoms in 48-72 hours
- Complete resolution with effective treatment

POSSIBLE COMPLICATIONS

- Stricture formation
- Pelvic inflammatory disease in women

URINARY INCONTINENCE
(Stress Incontinence, Urge Incontinence, Overflow Incontinence)

DESCRIPTION

Involuntary loss of urine (in an adult patient) from the urethra which is usually recognized by the patient as a problem or inconvenience

Involuntary loss of urine in children usually termed enuresis.

ETIOLOGY

Urge Incontinence (detrusor instability):
- Urinary tract infection

- Chronic cystitis
- Dementia
- Parkinson's disease
- Aging
- Stroke
- Irradiation of bladder

Conditions which mimic *urge incontinence*
◊ **D**ementia ◊ **I**nfection ◊ **A**trophic vaginitis ◊ **P**harmaceuticals (retention) ◊ **E**xcess urinary output ◊ **R**estricted mobility ◊ **S**tool impaction

Stress Incontinence (sphincter incompetence):
- Aging
- Pelvic floor muscle weakness
- Estrogen deficiency
- Perineal trauma
- Prostatic/pelvic surgery

Reflex Incontinence:
- Disc herniation
- Diabetes mellitus
- Neurologic tumors
- Spinal cord disease
- Multiple sclerosis

Overflow Incontinence:
- Prostatic enlargement
- Medications (e.g., antidepressants, anticholinergics)
- Outflow tract obstruction
- Diabetic neuropathy

Functional Incontinence:
- Severe mental illness
- Sedating medications
- Physical or mental disability

***Mixed incontinence* is stress incontinence coupled with urge incontinence.**

INCIDENCE

- 5-15% of elderly in the community
- Approximately 12 million in the United States
- Up to 50% of nursing home residents
- Female > Male

RISK FACTORS

- Increasing age in men and women
- Declining estrogen levels
- Multiparity
- Dementia
- Diabetes mellitus
- Spinal cord injury/lesion, other neurological conditions
- Prostatic hypertrophy
- CVA
- Certain medications (e.g., diuretics)
- Immobility

ASSESSMENT FINDINGS

- Involuntary loss of urine
- Urinary urgency
- Burning with urination
- Perineal irritation
- Pelvic exam: may detect GU pathology
- Rectal exam: may demonstrate prostatic pathology, fecal impaction
- Abdomen: may palpate distended bladder

DIFFERENTIAL DIAGNOSIS

- Urinary tract infection
- Effect of medications
- Undiagnosed diabetes, BPH, STD
- Psychiatric illness

DIAGNOSTIC STUDIES

- Voiding diary for 2-3 days indicating when incontinent episodes occur
- Urinalysis: normal unless some underlying condition is present
- BUN, creatinine
- Post-voiding residual volume measurement
- Voiding cystourethrogram or uroflowmetry when obstruction is suspected

PREVENTION

- Kegel exercises, especially following childbirth
- Regular
- Treatment of prostatic hyperplasia

NONPHARMACOLOGIC MANAGEMENT

- Treat underlying problem if present

- Use of a voiding diary for 3 days to provide information about the patient's voiding habits
- Good perineal hygiene
- Regular emptying of bladder even if no urge is sensed
- Kegel exercises
- Intermittent self-catheterization for urinary retention
- Use of incontinence pads, vaginal cones in women
- Condom catheters in male patients
- Dietary/medication modifications (e.g., caffeine restriction, avoidance of alcohol, etc.)
- Biofeedback
- Surgery in selected patients (e.g., TURP, bladder suspension)
- Treat constipation

PHARMACOLOGIC MANAGEMENT

URGE INCONTINENCE		
AGENT	ACTION	COMMENTS
Anticholinergics *Example:* oxybutynin (Ditropan®) tolterodine (Detrol®) trospium (Sanctura®)	Urgency and frequency is decreased by inhibiting muscarinic activity of acetylcholine on smooth muscle. Bladder contraction is mediated by cholinergic muscarinic receptor stimulation.	Dry mouth, blurred vision are common side effects. Contraindicated in patients with urinary retention, narrow angle glaucoma, and GI obstruction. May produce heat in tolerance, constipation. May worsen gastric reflex. Monitor for dry interactions especially with tolterodine. Cautious use in the elderly, renal and hepatic dysfunction.

OVERFLOW INCONTINENCE		
AGENT	ACTION	COMMENTS
Alpha adrenergic antagonists *Example:* terazosin (Hytrin®) doxazosin (Cardura®) tamsulosin (Flomax®)	Blockade of the alpha adrenergic receptors causes relaxation of smooth muscle in the prostate and neck of the bladder	May cause orthostatic hypotension. Cautious use in patients with cardiac or cerebrovascular diseases. Contraindicated in patients taking Levitra® and Cialis®.
Antiandrogenic agents *Examples:* finasteride (Proscar®) dutasteride (Avodart®)	Inhibit conversion of testosterone to the androgen, DHT. Enlargement of the prostate gland is caused by DHT.	Hormones may cause impotence. At least 6-12 months are needed to adequately assess benefit of therapy. Pregnant patients should never handle crushed or broken tablets. PSA will decrease while taking this drug.

STRESS INCONTINENCE		
AGENT	ACTION	COMMENTS
Minimal benefit from medications, but consider: pseudoephedrine (Sudafed®), phenylpropanolamine (OMA del®), or imipramine (Tofranil®)		

PREGNANCY/LACTATION CONSIDERATIONS

- Stress incontinence may occur in pregnancy
- Should be treated non-pharmacologically with Kegel exercises, good hygiene, frequent voiding, and use of incontinence pads

CONSULTATION/REFERRAL

- Refer to urologist when refractory to initial medication measures or lifestyle modification
- Refer if neurological abnormalities present

FOLLOW-UP

- Frequent visits for assessment of therapy and support
- Assess BP in men on alpha blockers
- Ophthalmologist for measurement of intraocular pressure in patients with family history of glaucoma

EXPECTED COURSE

- Variable prognosis depending on underlying cause, but good improvement seen with medication management for urge and overflow incontinence
- Stress incontinence best managed (eradicated) with surgical intervention

POSSIBLE COMPLICATIONS

- Intolerable side effects from medication
- Urinary tract infection
- Hydronephrosis
- Renal failure
- Skin excoriation and breakdown
- Social isolation
- Depression and/or anxiety

ENURESIS
(Bed-wetting)

DESCRIPTION

Involuntary urination beyond the age of 5 years in children; nocturnal enuresis is defined as 2 episodes weekly of bedwetting having occurred for 3 months or more

TERMS

Nocturnal enuresis	Most common form, occurs during sleep
Diurnal enuresis	Incontinence during waking hours
Primary enuresis	Child who has never achieved continence
Secondary enuresis	Child who has return of involuntary urination after achieving continence

ETIOLOGY

- Multifactorial
- Inheritance plays a role (75% of patients with enuresis have/had a first degree relative with enuresis)
- Other contributing factors may be:
  - ◊ Lack of normal increase in nocturnal ADH secretion
  - ◊ Reduced bladder capacity
  - ◊ Food allergies
  - ◊ Disorders of the genitourinary or nervous system (3-4 %)
  - ◊ Psychological factors may play a role
- Causes of secondary enuresis may be:
  - ◊ Bacteriuria
  - ◊ Inability to concentrate urine due to insufficient ADH or renal tubular defect
  - ◊ Glucosuria
  - ◊ Pelvic mass
  - ◊ Spinal cord malformation

INCIDENCE

- Approximately 10% of children

- Occurs in 40% of 3 year olds, 10% of 6 year olds, 3% of 12 year olds, and 1% of 18 year olds
- Male > Females (2:1)

RISK FACTORS

- History of at least one parent having been enuretic
- First born child
- Dysfunctional family, stressful life events for children
- Institutionalized children

ASSESSMENT FINDINGS

- Inability to keep from urinating while asleep at least once/month
- Wetting may occur during daytime
- Stress factors may be present

DIFFERENTIAL DIAGNOSIS

- Diabetes insipidus
- Diabetes mellitus
- Renal tubular defects
- Spinal cord malformations or tumors, especially seen with secondary and diurnal enuresis
- Urinary tract infection
- Genitourinary or neurologic anomalies

DIAGNOSTIC STUDIES

- Urinalysis
- Urine culture if infection present
- Pregnancy test if indication present
- If enuresis complicated by severe voiding dysfunction, encopresis, or abnormal neurologic exam consider:
    - ◊ Renal ultrasound
    - ◊ Intravenous pyelogram
    - ◊ Voiding cystourethrogram

NONPHARMACOLOGIC MANAGEMENT

- Counseling and behavior modification if enuresis due to apparent stressor or family dysfunction
- Positive reinforcement and praise for dry nights
- No fluids within 2 hours of bedtime
- Avoidance of stimulants before bedtime (caffeinated drinks, chocolate, spicy foods, etc.)
- Voiding immediately before bedtime
- No punishment of child for enuresis
- Child should not be made to feel guilty
- Bed-wetting alarms (70% rate of success)
- Bladder capacity and stretching exercises

Bed wetting alarms have a higher success rate than medications for eradication of enuresis.

PHARMACOLOGIC MANAGEMENT

- Tricyclic antidepressants at bedtime: imipramine (Tofranil®) or amitriptyline (Elavil®)
- Desmopressin (DDAVP®) is especially useful in older children for sleep-over with peers

Most cases resolve spontaneously.

CONSULTATION/REFERRAL

- Presence of emotional problem may require referral
- Neurological or genitourinary dysfunction requires referral to specialist

FOLLOW-UP

- Frequent visits for support and encouragement

EXPECTED COURSE

- Self-limiting problem
- Eventual resolution as child ages

HEMATURIA

DESCRIPTION

The presence of blood in an uncontaminated specimen of urine detected by dipstick, microscopic examination, or the naked eye

Microscopic hematuria occurs when 3000-4000 RBCs/minute are excreted in the urine. Macroscopic hematuria occurs when the rate exceeds 1 million/minute.

ETIOLOGY

Adults:

- Malignant neoplasms in the GU tract
- Infection
- Renal calculi
- Coagulopathy
- Glomerular disease
- Hydronephrosis
- Polycystic kidneys
- Trauma
- Medications (e.g., heparin, warfarin, aspirin)
- Benign prostatic hyperplasia
- Exercise-induced

Children:

- Urinary tract infection
- Perineal or urethral irritation
- Sickle cell disease
- Trauma

ASSESSMENT FINDINGS

- May be associated with pain
- May be intermittent or persistent
- Assessment findings consistent with underlying problem

DIFFERENTIAL DIAGNOSIS

- Urinary tract infection
- Polycystic kidney disease
- Neoplasm
- Lupus erythematosus
- Renal calculi
- Benign prostatic hyperplasia
- Wilm's tumor
- Sickle cell disease
- Drugs (e.g., heparin, warfarin, aspirin)
- Hemophilia
- Thrombocytopenia purpura
- Glomerulonephritis
- Epididymitis
- Vaginal bleeding
- Presence of pigment from various sources (e.g., porphyria, foods, medications)
- Strenuous exercise and long-distance running
- Fever
- Trauma
- False positive urine dipstick from some confounding substance

DIAGNOSTIC STUDIES

- Urinalysis: RBCs, RBC casts
- BUN, creatinine
- CBC to assess for anemia
- 24-hour urine specimen (to quantify RBC loss)
- IVP (good initial test)
- Renal ultrasound (differentiates cysts from solid masses), cystoscopy
- Renal biopsy
- CT scan (best to assess/identify renal masses or stone)
- MRI (evaluates renal masses, expensive)
- Sickle cell assessment
- Other specific tests as indicated

A cast is a mucoprotein formed in the renal tubules. An RBC cast is one which contains trapped RBCs. The presence of an RBC cast indicates glomerular injury and may be seen in freshly voided specimens.

MANAGEMENT

- Dependent on underlying etiology

CONSULTATION/REFERRAL

- Need consultation with referral to urologist/nephrologist depending on diagnostic work-up

FOLLOW-UP

- Repeat urinalysis within 4-6 weeks if uncomplicated urinary tract infection

EXPECTED COURSE

- Dependent on underlying etiology

POSSIBLE COMPLICATIONS

- Dependent on underlying etiology

UROLITHIASIS
(Urinary Tract Stones)

DESCRIPTION

Stones in the urinary tract generally composed of calcium (most common), uric acid, cystine, magnesium, aluminum, phosphate, etc.

ETIOLOGY

- Supersaturation of urine with stone-forming salts
- Cause of this phenomenon is multifactorial and dependent on type of stone

Calcium oxalate/calcium phosphate stones are most common (65-85% incidence).

INCIDENCE

- Male > Female (4:1)
- 2-5% of the population may have urolithiasis during their lifetime

RISK FACTORS

- Renal tubular acidosis
- Alkaline pH of urine
- Cystinuria
- Genetic defects
- Low water intake or high Vitamin C or D consumption
- Calcium supplementation
- Thiazide diuretic use, gout
- High animal protein diet
- Sedentary lifestyle

ASSESSMENT FINDINGS

- Sudden onset of back and flank pain (usually severe) that waxes and wanes
- Pain may radiate to groin, testicles, suprapubic area, and labia
- Costovertebral angle tenderness
- Hematuria
- Dysuria
- Urinary frequency
- Diaphoresis
- Restlessness
- Tachycardia
- Tachypnea
- Chills and fever if infection secondary to obstruction
- Nausea and/or vomiting

If stone is very large or unable to move outside the kidney, patient may be asymptomatic. Eventually, the stone will move or the patient will develop an infection.

DIFFERENTIAL DIAGNOSIS

- Acute peritonitis
- Pyelonephritis
- Acute appendicitis
- Abdominal aortic aneurysm
- Colitis, diverticulitis
- Salpingitis, other GYN disorder
- Cholecystitis
- Peptic ulcer disease
- Pancreatitis

DIAGNOSTIC STUDIES

- Urinalysis: hematuria, pyuria may or may not be present
- CBC: within normal limits
- BUN, creatinine, metabolic panel

- Urine culture: may be positive if obstruction to urinary flow has occurred
- 24-hour urine collection for calcium, uric acid, magnesium, oxalate, citrate, and creatinine if recurrent problem
- Stone analysis
- KUB x-ray
- Intravenous pyelogram (IVP)
- Ultrasonography, if cannot do IVP
- Spiral CT (most sensitive test and helpful in evaluating cause of pain if not due to a stone)

If urine pH is < 5.5, stone is likely uric acid in composition.
If urine pH is >7.5, stone is likely a "staghorn calculus". "Staghorn calculus" refers to the shape of the stone in the renal pelvis which forms as a result of high urinary pH. The stone is usually composed of magnesium ammonium nitrate (struvite).

PREVENTION

- Adequate fluids

NONPHARMACOLOGIC MANAGEMENT

- Low animal fat diet
- Increased fiber in diet
- Fluid intake to maintain urinary output at 2-3 L/day
- Strain urine for presence of stones for 72 hours after symptoms resolve
- Observation with periodic evaluation is recommended for initial treatment
- For larger stones > 6mm:
  - ◊ Extracorporeal shock wave lithotripsy
  - ◊ Ureteroscopy
  - ◊ Percutaneous nephrolithotomy
  - ◊ Open surgery for removal of the stone

Calcium stones:

- Restriction of:
  - ◊ Protein
  - ◊ Sodium
  - ◊ Dairy products
  - ◊ Calcium-rich foods
- Moderate calcium restriction (1000-1500 mg/day)

Uric acid stones:

- Alkalinization of urine for uric acid stones

There is a > 60% chance of passing a stone < 6 mm. If stone > 6mm, chance of passing stone is < 20%.

PHARMACOLOGIC MANAGEMENT

- Narcotic analgesics and NSAIDs for pain control
  - ◊ Hydrocodone/acetaminophen (Vicodin®)
  - ◊ Acetaminophen/codeine (Tylenol® #3)
  - ◊ Oxycodone/acetaminophen (Percocet®)
  - ◊ Ketorolac (Toradol®) intramuscular
  - ◊ Meperidine (Demerol®) intramuscular if pain refractory to oral medications
- Antiemetics, if nausea and vomiting present
- Allopurinol (Zyloprim®) for prevention of uric acid stones after acute episode past
- Thiazide diuretics for prevention of calcium stones
- Cellulose sodium phosphate (Calcibind®) in recalcitrant cases of calcium stones

CONSULTATION/REFERRAL

- Refer for hospitalization if:
  - ◊ Infection present
  - ◊ Stone >6 mm in diameter
  - ◊ Excessive nausea and vomiting present
  - ◊ Intractable pain
  - ◊ Gross hematuria
- Urological consult, if obstruction suspected or if symptoms persist >3-4 days
- Dietary consultation, if dietary modifications are planned

FOLLOW-UP

- Creatinine level weekly
- Parathormone level if stones are calcium
- Abdominal x-ray at 1-2 week intervals
- Monitor potassium levels and blood pressure in persons on hydrochlorothiazide (HCTZ®)

EXPECTED COURSE

- Up to 90% pass spontaneously
- Usually resolves within 4 weeks
- Recurrences common in up to 50% of patients within 5 years

POSSIBLE COMPLICATIONS

- Complete urinary obstruction
- Hydronephrosis
- Renal failure
- Infection

POSTSTREPTOCOCCAL GLOMERULONEPHRITIS

DESCRIPTION

Immune response to an infection which causes damage to the glomeruli; characterized by diffuse inflammatory changes in the glomeruli and clinically by gross hematuria

ETIOLOGY

- Follows infection of throat or skin with bacteria, usually *Streptococcus* sp. (Group A β-hemolytic)
- The patient typically develops an acute glomerulonephritis 1-3 weeks after a streptococcal infection

INCIDENCE

- 20 /100,000 cases annually in U.S.
- Most common in children between 2- 12 years of age

RISK FACTORS

- More common in children
- Recent streptococcal infection (e.g., pharyngitis or impetigo)

ASSESSMENT FINDINGS

- Skin or pharyngeal streptococcal infection within the past 2-3 weeks
- Hematuria, abrupt onset (100% exhibit)
- Oliguria/anuria
- Proteinuria
- Edema, particularly of face, hands, and feet
- Hypertension (82%)
- Malaise
- Fever
- Abdominal or flank pain

DIFFERENTIAL DIAGNOSIS

- Glomerulonephritis secondary to something other than Strep
- Systemic lupus erythematosus
- Anaphylactoid purpura
- Subacute bacterial endocarditis

DIAGNOSTIC STUDIES

- Antistreptolysin O (ASO): increased in 60-80% of cases
- Urinalysis: proteinuria, hematuria
- Throat and skin cultures: positive for streptococcal organism
- Total serum complement: decreased
- BUN/Creatinine

PREVENTION

- Early and aggressive treatment of streptococcal infections

It is unusual to have acute glomerulonephritis secondary to Strep more than once because immunity usually develops after the first episode.

NONPHARMACOLOGIC MANAGEMENT

- Treatment inpatient until edema and hypertension under control; followed as outpatient
- No-added salt diet
- Fluid restriction
- Dialysis may be needed

PHARMACOLOGIC MANAGEMENT

- Furosemide (Lasix®) for edema
- Penicillin or erythromycin if penicillin-allergic
- Hydralazine (Apresoline®) for control of hypertension if needed

CONSULTATION/REFERRAL

- Refer for inpatient management in the acute stage

FOLLOW-UP

- Depends on severity of illness
- Generally done by nephrologist

EXPECTED COURSE

- Usually self-limited
- Complete recovery in 95% of patients
- Resolution within 2-3 weeks
- Prognosis excellent in children; may have more morbidity in adults or in those with preexisting renal disease
- Proteinuria usually persists for up to 3 months, but may be present for up to 2 years

POSSIBLE COMPLICATIONS

- Glomerulonephritis which progresses to acute renal failure
- Persistence of abnormal urinalysis: hematuria, proteinuria
- Chronic renal failure is rare
- Nephrotic syndrome
- Congestive heart failure

RENAL INSUFFICIENCY

DESCRIPTION

Decrease in glomerular filtration rate (GFR) of the kidneys. Due to the difficulty of measuring GFR, another marker such as serum creatinine concentration or 24-hour urinary creatinine clearance may be used to define renal failure

ETIOLOGY

- Numerous etiologies: tubular, glomerular, and/or vascular in origin
- Uncontrolled hypertension, diabetes
- Infection
- Metabolic disease
- Collagen vascular disease
- Exposure to nephrotoxic substances or medications

INCIDENCE

- 100 million annually develop end-stage renal failure
- Incidence is greater in nonwhites
- Males > Females

ASSESSMENT FINDINGS

- May be asymptomatic until end-stage renal disease
- Normochromic, normocytic anemia
- Fatigue and weakness
- Pruritus
- Nausea and vomiting
- Hematuria and proteinuria
- Lethargy
- Increased skin pigmentation
- Impaired urine concentrating ability in early stages resulting in polydipsia, polyuria, and nocturia
- Oliguria in later stages of failure
- Hypertension
- Edema including pulmonary edema

DIAGNOSTIC STUDIES

- Urinalysis: hematuria, proteinuria, casts
- BUN: elevated
- Creatinine: elevated
- 24-hour urine creatinine: elevated
- Potassium: elevated
- Serum calcium: decreased
- Sodium level: increases as insufficiency worsens
- Phosphate level: increased
- Uric acid levels: increased
- CBC: anemia
- Impaired platelet function
- Bleeding studies: prolonged

GFR and Serum Creatinine Concentration Correlation with Renal Failure

	Males		*Females*	
	GFR	Creat Conc	GFR	Creat Conc
Normal renal function	130 ±15 ml/min	<1.3 mg/dl	120 ±15 ml/min	<1 mg/dl
Early renal failure	56-100 ml/min	1.3-1.9 mg/dl	56-100 ml/min	1-1.9 mg/dl
Mod renal failure	25-55 ml/min	2-4 mg/dl	25-55 ml/min	2-4 mg/dl
Severe renal failure	≤24 ml/min	>4 mg/dl	≤24 ml/min	>4 mg/dl

NONPHARMACOLOGIC MANAGEMENT

- Treatment of underlying renal disease
- Dietary intake of 35-45 kcal/kg/day
- Reduction of dietary protein intake to 0.5 g/kg/day of high quality protein
- Smoking cessation
- Fluid restriction when oliguria develops
- Sodium restriction of 4 grams/day when hypertension, oliguria, or congestive heart failure present
- Potassium restriction when patient becomes oliguric
- Restriction of uric acid if gout develops
- Peritoneal dialysis
- Hemodialysis
- Renal transplantation

Goal in treating contributing causes is to slow progression.

PHARMACOLOGIC MANAGEMENT

- Angiotensin converting-enzyme inhibitors are the drugs of choice for blood pressure control in renal insufficiency. Monitor potassium, BUN, creatinine levels CAREFULLY!
- Allopurinol (Zyloprim®) for prevention of gout
- Recombinant erythropoietin when patient becomes symptomatic from anemia
- Loop diuretic therapy (e.g., furosemide (Lasix®) for treatment of fluid overload

Thiazide diuretics are ineffective if GFR < 30 cc/min.

- Calcium citrate for correction of hyperphosphatemia
- Oral ferrous sulfate for iron deficiency anemia
- Multivitamin with folate
- Antiemetics
- Antihistamines for treatment of pruritus
- Dosages of medication which are excreted renally must be adjusted
- Avoid nephrotoxic drugs

ACE inhibitors are used to decrease proteinuria.

CONSULTATION/REFERRAL

- Early referral to nephrologist

FOLLOW-UP

- Must be followed closely with frequent visits and diagnostic testing

Many medications will require renal dose adjustment.

EXPECTED COURSE

- Largely determined by underlying renal disease
- Most patients develop end-stage renal failure within 1-5 years after initial diagnosis

POSSIBLE COMPLICATIONS

- Impotence and infertility
- Seizures
- Metabolic acidosis
- Coma
- Hypertension
- Hemorrhagic diathesis

Creatinine clearance (which closely correlates with GFR in most patients) can be estimated by using the following formula:
Creatinine clearance =

$$\frac{(\{140\text{-age in years}\} \times \text{lean body weight in kg})}{\text{plasma creatinine (mg/dL)} \times 72}$$

WILM'S TUMOR
(Nephroblastoma)

DESCRIPTION

Embryonal renal neoplasm that is the major cause of renal malignancy in children

ETIOLOGY

- Familial form is autosomal dominant trait

INCIDENCE

- 1 in 10,000 children < 16 years of age
- Most commonly occurs in children from infancy to age 15 years
- 2/3 of cases are in children <4 years old

RISK FACTORS

- Family member with Wilm's tumor

ASSESSMENT FINDINGS

- Usually asymptomatic
- Hematuria
- Abdominal mass
- Low grade fever
- Anemia
- Fatigue
- Anorexia
- Weight loss
- Associated anomalies: aniridia (absence of the iris of the eye), cryptorchidism, hypospadias, duplicated renal collecting systems, hemihypertrophy

DIFFERENTIAL DIAGNOSIS

- Neuroblastoma
- Hepatic tumors
- Sarcoma
- Abdominal mass

DIAGNOSTIC STUDIES

- Urinalysis: hematuria
- CBC: normocytic, normochromic anemia
- LDH: may be elevated
- KUB
- Abdominal ultrasound
- Chest x-ray
- CT scan of chest and abdomen
- MRI of abdomen

The chest is the usual site of recurrence of tumors or for metastasis. Therefore, it is prudent to order a chest x-ray and consider a chest CT.

PREVENTION

- Diagnostic work-up of children with associated anomalies

NONPHARMACOLOGIC MANAGEMENT

- Radiation therapy
- Radical nephrectomy

PHARMACOLOGIC MANAGEMENT

- Chemotherapy

CONSULTATION/REFERRAL

- Refer to pediatric oncologist and/or urologist upon diagnosis

EXPECTED COURSE

- Good prognosis with favorable histology and staging

POSSIBLE COMPLICATIONS

- Second malignancy

References

American Urological Association Ureteral Stones Clinical Guideline Panel. (1997). *Report on the management of ureteral calculi.* Baltimore: American Urological Association.

Bader, T.J. (2004). *OB/GYN secrets.* (Rev. 3rd ed.). St. Louis, MO: Mosby-Year Book.

Behrman, R.E., Kliegman, R.M., Arvin, A.M., & Nelson, W.E. (Eds.). (1995). *Nelson textbook of pediatrics* (15th ed.). Philadelphia: W.B. Saunders.

Bickley, L.S., & Szilagyi, P.G. (2003). *Bates' guide to physical examination and history taking* (8th ed.). Philadelphia: Lippincott Williams & Wilkins.

Branch, W.T. (2003). *Office practice of medicine* (4th ed.). Philadelphia: Saunders.

Burns, C.E., Brady, M.A., Blosser, C., Starr, N.B., & Dunn, A.M. (2004). *Pediatric primary care: A handbook for nurse practitioners* (3rd ed.). Philadelphia: W.B. Saunders.

Centers for Disease Control and Prevention. (2002). Sexually transmitted diseases treatment guidelines. *MMWR, 47*, RR-1.

Dambro, M.R. (2005). *Griffith's 5 minute clinical consult.* Philadelphia: Lippincott Williams & Wilkins.

Diokno, A., McCormick, K.A., Colling, J.A., et. al. (1992). *Urinary incontinence in adults.* Clinical practice guideline. AHCPR Pub. No. 92-0038. Rockville, MD: Agency for Health Care Policy and Research, Public Health Service, U.S. Department of Health and Human Services.

Gallo, M.L., Fallon, P.J., & Staskin, D.R. (1997). Urinary incontinence: Steps to evaluation, diagnosis, and treatment. *The Nurse Practitioner, 22*(2), 21-44.

Gambrell, R.C., & Blount, B.W. (1996). Exercise-induced hematuria. *American Family Physician, 53*, 905-911.

Gilber, D.N., Moellering, R.C., Eliopoulos, G.M., & Sande, M.A. (Eds.). (2004). *Sanford Guide to Antimicrobial Therapy* (34th ed.). Hyde Park, VT: Antimicrobial Therapy.

Goldaber, K.G. (1997). Urinary tract infection during pregnancy. *Hospital Medicine, 33*(5), 14-24.

Goroll, A. H., & Mulley, A. G., Jr. (Eds.). (2000). *Primary care medicine: Office evaluation and management of the adult patient* (4th ed.). Philadelphia: Lippincott Williams Wilkins.

Graber, M.A., & Lanternier, M.L. (Eds.) (2001). *The family practice handbook.* (4th ed.). St. Louis: Mosby.

Gray, M. (2005). Assessment and management of urinary incontinence. *The Nurse Practitioner, 30*(7), 32-43.

Hahn, R.G., Knox, L.M., & Forman, T.A. (2005). Evaluation of poststreptococcal illness. *American Family Physician, 71*, 1949-1954.

Hamilton, E.M. (1996). Management of upper and lower urinary tract infections in pregnant women. *Journal of the American Academy of Nurse Practitioners, 8*, 559-563.

Holcomb, S.S. (2005). Evaluating chronic kidney disease risk. *The Nurse Practitioner, 30*(4), 12-25.

Klausner, T.I. (2005). The best kept secret: Pelvic floor muscle therapy for urinary incontinence. *Advance for Nurse Practitioners, 13*(7), 43-48.

Kobrin, S., & Aradhye, S. (1997). Preventing progression and complications of renal disease. *Hospital Medicine, 33*(11), 11-40.

Mangion, S. (2000). *Physical diagnosis secrets.* Philadelphia: Hanley and Belfus.

Mehnert-Kay, S.A. (2005). Diagnosis and treatment of uncomplicated urinary tract infections. *American Family Physician, 72(3)*, 451-456.

Mold, J.W. (1996). Pharmacotherapy of urinary incontinence. *American Family Physician, 54*(2), 673-680.

Nygaard, I.E., & Johnson, J.M. (1996). Urinary tract infections in elderly women. *American Family Physician, 53*(1), 175-182.

Portis, A. J., & Sundaram, C. P. (2001). Diagnosis and initial management of kidney stones. *American Family Physician, 63,* 1329-1338.

Pye, S. (1999). Diagnosis and referral of Wilm's tumor. *The Nurse Practitioner, 24*(5), 121-27.

Rakel, R.E. (Ed.). (1998). *Essentials of family practice.* (2nd ed.). Philadelphia: W

Ransom, S.B., & McNeeley, S.G. (Eds.). (1997). *Gynecology for the primary care provider*. Philadelphia: WB Saunders.

Riley, K.E. (1997). Evaluation and management of primary nocturnal enuresis. *The Journal of the American Academy of Nurse Practitioners, 9*(1), 33-39.

Schwartz, M.W. (Ed.). (2002). *The 5 minute pediatric consult.* (2nd ed.) Philadelphia:

Ullom-Minnich, M. (1996). Diagnosis and management of nocturnal enuresis. *American Family Physician, 54*(7), 2259-2266.

Uphold, C.R., & Graham, M.V. (2003). *Clinical guidelines in family practice.* (4th ed.). Gainesville, FL: Barmarrae Books.

U.S. Preventive Services Task Force. (1996). *Guide to clinical preventive services.* (2nd ed.) Washington, D.C.: Office of Disease Prevention and Health Promotion, U.S. Government Printing Office.

Viera, A. J., & Larkins-Pettigrew, M. (2000). Practical use of the pessary. *American Family Physician, 61,* 2719-2726, 2729.

22

WOMEN'S HEALTH

Women's Health

MENSTRUAL CYCLE

NORMS

Age of menarche (1st menstrual cycle)	Average: 12-13 years Normal range: 10-16 years
Length of menstrual cycle	Average: 28 days
Length of menses	Normal range: 4-6 days
Blood loss with menses	25-60 ml/ cycle

The menstrual cycle includes two cycles occurring simultaneously: *ovarian* and *endometrial*. Below is a summary of the two cycles.

Ovarian Cycle

Timing in Cycle	Phase	Prominent Hormones	Description
Day 1-14	Follicular	Follicular-stimulating hormone (FSH) Estrogen	Maturation of ovarian follicle
Day 14	Ovulation	Luteinizing hormone(LH)	Ovulation occurs 36 hours after LH surge Basal body temperature elevation occurs
Day 15-28	Luteal	Progesterone Estrogen	Follicle becomes corpus luteum

Endometrial Cycle

Timing in Cycle	Phase	Prominent Hormones	Description
Day 1-5 (variable)	Menses (part of proliferative phase)	Prostaglandin	Endometrium sloughs if fertilization of ovum does not occur
Day 1-14	Proliferative	Estrogen	Endometrium proliferates
Day 14-28	Secretory	Progesterone	Endometrium thickens in preparation for implantation

ABNORMAL VAGINAL BLEEDING

DESCRIPTION

Vaginal bleeding that is not related to normal menses

TERMS

Menorrhagia (hyper menorrhagia)	Heavy or prolonged bleeding at normal intervals
Metrorrhagia	Intermenstrual bleeding, spotting or breakthrough
Polymenorrhea	Normal bleeding with menstrual interval <21 days
Oligomenorrhea	Menstrual interval >35 days
Hypomenorrhea	Decreased menstrual flow
Amenorrhea	Absence of menstrual bleeding

ETIOLOGY

- Anovulation is most frequent cause
- Multiple causes

Trauma:
- Tampon use
- Foreign body, especially in 4-8year olds
- IUD
- Sexual abuse

Pregnancy-related:
- Ectopic pregnancy
- Spontaneous abortion
- Placenta previa
- Abruptio placenta

Medications:
- Aspirin, NSAIDs, anticoagulants
- Oral contraceptives
- Tranquilizers
- Neuroleptics
- Corticosteroids
- Tamoxifen (Nolvadex®)
- Hormone replacement therapy

Reproductive tract origin:
- Dysfunctional uterine bleeding
- Endometriosis
- Uterine fibroids
- Carcinoma
- Ovarian cysts
- Inflammation and/or infection of the vagina, cervix, uterus, or adnexa

Systemic disease:
- Bleeding disorder
- Thyroid disease
- Adrenal disease
- Renal or hepatic disease

Other:
- Influence of maternal hormones on newborn
- Precocious puberty

INCIDENCE

- Common
- Approximately 40,000 new cases annually
- 50% occur after age 40 years

RISK FACTORS

- Anovulation
- Hormone replacement

ASSESSMENT FINDINGS

- Anemia
- Heavy bleeding during menstrual cycle
- Bleeding lasting > 7 days
- Frequent passage of clots during menses

DIFFERENTIAL DIAGNOSIS

- *See* Etiology

DIAGNOSTIC STUDIES

- hCG
- Cervical screening with cytology
- Wet prep of vaginal secretions
- CBC with platelet count to determine severity of blood loss
- STD testing
- Depending on history and physical:
  - ◊ TSH
  - ◊ Chemistry profile
  - ◊ Liver function tests
  - ◊ BUN and creatinine
  - ◊ Bleeding/clotting studies
  - ◊ Endometrial biopsy in perimenopausal and postmenopausal women
  - ◊ Ultrasonography if mass palpated or suspected

hCG should always precede evaluation of a female of menstruating age who presents with vaginal bleeding.

NONPHARMACOLOGIC MANAGEMENT

- Rule out pregnancy
- Removal of foreign bodies if present
- Hospitalization may be required if bleeding severe
- Surgical intervention may be required if bleeding severe: dilatation and curettage or hysterectomy in extreme cases

PHARMACOLOGIC MANAGEMENT

- Antibiotics as indicated for infection (sexually transmitted infections)

- Consider topical estrogen cream if vaginal atrophy present
- Iron replacement therapy for anemia
- For less severe bleeding:
  - ◊ Oral contraceptives
  - ◊ Medroxyprogesterone acetate (Provera®)
- Prostaglandin inhibitors (e.g., NSAIDs)
- Danazol (Danocrine®) may be indicated in some cases caused by dysfunctional uterine bleeding

CONSULTATION/REFERRAL

- Hospitalization may be required for severe bleeding
- Consult gynecologist if bleeding is moderate and cause is not evident or if bleeding is severe
- Consult hematologist if apparent cause is hematological

FOLLOW-UP

- Reevaluate in 1-2 weeks, review diagnostic studies with patient, and determine response to intervention
- Monitor hemoglobin and hematocrit if bleeding moderate to severe

EXPECTED COURSE

- Dependent on cause and severity of bleeding

POSSIBLE COMPLICATIONS

- Anemia

AMENORRHEA

DESCRIPTION

Primary	Absence of menses by age 14 years in the absence of secondary sexual characteristics By age 16 years regardless of appearance of secondary sexual characteristics
Secondary	Absence of menses for 6 months or three cycles after having at least one spontaneous menstrual period

ETIOLOGY

Primary:

- Gonadal dysgenesis
- Uterovaginal anomalies (e.g., imperforate hymen, uterine agenesis, Turner's syndrome)
- Hypothalamic/pituitary disorders
- Immature hypothalamic-pituitary axis
- Thyroid disease

Secondary:

- Pregnancy, breast feeding, menopause
- Prolactin-secreting adenoma
- Hypothalamic/pituitary disorders (stress, excessive weight loss, low BMI)
- Excessive exercise
- Polycystic ovarian disease (Stein-Leventhal syndrome)
- Anorexia nervosa
- Systemic lupus erythematosus
- Crohn's disease
- Sheehan's syndrome
- Diabetes mellitus, uncontrolled
- Systemic corticosteroids
- Use of danazol (Danocrine®)
- OCP
- Thyroid disease

The most common cause of amenorrhea is pregnancy.

INCIDENCE

- Primary: 0.3% of women
- Primary and secondary combined: 3.3% of women of childbearing age in the U.S.

RISK FACTORS

- Strenuous physical exercise (long distance runners, cyclists, gymnasts, dancers, etc.)
- Eating disorders
- Emotional crisis
- Extreme levels of stress

ASSESSMENT FINDINGS

- Absence of menses
- Temperature intolerance

- Signs and symptoms of pregnancy
- Signs of androgen excess (e.g., hirsutism)

DIAGNOSTIC STUDIES

- hCG
- TSH
- FSH
- Prolactin
- Blood glucose
- Chromosomal analysis if suspect abnormality (e.g., Turner's syndrome)

PREVENTION

- Maintenance of appropriate body mass index (BMI)
- Avoid overtraining

NONPHARMACOLOGIC MANAGEMENT

- Depends on etiology
- Correction of over- or underweight states

PHARMACOLOGIC MANAGEMENT

- Depends on etiology
- Progesterone challenge will result in withdrawal bleeding if pituitary-ovarian axis is intact and patient is NOT pregnant
- Oral contraceptives

CONSULTATION/REFERRAL

- Refer any patient with primary amenorrhea to obstetrician

FOLLOW-UP

- Discontinue hormone (oral contraceptives) therapy after 6 months to assess for menses

EXPECTED COURSE

- Dependent on underlying cause
- If due to pituitary-ovarian suppression, 99% will resume normal menses in 6 months

POSSIBLE COMPLICATIONS

- Infertility
- Vaginal dryness
- Vasomotor instability
- Osteoporosis
- Cardiovascular disease

DYSMENORRHEA

DESCRIPTION

Painful cramping associated with menstruation

ETIOLOGY

Primary:

- Increased prostaglandins cause platelet aggregation, vasoconstriction, and uterine contractions which increases the likelihood of uterine ischemia
- No underlying pathology

Secondary:

- Congenital anomaly of the uterus or vagina
- Pelvic infection, STDs
- Adenomyosis
- Endometriosis
- Pelvic tumors (e.g., leiomyomata)

INCIDENCE

- 40% of women of childbearing age in the U.S. have dysmenorrhea
- Primary*:* predominant age is teens to early twenties
- Secondary*:* predominant age is twenties and thirties

RISK FACTORS

Primary:

- Nulliparity
- Positive family history
- Cigarette smoking

Secondary:

- Pelvic infection or STDs
- Endometriosis

ASSESSMENT FINDINGS

- Pelvic cramping
- Sensation of heaviness in pelvis
- Malaise
- Headache
- Nausea, vomiting, diarrhea
- Back, thigh pain
- Urinary frequency

Primary:
- Occurs usually in first 2 days of menstruation
- Located in suprapubic area and radiates to back and thighs
- May be associated with diarrhea, nausea, and vomiting

Secondary:
- Pain may refer to area of underlying pathology

DIFFERENTIAL DIAGNOSIS

- Intrauterine polyps
- Presence of intrauterine device
- Pelvic/genital infection
- Endometriosis
- Uterine/ovarian tumors
- Adhesions
- Incomplete abortion
- Ectopic pregnancy
- Complication of pregnancy

Non gynecologic causes:
- Urinary tract infection
- Adhesions

In a diagnosis of primary dysmenorrhea, the physical and pelvic exams should always be normal.

DIAGNOSTIC STUDIES

Primary:
- None usually indicated

Secondary:
- WBC: elevated in infections
- Cervical cultures
- As history and physical indicate

NONPHARMACOLOGIC MANAGEMENT

Primary:
- Heating pad to abdomen
- Hot bath
- Exercise (raises endorphins)
- Pelvic exercises
- Relaxation therapy
- Low fat diet may help

PHARMACOLOGIC MANAGEMENT

Primary:
- NSAIDs at onset of menses or cramping and continued for duration of pain
- Oral contraceptives
- Vitamin B_1 and Vitamin E may be helpful

Secondary:
- As diagnosis indicates

Primary dysmenorrheal typically abates as patient ages or has children.

CONSULTATION/REFERRAL

- For primary dysmenorrhea, if no improvement after 6 months of therapy
- For secondary dysmenorrhea if unable to achieve improvement in symptoms after 3-6 months

FOLLOW-UP

- 2 months after initial diagnosis to evaluate treatment

EXPECTED COURSE

Primary:
- Improves with age and parity

Secondary:
- Likely to require therapy based on underlying cause

POSSIBLE COMPLICATIONS

Primary:
- Anxiety
- Depression

Secondary:
- Infertility from underlying pathology

PREMENSTRUAL SYNDROME (PMS) / PREMENSTRUAL DYSPHORIC DISORDER (PMDD)

DESCRIPTION

Group of symptoms that occurs most commonly during the luteal phase of the menstrual cycle (5-11 days before menses) and abates within 1-2 days of onset of menses. When primary symptoms are emotional, PMDD.

DSM IV criteria are used to diagnose PMDD.

ETIOLOGY

- Unknown
- Presumed multifactorial and hormonally influenced; worsened by stress
- Fluid imbalance and increased prostaglandins thought to play a role

INCIDENCE

- 20-90% of women experience some symptoms of PMS, but PMS occurs in only about 5% of women
- Most common in women 25-40 years of age

RISK FACTORS

- Caffeine intake
- Pre-existing depression
- High fluid and/or sodium intake
- Stress
- Increasing age
- History of postpartal depression or affective disorder

ASSESSMENT FINDINGS

- Irritability, fatigue
- Depression
- Insomnia
- Crying spells
- Mood swings/depressed mood
- Difficulty concentrating
- Edema
- Sleep disturbances
- Appetite changes (carbohydrate craving)
- Libido changes
- Breast tenderness
- Nervousness
- Headache
- Lethargy
- Food cravings

Symptoms disappear at menopause.

DIFFERENTIAL DIAGNOSIS

- Depression
- Anxiety disorder
- Marital discord
- Alcohol/drug abuse
- Eating disorder
- Dysmenorrhea

DIAGNOSTIC STUDIES

- None indicated except to rule out other disorders

NONPHARMACOLOGIC MANAGEMENT

- Menstrual diary for 2 menstrual cycles to establish pattern of symptoms
- Decrease sodium intake
- Limit/avoid alcohol, caffeine, highly processed foods, foods high in fat
- Diet high in complex carbohydrates and lower in protein may be beneficial
- Regular, daily exercise
- Smoking cessation
- Adequate sleep and rest
- Stress reduction techniques
- Support groups

PHARMACOLOGIC MANAGEMENT

- Vitamin and mineral supplementation, especially B_6, E, calcium, magnesium
- NSAIDs
- Oral contraceptives
- Diuretics such as spironolactone (Aldactone®) can be used cautiously if edema is present
- Antidepressants: SSRIs (fluoxetine, others)
- Anxiolytics such as buspirone (BuSpar®)

Avoid using spironolactone concomitantly with ACE inhibitors because of risk of hyperkalemia.

CONSULTATION/REFERRAL

- Refer if refractory to above treatments

FOLLOW-UP

- Reevaluate in 2 months and review diary, then every 3-6 months.

PMS symptoms can continue after hysterectomy.

EXPECTED COURSE

- Usually symptoms can be adequately controlled

POSSIBLE COMPLICATIONS

- Severe depression
- Social isolation

ABNORMAL PAP SMEAR
(Abnormal Cervical Cytology)

DESCRIPTION

Papanicolaou smears are used for the early detection of abnormal cervical cells. An abnormal Pap smear is defined as any classification of cervical cytology other than within normal limits

ETIOLOGY

Infection:
- Human papilloma virus (HPV)
- Herpes simplex virus
- Bacterial vaginosis
- Trichomoniasis
- Gonorrhea
- Chlamydia

Inflammation:
- Chemotherapy
- Radiation
- Use of intrauterine device
- DES exposure

Neoplasia:
- Vaginal
- Endometrial
- Cervical

The most common reason females have abnormal cervical cytology is from HPV infections.

INCIDENCE

- 13,000-14,000 new cases of cervical cancer in U.S. annually
- Sixth most common malignancy in women
- Average age of diagnosis of cervical cancer is 45 years

RISK FACTORS

- Early age of first sexual intercourse
- Multiple sexual partners
- Sexual partner with multiple sexual partners
- Cigarette smoking
- Previous abnormal Pap smear
- History of sexually transmitted disease
- Sexual partner with cancer of the penis
- Early age of first pregnancy (before age 18 years)
- Exposure to certain viruses: (herpes simplex, human papilloma virus)
- Immunocompromised state
- African-American ancestry
- Low socioeconomic status
- DES exposure in utero

ASSESSMENT FINDINGS

- Asymptomatic
- Vaginal discharge, especially if infectious etiology
- Vaginal bleeding
- External lesions related to HPV

PREVENTION

- Delaying onset of sexual activity
- Mutual monogamy
- Use of condom if non monogamous relationship
- Routine screening with PAP smear every 1-3 years depending on risk factors

SCREENING RECOMMENDATIONS

- 3 years after onset of initial sexual activity or age 21 years, which ever occurs first
- Annually times three, and then if all three are normal then interval may be lengthened *if* patient is low risk for cervical cancer
- Interval should not be longer than 3 years
- U.S. Preventive Task Force recommends that screening stop at age 65 years, if all previous Pap smears have been negative

BETHESDA SYSTEM OF REPORTING PAP SMEARS

- Section I: Specimen adequacy section
  - ◊ Should be satisfactory for evaluation

Common causes of unsatisfactory specimens are scant number or no cervical cells present, poor fixation, the presence of foreign material, obscuring inflammation, obscuring blood, or excess cytolysis.

- Section II: General categorization section
  - ◊ Negative for intraepithelial lesion or malignancy
  - ◊ Epithelial cell abnormalities
    - * Atypical squamous cells (ACS)
    - * Atypical squamous cells of undetermined origin (ASCUS)
    - * Atypical cells cannot exclude high grade SIL (ASC-H)
    - * Low grade squamous intraepithelial lesion (LSIL)
    - * High grade squamous intraepithelial lesion (HSIL)
  - ◊ Glandular Cells
    - * Atypical glandular cells (AGS) (these favor neoplastic process)
    - * Endocervical adenocarcinoma in situ

Thin Prep® is a method used to improve sensitivity of the sampling process by dispersing cervical cells in a fluid medium. It is more expensive than traditional methods.

MANAGEMENT

Specimen inadequacy:

- Unsatisfactory for evaluation
  - ◊ Repeat Pap smear

Colposcopy and biopsy recommended for the following

- HSIL on initial PAP
- ASC or ASCUS on two PAPs 4-6 months apart
- ASC-H
- Any cervical or vaginal lesion that is visible to the naked eye
- Atypical endocervical cells

PREGNANCY CONSIDERATIONS

- If conization is indicated, delay until after delivery.

EXPECTED COURSE

- Depends on categorization of lesion

CERVICAL CANCER

DESCRIPTION

Malignancy of the cervix usually originating at the squamocolumnar junction

ETIOLOGY

- Probable relation to viral infections
- Human papilloma virus (HPV) type 16, 18, 31, 33, and 35 implicated in many cases

INCIDENCE

- 4800 deaths annually

RISK FACTORS

- Infection with HPV (current or previous)
- HIV infection
- Cigarette smoking
- Multiple sexual partners
- Early age of first sexual intercourse
- DES exposure in utero
- Immunocompromised state

ASSESSMENT FINDINGS

- Often asymptomatic
- Irregular vaginal bleeding
- Postcoital vaginal bleeding
- Dyspareunia
- Pelvic pain
- Enlarged cervix

DIFFERENTIAL DIAGNOSIS

- Severe cervicitis
- Cervical polyp
- Endometrial carcinoma
- Metastatic cancer

DIAGNOSTIC STUDIES

- Pap smear
- LEEP (loop electrosurgical excision procedure)
- Colposcopy with endocervical biopsy

A common finding is invasive squamous cell carcinoma or invasive adenocarcinoma.

PREVENTION

- Screening for cervical cytology starting at age 21 years or after being sexually active for 3 years. If woman is low risk, (mutually monogamous) consider screening every 2-3 years *after* 3 consecutive negative screens. Women at high risk should continue to be screened annually.
- Smoking cessation
- Barrier contraceptive method and spermicides during intercourse

NONPHARMACOLOGIC MANAGEMENT

- Surgical intervention:
  - ◊ Hysterectomy
  - ◊ Cone biopsy
  - ◊ Lymph node dissection
  - ◊ Pelvic exenteration
- Radiation therapy

PHARMACOLOGIC MANAGEMENT

- Fluorouracil, cisplatin, hydroxyurea, others as supplemental therapy to radiation

PREGNANCY/LACTATION CONSIDERATIONS

- Can occur in pregnancy
- Choice of therapy dependent on stage of malignancy and gestational age of fetus

CONSULTATION/REFERRAL

- Surgical/oncology physician referral

FOLLOW-UP

- Physical exam and Pap smear after initial diagnosis and treatment:
  - ◊ Every three months for 1-2 years
  - ◊ Every six months until 5 years
  - ◊ Annually after 5 years

EXPECTED COURSE

Five-year survival:

- Stage 0 (carcinoma in situ): >99%
- Stage I (confined to uterus): 90%
- Stage II (invasion beyond uterus, but not to pelvic wall or lower third of vagina): 50-70%
- Stage III (invasion to pelvic wall, lower third or vagina, or causes hydronephrosis): 40%-60%
- Stage IV (invasion of bladder, rectum, or beyond true pelvis): 20%

POSSIBLE COMPLICATIONS

- Recurrence
- Ureteral fistula
- Rectovaginal fistula
- Hydronephrosis
- Uremia

Common signs of recurrence of cervical cancer are weight loss, pelvic or thigh pain, and edema in the lower extremities.

ATROPHIC VAGINITIS
(ESTROGEN DEFICIENT VULVOVAGINITIS)

DESCRIPTION

Thinning and atrophy of vaginal tissue resulting in friability and associated with urinary incontinence

ETIOLOGY

- Estrogen deficiency secondary to:
  - ◊ Menopause (natural or surgically induced)
  - ◊ Oophorectomy
  - ◊ Pelvic radiation

INCIDENCE

- Common in postmenopausal women especially if not on hormone replacement therapy

ASSESSMENT FINDINGS

- Vaginal dryness, atrophy, absence or decreased vaginal rugae
- Pruritus
- Blood-tinged vaginal discharge
- Bleeding after intercourse
- Erythematous and petechial patches on vaginal mucosa
- Dyspareunia

Another name used to describe atrophic vaginitis is urogenital atrophy. Urinary incontinence is commonly seen accompanying decreased estrogenic states.

DIFFERENTIAL DIAGNOSIS

- Candida vaginitis
- Bacterial vaginosis
- Trichomoniasis or another STD

DIAGNOSTIC STUDIES

- Wet prep: normal vaginal flora
- FSH level to confirm menopause: increased in menopause
- Estradiol level to measure circulating estrogen level: decreased in menopause
- Pap smear and mammogram before initiation of estrogen therapy

PREVENTION

- Hormone replacement therapy in estrogen deficient states is a personal decision which should be made after consultation with a health care provider

Average age of menopause is 52.5 years.

NONPHARMACOLOGIC MANAGEMENT

- Water-soluble lubricants before intercourse
- Cool baths and compresses for discomfort
- Cotton underwear

PHARMACOLOGIC MANAGEMENT

- Consider low dose oral estrogen daily
- Progesterone should be added in women who have not had hysterectomy
- Conjugated estrogen vaginal cream may be used for vaginal symptoms

Estrogen replacement is absolutely contraindicated in patients with history of breast cancer, undiagnosed vaginal bleeding, carcinoma, and/or active liver disease.

Lactation can produce a hypoestrogenic state and thus, dyspareunia or other symptoms of vaginal dryness may prevail. Use of vaginal lubricants may provide symptomatic relief. Symptoms usually resolve once breastfeeding is stopped.

CONSULTATION/REFERRAL

- Not usually required

FOLLOW-UP

- Reevaluate 1-2 months after beginning drug therapy
- Annual physical examination

EXPECTED COURSE

- Symptoms should resolve in 1-2 months after treatment instituted
- Most will be relieved by estrogen replacement therapy

POSSIBLE COMPLICATIONS

- Secondary infections
- Vaginal fissures or ulcerations

VULVOVAGINAL CANDIDIASIS
(Monilial Vulvovaginitis)

DESCRIPTION

Vulvovaginal infection, not considered a sexually transmitted disease

ETIOLOGY

- *Candida albicans* most common, but may be caused by other organisms (e.g., *C. glabrata*, *C. tropicalis*)
- Occurs when a change in the balance of microorganisms of the vagina allows proliferation of yeast

INCIDENCE

- Very common in women from menarche to menopause
- Accounts for 33% of all vaginal infections
- 13 million cases reported annually in the U.S.
- Rare in children

RISK FACTORS

- Recent antibiotic therapy
- Immunocompromised states, recent corticosteroid use
- Pregnancy
- Hypothyroidism, diabetes
- Anemia, especially iron deficiency
- Oral contraceptives
- Wearing tight-fitting, synthetic (non-cotton) clothing
- Previous candidal vulvovaginitis
- Obesity

ASSESSMENT FINDINGS

- Thick, white, curd-like vaginal discharge
- Thick, white patches on vaginal mucosa
- Vulvar itching, erythema, edema
- Dyspareunia
- Usually no malodor
- Dysuria

DIFFERENTIAL DIAGNOSIS

- Bacterial vaginosis
- Gonorrhea
- Chlamydial infection
- Atrophic vaginitis
- Allergic reaction
- Trichomoniasis
- Pinworm vaginitis, especially in children
- Vaginal foreign body

DIAGNOSTIC STUDIES

- 10% KOH prep: budding yeast and pseudohyphae
- Vaginal secretions pH: ≤4.5
- Blood glucose if diabetes suspected
- HIV if suspect immunocompromise is underlying problem

PREVENTION

- Good perineal hygiene
- Cotton underwear
- Sleeping without underwear
- Avoid tight fitting clothing, especially jeans
- Weight loss if indicated
- Management of elevated glucose
- Frequent change of tampons and use of pad at night
- Use of unscented, mild soap
- Avoid frequent douching
- Consider screening and treating sexual partner if female has recurrent infection

Growth of yeast is facilitated in a warm, dark, moist environment.

NONPHARMACOLOGIC MANAGEMENT

- Refrain from sexual intercourse until symptoms resolved
- Creams and/or suppositories used for treatment may weaken latex condoms and diaphragms
- Good perineal hygiene
- Treatment of male sexual partner is not indicated unless balanitis present

PHARMACOLOGIC MANAGEMENT

- Many medications available
- Fluconazole (Diflucan®) orally *OR*
- Miconazole nitrate (Monistat®) vaginal suppository or cream *OR*
- Butoconazole nitrate (Femstat®) vaginal cream *OR*
- Terconazole (Terazol®) vaginal suppository or cream

Terconazole is a good choice for atypical yeast.

PREGNANCY/LACTATION CONSIDERATIONS

- Increased risk during pregnancy due to elevated levels of glycogen and reproductive hormones
- Only topical azole therapies should be used during pregnancy
- Treat for 7-14 days during pregnancy
- The triazole, fluconazole (Diflucan®) and itraconazole (Sporanox®), and possibly ketoconazole (Nizoral®), are excreted in breast milk and should be avoided during lactation

CONSULTATION/REFERRAL

- None usually needed

FOLLOW-UP

- None usually needed
- Treat sexual partner if infections are frequent or recalcitrant to therapy
- Culture if infection recurs 3 or more times annually

EXPECTED COURSE

- Complete resolution
- Recurrences common

POSSIBLE COMPLICATIONS

- Secondary bacterial infection

BARTHOLIN'S GLAND CYST/ABSCESS

DESCRIPTION

Obstruction of the major duct of Bartholin's gland resulting in cyst formation. Infection and obstruction of the duct will lead to an abscess.

ETIOLOGY

- Mechanical irritation from tight fitting undergarments resulting in chronic inflammation
- STDs

RISK FACTORS

- Vulvovaginal infection
- Poor perineal hygiene

ASSESSMENT FINDINGS

- Firm labia mass or cyst
- Pain, erythema, induration
- Edema of labia minora
- Low grade fever

DIFFERENTIAL DIAGNOSIS

- Sebaceous cyst
- Malignancy

DIAGNOSTIC STUDIES

- None usually indicated unless other infection suspected
- Culture and sensitivity of cyst contents
- Culture for STDs especially, *Neisseria gonorrhoeae*

PREVENTION

- Good perineal hygiene
- Early treatment

NONPHARMACOLOGIC MANAGEMENT

- Application of local moist heat
- Warm sitz baths
- Incision and drainage of fluctuant abscess
- No treatment needed if only 1-2 mm and patient is asymptomatic

Goal is to facilitate drainage of cyst contents. Warm baths provide comfort and may help to facilitate drainage.

PHARMACOLOGIC MANAGEMENT

- Base on culture and sensitivity, but consider trimethoprim-sulfamethoxazole, quinolone
- Analgesics

CONSULTATION/REFERRAL

- Consider referral to surgeon or gynecologist if large and initial treatment ineffective

FOLLOW-UP

- Reevaluate in 7-10 days

EXPECTED COURSE

- Complete resolution with conservative treatment is usual

POSSIBLE COMPLICATIONS

- Cellulitis of surrounding tissue

POLYCYSTIC OVARIAN DISEASE (Stein-Leventhal Syndrome)

DESCRIPTION

Chronic, complex endocrine disorder associated with oligo-ovulation and/or anovulation; characterized by formation of cysts in the ovaries

ETIOLOGY

- Hypothalamic suppression
- Pituitary suppression
- Disharmonious gonadotropin and estrogen production
- Inability of the ovary to respond to gonadotrophic stimulation
- Increased androgen production from the adrenals or ovaries

INCIDENCE

- Leading cause of oligomenorrhea and/or amenorrhea in premenopausal women
- 6% of premenopausal women

RISK FACTORS

- Endometrial hyperplasia
- Obesity, diabetes mellitus
- Infertility

ASSESSMENT FINDINGS

- Onset occurs at onset of menses or months to years after the onset of menses
- Hyperinsulinemia
- Hyperandrogenism
    - ◊ Hirsutism
    - ◊ Acne
    - ◊ Seborrhea
    - ◊ Alopecia
    - ◊ Voice changes
    - ◊ Hypertrophy of the clitoris
- Irregular menstrual cycles
- Amenorrhea
- Infertility
- Asymptomatic in majority of patients
- Enlarged ovaries

PCOS should be suspected in females who are overweight, have infrequent menses, hirsutism, and infertility.

DIFFERENTIAL DIAGNOSIS

- Cushing's syndrome

- Endocrine tumor: androgen-producing ovarian or adrenal tumor
- Prolactin-producing pituitary adenoma
- Adult-onset adrenal hyperplasia
- HAIR-An syndrome (includes ***h***yper***a***ndrogenism, ***i***nsulin ***r***esistance, ***a***canthosis ***n***igricans)
- Endometrial carcinoma

DIAGNOSTIC STUDIES

- Pregnancy test
- LH/FSH ratio: $\geq$2.5:1
- Testosterone: increased
- Prolactin level: elevated
- Doppler ultrasound of ovaries: multiple cysts on the ovaries ("string of pearls")
- Fasting insulin level: increased

NONPHARMACOLOGIC MANAGEMENT

- Weight loss if overweight
- Stress management
- Hair removal therapy

PHARMACOLOGIC MANAGEMENT

If pregnancy not desired:

- Low dose oral contraceptives *OR*
- Medroxyprogesterone acetate (Depo-Provera®) 12-14 days/month

If pregnancy desired:

- Metformin daily
- Clomiphene citrate (Clomid®) *OR*
- Menotropins (Pergonal®) *OR*
- Bromocriptine (Parlodel®)

Consider referring patients who desire pregnancy and treatment to stimulate release of ova from ovaries.

FOLLOW-UP

- Frequent monitoring

POSSIBLE COMPLICATIONS

- Endometrial, breast, ovarian cancer
- Hyperlipidemia, hyperinsulinemia, hyperglycemia
- Insulin resistance
- Diabetes mellitus
- Cardiovascular disease
- Infertility

BENIGN OVARIAN TUMORS

DESCRIPTION

Nonmalignant tumor of the ovary; may be solid or cystic

ETIOLOGY

- Unknown
- Endometriosis
- Physiologic cysts

Many different types of cells in the ovaries and so they are susceptible to benign and malignant tumors.

INCIDENCE

- Unknown

RISK FACTORS

- Age: post-menopausal

ASSESSMENT FINDINGS

- Asymptomatic in most cases
- Pain, abdominal or lower back
- Abdominal distention
- Bowel and/or bladder pressure

DIFFERENTIAL DIAGNOSIS

- Malignant tumor of the ovary
- Polycystic ovary
- Ectopic pregnancy
- Uterine tumors
- Urinary tract infection
- PID with tubo-ovarian abscess

DIAGNOSTIC STUDIES

- Pregnancy test
- Urinalysis
- CA-125: <35 μg /ml
- Pelvic ultrasound

PREVENTION

- Risk may be decreased by use of oral contraceptives

Physical and pelvic exam, along with history play important role in diagnosis.

NONPHARMACOLOGIC MANAGEMENT

- Surgical removal of tumor

PHARMACOLOGIC MANAGEMENT

- Oral contraceptives in premenopausal women for physiologic cysts may help resolve more rapidly

CONSULTATION/REFERRAL

- Gynecologic/surgical consultation to assist with diagnosis if needed

FOLLOW-UP

- Annual examination

EXPECTED COURSE

- Complete cure

POSSIBLE COMPLICATIONS

- Torsion
- Rupture
- Hemorrhage

OVARIAN CANCER

DESCRIPTION

A malignancy of the ovaries with origins in the epithelium, stroma, or germ cells

Ovarian cancer is the leading cause of gynecological death in women.

ETIOLOGY

- Unknown

INCIDENCE

- 26,500 new cases annually
- Causes 14,500 deaths annually in U.S.
- 4th leading cause of cancer death in women
- Usual age: 40-75 years of age

The incidence of ovarian cancer has not decreased in the last 6 decades.

RISK FACTORS

- History of breast cancer especially before age 40
- Nulliparity or low parity
- Pregnancy after age 30 years
- Family history in first-degree or second-degree relatives
- Increasing age
- Presence of BRCA-1, BRCA-2 genes

ASSESSMENT FINDINGS

- Bloating
- Dyspepsia
- Abdominal pressure, fullness, or pain
- Irregular vaginal bleeding
- Ascites
- Pelvic mass
- Dyspareunia
- Weight loss
- Vaginal discharge

DIFFERENTIAL DIAGNOSIS

- GI malignancy
- Uterine fibroid
- Other gynecologic malignancy
- Irritable bowel syndrome

- Inflammatory bowel syndrome

DIAGNOSTIC STUDIES

- Ultrasound of pelvis
- Surgical exploration
- CA-125 (normal < 35 u/ml) possibly helpful but not a good screening tool

CA-125 may be elevated in benign ovarian conditions, endometriosis, liver disease, CHF. Therefore, this test lacks specificity.

PREVENTION

- Oral contraceptives have role in prevention
- Multiparity
- Women who have breastfed their infants have lower rates of ovarian cancer

Women with a history of breast cancer before age 40 should be screened at least annually for ovarian cancer because the risk of ovarian cancer is 17- fold more than in women without breast cancer.

NONPHARMACOLOGIC MANAGEMENT

- Surgery
  - ◊ Total abdominal hysterectomy for epithelial malignancies
  - ◊ Salpingo-oophorectomy for germ cell cancers
- Radiation therapy

PHARMACOLOGIC MANAGEMENT

- Chemotherapy

CONSULTATION/REFERRAL

- Refer for surgical/oncological evaluation and treatment

FOLLOW-UP

- Follow with CA-125 for response to therapy (a 7 – fold decrease in CA-125 suggests good response to therapy)

EXPECTED COURSE

Five-year survival rates:

- Stage I (limited to ovaries): 80%
- Stage II (confined to pelvis): 60%
- Stage III (involvement of regional lymph nodes or upper abdomen): 15-30%
- Stage IV (distant or visceral metastasis): 10%

POSSIBLE COMPLICATIONS

- Adverse effects of treatment
- Ascites

CONTRACEPTION

Combined Oral Contraceptives

DESCRIPTION

Oral contraceptive containing both estrogen and progestin

MECHANISM OF ACTION

- Suppresses pituitary gonadotropins (FSH and LH) which inhibits ovulation

EFFECTIVENESS

- Theoretical effectiveness rate of 99.7%
- Actual effectiveness is 90-96%

ADVANTAGES

- Very reliable temporary method of contraception when used properly
- No interference with sexual activity
- Health-related benefits
  - ◊ Decreased menstrual flow and diminished reports of dysmenorrhea
  - ◊ Improvement of acne
  - ◊ Regularity of menses
  - ◊ Protection against anemia

DISADVANTAGES

- May cause life-threatening or serious complications
  - ◊ Thrombophlebitis/thromboembolism

- ◊ Hepatocellular adenomas
- ◊ Stroke
- ◊ Gallbladder disease
- ◊ Hypertension
- Must remember to take pill every day
- Provide no protection against STDs
- May decrease milk production in lactating women

SIDE EFFECTS

- Nausea
- Breast fullness and/or tenderness
- Cyclic weight gain and fluid retention
- Breakthrough bleeding, especially in first three months of use
- Decreased menstrual flow and/or amenorrhea
- Fatigue
- Acne
- Mild headaches
- Increased appetite

ABSOLUTE CONTRAINDICATIONS

- History of, or current thrombophlebitis, or thromboembolic disorder
- CVA
- Age >35 years and hypertensive or diabetic
- Migraine with aura
- LDL > 160 or Trigs > 250
- Ischemic heart disease or coronary artery disease
- Known or suspected breast cancer
- Diabetes with vascular complications
- Known or suspected estrogen-dependent neoplasia
- Pregnancy, known or suspected
- Hepatic adenomas
- Undiagnosed gynecologic bleeding
- Uncontrolled hypertension
- Active liver disease

RELATIVE CONTRAINDICATIONS

- Over 35 years old and a heavy smoker
- Migraine headaches that start after initiation of oral contraceptives
- Hypertension with resting diastolic blood pressure ≥90 mm Hg; or resting systolic ≥140 mm Hg on three separate visits; or a diastolic ≥110 mm Hg on a single visit
- Diabetes mellitus
- Elective major surgery requiring immobilization within next 4 weeks
- Sickle cell anemia
- Lactation
- Active gall bladder disease
- Congenital hyperbilirubinemia (Gilbert's disease)
- Age >50 years
- Conditions that make it difficult for a woman to take pills consistently and correctly (e.g., mental retardation, psychiatric illness, substance abuse)
- Family history of hyperlipidemia
- Family history of death of a parent or sibling from myocardial infarction before age 50 years

DIAGNOSTIC STUDIES

Before prescribing:

- Pap smear
- Pregnancy test
- STD screening as indicated
- Lipid profile

PATIENT EDUCATION

- Danger signs of OC's: *ACHES*
  A: severe abdominal pain (may be indicative of hepatic tumors)
  C: severe chest pain or shortness of breath
  H: severe headache
  E: eye problems (blurred vision, flashing lights, or blindness)
  S: severe leg pain
- Oral contraceptives do not provide STD prevention
- Smoking cessation
- Maintenance of ideal body weight
- Exercise program
- Must use back-up method if on any of these medications:
  - ◊ Rifampin
  - ◊ Barbiturates
  - ◊ Phenytoin (Dilantin®)
  - ◊ Phenylbutazone
  - ◊ Griseofulvin (Fulvicin®)
  - ◊ Ampicillin
  - ◊ Tetracycline
  - ◊ Carbamazepine (Tegretol®)
- Pill should be taken each day at same time

- If one pill is missed, take missed pill as soon as remembered. If not remembered until time for next pill, take two pills.
- If two consecutive pills are missed, take two pills per day for the next two days, and then resume one pill per day. Use vaginal spermicide and condoms for remainder of cycle.
- 50% of patients have breakthrough bleeding during the first 3 months on oral contraceptives, but then usually abates. Breakthrough bleeding does not indicate decrease in effectiveness of pills.

FOLLOW-UP

- Evaluate 3 months after beginning pills then annually
- Check weight and blood pressure after 3 months on pills
- Breast examination and Pap smear annually

Progestin-only Oral Contraceptive (Mini-Pill)

DESCRIPTION

Oral contraceptive that contains no estrogen, only progestin

MECHANISM OF ACTION

- Suppression of ovulation
- Creation of a thin, atrophic endometrium
- Thickening of cervical mucous making sperm penetration difficult

EFFECTIVENESS

- 97-99% rate of effectiveness
- Failure rate highest in women younger than 40 years
- Rate nearly 100% in lactating women

ADVANTAGES

- May be used in lactating women, does not alter quality or quantity of breast milk
- May be used in women with cardiovascular risk factors
- Health benefits similar to combined oral contraceptives: protection against developing endometrial cancer and decreased risk of pelvic inflammatory disease
- Decreased menstrual cramps
- Less heavy bleeding and shorter menses
- Decreased premenstrual syndrome symptoms
- Decreased breast tenderness

DISADVANTAGES

- Increased chance of ectopic pregnancy
- Must be taken each day at same time
- Missing only one pill will substantially increase risk of pregnancy
- Menstrual cycle changes

SIDE EFFECTS

Serious:

- Same as combined oral contraceptives

Other:

- Functional ovarian cysts
- Menstrual cycle changes including spotting, breakthrough bleeding, prolonged cycles, and amenorrhea

INDICATIONS

- Women who experience unacceptable estrogen-related side effects (e.g., GI upset, breast tenderness, or decreased libido)
- Women who have developed severe headaches or hypertension while on combined oral contraceptives
- Women who have an absolute or relative contraindication to estrogen and combined oral contraceptives
    - ◊ Age over 40 years
    - ◊ History of severe headaches
    - ◊ Stable hypertension
    - ◊ Well-controlled diabetes
    - ◊ Chloasma
    - ◊ Mental depression
    - ◊ Lactation

CONTRAINDICATIONS

- Active thrombophlebitis or thromboembolic disorder
- History of myocardial infarction, ischemic heart disease, or coronary artery disease
- Known or suspected breast cancer
- Pregnancy, known or suspected
- Liver disease

- Undiagnosed gynecologic bleeding
- Medical condition which is worsened by fluid retention (e.g., CHF, mitral stenosis, pulmonary hypertension)
- Use of rifampin, barbiturates, phenytoin, carbamazepine, and/or phenylbutazone

DIAGNOSTIC STUDIES

Before prescribing:
- Pap smear
- STD screening as indicated
- Pregnancy test

PATIENT EDUCATION

- If changing from combined to mini pills, start pill on first day of menses or anytime during combined oral contraceptive cycle
- If no history of unprotected postpartal intercourse and not currently taking oral contraceptives, start mini-pills immediately
- Use backup method for one month following initiation of pills
- If pill is taken more than 3 hours late, use back-up method for remainder of pill pack
- If one pill is missed, take it as soon as possible
- If more than one pill is missed, the chance of pregnancy is great. A back-up method should be used for remainder of pill pack.
- Most women will experience irregular menstrual bleeding with spotting, breakthrough bleeding, prolonged cycles, and/or amenorrhea

FOLLOW-UP

- Evaluate 3 months after beginning pills then annually
- Notify health care provider when discontinuing breastfeeding

Diaphragm

DESCRIPTION

Dome-shaped latex cup with a flexible spring rim which is filled with spermicide and placed in the upper vagina to cover the cervix completely

MECHANISM OF ACTION

- The latex dome forms a barrier between the cervix and semen, preventing sperm from entering the uterus. The spermicidal cream or jelly is used with the diaphragm for additional protection, killing any sperm that accidentally slip past the rim of the diaphragm.

EFFECTIVENESS

- About 82%
- 94% with consistent, perfect use

ADVANTAGES

- Helpful in prevention of STDs
- No serious side effects
- Insertion may be incorporated into foreplay
- Decreased incidence of cervical neoplasia

DISADVANTAGES

- Must be used each time intercourse occurs
- May be embarrassing for women who dislike touching their genitals
- May be considered "messy" by some women
- Decreased effectiveness with increased frequency of intercourse
- Must be refitted if change in weight and after delivery or cervical surgery

SIDE EFFECTS

- May be uncomfortable once inserted
- Recurrent bladder infections
- Possible allergic reaction to latex and/or spermicide
- Foul smelling, profuse vaginal discharge if diaphragm forgotten or left in place too long
- Toxic shock syndrome
- Vaginal trauma or ulceration caused by excessive rim pressure or prolonged wear

CONTRAINDICATIONS

- Latex allergy
- Allergy to spermicide
- History of toxic shock syndrome
- History of frequent UTI
- Abnormalities of uterine anatomy that prevent a satisfactory fit:
  - ◊ Uterine prolapse

  - ◊ Extreme uterine retroversion
  - ◊ Vaginal septum
  - ◊ Severe cystocele or rectocele
- Inability of patient or partner to learn correct insertion technique
- Full-term pregnancy delivered within the past 6 weeks

DIAGNOSTIC STUDIES

- Pap smear
- STD screening

PATIENT EDUCATION

- Proper insertion and removal
- May insert diaphragm up to six hours prior to intercourse
- Remove diaphragm 6-8 hours after intercourse
- Always use diaphragm with spermicidal cream/jelly
- Return for refitting if weight gain of 10-20 lbs, after pregnancy, and after pelvic surgery
- Periodic inspection of integrity of diaphragm
- Signs and symptoms of toxic shock syndrome
- To decrease risk of toxic shock syndrome:
  - ◊ Do not use diaphragm during menses
  - ◊ Do not wear diaphragm longer than 24 hours
  - ◊ Wash hands carefully before inserting or removing diaphragm

FOLLOW-UP

- 1-3 weeks return with diaphragm in place for evaluation of proper position and size
- Annual examination

Male Condoms

DESCRIPTION

Latex or rubber sheath used to cover the penis during intercourse; may be used with or without spermicide

MECHANISM OF ACTION

- Mechanical barrier which prevents sperm from entering cervix

EFFECTIVENESS

- 88-98% in prevention of pregnancy

ADVANTAGES

- Most effective method for preventing the spread of STDs including HIV
- Relatively inexpensive
- Easily attainable, do not require prescription

DISADVANTAGES

- May decrease sexual pleasure for either partner
- Putting on condom may interrupt foreplay
- Possibility of breakage

CONTRAINDICATIONS

- Latex allergy
- Allergy to spermicide

PATIENT EDUCATION

- Use spermicide to increase effectiveness of condom
- Proper usage: place on erect penis before penis comes into contact with vulvar area; leave about $^1/_2$ inch space at end of condom; after intercourse, hold onto condom as the penis is withdrawn
- Condoms should be used only once
- Condoms should not be kept in a wallet, glove compartment of a car, or other warm area that may cause deterioration of the rubber
- Avoid use of oil-based vaginal creams or lubricants that may weaken condoms (e.g., petroleum jelly, antifungals)

Natural Family Planning

DESCRIPTION

Method of determining days of each month when it is most likely for a woman to be fertile and then, abstaining from intercourse during that time. Use of basal body temperature tracking and assessment of cervical mucous greatly increases effectiveness of this method over the old rhythm-type calendar method.

EFFECTIVENESS

- Theoretical effectiveness is 87%
- Actual effectiveness is 79%

ADVANTAGES

- Involves no chemicals or devices
- Few religious objections to its use
- Low cost

DISADVANTAGES

- May require long periods of abstinence
- No protection against STDs

CONTRAINDICATIONS

- Irregular intervals between menses
- History of anovulatory cycles
- During the perimenopausal period

Intrauterine Device (IUD)

DESCRIPTION

Device made of copper or other material that is placed and retained within the uterine cavity

- Two types available in the U.S.:
  - ◊ Progestasert®: contains progesterone
  - ◊ ParaGard Copper T380A®: contains copper

MECHANISM OF ACTION

- Not exactly known. Hypotheses are:
  - ◊ Increased motility of ovum in fallopian tubes
  - ◊ Inflammatory effects on the endometrium
  - ◊ Local foreign body inflammatory response that interferes with sperm survival, motility, and/or capacitation
  - ◊ The copper in the ParaGard® interferes with estrogen uptake and its effect on the endometrium
  - ◊ The progesterone in Progestasert® thickens cervical mucus, blocking entry to uterine cavity

EFFECTIVENESS

- Progestasert®: 98%
- ParaGard®: 99.2%

ADVANTAGES

- No action required for contraception
- IUD not detectable during intercourse
- No systemic effect on hormones
- Long-term contraception
- Cost-effective if used long-term
- Good choice for lactating women: no effect on milk production and if using ParaGard®, no hormone secreted in milk

DISADVANTAGES

- 2-5% of patients spontaneously expel IUD
- Limited population of women are candidates
- Do not protect against STDs

SIDE EFFECTS

- Abdominal infection or adhesions
- Sepsis
- Cervical infection or erosion
- Ovarian cysts
- Ectopic pregnancy
- Embedment of IUD in uterine tissue
- Infertility
- Spotting between periods
- Dysmenorrhea
- Pregnancy
- Prolonged or heavy menstrual flow

INDICATIONS

- Contraception in women who have had at least one full-term pregnancy
- Women who are in a stable, mutually monogamous sexual relationship
- Women aged 21 years or older
- No history of PID
- Desire for long-term contraception

CONTRAINDICATIONS

- <6 weeks postpartum
- <2 weeks postabortion
- History of pelvic inflammatory disease
- Multiple sexual partners or sexual partner of person with multiple sexual partners
- Acute or subacute infection of cervix, uterus, fallopian tubes, postpartal endometritis or infected abortion

- Cancer of the uterus, cervix, or fallopian tubes
- Untreated dysplasia on recent Pap smear
- Undiagnosed gynecologic bleeding
- Current abnormal vaginal discharge or infection
- Current or suspected pregnancy
- Immunocompromised state
- Abnormal uterine cavity
- Current genital actinomycosis
- Active herpes simplex virus
- Valvular heart disease

ParaGard®:
- Wilson's disease
- Allergy to copper, if copper device is used

Progestasert®:
- Presence of, or history of, STDs (e.g., chlamydia or gonorrhea)
- History of pelvic surgery that may be associated with increased risk of ectopic pregnancy (e.g., surgery on fallopian tubes, endometriosis)
- History of ectopic pregnancy or condition that predisposes to ectopic pregnancy
- Incomplete involution after abortion or birth
- Factors predisposing to patient to PID

DIAGNOSTIC STUDIES

Before insertion:
- Pap smear
- Hematocrit
- STD screening (HIV, gonorrhea, chlamydia)
- Pregnancy test
- Vaginal wet prep

PATIENT EDUCATION

- Complications of IUD use
- Barrier method of contraception until reevaluation after next menses
- Monthly string checks after menses and notify health care provider if cannot locate
- Progestasert® needs to be changed every year, ParaGard® every 10 years
- Educate about signs and symptoms of infection
- Warning signs associated with IUD use:
    - ◊ Late or missed period
    - ◊ Abdominal pain
    - ◊ Fever or chills
    - ◊ Delayed period, followed by scanty or irregular bleeding
    - ◊ Exposure to STD
    - ◊ Foul smelling vaginal discharge
    - ◊ Genital lesion
    - ◊ Fever with vaginal discharge
    - ◊ Severe or prolonged menstrual bleeding
    - ◊ String disappearance
    - ◊ Dyspareunia

FOLLOW-UP

- Evaluate after next menses, then annually
- Pregnancy test if amenorrheic

Medroxyprogesterone Acetate (Depo-Provera®)

DESCRIPTION

Injectable progestin which is administered intramuscularly is slowly released and provides contraception for thirteen weeks

MECHANISM OF ACTION

- Suppression of ovulation
- Creation of a thin, atrophic endometrium
- Thickening of cervical mucous making sperm penetration difficult

EFFECTIVENESS

- 99.7% effective in pregnancy prevention

ADVANTAGES

- No increased risk of thromboembolism, hypertension, and other estrogenic side effects
- Decreased or no menstrual flow or cramping
- 13 week period of effectiveness
- No effect on milk production in lactating women

DISADVANTAGES

- Fertility may not return for up to two years following last injection, but most women will be fertile within 12 months
- Requires injection for administration

SIDE EFFECTS

- Side effects of menstrual changes: amenorrhea, irregular spotting or bleeding, or heavy vaginal bleeding
- Headaches
- Weight changes, especially gain
- Libido changes
- Depression
- Dizziness

CONTRAINDICATIONS

- Undiagnosed gynecologic bleeding
- Suspected or confirmed pregnancy
- Breast cancer
- Active thrombophlebitis
- Active liver disease
- Active gallbladder disease
- Coronary artery disease
- History of CVA
- Known sensitivity to medroxyprogesterone

DIAGNOSTIC STUDIES

Before administering:

- Pap smear
- Pregnancy test
- STD screening as indicated

PATIENT EDUCATION

- Side effect profile of drug
- Menses may not return for three to 12 months following last Depo-Provera® injection
- Change of contraceptive method 6-18 months before attempting pregnancy
- Use of barrier method for prevention of STDs

FOLLOW-UP

- Repeat injections every 13 weeks
- Annual examination
- Hematocrit or hemoglobin if history of heavy or persistent menstrual bleeding
- Pregnancy test if no regular menses and/or symptoms of pregnancy are present

Norplant®

DESCRIPTION

Contraceptive system made of six silastic capsules which are inserted into the subcutaneous tissue of the upper arm. The capsules slowly release levonorgestrel to provide contraception for up to 5 years.

MECHANISM OF ACTION

- Suppression of ovulation
- Creation of a thin, atrophic endometrium
- Thickening of cervical mucous making sperm penetration difficult

EFFECTIVENESS

- 99.8% effective in pregnancy prevention

ADVANTAGES

- Does not require patient compliance
- Less menstrual cramping

DISADVANTAGES

- Menstrual changes: amenorrhea or irregular periods, may be heavier or lighter than usual. These usually resolve in 6-8 months.

SIDE EFFECTS

- Depression
- Leg cramps
- Dizziness
- Allergy
- Decreased libido

CONTRAINDICATIONS

- Undiagnosed gynecologic bleeding
- Known or suspected pregnancy
- Active thrombophlebitis or thromboembolic disease
- Active liver disease
- History of myocardial infarction or CVA
- Known or suspected carcinoma of the breast, uterus, or ovaries
- Use of rifampin, barbiturates, phenytoin, carbamazepine, and/or phenylbutazone
- Idiopathic intracranial hypertension

DIAGNOSTIC STUDIES

Before inserting:
- Pap smear
- Hematocrit and hemoglobin
- STD screening
- Pregnancy test

PATIENT EDUCATION

- Protection from pregnancy begins 24 hours after insertion
- May be removed at any time
- Removal in five years is mandatory, but new system may be inserted at that time if desired
- Danger signs:
  - ◊ Severe lower abdominal pain
  - ◊ Heavy vaginal bleeding
  - ◊ Signs of infection at site of insertion
  - ◊ Expulsion of capsule
  - ◊ Migraines or any severe headaches
  - ◊ Chest pain
  - ◊ Shortness of breath
  - ◊ Jaundice
  - ◊ Severe nausea and/or vomiting

FOLLOW-UP

- Inspection of insertion site one week after insertion
- Pregnancy test if amenorrheic and/or symptoms of pregnancy present
- Annual examination
- Removal in five years

Spermicides

DESCRIPTION

Spermicidal product (usually nonoxynol-9) placed in the vagina for contraceptive purposes; can be used alone or with condom or diaphragm

MECHANISM OF ACTION

Composed of chemicals which are toxic to sperm

EFFECTIVENESS

- 80-85% when used alone
- 99% when used with condom

ADVANTAGES

- Helps prevent STDs, especially gonorrhea and chlamydia
- Easily attainable over-the-counter
- Provides lubrication
- Relatively inexpensive
- Can serve as back up method of other contraceptive
- Does not affect milk production in lactating women

DISADVANTAGES

- Some women consider the use of foam "messy"
- Must be consistently used with each act of intercourse
- High user-failure rate

SIDE EFFECTS

- Irritation or burning
- Temporary skin irritation on vulva or penis

CONTRAINDICATIONS

- Allergy to product

DIAGNOSTIC STUDIES

- Pap smear
- STD screening

PATIENT EDUCATION

- Proper usage: place a full applicator of spermicide deep into the vagina while in supine position
- Spermicide should remain in vagina for 8 hours following intercourse
- No douching within 8 hours after intercourse
- Increased efficacy with barrier method (e.g., diaphragm or condom)
- Wash applicator with soap and water at each use
- Additional spermicide and fresh condom for subsequent acts of intercourse

FOLLOW-UP

- Annual examination

Emergency Contraception

DESCRIPTION

Use of a birth control method after sexual intercourse has occurred

EFFECTIVENESS

- 75% effective in preventing pregnancy if taken within 72 hours of intercourse

MECHANISM OF ACTION

- Inhibit or delay ovulation
- May inhibit fertilization or implantation of a fertilized egg

ADVANTAGES

- Back up method for barrier method failure (e.g., torn diaphragm, condom) and missed oral contraceptives
- May use this method more than once in a cycle
- No reports of teratogenic effects when emergency contraception failed

DISADVANTAGES

- Health care providers not familiar with use
- 72-hour window for use

SIDE EFFECTS

- Nausea
- Vomiting

INDICATIONS

- Women who have had unprotected intercourse within the past 72 hours and do not desire pregnancy

CONTRAINDICATIONS

- Same as combined oral contraceptives

DIAGNOSTIC STUDIES

- Pregnancy test before administering

PATIENT EDUCATION

- The first dose of pills must be taken within 72 hours of intercourse and the second dose must be taken 12 hours after the first (*see* Sexual Abuse)
- Danger signs (as above in combined oral contraceptives)
- Take antiemetic one hour before ingestion of emergency oral contraceptive
- Need for routine contraceptive and health care

FOLLOW-UP

- If no menstrual bleeding within 3 weeks of emergency oral contraception
- If menstrual bleeding less than 2 days duration
- If development of early pregnancy signs: breast tenderness, fatigue, loss of appetite
- Pregnancy test if any of the above are present

MENOPAUSE

DESCRIPTION

Cessation of menstrual cycle for 12 months; premature menopause is defined as occurring before age 40 years

ETIOLOGY

- Physiologic due to depletion of follicles in ovaries and decreased estrogen synthesis and resultant stoppage of menses
- Surgical
- Medical due to administration of medications for treatment of breast cancer and endometriosis

INCIDENCE:

- 30-40 million women in the U.S. with the number growing
- 10% by age 38 years
- 20% by age 43 years
- 50% by age 48 years
- 90% by age 54 years

- 100% by age 58 years
- Surgical menopause is present in 25-33% of women by age 55 years

ASSESSMENT FINDINGS

- Cycles become farther and farther apart and irregular with eventual cessation of menses
- Vasomotor instability (hot flashes, night sweats): 85% of women experience
- Depression
- Nervousness
- Headache
- Fatigue
- Palpitations
- Paresthesias
- Insomnia
- Vaginal atrophy (mucosa appears thin, pale, friable)
- Decrease in vaginal lubrication resulting in itching, discharge, bleeding, dyspareunia, increased risk of urethritis
- May have decreased libido

DIFFERENTIAL DIAGNOSIS

- Pregnancy
- Diabetes mellitus
- Thyroid disease
- Hyperparathyroidism
- Polycystic ovarian disease
- Pituitary adenoma
- Hypothalamic dysfunction

DIAGNOSTIC STUDIES

- Usually none required to diagnose
- FSH: elevated $\geq$40 mIU/ml
- LH: >30 mIU/ml FSH:LH ratio: >1
- Progesterone challenge: absence of withdrawal bleeding suggests menopause
- Pap smear
- Mammogram
- Bone density measurement in high-risk patients

NONPHARMACOLOGIC MANAGEMENT

- Avoid factors which precipitate vasomotor instability (e.g., hot drinks, alcohol, caffeine, stress, warm environment, and overdressing)
- Wear layered clothing
- Smoking cessation
- Regular exercise program to promote feeling of well-being and prevention of osteoporosis
- Weight bearing exercise to prevent osteoporosis
- Kegel exercises
- Self-breast examination monthly
- Use of contraceptive during perimenopausal period unless pregnancy desired
- Low fat, high calcium diet

PHARMACOLOGIC MANAGEMENT

- Hormone replacement therapy should be carefully considered
    - ◊ oral
    - ◊ transdermal
- Estrogen alone if uterus removed
- Estrogen with progestin if uterus intact
- Calcium supplement

Estrogen therapy should not be used in patients with history of breast cancer, undiagnosed vaginal bleeding, known or suspected pregnancy, active thrombosis or thrombophlebitis, endometrial adenocarcinoma, and/or active liver disease.

CONSULTATION/REFERRAL

- Cardiologist referral for signs/symptoms of cardiovascular disease

FOLLOW-UP

- Reevaluate 1-2 months after beginning drug therapy for effectiveness of therapy
- Mammogram every 1-2 years between ages 40-49 years then annually after age 50 years
- Pap smear annually

EXPECTED COURSE

Without hormone replacement:
- Gradual disappearance of vasomotor symptoms over years
- Development of osteoporosis and cardiovascular disease

With hormone replacement:
- Minimal effects of estrogen depletion

Women who experience early menopause are at increased risk of osteoporosis and so should be screened and treated if necessary.

POSSIBLE COMPLICATIONS

- Stress incontinence
- Osteoporosis
- Cardiovascular disease

BREAST CANCER

DESCRIPTION

Malignant tumor of the breast occurring primarily in women but may occur in men

ETIOLOGY

- 20% of patients have a family history
- Etiology is otherwise unknown

The presence of BRCA 1 and BRCA 2 genes are strongly associated the development of breast cancer.

INCIDENCE

- 1 in 8 women in the US will develop breast cancer at some time
- >150,000 new cases annually
- Account for 50,000 deaths annually
- Females > Males

77% of women with breast cancer are over age 50 years.

RISK FACTORS

- Age, median age at time of diagnosis is 54 years
- History of previous breast cancer
- Family history of breast cancer in first-degree relative
- Early menarche (≤11 years)
- Onset of menopause after age 55 years
- Nulliparity
- First term pregnancy after age 30 years
- Obesity in postmenopausal women
- Ashkenazi Jewish descent
- Presence of BRCA1 or BRCA2 gene
- Controversial risk factors:
    - ◊ Estrogen use
    - ◊ High dietary fat
    - ◊ High alcohol use
    - ◊ Obesity

ASSESSMENT FINDINGS

- Painless, firm, fixed mass
- No changes in mass with menstruation
- Spontaneous nipple discharge that is usually clear
- Dimpling of skin (*peau d'orange* appearance)
- Nipple retraction
- Increased vascular pattern of breast
- Significant asymmetry of breasts
- Axillary, supraclavicular, and/or infraclavicular lymph node enlargement
- Skin ulcerations
- Scaly lesions of nipple (Paget's disease)

DIFFERENTIAL DIAGNOSIS

- Fibrocystic breast disease
- Intraductal papilloma
- Fibroadenoma
- Mastitis

DIAGNOSTIC STUDIES

- Mammography
- Ultrasound of breast to differentiate fluid-filled cyst from solid mass
- Fine needle aspiration biopsy
- Open biopsy

PREVENTION

- Baseline mammography by age 35 years; every 1-2 years between ages 40-49 years; then every 1 year after age 50 years. Women who have higher than average risk for breast cancer may need more frequent mammography.
- Monthly self-breast examinations

NONPHARMACOLOGIC MANAGEMENT

- Lumpectomy
- Mastectomy
- Radiation therapy

- Assessment of estrogen receptors in tumor
- Baseline bone scan, chest x-ray, liver scan

A breast mass in conjunction with a normal mammogram is NOT normal. An ultrasound must be performed.

PHARMACOLOGIC MANAGEMENT

- Hormone therapy with agent such as tamoxifen (Nolvadex®)
- Chemotherapy, radiation

CONSULTATION/REFERRAL

- Refer all palpable masses to surgeon for evaluation and biopsy if indicated

FOLLOW-UP

- Mammogram at least annually
- Bone scan with development of bone pain or elevated alkaline phosphate

EXPECTED COURSE

10-year survival rates:

- Noninvasive (tumors <1 cm with no axillary node involvement): 95%
- Stage I (tumors >1 cm with no axillary node involvement): 90%
- Stage II (tumors <5 cm or axillary node involvement): 40%
- Stage III (tumors >5 cm or with chest wall or skin extension, inflammatory changes, or supraclavicular involvement): 15%
- Stage IV (metastatic): 0%

POSSIBLE COMPLICATIONS

- Postoperative lymphedema
- Limited shoulder movement after surgery
- Side effect of chemotherapy: nausea, vomiting, alopecia, leukopenia, stomatitis, fatigue
- Radiation side effects: skin reactions

FIBROCYSTIC BREAST DISEASE (Benign Breast Disease)

DESCRIPTION

Benign breast disorder

ETIOLOGY

- Unknown
- Possible causes:
  - ◊ Luteal phase defect
  - ◊ Increased estrogen
  - ◊ Hyperprolactinemia
  - ◊ Hypersensitivity to estrogen
  - ◊ Sensitivity to methylxanthines
  - ◊ Dietary fat intake

INCIDENCE

- 50% of women in the U.S. have fibrocystic breast disease to some extent

RISK FACTORS

- None definitively known
- Possibly ingestion of methylxanthines (e.g., caffeine-containing beverages, chocolate)

ASSESSMENT FINDINGS

- Asymptomatic
- Palpation of smooth, movable masses
- Breast pain or tenderness which diminishes after menses
- Breast engorgement
- Breast thickening
- Worsening of symptoms premenstrually
- Nipple discharge of varying color and consistency

Mastoplasia is thickening of the breast tissue in a rope-like manner that predominates during the menstrual cycle.

DIFFERENTIAL DIAGNOSIS

- Breast cancer
- Chest wall syndrome
- Neuralgia
- Intraductal papilloma
- Fibroadenoma
- Mastitis

DIAGNOSTIC STUDIES

- Prolactin level
- TSH
- Mammogram
- Ultrasound of breast differentiates cysts from solid masses
- Needle or open biopsy

NONPHARMACOLOGIC MANAGEMENT

- Evaluate to rule out malignancy
- Reassurance
- Cold compresses
- Supportive brassiere
- Wearing brassiere 24 hours may help
- Sodium restriction 10 days before onset of menstruation
- Decrease or eliminate caffeine
- Biopsy often needed to differentiate from malignant mass

PHARMACOLOGIC MANAGEMENT

- Spironolactone (Aldactone®) for swelling and pain premenstrually
- Vitamin B_6, E
- Oral contraceptives
- Danazol (Danocrine®) or bromocriptine (Parlodel®) may be used for more severe disease

PREGNANCY/LACTATION CONSIDERATIONS

- No known effect on lactation

CONSULTATION/REFERRAL

- Refer to surgeon for evaluation of especially painful masses or any abnormalities on mammogram or ultrasound

FOLLOW-UP

- Mammogram by age 35, every 1-2 years between ages 40-49 years, and annually after age 50 years

EXPECTED COURSE

- Benign but chronic condition

POSSIBLE COMPLICATIONS

- May have an increased risk of malignancy if atypical hyperplasia is present on biopsy.

FIBROADENOMA

DESCRIPTION

A benign tumor containing fibrous tissue which occurs in the breast

ETIOLOGY

- Unknown, thought to be hormonally induced

INCIDENCE

- Most common benign tumor in the female breast
- Occurs most in ages 20-30 years

ASSESSMENT FINDINGS

- Single, nontender, and firm mass
- Multiple lesions in 10-15% of cases
- Freely movable
- No change in mass with menstrual cycle
- No nipple discharge

DIFFERENTIAL DIAGNOSIS

- Fibrocystic breast disease
- Intraductal papilloma
- Breast cancer
- Other benign breast disease

DIAGNOSTIC STUDIES

- Mammography
- Ultrasound to differentiate fluid-filled cyst from solid mass
- Fine needle aspiration biopsy
- Open biopsy

NONPHARMACOLOGIC MANAGEMENT

- Surgical excision (elective)

PREGNANCY/LACTATION CONSIDERATIONS

- Pregnancy stimulates growth
- No known effect on lactation

CONSULTATION/REFERRAL

- Surgical referral for excision

FOLLOW-UP

- None needed

EXPECTED COURSE

- Complete resolution after surgical removal without recurrence

POSSIBLE COMPLICATIONS

- Postoperative infection

INTRADUCTAL PAPILLOMA

DESCRIPTION

Benign tumor within the ductal system of the breast

ETIOLOGY

- Unknown
- Thought to be due to overgrowth of ductal epithelium

INCIDENCE

- Usually occurs perimenopausally during ages 40-50 years

ASSESSMENT FINDINGS

- Bloody or serous nipple discharge
- Usually unilateral unless multiple ducts involved

DIFFERENTIAL DIAGNOSIS

- Breast cancer
- Galactorrhea

DIAGNOSTIC STUDIES

- Mammography
- Ultrasound to differentiate fluid-filled cyst from solid mass

NONPHARMACOLOGIC MANAGEMENT

- Surgical excision

PREGNANCY/LACTATION CONSIDERATIONS

- Removal does not affect ability to breastfeed

CONSULTATION/REFERRAL

- Surgical consult for excision

FOLLOW-UP

- None indicated

EXPECTED COURSE

- Complete resolution after surgical removal without recurrence

References

American College of Obstetricians and Gynecologists. (1996). *ACOG practice patterns: Emergency oral contraception (No. 3).* Washington, D.C.: ACOG.

Arnold, G. J., & Neiheisel, M. B. (1997). A comprehensive approach to evaluating nipple discharge. *The Nurse Practitioner, 22*, 96-111.

Bader, T.J. (2004). *OB/GYN secrets* (Rev. 3rd ed.). St. Louis, MO: Mosby-Year Book.

Brotzman, G.L., & Julian, T.M. (1996). The minimally abnormal Papanicolaou smear. *American Family Physician, 53*, 1154-1162.

Burns, C.E., Brady, M.A., Blosser, C., Starr, N.B., & Dunn, A.M. (2004). *Pediatric primary care: A handbook for nurse practitioners* (3rd ed.). Philadelphia: W.B. Saunders.

Canavan, T. P., & Doshi, N. R. (2000). Cervical cancer. *American Family Physician*, 61(5): 1369-1376.

Centers for Disease Control and Prevention. (2002). Sexually transmitted diseases treatment guidelines. *MMWR, 47*, (RR-1).

Corwin, E. J. (1997). Endometriosis: Pathophysiology, diagnosis, and treatment. *The Nurse Practitioner, 22*(10), 35-55.

Cullins, V. E., Dominguez, L., Guberski, T., et al. (1999). Treating vaginitis. *The Nurse Practitioner, 24*(10), 46-63.

Dambro, M.R. (2005). *Griffith's 5 minute clinical consult.* Philadelphia: Lippincott Williams & Wilkins.

Finkel, M. L., Cohen, M., Mahoney, H. (2001). Treatment options for the menopausal women. *The Nurse Practitioner, 26*(2), 5-15.

Graber, M.A., & Lanternier, M.L. (Eds.) (2001). *The family practice handbook.* (4th ed.). St. Louis: Mosby.

Goroll, A. H., & Mulley, A. G., Jr. (Eds.). (2000). *Primary care medicine: Office evaluation and management of the adult patient* (4th ed.). Philadelphia: Lippincott Williams Wilkins.

Hammond, C. B. (1997). Management of menopause. *American Family Physician, 55*, 1667-1674.

Hatcher, R. A., Trussell, J., Stewart, F., Nelson, A.L., Cates, W. Jr., & Kowal, D., (2004). *Contraceptive technology* (Rev. 18th ed.). New York: Ardent Media.

Knutson, C. (1997). A new generation of IUD use: Taking a fresh look at an old contraceptive. *Advance for Nurse Practitioners, 5*(1), 22-31.

Marantidies, D. (1997). Management of polycystic ovary syndrome. *The Nurse Practitioner, 22*(12), 34-41.

Mashburn, J., & Scharbo-DeHaan, M. (1997). A clinician's guide to Pap smear interpretations. *The Nurse Practitioner, 22*(4), 115-143.

Morgan, K.W., & Deneris, A. (1997). Emergency contraception: Preventing unintended pregnancy. *The Nurse Practitioner, 22*(11), 34-48.

Morrison, E. H. (1997). Controversies in women's health maintenance. *American Family Physician, 55*(4), 1283-1289.

Nordenberg, T. (2000). Protecting against unintended pregnancy: A guide to contraceptive choices. *FDA Consumer.*

Rakel, R.E. (1998). *Essentials of family practice.* (2nd ed.). Philadelphia: WB Saunders.

Ransom, S. B., & McNeeley, S. G. (1997). *Gynecology for the primary care provider.* Philadelphia: W.B. Saunders.

Scharbo-DeHaan, M. (1996). Hormone replacement therapy. *The Nurse Practitioner, 21* (Suppl. 2), 1-13.

Shaw, C. R. (1997). The perimenopausal hot flash: Epidemiology, physiology, and treatment. *The Nurse Practitioner, 22*(3), 55-66.

Shepherd, J. C., & Fried, R. A. (1995). Preventing cervical cancer: The role of the Bethesda system. *American Family Physician, 51*, 434-440.

South-Paul, J. E. (2001). Osteoporosis: Part II. Nonpharmacologic and pharmacologic treatment. *American Family Physician, 63,* 1121-1128.

Speroff, L., & Darney, P. (2005). *A clinical guide for contraception* (4th ed.). Philadelphia: Lippincott Williams & Wilkins.

Strickland, K., & Dempster, J. S. (1996). The primary care management of leiomyoma-induced abnormal uterine bleeding. *Journal of the American Academy of Nurse Practitioners, 8*, 541-545.

Tobin, M. J. (1995). Vulvovaginal candidiasis. *American Family Physician, 51*, 1715-1720.

Treinen, A. D. (1997). Breast cancer screening. *Advance for Nurse Practitioners, 5*(5), 17-23.

Uphold, C.R., & Graham, M.V. (2003). *Clinical guidelines in family practice.* (4th ed.). Gainesville, FL: Barmarrae Books.

U.S. Preventive Services Task Force. (1996). *Guide to clinical preventive services.* (2nd ed.) Washington, D.C.: Office of Disease Prevention and Health Promotion, U.S. Government Printing Office.

Wehrle, K. E. (1996). Perfect timing for a healthy life: What to expect during perimenopause. *Advance for Nurse Practitioners, 4*(11), 18-27.

Zuber, T. J. (2001). Endometrial biopsy. *American Family Physician, 63,* 1131-1135, 1137-1138, 1139-1141.

Index